COMPUTED TOMOGRAPHY
for TECHNOLOGISTS

A Comprehensive Text

COMPUTED TOMOGRAPHY
for TECHNOLOGISTS

A Comprehensive Text

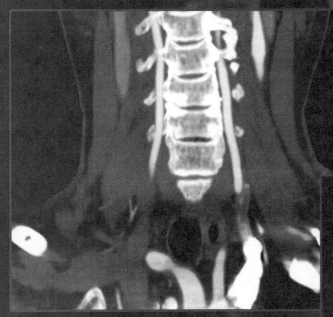

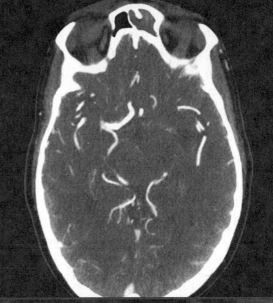

LOIS E. ROMANS, RT, (R)(CT)

Wolters Kluwer | Lippincott Williams & Wilkins
Health

Philadelphia • Baltimore • New York • London
Buenos Aires • Hong Kong • Sydney • Tokyo

Acquisitions Editor: Pete Sabatini
Product Director: Eric Branger
Product Manager: Amy Millholen
Marketing Manager: Allison Powell
Compositor: SPi Technologies
Printer: C&C Offset - China

Printed in China

Library of Congress Cataloging-in-Publication Data
Romans, Lois E.
  Computed tomography for technologists : a comprehensive text / Lois E. Romans.
     p. ; cm.
  Includes bibliographical references and index.
  ISBN 978-0-7817-7751-3 (alk. paper)
  1. Tomography—Textbooks. 2. Medical technologists. I. Title.
  [DNLM: 1. Tomography, X-Ray Computed. WN 206 R758c 2011]
  RC78.7.T6R659   2011
  616.07'57—dc22

                                                          2009045125

The publishers have made every effort to trace the copyright holders for borrowed material. If they have inadvertently overlooked any, they will be pleased to make the necessary arrangements at the first opportunity.

To purchase additional copies of this book, call our customer service department at **(800) 638-3030** or fax orders to (301) 824-7390. International customers should call **(301) 714-2324.**

Visit Lippincott Williams & Wilkins on the Internet: http://www.LWW.com.
Lippincott Williams & Wilkins customer service representatives are available from 8:30 am to 6:00 pm, EST.

  12 13 14
  4 5 6 7 8 9 10

To my husband, Ken, and my daughters, Ashleigh,
Chelsea, and Abigail

Preface

Since its inception in the early 1970s, computed tomography (CT) has made an enormous impact in diagnostic imaging. Over the years, improvements in both CT hardware and software have resulted in advances in all its major features including image resolution, temporal resolution, and reconstruction speed. In just over 30 years, technological innovation has taken us from scanners that employed a single x-ray detector and took several minutes to acquire a single cross-sectional slice to scanners that employ multiple rows of detectors, in both x and y directions and can acquire more than 100 cross-sectional slices in less than a second. In 1972, scan time per slice was 300 seconds; by 2005, it had decreased to just 0.005 seconds! This technologic evolution has opened the door to new and varied uses for CT, from assessing coronary disease to colorectal screening. In some cases, new indications for CT exams may replace other, more invasive procedures; in other situations, such as that of appendicitis, they offer clinicians an alternative approach when a diagnosis is problematic. As the scope and practice of CT expands, so must the knowledge of technologists working in the field. Although the establishment of guidelines and protocols are most often the purview of radiologists, in the course of their work technologists must make myriad decisions that affect the quality of an exam. Such decisions can only be appropriately made if technologists have an adequate foundation in each of the key content areas of CT. The goal of this book is to provide a centralized resource for the CT technologist to gain the knowledge necessary to consistently provide excellent patient care that will result in high quality CT exams. This text will also provide the reader the information necessary to successfully sit for the advanced level certification exam offered by The American Registry of Radiologic Technologists (ARRT). This text is also appropriate for radiography students taking a CT course.

By identifying three major content categories, the ARRT has provided a framework to allow the assessment of the knowledge and skills that underlie a technologist's decision-making process. This text is organized in accordance to the categories identified by the ARRT. Each major section covers one of the ARRT-designated content areas, namely physics and instrumentation, patient care, and imaging procedures. However, the categorization of topics is far from clear-cut. For instance, a question regarding the appropriate type and dose of iodinated contrast for a given procedure could just as easily fall under the category of patient care as that of imaging procedures. Since topic categories often overlap, many subjects will appear in more than one section of the book, most likely with a slightly different perspective. Using the example above to illustrate, in the section on patient care, contrast media is covered from a global standpoint and includes such things as its characteristics and types. In the section on imaging procedures, the topic of contrast media arises again, this time in regards to why certain agents are preferred for certain types of procedures.

Having worked as a technologist for over 20 years, I have approached this text with a technologist's (not a physicist's or a radiologist's) perspective. The focus is on caring for patients and creating quality exams, with just enough physics so that everything makes sense. It is apparent from the content specifications of the advanced level CT certification exam that the ARRT shares my philosophy. Seventy percent of the questions contained on the exam relate to exam protocols and patient care.

The ability to accurately identify cross-sectional anatomy is an important aspect of the technologist's job and comprises a significant portion of the ARRT certification exam. The anatomy section included in this text is intended only as an introduction to cross-sectional anatomy; the images included should give the reader an idea of the level of anatomic detail with which the technologist is expected to become familiar. Many excellent texts currently exist that provide a full range of cross-sectional images, should the reader wish to continue their studies.

Many individuals are looking for a "cookbook" of exam protocols. There are two main problems with creating such a cookbook. First, there are no universally accepted protocols that could be considered the standard of care in the field. Protocols are as varied as the professionals that use them, with adjustments made for the type of patient, the type of scanner, and the preferences of the radiologists. The other main barrier to a cookbook approach is that the rapid advancements in the field of radiology make any such document obsolete before the ink dries. With that caveat, in each main anatomic category I have included a few exam protocols, in many cases ones that we use at the University of Michigan. These are intended as a frame of reference only with the expectation that protocols must constantly evolve to keep up with new developments in the field.

The companion website for instructors contains valuable teaching resources to complement the text. Instructor resources on thePoint include PowerPoint slides for each chapter, an image bank containing all images found in the book, and situational judgment questions.

Lois E. Romans, RT, (R)(CT)
University of Michigan Health Systems
Ann Arbor, Michigan

User's Guide

This User's Guide introduces you to the helpful features of *Computed Tomography for Technologists: A Comprehensive Text* that enable you to quickly master new concepts and put your new skills into practice.

Chapter features to increase understanding and enhance retention of the material include:

Key terms help you focus on the most important concepts as you progress through the chapter.

Key Concepts Boxes present important information for readers to remember (exam material).

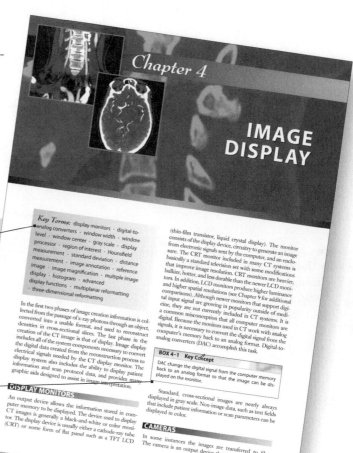

Clinical Application Boxes use real-life scenarios to illustrate and explain concepts.

Review Questions at the end of each chapter promote a deeper understanding of fundamental concepts by encouraging analysis and application of information presented.

Recommended Reading or References provide the opportunity to expand on the knowledge gained from the chapter.

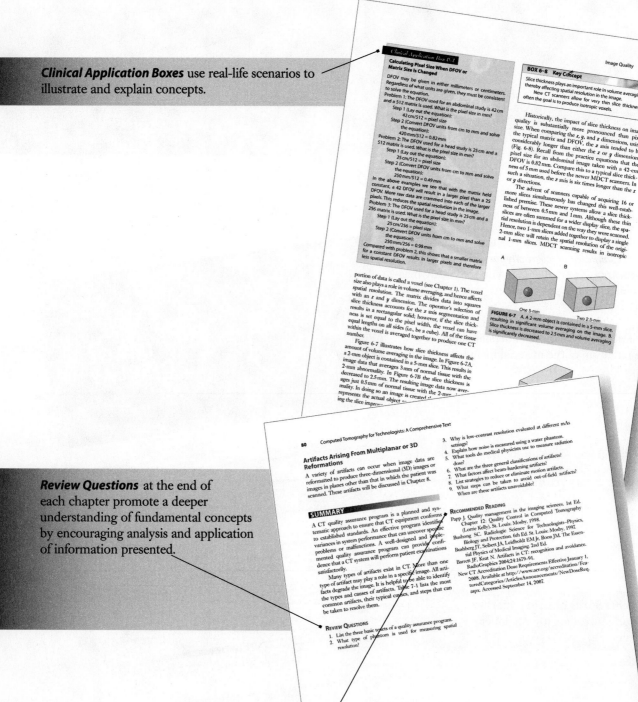

Clinical Application Box 6-1

Calculating Pixel Size When DFOV or Matrix Size Is Changed

DFOV may be given in either millimeters or centimeters. Regardless of what units are given, they must be consistent to solve the equation.

Problem 1: The DFOV used for an abdominal study is 42 cm and a 512 matrix is used. What is the pixel size in mm?

Step 1 (Lay out the equation):
42 cm/512 = pixel size

Step 2 (Convert DFOV units from cm to mm and solve the equation):
420 mm/512 = 0.82 mm

Problem 2: The DFOV used for a head study is 25 cm and a 512 matrix is used. What is the pixel size in mm?

Step 1 (Lay out the equation):
25 cm/512 = pixel size

Step 2 (Convert DFOV units from cm to mm and solve the equation):
250 mm/512 = 0.49 mm

In the above examples we see that with the matrix held constant, a 42 DFOV will result in a larger pixel than a 25 DFOV. More raw data are crammed into each of the larger pixels. This reduces the spatial resolution in the image.

Problem 3: The DFOV used for a head study is 25 cm and a 256 matrix is used. What is the pixel size in mm?

Step 1 (Lay out the equation):
25 cm/256 = pixel size

Step 2 (Convert DFOV units from cm to mm and solve the equation):
250 mm/256 = 0.98 mm

Compared with problem 2, this shows that a smaller matrix for a constant DFOV results in larger pixels and therefore less spatial resolution.

portion of data is called a voxel (see Chapter 1). The voxel size also plays a role in volume averaging, and hence affects spatial resolution. The matrix divides data into squares with an *x* and *y* dimension. The operator's selection of slice thickness accounts for the *z* axis segmentation and results in a rectangular solid; however, if the slice thickness is set equal to the pixel width, the voxel can have equal lengths on all sides (i.e., be a cube). All of the tissue within the voxel is averaged together to produce one CT number.

Figure 6-7 illustrates how slice thickness affects the amount of volume averaging in the image. In Figure 6-7A, a 2-mm object is contained in a 5-mm slice. This results in image data that averages 3 mm of normal tissue with the 2-mm abnormality. In Figure 6-7B the slice thickness is decreased to 2.5 mm. The resulting image data now averages just 0.5 mm of normal tissue with the 2-mm abnormality. In doing so an image is created that more closely represents the actual object ... decreasing the slice improv...

BOX 6-8   Key Concept

Slice thickness plays an important role in volume averaging, thereby affecting spatial resolution in the image. New CT scanners allow for very thin slice thickness; often the goal is to produce isotropic voxels.

Historically, the impact of slice thickness on image quality is substantially more pronounced than pixel size. When comparing the *x*, *y*, and *z* dimensions, using the typical matrix and DFOV, the *z* axis tended to be considerably longer than either the *x* or *y* dimensions (Fig. 6-8). Recall from the practice equations that the pixel size for an abdominal image taken with a 42-cm DFOV is 0.82 mm. Compare this to a typical slice thickness of 5 mm used before the newer MDCT scanners. In such a situation, the *z* axis is six times longer than the *x* or *y* directions.

The advent of scanners capable of acquiring 16 or more slices simultaneously has changed this well-established premise. These newer systems allow a slice thickness of between 0.5 mm and 1 mm. Although these thin slices are often summed for a wider display slice, the spatial resolution is dependent on the way they were scanned. Hence, two 1-mm slices added together to display a single 2-mm slice will retain the spatial resolution of the original 1-mm slices. MDCT scanning results in isotropic

A   B

One 5-mm   Two 2.5-mm

FIGURE 6-7   A, A 2-mm object is contained in a 5-mm slice, resulting in significant volume averaging on the image. B, Slice thickness is decreased to 2.5 mm and volume averaging is significantly decreased.

Artifacts Arising From Multiplanar or 3D Reformations

A variety of artifacts can occur when image data are reformatted to produce three-dimensional (3D) images or images in planes other than that in which the patient was scanned. These artifacts will be discussed in Chapter 8.

SUMMARY

A CT quality assurance program is a planned and systematic approach to ensure that CT equipment conforms to established standards. An effective program identifies variances in system performance that can uncover specific problems or malfunctions. A well-designed and implemented quality assurance program can provide confidence that a CT system will perform patient examinations satisfactorily.

Many types of artifacts exist in CT. More than one type of artifact may play a role in a specific image. All artifacts degrade the image. It is helpful to be able to identify the types and causes of artifacts. Table 7-1 lists the most common artifacts, their typical causes, and steps that can be taken to resolve them.

REVIEW QUESTIONS

1. List the three basic tenets of a quality assurance program.
2. What type of phantom is used for measuring spatial resolution?

3. Why is low-contrast resolution evaluated at different mAs settings?
4. Explain how noise is measured using a water phantom.
5. What tools do medical physicists use to measure radiation dose?
6. What are the three general classifications of artifacts?
7. What factors affect beam-hardening artifacts?
8. List strategies to reduce or eliminate motion artifacts.
9. What steps can be taken to avoid out-of-field artifacts? When are these artifacts unavoidable?

RECOMMENDED READING

Papp J. Quality management in the imaging sciences. 1st Ed. Chapter 12: Quality Control in Computed Tomography (Lorrie Kelly). St. Louis: Mosby, 1998.

Bushong SC. Radiologic Science for Technologists–Physics, Biology and Protection. 6th Ed. St. Louis: Mosby, 1997.

Bushberg JT, Seibert JA, Leidholdt EM Jr, Boon JM. The Essential Physics of Medical Imaging. 2nd Ed.

Barrett JF, Keat N. Artifacts in CT: recognition and avoidance. RadioGraphics 2004;24:1679–91.

New CT Accreditation Dose Requirements Effective January 1, 2008. Available at http://www.acr.org/accreditation/FeaturedCategories/ArticlesAnnouncements/NewDoseReq. aspx. Accessed September 14, 2007.

Examples of Exam Protocols are included for each major anatomical area.

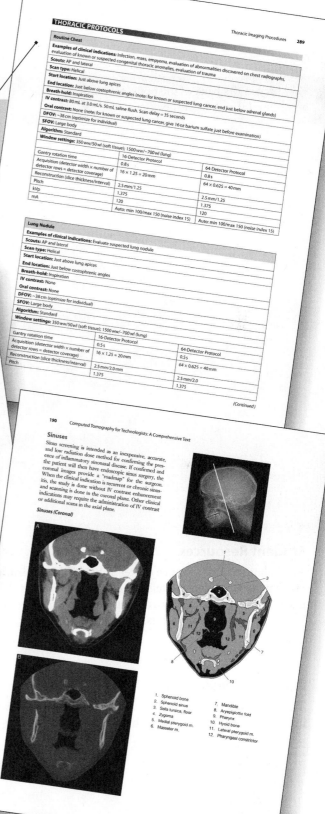

CT cross-sectional slices accompanied by shaded diagrams and a reference image are featured in the Cross-Sectional Anatomy section of the book.

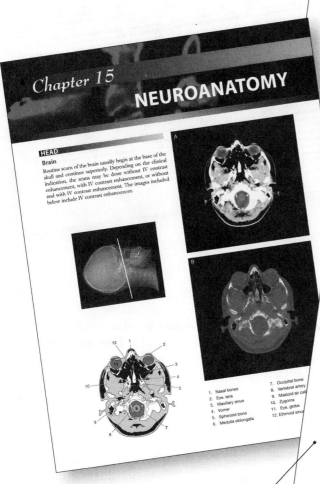

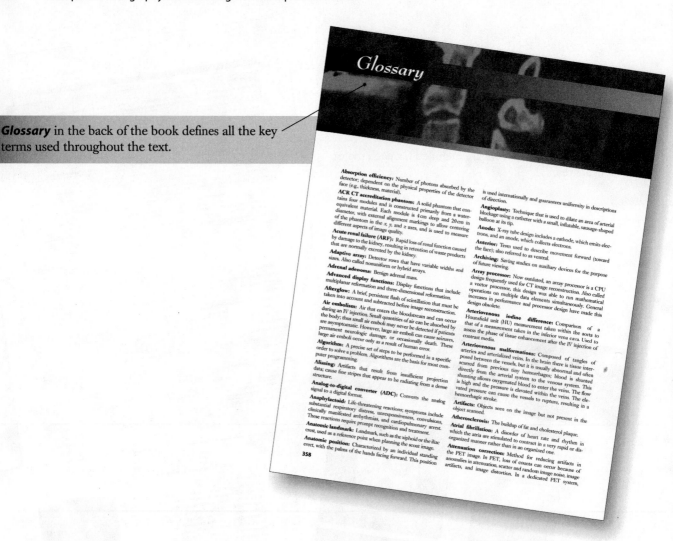

Glossary in the back of the book defines all the key terms used throughout the text.

Student Resources

The online student resource center at **http://thePoint.lww.com/RomansCT** reinforces what you learn in the text. Student resources include full text online, PowerPoint slides, and the protocol tables from the book containing localizer images to guide technologists in setting the scan range of each specific study. See the inside front cover for details on how to access these resources.

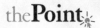

Instructor Resources

The online instructor resources available for use with *Computed Tomography for Technologists: A Comprehensive Text* include PowerPoints, an image bank, and situational judgment questions.

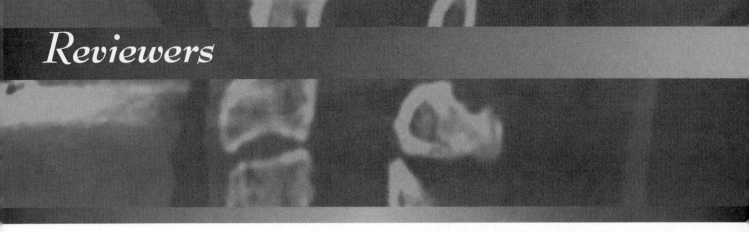

Reviewers

The publisher, author, and editors gratefully acknowledge the valuable contributions made by the following professionals who reviewed this text:

Matthew G. Aagesen
Musculokeletal Fellow
University of Michigan Health System
Ann Arbor, MI

Jeff L. Berry, MS, RT (R) (CT)
Radiography Program Director
Department of Medical Imaging & Radiation Sciences
University of Oklahoma Health Sciences Center
Oklahoma City, OK

Jonathan R. Dillman, M.D
Abdominal Radiology Fellow
University of Michigan Health System
Ann Arbor, MI

Lois Doody, MEd
Instructor
Medical Radiography Program
BCIT
Vancouver, BC

John W. Eichinger, MSRS, (R)(CT) ARRT
Program Director-Radiologic Technology
Technical College of the Lowcountry
Beaufort, South Carolina

James H. Ellis, M.D., F.A.C.R.
Professor of Radiology
University of Michigan Health System
Ann Arbor, MI

Frances Gilman, MS, RT, R, CT, MR, CV, ARRT
Assistant Professor and Chair
Department of Radiologic Sciences
Thomas Jefferson University
Philadelphia, PA

Ella A. Kazerooni, M.D., F.A.C.R.
Professor of Radiology
Director, Cardiothoracic Radiology
University of Michigan Health System
Ann Arbor, MI

Kathleen Lowe, RTR, RTMR, BappSc
Faculty Diagnostic Imaging
Dawson College
Westmount, Quebec
Canada

Leanna B. Neubrander, BS, RT (R) (CT)
Instructor, Department of Radiologic Sciences
Florida Hospital College of Health Sciences
Orlando, FL

Dr. Saabry Osmany
Department of Nuclear Medicine and PET
Singapore General Hospital
Singapore

Deena Slockett, MBA, RT (R), (M)
Associate Professor, FHCHS
Program Coordinator, Department of Radiologic
Sciences
Orlando, FL

Suzette Thomas-Rodriguez, BS (Medical Imaging), ARRT(R) (CT) (MRI)
Senior Lecturer
Department of Radiological Sciences
College of Science Technology and Applied Arts of
   Trinidad & Tobago (COSTAATT)
Port-of-Spain
Trinidad

Amit Vyas
Neuroradiology Fellow
University of Michigan Health System
Ann Arbor, MI

Bettye G. Wilson, MAEd, ARRT(R) (CT), RDMS, FASRT
Associate Professor of Medical Imaging and Therapy
University of Alabama at Birmingham
School of Health Professions
Birmingham, AL

Acknowledgments

I cannot overstate the contributions of Dr. James Ellis from the University of Michigan Radiology Department. I routinely handed him a sow's ear and he unfailingly amazed me by returning a silk purse. His meticulous review went far beyond my wildest expectation. His thoughtful suggestions and patient guidance improved every aspect of the manuscript. Special thanks to Dr. Saabry Osmany for his help in editing the chapter on PET/CT and for supplying PET/CT images. I gratefully acknowledge the expertise of diagnostic physicists Emmanuel Christodoulou and Mitch Goodsitt, who helped me make sense of the complex data available on radiation dose. Thanks to my dear friend and fellow technologist, Renee Maas for support, encouragement and willingness to be my model when I needed photographs of a patient in a scanner. Thanks to 3D lab technologist Melissa Muck, who supplied outstanding images for the chapter on post-processing techniques. My gratitude to the many CT technologists at the University of Michigan that helped me to find just the right images: Ronnie Williams, Ricky Higa, John Rowe and Eric Wizauer. Thanks to Lisa Modelski for keeping me organized. Finally, my thanks to the exceptionally talented artist, Jonathan Dimes, who listened to my ramblings and somehow produced exactly what was in my mind's eye.

Table of Contents

Preface   vii

User's Guide   ix

Reviewers   xiii

Acknowledgments   xv

SECTION I: Physics and Instrumentation

CHAPTER 1   Basic Principles of CT   03

CHAPTER 2   Data Acquisition   14

CHAPTER 3   Image Reconstruction   23

CHAPTER 4   Image Display   31

CHAPTER 5   Methods of Data Acquisition   40

CHAPTER 6   Image Quality   58

CHAPTER 7   Quality Assurance   71

CHAPTER 8   Post-Processing   81

CHAPTER 9   Data Management   93

SECTION II: Patient Care

CHAPTER 10   Patient Communication   103

CHAPTER 11   Patient Preparation   110

CHAPTER 12   Contrast Agents   120

CHAPTER 13   Injection Techniques   142

CHAPTER 14   Radiation Dosimetry in CT   165

SECTION III: Cross-Sectional Anatomy

CHAPTER 15   Neuroanatomy   183

CHAPTER 16   Thoracic Anatomy   204

CHAPTER 17   Abdominopelvic Anatomy   214

CHAPTER 18   Musculoskeletal Anatomy   224

SECTION IV: Imaging Procedures and Protocols

CHAPTER 19   Neurologic Imaging Procedures   239

CHAPTER 20   Thoracic Imaging Procedures   267

CHAPTER 21 Abdomen and Pelvis Imaging Procedures   300
CHAPTER 22 Musculoskeletal Imaging Procedures   335
CHAPTER 23 Interventional CT and CT Fluoroscopy   345
CHAPTER 24 PET/CT Fusion Imaging   348
             Glossary   358
             Index   371

Section I

PHYSICS and INSTRUMENTATION

CHAPTER 1 • Basic Principles of CT

CHAPTER 2 • Data Acquisition

CHAPTER 3 • Image Reconstruction

CHAPTER 4 • Image Display

CHAPTER 5 • Methods of Data Acquisition

CHAPTER 6 • Image Quality

CHAPTER 7 • Quality Assurance

CHAPTER 8 • Post-Processing

CHAPTER 9 • Data Management

INTRODUCTION

The cornerstone of a technologist's responsibility is to produce consistently high-quality examinations while ensuring the safety and well-being of patients. Educational content for the CT technologist must be evaluated with that goal in mind. It is not necessary that a technologist's understanding of CT physics rival that of a medical physicist. I believe in the concept expressed in the phrase, "You don't have to know how to build a car to be a good driver." However, understanding the physical aspects of CT technology allows the technologist to identify deficiencies in images and to take appropriate corrective actions, just as understanding the basics of auto mechanics will help a driver know whether their car simply needs gas or whether a trip to the repair shop is warranted. The physics presented in this section will allow technologists to move past the rote learning of examination protocols and allow them to grasp why we do what we do. They will understand the connection between the choices they make selecting scan parameters and the radiation dose delivered to the patient. It will not prepare them for a career as a physicist. For those readers who desire a more in-depth understanding of CT physics, there are many textbooks from which to choose.

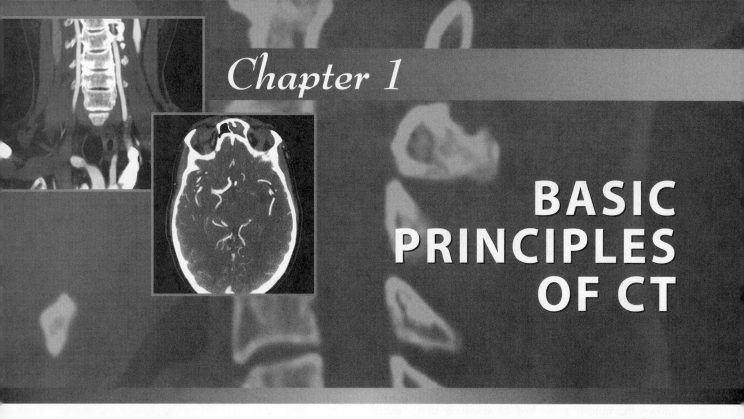

Chapter 1

BASIC PRINCIPLES OF CT

Key Terms: spatial resolution • low-contrast resolution • temporal resolution • Z axis • collimators • pixel • voxel • matrix • beam attenuation • low attenuation • high attenuation • linear attenuation coefficient • positive contrast agents • negative contrast agents • Hounsfield units • polychromatic x-ray energy • artifacts • beam-hardening artifacts • cupping artifacts • volume averaging • partial volume effect • raw data • scan data • Image reconstruction • prospective reconstruction • retrospective reconstruction • step-and-shoot scanning • spiral/helical scanning • multidetector row CT scanning • imaging planes • anatomic position • anterior • ventral • posterior • dorsal • Inferior • caudal • superior • distal • proximal • transverse plane • longitudinal plane • sagittal plane • coronal plane • oblique plane • kinetic energy • gantry • anode • focal spot • tube current • heat capacity • heat dissipation • data acquisition system • view • central processing unit • display processor

BACKGROUND

Conventional radiographs depict a three-dimensional object as a two-dimensional image. This results in over-lying tissues being superimposed on the image, a major limitation of conventional radiography. Computed tomography (CT) overcomes this problem by scanning thin sections of the body with a narrow x-ray beam that rotates around the body, producing images of each cross section. Another limitation of the conventional radiograph is its inability to distinguish between two tissues with similar densities. The unique physics of CT allow for the differentiation between tissues of similar densities.

The main advantages of CT over conventional radiography are in the elimination of superimposed structures, the ability to differentiate small differences in density of anatomic structures and abnormalities, and the superior quality of the images.

TERMINOLOGY

The word tomography has as its root *tomo,* meaning to cut, section, or layer from the Greek *tomos* (a cutting). In the case of CT, a sophisticated computerized method is used to obtain data and transform them into "cuts," or cross-sectional slices of the human body.

The first scanners were limited in the ways in which these cuts could be performed. All early scanners produced axial cuts; that is, slices looked like the rings of a tree visualized in the cut edge of a log. Therefore, it was common to refer to older scanning systems as computerized axial tomography, hence the common acronym, CAT scan.

Newer model scanners offer options in more than just the transverse plane. Therefore, the word "axial" has been dropped from the name of current CT systems. If the old acronym CAT is used, it now represents the phrase computer-assisted tomography.

The historic evolution of CT, although interesting, is beyond the scope of this text. However, for clarity, a few key elements in the development of CT are mentioned here.

Although all CT manufacturers began with the same basic form, each attempted to set their scanners apart in the marketplace by adding features and functionality to the existing technology. As each feature was developed, each manufacturer gave the feature a name. For this reason, the same feature may have a variety of different names, depending on the manufacturer. For example, the preliminary image each scanner produces may be referred to as a "topogram" (Siemens), "scout" (GE Healthcare), or "scanogram" (Toshiba). Another well-known example is a method of scanning that, generically, is referred to as continuous acquisition scanning; this method can also be called "spiral" (Siemens), "helical" (GE Healthcare), or "isotropic" (Toshiba) scanning. In many cases, the trade name of the function is more widely recognized than the generic term. This text refers to each function by the name that best describes it or by the term that is most widely used. Once one understands what each operation accomplishes, switching terms to accommodate scanners is simple.

CT image quality is typically evaluated using a number of criteria:

- Spatial resolution describes the ability of a system to define small objects distinctly.
- Low-contrast resolution refers to the ability of a system to differentiate, on the image, objects with similar densities.
- Temporal resolution refers to the speed that the data can be acquired. This speed is particularly important to reduce or eliminate artifacts that result from object motion, such as those commonly seen when imaging the heart.

These aspects of image quality will be explained more fully in Chapter 6.

COMPUTED TOMOGRAPHY DEFINED

Computed tomography uses a computer to process information collected from the passage of x-ray beams through an area of anatomy. The images created are cross-sectional. To visualize CT, the often-used loaf of bread analogy is useful. If the patient's body is imagined to be a loaf of bread, each CT slice correlates to a slice of the bread. The crust of the bread is analogous to the skin of the patient's body; the white portion of the bread, the patient's internal organs.

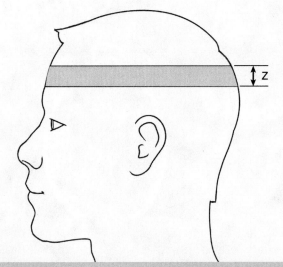

FIGURE 1-1 The thickness of the cross-sectional slice is referred to as its Z axis.

The individual CT slice shows only the parts of the anatomy imaged at a particular level. For example, a scan taken at the level of the sternum would show portions of lung, mediastinum, and ribs, but would not show portions of the kidneys and bladder. Computed tomography requires a firm knowledge of anatomy, in particular the understanding of the location of each organ relative to others.

Each CT slice represents a specific plane in the patient's body. The thickness of the plane is referred to as the Z axis. The Z axis determines the thickness of the slices (Fig. 1-1). The operator selects the thickness of the slice from the choices available on the specific scanner. Selecting a slice thickness limits the x-ray beam so that it passes only through this volume; hence, scatter radiation and superimposition of other structures are greatly diminished. Limiting the x-ray beam in this manner is accomplished by mechanical hardware that resembles small shutters, called collimators, which adjust the opening based on the operator's selection.

The data that form the CT slice are further sectioned into elements: width is indicated by X, while height is indicated by Y (Fig. 1-2). Each one of these two-dimensional squares is a pixel (picture element). A composite of thousands of pixels creates the CT image that displays on the CT monitor. If the Z axis is taken into account, the result is a cube, rather than a square. This cube is referred to as a voxel (volume element).

A matrix is the grid formed from the rows and columns of pixels. In CT, the most common matrix size is 512. This size translates to 512 rows of pixels down and 512 columns of pixels across. The total number of pixels in a matrix is the product of the number of rows and the number of columns, in this case 512 × 512 (262,144). Because the outside perimeter of the square is held constant, a larger matrix size (i.e., 1,024 as opposed to 512)

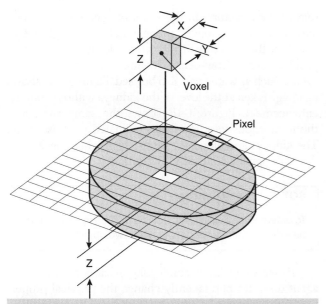

FIGURE 1-2 The data that form the CT slice are sectioned into elements.

will contain smaller individual pixels. Each pixel contains information that the system obtains from scanning.

BEAM ATTENUATION

The structures in a CT image are represented by varying shades of gray. The creation of these shades of gray is based on basic radiation principles. An x-ray beam consists of bundles of energy known as photons. These photons may pass through or be redirected (i.e., scattered) by a structure. A third option is that the photons may be absorbed by a given structure in varying amounts, depending on the strength (average photon energy) of the x-ray beam and the characteristics of the structure in its path. The degree to which a beam is reduced is a phenomenon referred to as attenuation.

BOX 1–1   Key Concept

The degree to which an x-ray beam is reduced by an object is referred to as *attenuation*.

In conventional film-screen radiography, the x-ray beam passes through the patient's body and exposes the photographic film. Similarly, in CT, the x-ray beam passes through the patient's body and is recorded by the detectors. The computer then processes this information to create the CT image. In both cases, the quantities of x-ray photons that pass through the body determine the shades of gray on the image.

By convention, x-ray photons that pass through objects unimpeded are represented by a black area on the image. These areas on the image are commonly referred to as having low attenuation. Conversely, an x-ray beam that

is completely absorbed by an object cannot be detected; the place on the image is white. An object that has the ability to absorb much of the x-ray beam is often referred to as having high attenuation. Areas of intermediate attenuations are represented by various shades of gray.

The number of the photons that interact depends on the thickness, density, and atomic number of the object. Density can be defined as the mass of a substance per unit volume. More simply, density is the degree to which matter is crowded together, or concentrated. For example, a tightly packed snowball has a higher density than a loosely packed one. Dense elements, those with a high atomic number, have many circulating electrons and heavy nuclei and, therefore, provide more opportunities for photon interaction than elements of less density.

To better understand how these physical properties of an object affect the degree of beam attenuation, envision a single x-ray photon passing through an object. The more atoms in its path (the greater the object's thickness and density), the more likely that an atom in the object will interact with the photon. Similarly, the more electrons, neutrons, and protons in each atom, the higher the likelihood of photon interaction. Therefore, the number of photons that interact increases with the density, thickness, and atomic number of the object (Fig. 1-3).

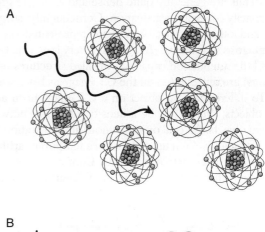

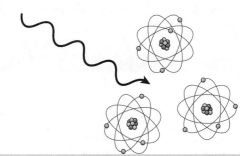

FIGURE 1-3 The relative number of photons that interact increases with the increased density, thickness, and atomic number of the object. In (A), the object in the path of the photon is thicker, denser, and composed of heavier atoms than that of the object depicted in (B); hence, the photon is much more likely to be attenuated in (A).

The amount of the x-ray beam that is scattered or absorbed per unit thickness of the absorber is expressed by the linear attenuation coefficient, represented by the Greek letter μ. For example, if a 125-kVp x-ray beam is used, the linear attenuation coefficient for water is approximately $0.18\,cm^{-1}$ (the unit cm^{-1} indicates per centimeter). This means that about 18% of the photons are either absorbed or scattered when the x-ray beam passes through 1 cm of water (Table 1-1).

In general, the attenuation coefficient decreases with increasing photon energy and increases with increasing atomic number and density. It follows that if the kVp is kept constant, the linear attenuation coefficient will be higher for bone than it would be for lung tissue. This corresponds with what we commonly see in practice. That is, bone attenuates more of the x-ray beam than does lung, allowing fewer photons to reach the CT detectors. Ultimately, this results in an image in which bone is represented by a lighter shade of gray than that representing lung.

Differences in linear attenuation coefficients among tissues are responsible for x-ray image contrast. In CT, the image is a direct reflection of the distribution of linear attenuation coefficients. For soft tissues, the linear attenuation coefficient is roughly proportional to physical density. For this reason, the values in a CT image are sometimes referred to as density.

Metals are generally quite dense and have the greatest capacity for beam attenuation. Consequently, surgical clips and other metallic objects are represented on the CT image as white areas. Air (gas) has very low density, so it has little attenuation capacity. Air-filled structures (such as lungs) are represented on the CT image as black areas.

To differentiate an object on a CT image from adjacent objects, there must be a density difference between the two objects. An oral or intravenous administration of a contrast agent is often used to create a temporary artificial density difference between objects. Contrast agents fill a structure with a material that has a different density than that of the structure. In the cases of agents that contain barium sulfate and iodine, the material is of a higher density than the structure. These are typically referred to as positive agents. Low-density contrast agents, or negative agents, such as water, can also be used. Figure 1-4 A shows an image taken at the level of the kidneys without contrast enhancement. Figure 1-4B shows the same slice after the intravenous injection of an iodinated contrast agent. The kidneys and blood vessels are highlighted because of the high-density contrast they contain.

BOX 1-2   Key Concept

To differentiate adjacent objects on a CT image, there must be a density difference between the two objects.

Patients may find it comforting to learn that a contrast agent does not permanently change the physical properties of the structure containing it. A helpful analogy may be that of a glass of water viewed from a distance. Because the water is clear, it is difficult to see the outline of the glass clearly. If coloring is added to the water, the outline of the glass becomes more visible. The actual glass is not changed; when the colored water is replaced by clear water, the glass reverts to its former appearance. Similarly, the administration of oral or intravenous contrast agents does not change the lining of the gastrointestinal tract or the blood vessels. Rather, these agents simply fill the structures with a higher-density fluid so that their margins can be visualized on the CT image.

HOUNSFIELD UNITS

How can the degree of attenuation be measured so that comparisons are possible? In conventional film-screen radiography, only subjective means are available. That is, we must determine visually the shades of gray and surmise the densities of the structures in the patient; hence, if on a chest x-ray image we were to see a circular area of lighter gray in a lung, we would compare the shade of gray to those of other known objects on the image.

In CT, we are better able to quantify the beam attenuation capability of a given object. Measurements are expressed in Hounsfield units (HU), named after Godfrey Hounsfield, one of the pioneers in the development of CT. These units are also referred to as CT numbers, or density values.

BOX 1-3   Key Concept

Hounsfield units quantify the degree that a structure attenuates an x-ray beam.

Hounsfield arbitrarily assigned distilled water the number 0 (Fig. 1-5). He assigned the number 1000 to dense bone and −1000 to air. Objects with a beam

---

TABLE 1-1   Linear Attenuation Coefficients (cm^{-1}) at 125 kVp for Various Tissues

Tissue	Linear Attenuation Coefficient (cm^{-1})
Air	0.0003
Fat	0.162
Water	0.180
Cerebrospinal fluid	0.181
White matter	0.187
Gray matter	0.184
Blood	0.182
Dense bone	0.46

Reprinted with permission from Bushong S. Radiologic Science for Technologists: Physics, Biology, and Protection. St. Louis: Mosby, 1993:420.

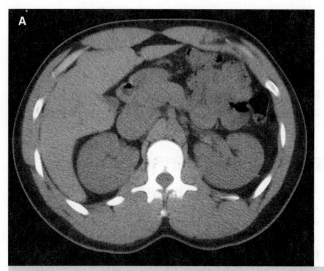
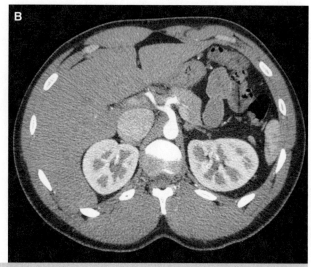

FIGURE 1-4   In (A), the slice has been taken at the level of the kidneys without contrast enhancement. Note the difficulty in differentiating blood vessels from surrounding structures. In (B), the slice has been taken after the administration of intravenous contrast media.

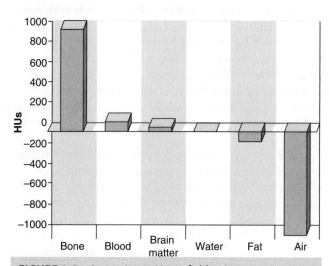

FIGURE 1-5   Approximate Hounsfield units.

attenuation less than that of water have an associated negative number. Conversely, substances with an attenuation greater than that of water have a proportionally positive Hounsfield value. The Hounsfield unit of naturally occurring anatomic structures fall within this range of 1000 to −1000. The Hounsfield unit value is directly related to the linear attenuation coefficient: 1 HU equals a 0.1% difference between the linear attenuation coefficient of the tissue as compared with the linear attenuation coefficient of water.

Using the system of Hounsfield units, a measurement of an unknown structure that appears on an image is taken and compared with measurements of known structures. It is then possible to approximate the composition of the unknown structure.

For example, a slice of abdomen shows a circular low-attenuation (dark) area on the left kidney. By taking a density reading of this area, it is discovered to measure 4 HU. It can then be assumed that it is fluid-filled (most likely a cyst). It is important to keep in mind that the reading for the assumed cyst is not exact. In this example, it is suspected that the mass is fluid because its measurement is close to that of pure water. The difference of 4 units could be caused by impurities in the cyst; it is not likely that a cyst would consist of pure water. Factors that contribute to an inaccurate Hounsfield measurement include poor equipment calibration, image artifacts, and volume averaging.

POLYCHROMATIC X-RAY BEAMS

All x-ray beam sources for CT and conventional radiography produce x-ray energy that is polychromatic. That is, the x-ray beam comprises photons with varying energies. The spectrum ranges from x-ray photons that are weak to others that are relatively strong. It is important to understand how this basic property affects the image. Low-energy x-ray photons are more readily attenuated by the patient. The detectors cannot differentiate and adjust for differences in attenuation that are caused by low-energy x-ray photons. To the detectors, any x-ray photon that reaches the detector is treated identically, whether it began with high or low energy (Fig. 1-6).

This phenomenon can produce artifacts. Artifacts are objects seen on the image but not present in the object scanned. Artifacts always degrade the image quality. Artifacts that result from preferential absorption of the low-energy photons, which leaves higher-intensity photons to strike the detector array, are called beam-hardening

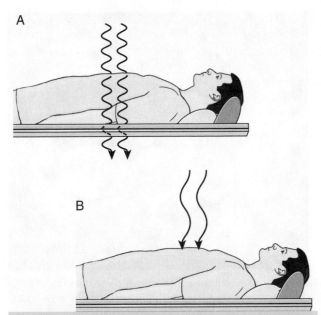

A

B

FIGURE 1-6 In (A), the photon has a higher energy and is able to penetrate the object. In (B), the photon is much weaker, and even though the object is identical, it is attenuated. The system is unable to adjust for difference in photon strength; instead, it displays the object in (B) as if it were composed of tissue of a higher density.

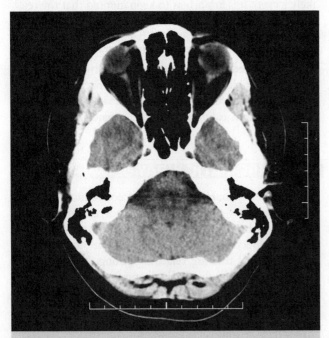

FIGURE 1-7 Streak artifacts arising from the dense petrous bones are a result of beam-hardening.

artifacts. This effect is most obvious when the x-ray beam must first penetrate a dense structure, such as the base of the skull. Beam-hardening artifacts appear as dark streaks or vague areas of decreased density, sometimes called cupping artifacts (Fig. 1-7).

Filtering the x-ray beam with a substance, such as Teflon or aluminum, helps to reduce the range of x-ray energies that reach the patient by eliminating the photons with weaker energies. It makes the x-ray beam more homogeneous. Creating a beam intensity that is more uniform improves the CT image by reducing artifacts. Additionally, filtering the soft (low-energy) photons reduces the radiation dose to the patient.

VOLUME AVERAGING

All CT examinations are performed by obtaining data for a series of slices through a designated area of interest. The nature of the anatomy and the pathology suspected determines how the examination is performed. Scanners allow the technologist to select slice thickness, and these scanners vary in the thickness choices available.

In general, the smaller the object being scanned, the thinner the CT slice required. Again, the loaf of bread analogy is helpful. This time, though, it is raisin bread. As the loaf is sliced and examined, some slices contain raisins and others do not. If the slices are thick, it increases the possibility that even though a given slice contains a raisin, it will be obscured by the bread. If the slices are thin, the likelihood of missing a raisin decreases, but the total number of slices increases. Continuing the analogy and switching to rye bread, in which small caraway seeds are being sought, one can easily understand how the slice thickness must be adjusted depending on the object being examined.

Thicker CT slices increase the likelihood of missing very small objects. For example if 10-mm slices are created, and the area of pathologic tissue measures just 2 mm, normal tissue represents 8 mm and is averaged in with the pathologic tissue, potentially making the pathologic tissue less apparent on the image, in a fashion similar to the raisins in the bread. This process is referred to as volume averaging, or partial volume effect. Therefore, if an area scanned produces images that are suspicious for a mass, but not definitive, creating thinner slices of the same area may be useful.

BOX 1–4   Key Concept

The process in CT by which different tissue attenuation values are averaged to produce one less accurate pixel reading is called *volume averaging*.

Why do some scanning protocols use thicker cuts? Modern scanners acquire data very quickly and have the capability of creating slices thinner than 1 mm. However, thinner slices result in a higher radiation dose to the patient. In addition, if the area to be scanned is large, a huge number of slices are produced. Scanning procedures are designed to provide the image quality necessary for diagnosis at an acceptable radiation dose. Generally, if the structures being investigated are very small (coronary arteries, for example) and the region to be scanned is not extensive (the heart versus the entire abdomen), then slice thickness can be quite thin. Conversely, scan protocols that span a longer anatomic region (such as the abdomen and pelvis) typically use a slice thickness of 5 to 7 mm. In addition, spiral-scanning techniques have allowed options for using data sets to retrospectively adjust the slice thickness when circumstances dictate. This technique will be discussed more fully in subsequent chapters.

The Z axis, which is defined by the slice thickness, has a significant effect on the degree of volume averaging that is present on the image. In addition, the X and Y dimensions of the pixel also affect the likelihood of volume averaging. The larger the X and Y dimensions (i.e., the larger the pixel), the more chance that the pixel will contain tissues of different densities. Because the Hounsfield unit of a single pixel is the average of all data measurements within that pixel, this type of averaging can lead to inaccuracies in the image. For example, imagine a pixel that contains equal parts calcium (measuring 600 HU) and lung tissue (measuring −600 HU). The resulting density of the specific pixel is the average of the two tissues, or 0 HU. In this case, the image pixel does not accurately reflect either the calcium or the lung tissue. Using a small pixel size reduces the likelihood of volume averaging by limiting the amount of data to be averaged. Pixel size is determined by the matrix size and the field of view selected for display (more on this in Chapter 6).

RAW DATA VERSUS IMAGE DATA

All of the thousands of bits of data acquired by the system with each scan are called raw data. The terms scan data and raw data are used interchangeably to refer to computer data waiting to be processed to create an image. Raw data have not yet been sectioned to create pixels; hence, Hounsfield unit values have not yet been assigned. The process of using the raw data to create an image is called image reconstruction. Once raw data have been processed so that each pixel is assigned a Hounsfield unit value, an image can be created; the data included in the image are now referred to as image data (see Chapter 3). The reconstruction that is automatically produced during scanning is often called prospective reconstruction. The same raw data may be used later to generate new images. This process is referred to as retrospective reconstruction.

SCAN MODES DEFINED

Step-and-Shoot Scanning

The scanning systems of the 1980s operated exclusively in a "step-and-shoot" mode. In this method 1) the x-ray tube rotated 360° around the patient to acquire data for a single slice, 2) the motion of the x-ray tube was halted while the patient was advanced on the CT table to the location appropriate to collect data for the next slice, and 3) steps

one and two were repeated until the desired area was covered. The step-and-shoot method was necessary because the rotation of the x-ray tube entwined the system cables, limiting rotation to 360°. Consequently, gantry motion had to be stopped before the next slice could be taken, this time with the x-ray tube moving in the opposite direction so that the cables would unwind. Although the terms are imprecise, this method is commonly referred to as axial scanning, conventional scanning, or serial scanning.

Helical (Spiral) Scanning

Many technical developments of the 1990s allowed for the development of a continuous acquisition scanning mode most often called spiral or helical scanning. Key among the advances was the development of a system that eliminated the cables and thereby enabled continuous rotation of the gantry. This, in combination with other improvements, allowed for uninterrupted data acquisition that traces a helical path around the patient.

Multidetector Row CT Scanning

The first helical scanners emitted x-rays that were detected by a single row of detectors, yielding one slice per gantry rotation. This technology was expanded on in 1992 when scanners were introduced that contained two rows of detectors, capturing data for two slices per gantry rotation. Further improvements equipped scanners with multiple rows of detectors, allowing data for many slices to be acquired with each gantry rotation.

Each of these scanning modes will be explored further in Chapter 5.

IMAGING PLANES

Understanding the intricacies of CT scanning requires familiarity with imaging planes. The bread slicing analogy presented earlier helps explain body planes. A brief review of the directional terms used in medicine may also make a discussion of body planes easier to understand.

All directional terms are based on the body being viewed in the anatomic position. This position is characterized by an individual standing erect, with the palms of the hands facing forward (Fig. 1-8). This position is used internationally and guarantees uniformity in descriptions of direction.

The terms anterior and ventral refer to movement forward (toward the face). Posterior and dorsal are equivalent terms used to describe movement toward the back surface of the body.

Inferior refers to movement toward the feet (down) and is synonymous with caudal (toward the tail or, in humans, the feet). Superior defines movement toward the head (up) and is used interchangeably with the term cranial or cephalic. Lateral refers to movement toward the sides of the body. Inversely, medial refers to movement toward the midline of the body.

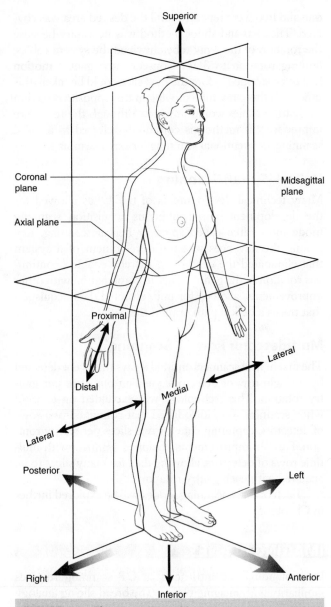

FIGURE 1-8   The anatomic position.

divides the body into right and left sections. The sagittal plane that is located directly in the center, making left and right sections of equal size, is appropriately referred to as the median, or midsagittal, plane. A parasagittal plane is located to either the left or the right of the midline. Axial planes are cross-sectional planes that divide the body into upper and lower sections. Oblique planes are sheets of glass that are slanted and lie at an angle to one of the three standard planes (Fig. 1-10).

Changing the image plane shows the same structures in a new perspective. The loaf of bread analogy can help to explain this change. For example, if a coin is baked within the bread and lies standing on edge in the loaf, a sharp knife cutting through the bread lengthwise will show the coin as a flat, rectangular density. However, if the bread is restacked and cut in an axial plan, the coin appears circular (Fig. 1-11).

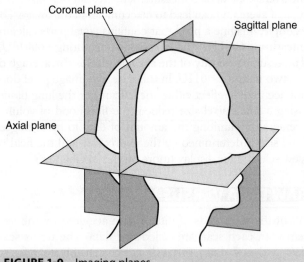

FIGURE 1-9   Imaging planes.

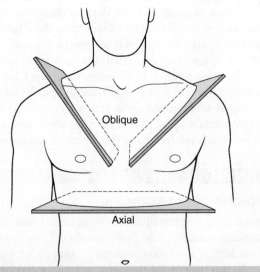

FIGURE 1-10   Oblique planes lie at an angle to one of the standard planes.

The terms distal and proximal are most often used in referring to extremities (limbs). Distal (away from) refers to movement toward the ends. The distal end of the forearm is the end to which the hand is attached. Proximal (close to), which is the opposite of distal, may be defined as situated near the point of attachment. For example, the proximal end of the arm is the end at which it attaches to the shoulder.

To help visualize the imaginary body planes, it is helpful to think of large sheets of glass cutting through the body in various ways. All sheets of glass that are parallel to the floor are called horizontal, or transverse, planes. Those that stand perpendicular to the floor are called vertical, or longitudinal, planes (Fig. 1-9).

A sheet of glass that divides the body into anterior and posterior sections is the coronal plane. The sagittal plane

The image plan can be adjusted by positioning the patient, gantry, or both to permit scanning in the desired plane or by reformatting the image data (see Chapter 8). Scanning in the desired planes produces better images than reformatting existing data, although advances in CT technology have reduced the quality difference.

Changing the image plane in CT provides additional information in a fashion similar to the coin within the bread. Changing the image plane from axial to coronal is indicated for two distinct reasons. The primary reason is when the anatomy of interest lies vertically rather than horizontally. The ethmoid sinuses are an example of this principle. Because the ethmoid turbinates lie predominately in the vertical plane, images taken in an axial plane show only sections of the anatomy, with no view of the entire ethmoid complex (Fig. 1-12A). In Figure 1-12B, the images are taken in the coronal plane, which is more suitable for displaying the ethmoid sinus structures and more readily shows an obstruction.

In the case of the sinuses, it is relatively easy to change the patient's position so that images can be acquired coronally. Obviously, this practice is not possible with all areas of the anatomy that may benefit from coronal imaging, for example, the pelvis. Because fat planes in the pelvis often run obliquely or parallel to the transverse plane, in some cases, images obtained in the coronal plane may be superior to those obtained in the axial plane. However, scanning in the coronal plane is not common because of the difficulty of positioning the pelvis. In this case, reformatting image data from an axial into a coronal plane may prove useful.

The second indication for scanning in a different plane is to reduce artifacts created by surrounding structures. For this reason, the coronal plane is preferred for scanning the pituitary gland. In the axial plane, the number of streak artifacts and the partial volume effect are greater than in the coronal plane.

Most scans are performed in the axial plane, but many head protocols require coronal scans.

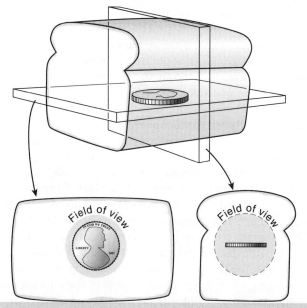

FIGURE 1-11 The imaging plane will affect the way that an area of anatomy is represented on the cross-sectional slice.

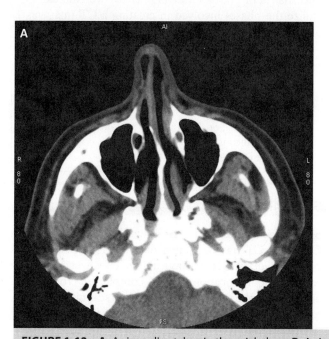
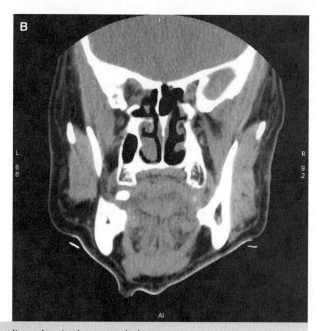

FIGURE 1-12 **A.** A sinus slice taken in the axial plane. **B.** A sinus slice taken in the coronal plane.

OVERVIEW OF CT SYSTEM OPERATION

Scanners vary widely in their mechanical makeup, and the ideal configuration and composition of detectors and tube are hotly debated topics within the industry. Each manufacturer claims that its scanner design is the best. Unfortunately, it is impossible to state unequivocally which set of design factors produces the best overall CT scanner. Fortunately, it is not essential that a technologist understand the precise makeup of each type of scanner available to perform high-quality studies. This section provides a basic understanding of how a CT image is created.

X-ray photons are created when fast-moving electrons slam into a metal target. The kinetic energy (the energy of motion) of the electrons is transformed into electromagnetic energy.

BOX 1–5   Key Concept

X-rays are produced when a substance is bombarded by fast-moving electrons.

In a CT system, the components that produce x-ray beams are housed in the gantry. The x-ray tube contains filaments that provide the electrons that create x-ray photons. This is accomplished by heating the filament until electrons start to boil off, hovering around the filament in what is known as a space cloud. The generator produces high voltage (or kV) and transmits it to the x-ray tube. This high voltage propels the electrons from the x-ray tube filament to the anode. The area of the anode where the electrons strike and the x-ray beam is produced is the focal spot. The quantity of electrons propelled is controlled by the tube current and is measured in thousandths of an ampere, milliamperes (mA). The electrons then strike the rotating anode target and disarrange the electrons in the target material. The result is the production of heat and x-ray photons. The vast majority (generally more than 99%) of the kinetic energy of the projectile electrons is converted to thermal energy. To spread the heat over a larger area, the target rotates. Increasing the voltage increases the energy with which the electrons strike the target and, hence, increases the intensity of the x-ray beam. The intensity of the x-ray beam is controlled by the kVp setting.

The ability of the tube to withstand the resultant heat is called its heat capacity, whereas its ability to rid itself of the heat is its heat dissipation. The length and frequency of scans are determined in part by the tube's heat capacity and dissipation rate.

The x-ray photons that pass through the patient strike the detector. If the detector is made from a solid-state scintillator material, the energy of the x-ray photons detected is converted to light. Other elements in the detector, usually a photodiode, convert the light levels into an electric current. On older CT systems, detectors are sometimes of the xenon gas variety. In this case, the striking photon ionizes the xenon gas. These ions are accelerated by the high voltage on the detector plates.

Regardless of the detector material, each detector cell is sampled and converted to a digital format by the data acquisition system (DAS). Each complete sample is called a view. The digital data from the DAS are then transmitted to the central processing unit (CPU). The CPU is often referred to as the brain of the CT scanner.

The reconstruction processor takes the individual views and reconstructs the densities within the slice. To create an image, information from the DAS must be translated into a matrix. To do so, the system assigns each pixel in the matrix one value, or density number. This density number, in Hounsfield units, is the average of all attenuation measurements for that pixel. These digitized data are then sent to a display processor that converts them into shades that can be displayed on a computer monitor.

Although there is wide variation in the design of scanners, they share some characteristics. The CT process can be broken down into three general segments: data acquisition, image reconstruction, and image display. In the first segment, the x-ray photons are created and directed through the patient, where either they are absorbed or they penetrate the patient to strike the CT system's detectors. The goal of this phase is to acquire the information. In the second segment, the data are sorted so that each pixel has one associated Hounsfield value. The goal of this phase is to use the information collected in the previous segment and prepare it for display. In the final phase of creating the CT image, the processed data are converted into shades of gray for viewing. Therefore, one can generalize the phases involved in creating a CT image as 1) obtaining data, 2) using data, and 3) displaying data.

BOX 1–6   Key Concept

The CT process can be broken down into three main segments:

Data Acquisition → Get Data
Image Reconstruction → Use Data
Image Display → Display Data

SUMMARY

Since its introduction by Godfrey Hounsfield and Allan Cormack, CT has continued to evolve. New techniques cover a wide variety of applications. However, with such technologic innovation comes complexity. To develop and practice the most safe and effective scanning methods, radiologic technologists must first understand the physical principles that make up the foundation of CT.

REVIEW QUESTIONS

1. What are the main advantages of CT over conventional radiography?
2. What defines the Z axis?
3. Define pixel, voxel, and matrix.
4. Explain beam attenuation. What determines a structure's ability to attenuate the x-ray beam?
5. What unit quantifies a structure's ability to attenuate the x-ray beam?
6. What is the relationship between Hounsfield units and the linear attenuation coefficient?
7. What are image artifacts?
8. Why does the slice thickness vary among examination protocols?
9. What is the anatomic position?
10. How are x-ray photons produced?

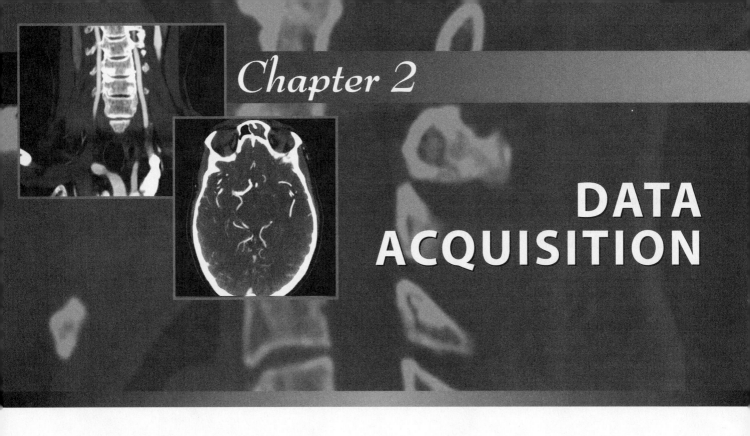

Chapter 2

DATA ACQUISITION

Key Terms: gantry aperture • high-frequency generator • power capacity • slip rings • cooling systems • focal spot size • compensating filters • bow tie filters • prepatient collimators • predetector collimators • detector • detector array • reference detectors • detector efficiency • afterglow • capture efficiency • absorption efficiency • response time • dynamic range • detector spacing • detector aperture • third-generation design • ring artifacts • fourth-generation design • electron beam imaging • data-acquisition system • analog-to-digital converter • sampling rate • table incrementation • anatomic landmark • scannable range • table referencing

CT scanners are complex, with many different components involved in the process of creating an image. Adding to the complexity, different CT manufacturers often modify the design of various components. To understand how a CT system works it is important to understand the basic function of each component, and some of the major variations in their design. From a broad perspective, all makes and models of CT scanners are similar in that they consist of a scanning gantry, x-ray generator, computer system, operator's console, and physician's viewing console. Although hard-copy filming has largely been replaced by workstation viewing and electronic archiving, most CT systems still include a laser printer for transferring CT images to film.

To help simplify the process, CT can be broken down into three segments: data acquisition, image reconstruction, and image display. This chapter will examine the components involved in the first of these three segments.

Data are acquired when x-rays pass through a patient to strike a detector and are recorded. The major components that are involved in this phase of image creation are the gantry and the patient table (Fig. 2-1).

GANTRY

The gantry is the ring-shaped part of the CT scanner. It houses many of the components necessary to produce and detect x-rays (Fig. 2-2). Components are mounted on a rotating scan frame. Gantries vary in total size as well as in the diameter of the opening, or aperture. The range of aperture size is typically 70 to 90 cm. The CT gantry can be tilted either forward or backward as needed to accommodate a variety of patients and examination protocols. The degree of tilt varies among systems, but ±15° to ±30° is usual. The gantry also includes a laser light that is used to position the patient within the scanner. Control panels located on either side of the gantry opening allow the technologist to control the alignment lights, gantry tilt, and table movement. In most scanners, these functions may also be controlled via the operator's console. A microphone is embedded in the gantry to allow communication between the patient and the technologist throughout the scan procedure.

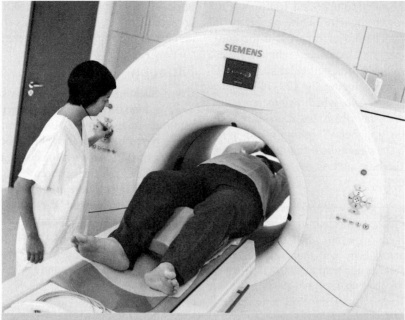

FIGURE 2-1 The gantry and patient table are major components of a CT image system. (Courtesy of Siemens AG.)

> **BOX 2-1   Key Concept**
>
> The gantry houses many of the components necessary to produce and detect x-rays. Components are mounted on a rotating scan frame.

Slip Rings

Early CT scanners used recoiling system cables to rotate the gantry frame. This design limited the scan method to the step-and-shoot mode and considerably limited the gantry rotation times. Current systems use electromechanical devices called slip rings. Slip rings use a brush-like apparatus to provide continuous electrical power and electronic communication across a rotating surface. They permit the gantry frame to rotate continuously, eliminating the need to straighten twisted system cables.

> **BOX 2-2   Key Concept**
>
> Slip rings permit the gantry frame to rotate continuously, making helical scan modes possible.

Generator

High-frequency generators are currently used in CT. They are small enough so that they can be located within the gantry. Highly stable three-phase generators have also been used, but because these are stand-alone units located near the gantry and require cables, they have become obsolete.

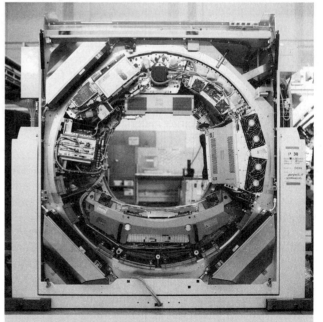

FIGURE 2-2 The gantry houses many of the components necessary to produce and detect x-rays. The gantry cover is removed on this third-generation scanner configuration to reveal the components necessary for data acquisition, including the x-ray tube and detector array. Image courtesy of Siemens AG.

Generators produce high voltage and transmit it to the x-ray tube. The power capacity of the generator is listed in kilowatts (kW). The power capacity of the generator determines the range of exposure techniques (i.e., kV and mA settings) available on a particular system. CT generators produce high kV (generally 120–140 kV) to increase the intensity of the beam, which will increase the penetrating ability of the x-ray beam and thereby reduce patient dose. In addition, a higher kV setting will help to reduce the heat load on the x-ray tube by allowing a lower mA setting. Reducing the heat load on the x-ray tube will extend the life of the tube.

BOX 2–3   Key Concept

High kV is used to increase the intensity of the beam, increasing its penetrating ability and thereby reducing patient dose. High kV settings also help to reduce the heat load on the x-ray tube by allowing a lower mA setting.

Cooling Systems

Cooling mechanisms are included in the gantry. They can take different forms, such as blowers, filters, or devices that perform oil-to-air heat exchange. Cooling mechanisms are important because many imaging components can be affected by temperature fluctuation.

X-ray Source

X-ray tubes produce the x-ray photons that create the CT image. Their design is a modification of a standard rotating anode tube, such as the type used in angiography. Tungsten, with an atomic number of 74, is often used for the anode target material because it produces a higher-intensity x-ray beam. This is because the intensity of x-ray production is approximately proportional to the atomic number of the target material. CT tubes often contain more than one size of focal spot; 0.5 and 1.0 mm are common sizes. Just as in standard x-ray tubes, because of reduced penumbra small focal spots in CT tubes produce sharper images (i.e., better spatial resolution), but because they concentrate heat onto a smaller portion of the anode they cannot tolerate as much heat.

An enormous amount of stress is placed on the CT tube. Scanning protocols often require multiple long exposures performed on numerous patients per day. A CT tube must be designed to handle such stress. The way a tube dissipates the heat that is created during x-ray production is critical. All manufacturers list generator and tube cooling capabilities in their product specifications. These specifications usually list the system generator's maximum power in kW. Also listed is the anode heat capacity in million heat units (MHU) and the maximum anode heat dissipation rate in thousand heat units (KHU). These specifications can be helpful in comparing various CT systems. It is important to remember that these values represent the upper limit of tube performance. It is also important to compare the length of protocols that the tube will allow and how quickly they can be repeated.

Filtration

Compensating filters are used to shape the x-ray beam. They reduce the radiation dose to the patient and help to minimize image artifact. As mentioned in Chapter 1, radiation emitted by CT x-ray tubes is polychromatic. Filtering the x-ray beam helps to reduce the range of x-ray energies that reach the patient by removing the long-wavelength (or "soft") x-rays. These long-wavelength x-rays are readily absorbed by the patient, therefore they do not contribute to the CT image but do contribute to the radiation dose to the patient. In addition, creating a more uniform beam intensity improves the CT image by reducing artifacts that result from beam hardening.

BOX 2–4   Key Concept

Filtering the x-ray beam helps to reduce the radiation dose to the patient and improves image quality.

Different filters are used when scanning the body than when scanning the head. Human body anatomy typically has a round cross section that is thicker in the middle than in the periphery. Hence, body-scanning filters are used to reduce the beam intensity at the periphery of the beam, corresponding to the thinner areas of a patient's anatomy. Because of their shape they are often referred to as bow tie filters (Fig. 2-3).

Collimation

Collimators restrict the x-ray beam to a specific area, thereby reducing scatter radiation. Scatter radiation reduces image quality and increases the radiation dose to the patient. Reducing the scatter improves contrast resolution and decreases patient dose. Collimators control the slice thickness by narrowing or widening the x-ray beam.

The source collimator is located near the x-ray source and limits the amount of x-ray emerging to thin ribbons. Because it acts on the x-ray beam before it passes through the patient it is sometimes referred to as prepatient collimation. The source collimator affects patient dose and determines how the dose is distributed across the slice thickness (i.e., dose profile). The source collimator resembles small shutters with an opening that adjusts, dependent on the operator's selection of slice thickness. In MDCT systems, slice thickness is also influenced by the detector element configuration (see Chapter 5). Scanners vary in the choices of slice thickness available. Choices range from 0.5 to 10 mm.

Some CT systems also use predetector collimation. This is located below the patient and above the detector array. Because this collimator shapes the beam after it has

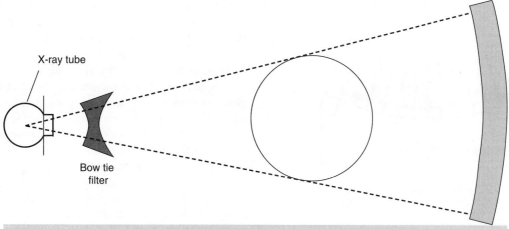

X-ray tube

Bow tie
filter

FIGURE 2-3 Filtering shapes the x-ray beam intensity. Removing low-energy x-rays minimizes patient exposure and produces a more uniform beam.

passed through the patient it is sometimes referred to as postpatient collimation. The primary functions of predetector collimators are to ensure the beam is the proper width as it enters the detector and to prevent scatter radiation from reaching the detector.

Detectors

As the x-ray beam passes through the patient it is attenuated to some degree. To create an x-ray image we must collect information regarding the degree to which each anatomic structure attenuated the beam. In conventional radiography we used a film-screen system to record the attenuation information. In CT, we use detectors to collect the information. The term detector refers to a single element or a single type of detector used in a CT system. The term detector array is used to describe the entire collection of detectors included in a CT system. Specifically, the detector array comprises detector elements situated in an arc or a ring, each of which measures the intensity of transmitted x-ray radiation along a beam projected from the x-ray source to that particular detector element. Also included in the array are elements referred to as reference detectors that help to calibrate data and reduce artifacts.

The scan field of view determines the size of the fan beam, which, in turn, determines the number of detector elements that collect data. Scan field of view is discussed in more detail in Chapter 3.

Detectors can be made from different substances, each with their own advantages and disadvantages. The optimal characteristics of a detector are as follows: 1) high detector efficiency, defined as the ability of the detector to capture transmitted photons and change them to electronic signals; 2) low, or no, afterglow, defined as a brief, persistent flash of scintillation that must be taken into account and subtracted before image reconstruction; 3) high scatter suppression; and 4) high stability, which

allows a system to be used without the interruption of frequent calibration.

Overall detector efficiency is the product of a number of factors. These are 1) stopping power of the detector material; 2) scintillator efficiency (in solid-state types); 3) charge collection efficiency (in xenon types); 4) geometric efficiency, defined as the amount of space occupied by the detector collimator plates relative to the surface area of the detector; and 5) scatter rejection.

Other terms are sometimes used to describe aspects of a detector's efficiency. Capture efficiency refers to the ability with which the detector obtains photons that have passed through the patient. Absorption efficiency refers to the number of photons absorbed by the detector and is dependent on the physical properties of the detector face (e.g., thickness, material). Response time is the time required for the signal from the detector to return to zero after stimulation of the detector by x-ray radiation so that it is ready to detect another x-ray event. The detector response is generally a function of the detector design. Dynamic range is the ratio of the maximum signal measured to the minimum signal the detectors can measure.

All new scanners possess detectors of the solid-state crystal variety. Detectors made from xenon gas have been manufactured but have largely become obsolete as their design prevents them from use in MDCT systems. However, because some xenon gas detector systems may still be in use on older models their design will be briefly discussed here.

Xenon Gas Detectors

Pressurized xenon gas fills hollow chambers to produce detectors that absorb approximately 60% to 87% of the photons that reach them. Xenon gas is used because of its ability to remain stable under pressure. Compared with the solid-state variety, xenon gas detectors are significantly

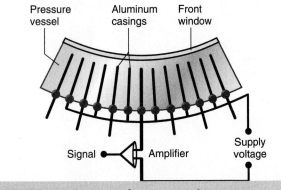

FIGURE 2-4   Structure of a xenon gas detector array.

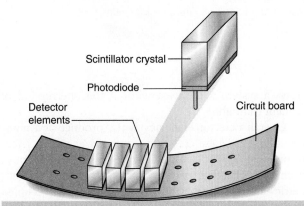

FIGURE 2-5   Structure of a solid-state detector array.

less expensive to produce, somewhat easier to calibrate, and are highly stable.

A xenon detector channel consists of three tungsten plates. When a photon enters the channel, it ionizes the xenon gas. These ions are accelerated and amplified by the electric field between the plates. The collected charge produces an electric current. This current is then processed as raw data. A disadvantage of xenon gas is that it must be kept under pressure in an aluminum casing. This casing filters the x-ray beam to a certain extent. Loss of x-ray photons in the casing window and the space taken up by the plates are the major factors hampering detector efficiency. Figure 2-4 demonstrates the basic structure of a xenon gas detector array.

Solid-State Crystal Detector

Solid-state detectors are also called scintillation detectors because they use a crystal that fluoresces when struck by an x-ray photon. A photodiode is attached to the crystal and transforms the light energy into electrical (analog) energy. The individual detector elements are affixed to a circuit board (Fig. 2-5). Solid-state crystal detectors have been made from a variety of materials, including cadmium tungstate, bismuth germinate, cesium iodide, and ceramic rare earth compounds such as gadolinium or yttrium. Because these solids have high atomic numbers and high

density in comparison to gases, solid-state detectors have higher absorption coefficients. They absorb nearly 100% of the photons that reach them. In addition, there is no loss in the front window, as in xenon systems. This increased absorption efficiency is the chief advantage of solid-state detectors. Solid-state detectors may produce a brief afterglow. However, this has been greatly reduced or eliminated in modern CT detectors. Solid-state detectors are more sensitive to fluctuation in temperature and moisture than the gas variety. Table 2-1 compares solid-state detectors to the xenon gas variety.

The relative placement, shape, and size of the detectors affect the amount of scatter radiation that reaches the image. A deep, narrow detector design will accept less scatter than short, wide detectors. Detectors are separated using spacing bars. This allows the detectors to be placed in an arc or circle. Detector spacing is measured from the middle of one detector to the middle of the neighboring detector and accounts for the spacing bar. Ideally, detectors should be placed as close together as possible, so all x-rays are converted to data. The size of the detector opening is called the aperture. A small detector is important for good spatial resolution and scatter rejection. Maximum utilization and small aperture are desirable. Figure 2-6 shows the relationship between detector arrangement and scatter acceptance.

Scanner Generation

The configuration of the x-ray tube to the detectors determines scanner generation. The first system produced by the now defunct EMI medical division had a design that is referred to as first generation. A thin x-ray beam passed linearly over the patient, and a single detector followed on the opposite side of the patient. The tube and detector were then rotated slightly, and the process was repeated until a 180° arc was covered. Scan times were very long. This design is no longer in use.

As new developments in scanning occurred, each new tube-detector design was referred to by a consecutive generation number. The second-generation design is one in which the x-ray beam also passed linearly across the patient before rotating. However, a fan-shaped x-ray beam was used, rather than the thin beam used with first-generation designs. Only part of the field of view could be covered

TABLE 2-1 Characteristics of Detectors	
Solid-State Crystal	**Pressurized Xenon Gas**
High photon absorption	Moderate photon absorption
Sensitive to temperature, moisture	Highly stable
Solid material	Low-density material (gas)
Can exhibit afterglow	No afterglow
No front window loss	Losses attributable to front window and the spaces taken up by the plates

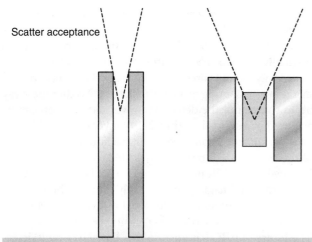

FIGURE 2-6 Detector spacing and aperture. **A.** The width and spacing of the detectors affect the amount of scatter that is recorded. **B.** Low scatter acceptance is desirable. Simple geometric principles affect scatter acceptance.

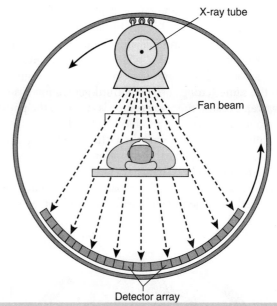

FIGURE 2-7 A third-generation scanner design is one in which the x-ray tube is placed opposite the detector array. Both the tube and the detector move in a circle within the gantry.

with this fan beam. A detector array was also incorporated in the second-generation design. Although scan times were shorter than that of the original design, they were still very long. This type of design is also no longer used.

BOX 2–5   Key Concept

The configuration of the x-ray tube to the detector determines scanner generation.

The next advance in CT technology brought the third-generation design. This design consists of a detector array and an x-ray tube that produces a fan-shaped beam that covered the entire field of view and a detector array (Fig. 2-7). Reference detectors are typically located at either end of the detector array to measure the unattenuated x-ray beam. The third-generation design made it no longer necessary to translate the beam and detector as both could move in a circle within the gantry. The rotating detector design allows all of the readings that make up a view to be recorded instantaneously and simultaneously. This greatly reduced scan times and helped to reduce artifact resulting from patient motion. An advantage of the third-generation system is that the tube is directly focused on the detector array (Fig. 2-8). The fixed relationship between the x-ray source and the detectors allow the beam to be highly collimated, which greatly reduces scatter radiation, thereby improving image quality. A disadvantage of the third-generation design (as compared with the fourth-generation design described in the next paragraph) is the more frequent occurrence of ring artifacts. Because the same bank of detectors is used repeatedly, even a very small misalignment of a single detector will result in visible ring artifact (more about artifacts in Chapter 7). Third-generation systems are sometimes referred to as rotate-rotate scanners. The third-generation

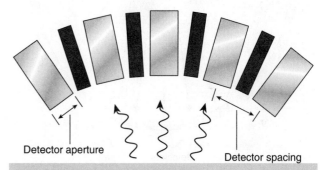

FIGURE 2-8 Third-generation systems allow the x-rays to be focused directly on the detector bank, which reduces the amount of scatter that reaches the detectors.

design is the most widely used configuration in the industry today. All new multidetector CT systems sold in the United States use the third-generation design.

Fourth-generation scanners use a detector array that is fixed in a 360° circle within the gantry. The tube rotates within the fixed detector array and produces a fan-shaped beam (Fig. 2-9). Although many more detector elements are included in this design, the number of detectors in use at any one time is controlled by the width of the beam. In the stationary detector design, the readings that make up a view are recorded consecutively during approximately one-fifth of the scan time. Because the emerging beam does not strike the detectors at exactly the same time, motion artifacts are more of a problem. Fourth-generation systems often use overscans to address this problem. An overscan is a tube arc greater than 360°. The use of an overscan technique will increase the radiation dose to the patient. In addition, because the tube is closer to the patient, the same milliampere-seconds (mAs) and kilovolt-peak (kVp) setting will produce a higher dose when a fourth-generation system is used (as compared with the same settings used in a third-generation system). However, because the x-ray source is closer to the patient, techniques necessary to produce an adequate image are generally somewhat lower than that used on a third-generation system. Fourth-generation scanners may also be called rotate-only systems.

Many variations of these basic designs have been introduced and then abandoned. The only other design currently in use is called electron beam imaging, also referred to as EBCT or ultrafast CT. It differs from conventional CT in a number of ways. This system, which was originally produced by Imatron, uses a large electron gun as its x-ray beam source. A massive anode target is placed in a semicircular ring around the patient. Neither the x-ray beam source nor the detectors move, and the scan can be acquired in a short time (Fig. 2-10). Invented in the 1980s, its superior speed compared with traditional CT scanners of the time made it particularly suited to cardiac imaging. However, shortfalls in spatial resolution kept EBCT from use in routine imaging, dramatically limiting the technology's clinical versatility. Additional drawbacks were high cost and difficulties obtaining insurance reimbursement. The future of EBCT is uncertain as the newer multidetector row technology applied to third-generation scanners has increased scanning speed so that they compare favorably with EBCT. Because of its many fundamental differences from CT and uncertainties regarding its future, electron beam imaging is not covered in this text.

Detector Electronics

X-ray photons that strike the detector must be measured, converted to a digital signal, and sent to the computer. This is accomplished by the data-acquisition system (DAS), which is positioned within the gantry near the detectors. Signals emitted from the detectors are analog (electric), whereas computers require digital signals. Therefore, one of the tasks of the DAS is to convert the analog signal to a digital format. This is accomplished with the aptly named analog-to-digital converter or ADC.

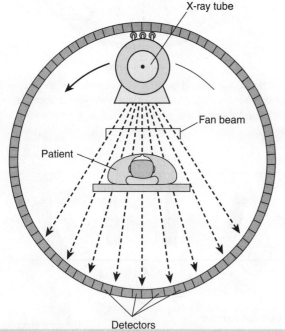

FIGURE 2-9 A fourth-generation scanner design uses a detector array that is fixed in a 360° circle within the gantry. The tube rotates within the gantry.

BOX 2–6   Key Concept

The data-acquisition system, or DAS, measures the number of photons that strikes the detector, converts the information to a digital signal, and sends the signal to the computer.

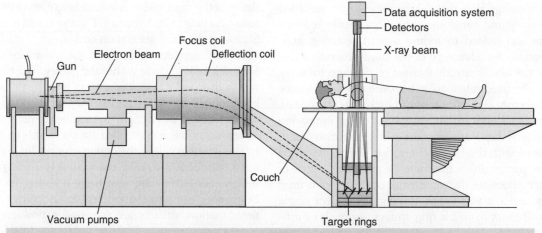

FIGURE 2-10   The design of EBCT scanners is fundamentally different from the design of other CT systems.

To measure the x-ray photons that have penetrated the patient, the detectors are sampled many times, as many as 1,000 times per second by the DAS. The number of samples taken per second from the continuous signal emitted from the detector is known as the sampling rate, sample rate, or sampling frequency. Artifacts, such as streaking, can appear on the image if the number of samples is insufficient.

PATIENT TABLE

The patient lies on the table (or couch, as it is referred to by some manufacturers) and is moved within the gantry for scanning. The process of moving the table by a specified measure is most commonly called incrementation, but is also referred to as feed, step, or index. Helical CT table incrementation is quantified in millimeters per second because the table continues to move throughout the scan. The degree to which a table can move horizontally is called the scannable range, and will determine the extent a patient can be scanned without repositioning.

A numeric readout of the table location relative to the gantry is displayed. When the patient is placed within the gantry, an anatomic landmark, such as the xiphoid or the iliac crest, is adjusted so that it lies at the scan point. At this level, the table is referenced, which means that the table position is manually set at zero by the technologist. Accurate table referencing helps to maintain consistency between examinations. For example, if a lesion is seen on an image that is 50 mm inferior* to the xiphoid landmark (zero point), the patient is removed from the gantry, and a ruler is used to measure 50 mm inferior from the xiphoid. This point provides an approximation of the location of the lesion. This system is also helpful if the scan will be repeated at a later date, exclusively through the area of interest determined on the earlier scan. For this reason, the setting of landmarks must be consistent among CT staff.

The specifications of tables vary, but all have certain weight restrictions. If the patient's weight exceeds the specified limits, scanning is often still possible. However, the table increments may not be as accurate. This problem affects small table increments more than those 5 mm or larger. On most scanners, it is possible to place the patient either head first or feet first, supine or prone. Patient position within the gantry depends on the examination being performed. Various attachments are available for specific types of scanning procedures. For example, attachments for direct coronal scanning of the head and for therapy planning are common.

---

*Most scanners refer to this point as −50, using numbers that are consecutively more negative as the scan progresses toward the feet. However, some systems reverse this numbering system. There are also systems that refer to this point as I50, meaning 50 mm inferior to the zero point.

SUMMARY

The first step in creating a CT image is to acquire data that result from the attenuation of the x-ray beam as it passes through the patient to strike the detector. The mechanisms housed within the gantry and the patient table are the components necessary for data acquisition. Figure 2-11 diagrams the basic data-acquisition scheme in CT.

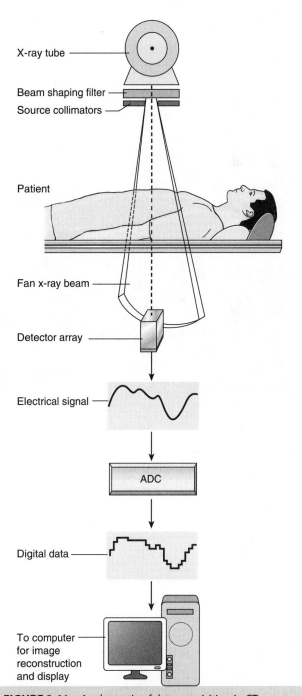

FIGURE 2-11 A schematic of data acquisition in CT.

REVIEW QUESTIONS

1. What are the major components used for data acquisition?
2. What advances in scanning were made possible by slip rings?
3. Name an advantage and a disadvantage to using a small focal spot.
4. What is the purpose of x-ray beam filtration?
5. Explain the function and purpose of source collimators.
6. List and define the optimal characteristics of a detector.
7. Why are solid-state detectors sometimes called scintillators?
8. Explain the fundamental difference between third- and fourth-generation CT systems.
9. Explain why ring artifacts are more common in CT systems with a third-generation design.
10. Why is an ADC a necessary part of the DAS?
11. Why is it important for all CT staff to set landmarks in the same way?

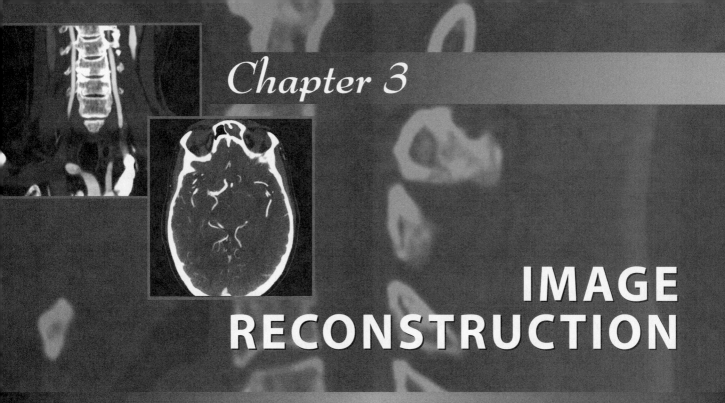

Chapter 3

IMAGE RECONSTRUCTION

Key Terms: algorithm · Fourier transform · discrete Fourier transform · fast Fourier transform · linear interpolation · hardware · software · hard disk, · archiving · input device · output device · central processing unit · memory · array processor · read-only memory · random access memory · write-once read-many times memory · serial access memory · raw data · scan data · prospective reconstruction · retrospective reconstruction · image data · ray · ray sum · view · attenuation profile · back projection · filter functions · convolution · scan field of view · isocenter · out-of-field artifacts · display field of view · image center · RAS coordinates

The data collected from the detectors must undergo many steps in the reconstruction process. This chapter examines how the acquired data are manipulated to produce a CT image.

RECONSTRUCTION TERMINOLOGY

Some of the terminology used to describe steps in the reconstruction process may be unfamiliar to the reader. Therefore, the first step in describing image reconstruction is to define common terms.

Algorithm

An algorithm is a finite set of unambiguous steps performed in a prescribed sequence to solve a problem. Algorithms are the basis for most computer programming. In CT, reconstruction algorithms are used by the computer to solve the many mathematical equations necessary for information from the detector array to be converted to information suitable for image display. Fortunately, understanding the specific mathematics involved is not necessary to grasp the process used for image reconstruction.

BOX 3–1   Key Concept

An algorithm is a precise set of steps to be performed in a specific order to solve a problem. Algorithms are the basis for most computer programming.

Fourier Transform

Developed by the 17th-century mathematician Baron Jean-Baptiste-Joseph Fourier, the Fourier transform is a method to study waves of many different sorts and also to solve several kinds of linear differential equations. Loosely speaking it separates a function into its frequency components. A rough analogy is a musical chord being separated into individual notes. More precisely, it is a technique for expressing a waveform as a weighted sum of sines and cosines. Computers generally rely on a version known as discrete Fourier transform (DFT). An efficient algorithm to compute DFT and its inverse is called fast Fourier transform (FFT). FFTs are of great importance to a wide variety of applications including acoustical and image analysis, and have been used in fields as varied as geologic surveying to actuarial analysis for the insurance industry.

Interpolation

Interpolation is a mathematical method of estimating the value of an unknown function using the known value on either side of the function. Linear interpolation is the simplest type and is frequently used in mathematics and science. Linear interpolation assumes that an unknown point falls along a straight line between two known points. Assume that point A is known to equal 0, and point C is known to equal 10. Linear interpolation allows us to assume that a point halfway between A and C will equal 5.

Many other forms of interpolation exist, such as polynomial, spline, and multivariate interpolation. The various interpolation methods can only be completely understood by examining the series of equations associated with each method. However, this level of comprehension is not necessary to understand the concept of image reconstruction.

BOX 3-2   Key Concept

Interpolation is a mathematical method of creating missing data.

EQUIPMENT COMPONENTS USED FOR IMAGE RECONSTRUCTION

Hardware and Software

A computer consists of both hardware and software. The hardware is the portion of the computer that can be physically touched. Software is instructions that tell the computer what to do and when to do it. Each time the x-ray tube is activated, information is gathered and fed into the system computer. The computer processes thousands of bits of data from each scan acquired to create the CT image. These data must be saved to a computer file so that the information will be available for use in the formation of an image. These stored data can later be retrieved and manipulated. The hard disk is the device within the computer that saves this information.

Hard Disk

The hard disk (or hard drive) is an essential component of all CT systems. The number of images that the hard disk can store varies according to the make and model of the scanner. It is important to remember than an enormous amount of information is collected for each image.

For example, a single image in a 512 matrix system consists of 262,144 pixels (512 × 512). The digitization requires 10 to 12 bits; an 8-bit byte is standard. Therefore, it takes 2 bytes to cover each pixel in the dynamic range. This requirement translates to 2 × 262,144 = 524,288

bytes, or 0.52 megabytes (MB). When a 1,024 matrix system is used, each image requires approximately 2 MB.

When hard disk space capacity is reached, existing data must be deleted before any new data can be acquired. Many facilities use a long-term storage device to save these data. Saving studies on auxiliary devices for possible future viewing is referred to as archiving. The many options available for archiving are discussed in Chapter 9.

Computer Components

The principal components in a computer are an input device, an output device, a central processing unit (CPU), and memory. Input and output devices are ancillary pieces of computer hardware designed to feed data into the computer or accept processed data from the computer. Examples of input devices are keyboard, mouse, touch-sensitive plasma screen, and CT detector mechanisms. Output devices include monitor, laser camera, printer, and archiving equipment such as optical disks or magnetic tape.

Central Processing Unit

The CPU is the component that interprets computer program instructions and sequences tasks. It contains the microprocessor, the control unit, and the primary memory. In the past the CPU design frequently used for CT image reconstruction was the array processor. Also called a vector processor, this design was able to run mathematical operations on multiple data elements simultaneously. Array processors were common in the scientific computing area throughout the 1980s and into the 1990s, but general increases in performance and processor design resulted in their elimination.

BOX 3-3   Key Concept

The central processing unit, or CPU, interprets computer program instructions and sequences tasks. It has been referred to as the "brain" of the CT system.

Computer Memory

The three principal types of solid-state memory are read-only memory (ROM), random access memory (RAM), and write-once read-many times (WORM) memory. Both ROM and RAM are part of the system's primary memory. Primary storage refers to the computer's internal memory. It is accessible to the CPU without the use of the computer's input/output channels. Primary memory is used to store data that are likely to be in active use. Primary storage is typically very fast.

ROM is imprinted at the factory and is used to store frequently used instructions such as those required for starting the system. RAM includes instructions that are frequently changed, such as the data used to reconstruct images. RAM is so named because all parts of it can be reached easily at random. RAM is very fast, but is also volatile, losing the stored data in the case of a power loss. The opposite of RAM is serial access memory (SAM), which stores data that can only be accessed sequentially (like a cassette tape). WORM refers to computer storage devices that can be written to once, but read from many times. These can be subdivided into two types: those that can be physically written to only once, such as CD-R (compact disk-recordable) and DVD-R (digital video disk-recordable), and those that have rewriting capabilities but use devices that prevent data already written on a tape from being rewritten, reformatted, or erased. The rationale for disabling rewrite functionality is to comply with regulatory standards, such as the Health Insurance Portability and Accountability Act (HIPAA).

BOX 3-4   Key Concept: How Computer Memory Works

- The computer is turned on.
- The computer loads data from ROM and performs tests to make sure all the major components are functioning properly. The computer loads the basic input/output system from ROM, providing information about things such as storage devices, start-up sequences, security, and ancillary device recognition.
- The computer loads the operating system (OS) from the hard disk into the system's RAM. The critical parts of the OS are maintained in RAM as long as the computer is on, allowing the CPU to have immediate access to the OS.
- When an application is opened, it is loaded in RAM. This temporary storage area allows the information to be more readily accessed by the CPU. Hence, the CPU gets the data it needs from RAM, processes it, and writes new data back to the RAM in a continuous cycle.
- When you save a file and close the application, the file is written to the specific storage device, and then it and the application are purged from RAM. If the files are not saved to a permanent storage device before being purged, they are lost.
- In CT systems, software instructs the computer to automatically save reconstructed images to a permanent storage device to prevent unintentional loss.

DATA TYPES

Raw Data

All of the thousands of bits of data acquired by the system with each scan are called raw data. The terms scan data and raw data are used interchangeably to refer to the data sitting in the computer waiting to be made into an image. The process of using raw data to create an image is called image reconstruction. The reconstruction that is automatically produced during scanning is often called prospective reconstruction. The same raw data may be used later to generate a new image. This process is referred to as retrospective reconstruction.

Because raw data include all measurements obtained from the detector array, a variety of images can be created from the same data. Because raw data requires a vast amount of hard disk space, CT systems offer limited disk space for the storage of raw data.

BOX 3-5   Key Concept

Raw data includes all measurements obtained from the detector array. Raw data storage requires much more computer storage space than that of image data.

Image Data

To form an image, the computer assigns one value (Hounsfield unit) to each pixel. This value, or density number, is the average of all attenuation measurements for that pixel. The two-dimensional pixel represents a three-dimensional portion of patient tissue. The pixel value represents the proportional amount of x-ray energy that passes through anatomy and strikes the detector. Once the data are averaged so that each pixel has one associated number, an image can be formed. The data included in this image are appropriately called image data. Image data require approximately one-fifth of the computer space needed for raw data. For this reason it is common for CT systems to accommodate many more image data files than they do raw data files.

If only image data are available, data manipulation is limited. Image data allow measurements such as Hounsfield units, standard deviation (see Chapter 4), and distance, but anything not seen on the image is unavailable for analysis.

BOX 3-6   Key Concept

Image data are those which result once the computer has processed the raw data. One Hounsfield unit value is assigned to each pixel.

OVERVIEW OF IMAGE RECONSTRUCTION

As the x-ray tube travels along its circular path, continuous x-ray energy is being generated. The path that the x-ray beam takes from the tube to the detector is referred to as a ray (Fig. 3-1A). The DAS reads each arriving ray and measures how much of the beam is attenuated. This measurement is called a ray sum. A complete set of ray sums is known as a view (Fig. 3-1B). A view can be compared with a person looking at an object. From only one angle, it is difficult to obtain a true understanding of the shape of the object. To obtain the most realistic picture of the object, it would be best to walk around and observe it from many angles. The observer's final evaluation of the object would involve all of his observations. The CT image is created in much the same way. Many views are needed to create an image.

The system accounts for the attenuation properties of each ray sum and correlates them with the position of the ray. The result of this type of correlation is called an attenuation profile. An attenuation profile is created for each view in the scan (Fig. 3-2). The information from all of the profiles is projected onto a matrix. This process of converting the data from the attenuation profile to a matrix is known as back projection (Fig. 3-3).

A

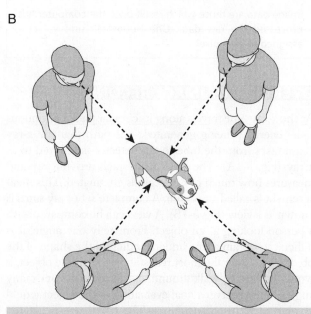

B

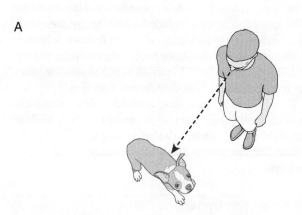

FIGURE 3-1 This figure depicts the concepts of ray (A) and view (B).

Filter Functions

There is a significant drawback to back projecting data onto a matrix: it produces streak artifacts in a star pattern on the image. To minimize these artifacts, a process called filtering is applied to the scan data before back projection occurs. The process of filtering is done through complicated mathematic steps. The process of applying a filter function to an attenuation profile is called convolution. Filtered back-projection algorithms use Fourier theory to reduce statistical noise and create an image that is pleasing to the eye.

Many different filters are available that use different algorithms depending on which parts of the data must be enhanced or suppressed. Some will "smooth" the data more heavily, by reducing the difference between adjacent pixels. This can help to reduce the appearance of artifacts but does so at the cost of reduced spatial resolution. Conversely, some filters accentuate the difference between neighboring pixels to optimize spatial resolution, but must make sacrifices in low contrast resolution. Because of their impact on image quality, filtering algorithms will be discussed again in Chapter 6. Depending on the manufacturer, the filter function may be referred to as algorithm, convolution filter, or kernel. Filter functions can only be applied to raw data (not image data). Therefore, to reconstruct an image using a

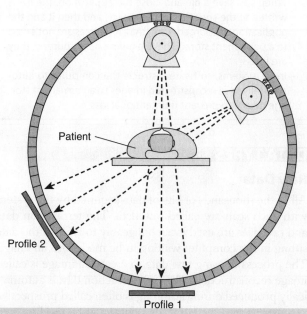

FIGURE 3-2 An attenuation profile is created for each view.

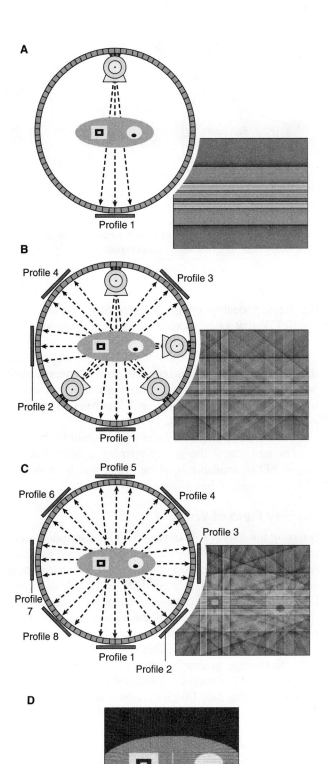

FIGURE 3-3 Data are converted from the attenuation profiles to a matrix with a process known as back projection. **A.** With only one back projection, not much information about the object scanned is revealed. **B.** With four back projections, some details start to emerge. **C.** With eight back projections, more details are visible. **D.** With 60 back projections, the image finally resembles the objects scanned.

different filter function, the raw data must be available for that image. It is important to differentiate reconstruction algorithms from merely setting a window width and level. Changing the window setting (which will be discussed in detail in the next chapter) merely changes the way the image is viewed. Changing the algorithm will change the way the raw data are manipulated to reconstruct the image.

Adaptive Statistical Iterative Reconstruction

Another method of image reconstruction has been recently introduced for use in CT image reconstruction known as iterative reconstruction. Although the iterative reconstruction method also uses a group of algorithms to reconstruct images from the projections of an object, it differs from the filtered back-projection method. There are a large variety of algorithms used, but each starts with an assumed image, computes projections from the image, compares it with the original projection data, and updates the image on the basis of the difference between the calculated and the actual projections. These are called adaptive statistical iterative reconstruction algorithms. Using these algorithms statistical noise profiles are used in an iterative manner to extract additional image clarity and suppress noise. This new advanced reconstruction technique can reduce image noise, thereby improving image quality by improving low-contrast detectability. Compared with standard filtered back-projection methods, this technique has been shown to reduce the radiation dose to the patient by as much as 50%.

Scan Field of View

Scan field of view (SFOV) is also called calibration field of view. Selecting the SFOV determines the area, within the gantry, from which the raw data are acquired (Fig. 3-4). By selecting a 25-cm SFOV, a technologist acquires data in a circular shape, with a diameter of 25 cm, lying in the absolute center, or isocenter, of the gantry. Because scan data are always acquired around the isocenter, the patient must be positioned in the center of the gantry. SFOV selection determines the number of detector cells collecting data (Fig. 3-5). The choices of SFOV vary among scanners. Typical choices are small (25 cm), which is used for the head; medium (35 cm), which is often used for the chest; and large (42–50 cm), which is used for the abdomen. On some systems, only two choices are available: half-field, which is used for the head, and full-field, which is used for everything else.

BOX 3-9   Key Concept

SFOV determines the area, within the gantry, from which the raw data are acquired.

A

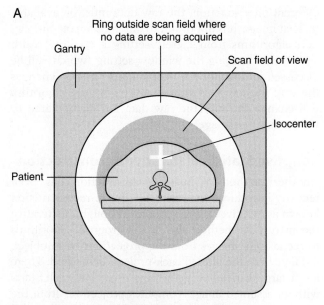

B

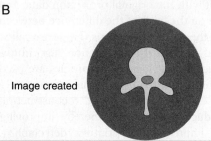

FIGURE 3-4   A. Raw data are collected within the scan field of view. **B.** Image data are confined to those displayed on the monitor.

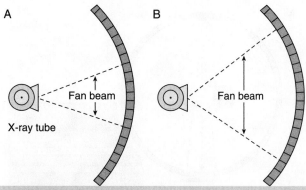

FIGURE 3-5   The selection of scan field of view determines the number of detector cells collecting data.

CT systems often incorporate other factors, in addition to size, into the SFOV selection. These factors include calibration vectors and types of image processing (head versus body). It is important to understand which factors are being included with which SFOV. For instance, if two small fields are available on a scanner, both offering a 25-cm scan size, how do they differ? Usually, the difference is related to associated image processing, which attempts to compensate for difficulties inherent when scanning specific anatomy. For instance, the small SFOV that is intended for head scanning may include special image processing that attempts to reduce the streak artifact commonly seen in the posterior fossa. Choices specific to each manufacturer are described in the product literature.

Anything outside the SFOV is not imaged because no data are collected beyond this circle.* To produce

the highest quality image, the operator should select the SFOV that comes closest to just encompassing the patient. It is important that no part of the patient lie outside the scan field. Parts of the patient located outside the SFOV may cause inaccuracies in the image, called out-of-field artifacts. These artifacts are manifest in the image as streaking, shading, and incorrect Hounsfield numbers.

Data are not acquired on everything within the gantry. For example, if the gantry opening is 70 cm but the largest SFOV available is 48 cm, there will be a ring in which data cannot be collected.

Display Field of View

Selecting the display field of view (DFOV; also called zoom or target) determines how much of the collected raw data is used to create an image. For example, if a lumbar spine is correctly scanned with a large SFOV to include the entire body, but the operator chooses to target the image so that the vertebrae occupy most of the screen, the rest of the patient's abdomen is not visualized on the image. The section that is visualized is the DFOV. Changing the DFOV will affect image quality by changing the pixel size (see Chapter 6). DFOV works in a manner similar to the zoom on a camera (Fig. 3-6). Imagine a viewer is looking at a grid through a camera lens and wishes to see the entire grid; she adjusts the lens of the camera to a corresponding point. If the viewer wishes to see a specific part of the grid more clearly, she adjusts the zoom of the camera lens to enlarge that part, even though other sections of the grid will no longer be visible.

BOX 3–10   Key Concept

The section of data selected for display on the image is called the DFOV.

To select the amount of raw data to be displayed on the CT image, the operator selects some number

---

*A few systems collect data outside the field of view, but apply calibration only to the selected scan field size. In these systems, anatomy just outside the SFOV will not cause significant artifacts.

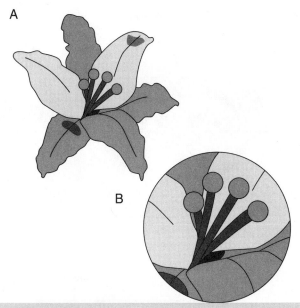

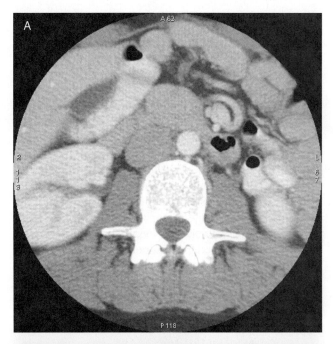

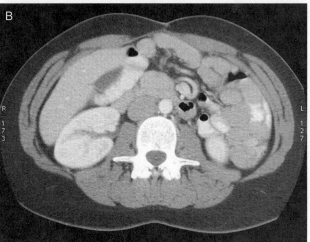

FIGURE 3-6 Selecting the display field of view determines how much of the raw data are used to create an image. Display field works like the zoom on a camera and can be used to show the entire area or to display a specific region of interest in greater detail.

(in either centimeters or millimeters depending on the scanner manufacturer) as the DFOV. Because the data selected for the DFOV are a subset of all the scan data available, the DFOV cannot be larger than the SFOV. (Refer to Clinical Application Box 3-1.)

FIGURE 3-7   **A.** Important parts of the anatomy are cut off in this image, displayed with a 25-cm field of view. Can it be corrected without rescanning? If the scan field of view was sufficient to encompass to all of the anatomy and the raw data are still available, a new image can be reconstructed using a larger field of view **(B)**. However, if the scan field of view was also 25 cm, then no other data were collected. The only solution would be to rescan the patient.

Clinical Application Box 3-1

Assume a scan of the body was performed on a large man using an appropriate body SFOV of 48 cm, but the operator mistakenly chose a 25-cm DFOV. The prospective images contain only the center portion of the patient's abdomen (Fig. 3-7A). However, because the SFOV was appropriate, data were collected that included the entire cross section of the patient's abdomen. Therefore, the raw data can be used to create a new set of images in which the DFOV is adjusted to encompass the entire area of interest (Fig. 3-7B). Of course, the retrospective images must be created while the raw data are still available.

In contrast, assume the scan was taken in error using a 25-cm SFOV (intended for a head scan) as well as a 25-cm DFOV. The prospective image that resulted would look similar to that of Figure 3-8A (there may be pronounced out-of-field artifact). However, in this situation no data were collected beyond those displayed, so the image could not be reconstructed with a larger DFOV.

Choosing the optimal display field improves the detectability of abnormalities. Selecting too large a DFOV makes the image appear unnecessarily small. In addition to the inherent difficulty in viewing smaller images, more data are included in each pixel and spatial resolution decreases (see Chapter 6). On the other hand, too small a DFOV may exclude necessary patient anatomy.

Image Center

To select the specific area within the SFOV that will be displayed on the image, the technologist must choose image coordinates. These are based on the standard Cartesian coordinates in math.* Some CT systems refer to these coordinates using the traditional *x* and *y*, whereas others have attempted to simplify the process by substituting directional coordinates. In these systems numbers are preceded by R (right), L (left), A (anterior), P (posterior), S (superior), and I (inferior). Directional coordinate systems have been called RAS systems, an acronym for **r**ight-left, **a**nterior-posterior, **s**uperior-inferior. Figure 3-8 diagrams how an image center would be adjusted using either traditional *x, y* values or RAS coordinates.

Software on modern scanners makes the process of selecting the correct image center simple. In most instances, the operator need only place a cursor on the localizer images to accurately set the center on the cross-sectional slices.

SUMMARY

Image reconstruction refers to the process whereby a computer manipulates data collected from the detectors to create a CT image. A basic understanding of the concepts common in computer science are helpful building blocks. These concepts include the use of algorithms, Fourier transform, and methods of interpolation. Similarly, the student should be aware of the function of the hardware and software used by CT systems.

Raw data include all attenuation measurements obtained from the detector array. Some of these raw data are used in the creation of the image. After the raw data are averaged and each pixel is assigned a Hounsfield number, an image can be reconstructed. The data that form this image are then referred to as image data.

SFOV refers to a selected circle in the center of the gantry. Raw data are acquired and calibrated for any object that lies within this circle. The entire scan circle or any portion of the circle may be selected to display on the monitor. The size of the circle that is displayed is called DFOV.

Once the computer has manipulated the raw data throughout the image reconstruction process, it is then ready to be displayed.

---

*In mathmatics the Carstesian coordinate system (also called **rectangular coordinate system**) is used to determine each point uniquely in a plane through two numbers, usually called the *x* coordinate and *y* coordinate of the point. To define the coordinates, two perpendicular directed lines (the *x* axis and the *y* axis) are specified.

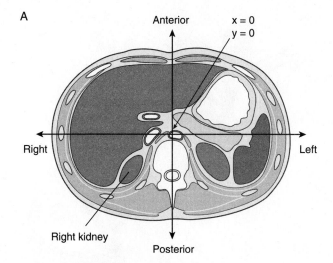

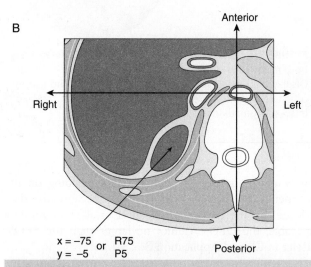

FIGURE 3-8   Raw data for an image are acquired at isocenter, where *x* = 0 and *y* = 0. If the patient is centered within the gantry and the display coordinates are not changed, the resulting image will be displayed as in **(A)**. However, if the image is to be displayed with the right kidney at the center, the image center must be adjusted. **B.** The new image center using traditional *x, y* coordinates is described as *x* = −75 and *y* = −5. In the RAS coordinate system the new center is described as R75 and P5.

Review Questions

1. Define algorithm and interpolation.
2. List the principal components in a computer. What is the function of each?
3. Explain how computer memory works. In what situation could scan data be lost?
4. What is the difference between raw data and image data?
5. Define the following terms: ray, ray sum, view, attenuation profile, back projection, and filter function.
6. What is the difference between SFOV and DFOV?
7. Explain how an image can be reconstructed with a different center.

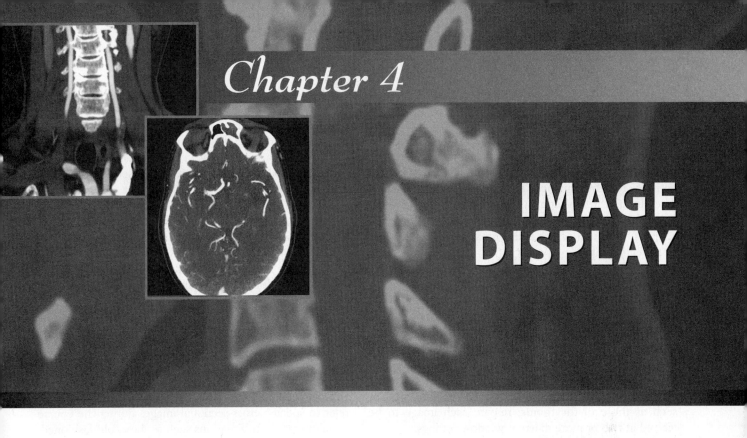

Chapter 4

IMAGE DISPLAY

In the first two phases of image creation information is collected from the passage of x-ray photons through an object, converted into a usable format, and used to reconstruct densities in cross-sectional slices. The last phase in the creation of the CT image is that of display. Image display includes all of the system components necessary to convert the digital data created from the reconstruction process to electrical signals needed by the CT display monitor. The display system also includes the ability to display patient information and scan protocol data, and provides many graphic aids designed to assist in image interpretation.

DISPLAY MONITORS

An output device allows the information stored in computer memory to be displayed. The device used to display CT images is generally a black-and-white or color monitor. The display device is usually either a cathode-ray tube (CRT) or some form of flat panel such as a TFT LCD (thin-film transistor, liquid crystal display). The monitor consists of the display device, circuitry to generate an image from electronic signals sent by the computer, and an enclosure. The CRT monitor included in many CT systems is basically a standard television set with some modifications that improve image resolution. CRT monitors are heavier, bulkier, hotter, and less durable than the newer LCD monitors. In addition, LCD monitors produce higher luminance and higher spatial resolutions (see Chapter 9 for additional comparisons). Although newer monitors that support digital input signal are growing in popularity outside of medicine, they are not currently included in CT systems. It is a common misconception that all computer monitors are digital. Because the monitors used in CT work with analog signals, it is necessary to convert the digital signal from the computer's memory back to an analog format. Digital-to-analog converters (DAC) accomplish this task.

BOX 4–1 Key Concept

DAC change the digital signal from the computer memory back to an analog format so that the image can be displayed on the monitor.

Standard, cross-sectional images are nearly always displayed in gray scale. Non-image data, such as text fields that include patient information or scan parameters can be displayed in color.

CAMERAS

In some instances the images are transferred to film. The camera is an output device that transfers the image from the monitor to the film. The camera used may be a multiformat camera, although most CT systems today include a laser camera. Multiformat cameras transfer the image displayed on the monitor to film. Laser cameras bypass the image on the display monitor and transfer data directly from the computer, bypassing the video system entirely, thereby significantly improving image quality. The film used in CT consists of a single emulsion that is sensitive to either the light-emission spectrum of the video screen phosphor (for the multiformat camera) or to the laser beam light.

WINDOW SETTINGS

The way an image is viewed on the computer monitor can be adjusted by changing the window width and window levels. At certain window settings, a slice of the thorax shows the lung parenchyma (Fig. 4-1A). At another setting, the same slice shows mediastinal detail and no longer displays the lung parenchyma (Fig. 4-1B). Many studies, such as those of the thorax, require each image to be viewed at two or more different window settings.

This section provides a technical explanation of window width and window levels. Although there are some guidelines for window settings, a substantial factor is personal preference. In the past, when a technologist's responsibilities included producing hard-copy film for the radiologist's interpretation, the subjective nature of window settings presented substantial challenges. Ideally, windows should be set so that the radiologist responsible for interpretation is satisfied. In practice, it was often impossible for a technologist to know which physician would be responsible for interpreting any given examination. Therefore, it was common practice for each imaging department

to have established window settings for filming each type of examination. It was well worth the radiologists' time to work closely with technologists in developing filming protocols to ensure that all parties understood exactly how the image is best displayed. It was also essential that technologists be allowed discretion in selecting window settings, because factors such as patient size and body composition have a pronounced effect. Optimal images cannot be achieved with standardized window widths and levels that do not consider influencing factors.

It is now common practice for radiologists to view studies from a computer workstation, thereby allowing them the freedom to adjust the window settings as they prefer. Although the creation of hard copies is no longer standard procedure for every examination, it is no less important today that technologists understand the impact of window settings. Obviously, technologists must appropriately view images as they are being created. In addition, there continue to be situations in which filmed images are still needed. One example is when a surgeon would like to refer to specific cross-sectional images during the course of an operation. In situations such as these, old-fashioned, polyester-based film is still the most practical method of viewing images. It is also important that the window be set correctly when images are saved onto a compact disk in a static format (these images are often called "screen-shots" because they capture the image exactly as is seen on the screen and do not allow for any further manipulation).

Gray Scale

In an ideal world, the image would be displayed with a different shade of gray for each Hounsfield unit represented. However, although there are more than 2,000 different Hounsfield values, the monitor can display only

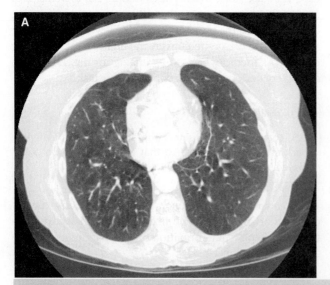 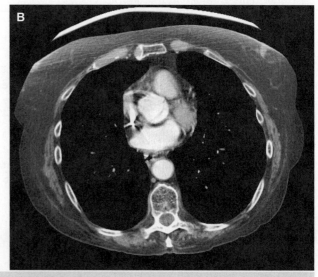

FIGURE 4-1   The effect of window settings on image appearance. **A.** This lung window provides good lung detail, but the mediastinum is completely white. **B.** The same slice displayed in a soft-tissue window provides good mediastinal detail, but the lungs are completely black.

Gray scale

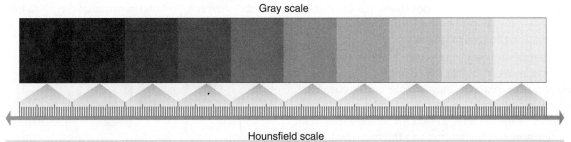

Hounsfield scale

FIGURE 4-2 The display processor assigns a group of Hounsfield unit to each shade of gray. In this simplified illustration, 10 different shades are available to display the 300 HU in the window width.

256 shades of gray. Even more limiting, the human eye can differentiate only a fraction of those shades–typically fewer than 40. As a general rule, the human eye cannot appreciate contrast differences of less than about 10%, whereas CT scanners can easily demonstrate differences of less than 1%. To overcome these inherent limitations, a gray scale is used in image display. In this system a display processor assigns a certain number of Hounsfield units (HU) to each level of gray. The number of Hounsfield units assigned to each level of gray is determined by the window width.

BOX 4–2   Key Concept

The gray scale is used to display CT images. This system assigns a certain number of Hounsfield units to each shade of gray.

As was explained in Chapter 1, the Hounsfield scale assigns 0 to the density of water. Correspondingly, −1,000 HU represents air and 1,000 HU represents a dense material such as bone. Values higher than 2,000 HU represent very dense materials, such as metallic dental fillings. By convention, the gray scale assigns higher Hounsfield unit values lighter shades of gray, whereas lower values are represented by darker shades.

Window Width

The window width determines the number of Hounsfield units represented on a specific image. The software assigns shades of gray to CT numbers that fall within the range selected. All values higher than the selected range appear white, and any value lower than the range appears black. By increasing the window width, usually referred to as "widening the width," more numbers are assigned to each shade of gray.

BOX 4–3   Key Concept

The window width determines the quantity of Hounsfield units represented as shades of gray on a specific image.

Level

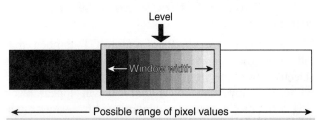

Possible range of pixel values

FIGURE 4-3 Window width assigns the quantity of pixel values to the gray scale. Window level determines the center pixel value in the gray scale.

Using a simplified scenario to demonstrate gray scale and window width, assume that we have 10 shades of gray available. We have selected 300 as our window width. Therefore, only 300 (of the more than 2,000 possible density values in our scale) will be represented on the image as a shade of gray. All others will be either black or white. In this example, 30 different Hounsfield units will be grouped together and represented by each shade of gray in the image (Fig. 4-2).

If the window width is set at 300, which 300 Hounsfield values, from all those possible, will be shown? Now that we have selected the *quantity* of Hounsfield units to be displayed by selecting the window width, we now need to determine the *range* of values to display.

Window Level

The window level selects the center CT value of the window width (Fig. 4-3). The terms window level and window center are often used interchangeably. The window level selects which Hounsfield numbers are displayed on the image.

BOX 4–4   Key Concept

The window level selects which Hounsfield values are displayed as shades of gray.

Answering the question posed in the previous paragraph, the particular Hounsfield units to be included in our image are entirely dependent on the window level selected. If 0 is chosen as the window level, the Hounsfield values that are represented as a shade of gray on this image will range from −150 to 150 (Fig. 4-4).

Now assume the width stays unchanged at 300, but the center is moved to 200. Determining the range of Hounsfield values requires only simple arithmetic. First, divide the window width in half. Next, subtract the quotient from the window level to determine the lower limit of the range, and add the quotient to the window level to determine the upper limit. The new range of Hounsfield numbers to be included in the gray scale is from 50 to 350 (Fig. 4-5).

Suggestions for Setting Window Width and Level

The software assigns shades of gray to CT numbers that fall within the range selected. All values higher than the selected range (in the current example, 350) will appear white, and any value lower than 50 will appear black (Fig. 4-6). If we increase the window width, a wider range of values will be included in the grayscale range; more values will be assigned to each shade of gray (Fig. 4-7).

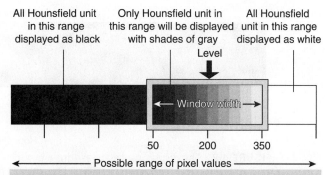

FIGURE 4-6 The software assigns shades of gray to CT numbers that fall within the range selected. All values higher than the selected range (in the current example, 350) will appear white, and any value lower than 50 will appear black.

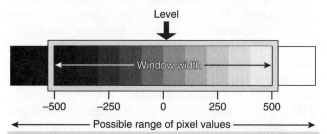

FIGURE 4-7 Widening the window width will include a wider range of values by placing more Hounsfield units into each shade of gray.

BOX 4–5   Key Concept

All values higher than those in the selected range will appear white on the image. All values lower than those in the selected range will appear black on the image.

The window level should be set at a point that is roughly the same value as the average attenuation number of the tissue of interest. For example, a window level setting that is intended to display lung parenchyma will be approximately −600 because air-filled lung tissue measures around −600 HU. The manipulation of window width and window level to optimize image contrast is referred to as windowing.

BOX 4–6   Key Concept

The window level should be set at a point that is roughly the same value as the average attenuation number of the tissue of interest.

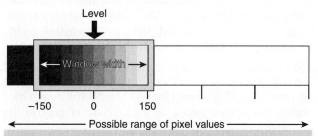

FIGURE 4-4 If the window width is 300 and 0 is chosen as the window level, the Hounsfield values that are represented as a shade of gray on this image will range from −150 to 150.

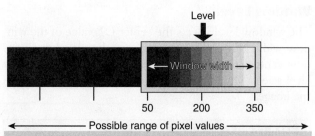

FIGURE 4-5 The width stays unchanged at 300, but the center is moved to 200. The new range of Hounsfield numbers to be included in the gray scale is from 50 to 350. Determining the range of Hounsfield values requires only simple arithmetic. First, divide the window width in half. Next, subtract the quotient from the window level to determine the lower limit of the range, and add the quotient to the window level to determine the upper limit.

In general, wide window widths (500–2,000 HU) are best for imaging tissue types that vary greatly, when the goal is to see all of the various tissues on one image. For example, in lung imaging, it is necessary to see low-density lung parenchyma as well as high-density, contrast-enhanced vascular structures. Wider window widths

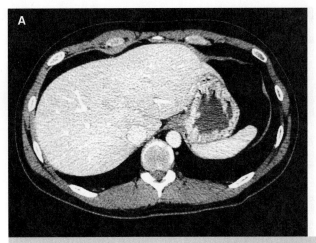 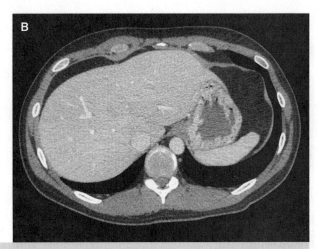

FIGURE 4-8   A. Image of the liver displayed with the department's "standard" window settings. **B.** Same cross-sectional slice is displayed with the window setting adjusted to better suit the patient.

encompass greater anatomic diversity, but subtle density discrimination is lost.

Because wider window width settings decrease image contrast, they suppress the display of noise on an image. For this reason, it is common practice to widen the window width when patients are obese or when there are metallic artifacts.

Tissue types with similar densities should be displayed in a lower, or narrow, window width (50–500 HU). This approach is best in the brain, in which there is not as much variation in CT numbers. The values can be spread out over the available gray scale so that two tissues with only a small density difference will be assigned separate shades and can therefore be differentiated by the viewer. Because narrow widths provide greater density discrimination and

contrast, using a narrow width when displaying the brain makes it possible to differentiate the white and gray matter of the brain.

Often systems provide the option of recording two different window settings, superimposed on one another, in a single image. This technique is known as dual window setting, or double window setting. Because many professionals find the superimposition of images to be confusing and distracting, the technique is infrequently used.

Table 4-1 provides some typical window settings for various examinations.

IMAGE DISPLAY OPTIONS

Region of Interest

A display function available on all scanners is that of defining an area on the image. This area is referred to as the region of interest (ROI). An ROI is most often circular, but may be elliptic, square, or rectangular, or may be custom drawn by the operator. Defining the size, shape, and location of the ROI is the first step in many display and measurement functions. Image magnification, obtaining an averaged Hounsfield measurement, and acquiring the standard deviation all demand defining an ROI.

Clinical Application Box 4-1

Window settings

Most facilities have a few window settings programmed into their CT systems. These are typically labeled with terms such as lung, abdomen, bone, and brain. Although these settings will not provide the optimal window setting for viewing all images in the various categories, they do provide an excellent starting point. For example, Figure 4-8A at the level of the liver is displayed with the department's programmed window setting: width 350, level 50. However, because of the patient's obesity, the image appears both grainy and light. Notice the improvement in Figure 4-8B, the same cross-sectional slice with the window width adjusted to 400 and the level lowered to 30.

Similarly, Figure 4-9A is an image of the neck displayed at the programmed window setting, width 300, level 50. Notice the diminished appearance of the streak artifact in Figure 4-9B when the window width is widened to 500.

BOX 4–7   Key Concept

Region of interest: an area on the image defined by the operator. Defining a region of interest is the first step in a number of image display and measurement functions.

Hounsfield Measurements and Standard Deviation

Hounsfield measurement is one of several valuable tools that aid in image interpretation. However, because

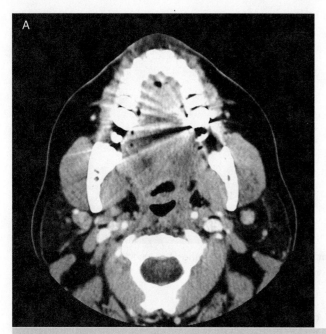 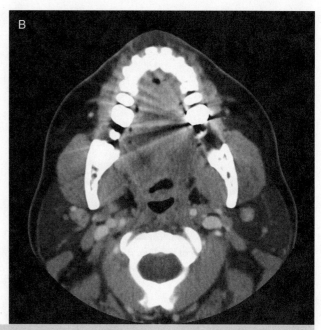

FIGURE 4-9   A. Image of the upper neck displayed with the department's "standard" window setting. **B.** Window width is adjusted to reduce the appearance of streak artifact caused from dental fillings.

TABLE 4-1   Typical Window Settings for Common CT Examinations

Examination	Width	Level
Head		
Posterior fossa	150	40
Brain	100	30
Temporal bone	2,800	600
Neck		
	250	30
Chest		
Mediastinum	350	50
Lung	1,500	−600
Abdomen		
Soft tissue	350	50
Liver (high contrast)	150	30
Pelvis		
Soft tissue	400	50
Bone	1,800	400
Spine		
Soft tissue	250	50
Bone	1,800	400

measurements may be negatively affected by volume averaging or image noise, caution should be used when Hounsfield values are used in the diagnosis of disease.

On most systems, a cursor (+) placed over an area reads out a measurement of that area. If a cursor is used, it is essential to understand that the subsequent measurement is only for the pixel covered by the cursor. If an ROI is first placed over an area, the reading is the average for all of the pixels within the ROI. If the ROI is accurately placed within the area of the suspected lesion, the averaged value is probably more accurate than the single-pixel reading.

A cursor measurement is effective when used as a rapid method of evaluating the density of a specific structure on an image. For example, if a cursor is placed over a known vascular area, such as the aorta, on the first image taken after the initiation of contrast media, this measure indicates whether the anatomy is actually contrast enhanced. If the measurement is 70 HU (indicating unenhanced blood) instead of the expected higher value of contrast-enhanced blood (90–160 HU), then a number of steps could be taken before the examination is continued. These steps may include checking the injection site for intravenous infiltration, checking the tubing for kinks or poor connections, and increasing the delay between injection and the start of scanning because the contrast material has not reached the desired areas of the anatomy. Injection techniques are discussed in Chapter 13.

ROI measurement should be used whenever the values will be considered in formulating a diagnosis. When an area is used, in addition to the averaged Hounsfield value of the pixels within the ROI, a standard deviation reading is given. This reading indicates the amount of CT number variance within the ROI. For example, if an area of interest has a Hounsfield value of 5 and the standard deviation is 0, what is known about the region? This standard deviation shows that there is no variation within the ROI; therefore, every pixel within the region has the value of 5 HU. If the standard deviation is not 0, but 20, all of the pixels within the ROI do not have an identical reading of 5 HU. The higher the standard deviation, the greater the variation among pixels within the region.[1] The standard deviation does not indicate the levels of the individual pixels. Factors that produce high standard deviation are 1) mixed attenuation

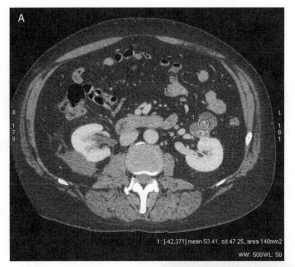

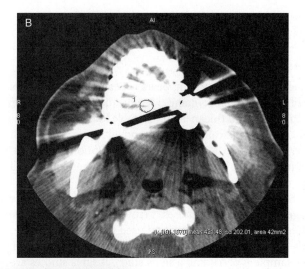

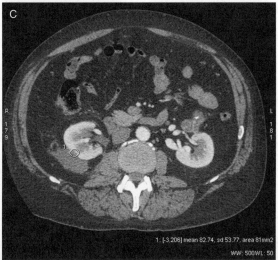

FIGURE 4-10 Factors that produce high standard deviations are mixed attenuation tissue with the ROI (e.g., calcium flecks within an organ (A)); an ROI that includes a streak artifact (B); and an ROI that is not inside the margins of the object being measured (C).

tissue within the ROI (Fig. 4-10A; e.g., calcium flecks within an organ); 2) an ROI that includes a streak artifact (Fig. 4-10B); and 3) an ROI that is not inside the margins of the object being measured (Fig. 4-10C; e.g., kidney cyst measured with an inappropriately large ROI that includes a section of the adjacent renal calyx, which is averaged in with the cyst). In the last two instances, the high standard deviation also reflects an inaccurate Hounsfield measurement.

---

[1]The standard deviation is the most widely used statistical measure of the spread or dispersion of a set of data. It is the positive square root of the variance. The standard deviation, like the variance, measures dispersion about the mean as center. However, the standard deviation has the same unit of measurement as the observation, whereas the unit of variance is the square of the unit of the observation. The standard deviation is always greater than or equal to zero. It is zero when all observations have the same value; this value is thus the mean, and so the dispersion is zero. The standard deviation increases as the dispersion increases (Mosteller FR, et al. Probability with Statistical Application, 2nd ed. 1970).

BOX 4–8   Key Concept

The amount of CT number variance within the region of interest is indicated by the standard deviation.

Distance Measurements

All CT systems allow distance measurements. This feature is helpful in reporting the size of the abnormality. It is also essential for the placement of a biopsy needle or drainage apparatus. The system calculates the distance between two deposited points in either centimeters or millimeters. Additionally, CT systems calculate the degree of angulation of the measurement line from the horizontal or vertical plane. A grid can also be placed over an entire image.

All CT images have a scale placed alongside the image for size reference. This feature allows a ruler to be placed along the scale, then subsequently placed along an area of diseased tissue in the patient. The CT distance scale is used in the same way as a scale of miles in a map key.

Image Annotation

Typical information that appears on each image includes facility name, patient name, identification number, date, slice number and thickness, pitch, table location, measurement scale, gray scale, and right and left indicators. Often other information is displayed as well. Optional information includes the addition of contrast enhancement and all scan parameter selections.

Software allows the operator to annotate specific images with words, phrases, arrows, or other markers. Whenever computer software is used to alter the position of an image, an explanatory annotation is recommended. An example is recording a sinus study. If sinus studies are typically obtained in a coronal position, with the patient lying prone, and a specific study must be done with the patient reversed in the supine coronal position, images are often reversed for filming. It is important to note this change to prevent any potential misdiagnoses because fluid appears to be floating to the top.

Reference Image

The reference image function displays the slice lines in corresponding locations on the scout image. This feature aids in localizing slices according to anatomic landmarks (Fig. 4-11).

Image Magnification

It is important to differentiate between image magnification and decreasing the field of view size. A decrease in display field of view increases the size of the displayed image. The result of both functions is an image that appears larger than the original. In each case, relevant clinical data may be easier to see because of the enlargement. However, image magnification uses only image data and does not improve resolution; it simply makes the existing image larger. In spite of this drawback, in many instances, simply magnifying the image data is appropriate. An example is the display of suspected abnormalities for measurement. Image magnification does not adversely affect the accuracy of Hounsfield unit or distance measurement. In fact, because magnifying the image may clarify the margins of the abnormality, allowing for more accurate cursor placement, measurement accuracy may improve.

BOX 4–9   Key Concept

Image magnification is NOT the same as decreasing the display field of view.

Image magnification should not be used when the image displayed on the monitor appears too small. This problem results from inappropriate DFOV size selection, and it should be corrected by using the raw data to reconstruct the entire study in the correct DFOV size. Image

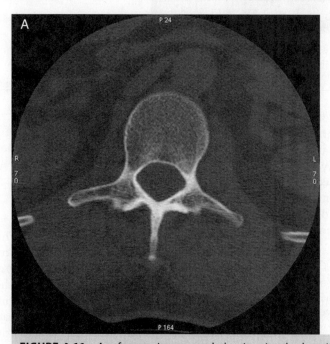
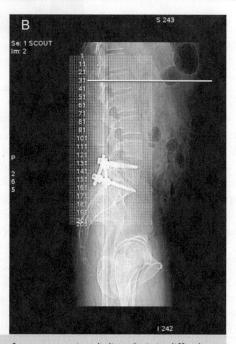

FIGURE 4-11   A reference image can help pinpoint the location of a cross-sectional slice. **A.** It is difficult to determine which lumbar vertebra is depicted in the cross-sectional image labeled as slice 36. Identifying slice 36 on the reference image **(B)** allows the viewer to determine that the cross-sectional image depicts the first lumbar vertebra.

resolution is improved if the image is enlarged using the raw data. However, if the raw data are not available, a less attractive alternative is to magnify each image in the study.

In summary, magnification is a useful tool that should be used on isolated images within a study. Magnification allows relevant clinical detail to be more easily seen and more accurately measured. However, magnification has inherent limitations and should not be used as an alternative to correct display field selection.

Multiple Image Display

The multiple image display function allows more than one image to be displayed in a single frame. It is often used as a method of saving film, particularly when copies are requested by the referring physician. The format (i.e., four images per frame, six images per frame) often varies with the manufacturer.

Histogram

A histogram is a graphical display showing how frequently a range of CT number occurs within an ROI (Fig. 4-12).

Advanced Display Functions

Conventional CT studies consist of several contiguous, typically axial images that are perpendicular to the long axis of the body. In many situations an alternative imaging plane may provide valuable information. In most cases, it is not possible to position the patient within the gantry in a way that will allow the direct imaging of other planes. This limitation of CT can be overcome by

image manipulation commonly referred to as multiplanar reformatting (MPR). This technique, along with three-dimensional reformatting, will be discussed in detail in Chapter 8.

SUMMARY

The display functions are the final step in creating the CT image. Analog monitors display the CT image. Therefore, the digital signal from the computer's memory must be converted back to an analog format.

Changing the window width broadens or narrows the range of visible CT numbers. Window width and window level determine which aspects of an image are displayed as shades of gray. The shade of gray that is assigned to a specific anatomic structure is related to the structure's beam attenuation. Higher Hounsfield values are represented by lighter shades of gray. The window width selects the range of Hounsfield units for a particular image, and the window level determines the center Hounsfield unit in this range. In general, the window level is set at roughly the same level as the Hounsfield value of the tissue of interest. Optimal window settings are highly subjective, and they vary dramatically within the field. Published window widths and centers are intended to serve as guidelines only. Patient conditions as well as personal preference make considerable adjustment necessary.

CT systems offer a variety of functions that allow images to be manipulated to facilitate diagnosis. Defining an ROI is the first step in many measurement and display functions. Hounsfield measurement, standard deviation, and distance measurement may offer valuable diagnostic information.

It is important to annotate images with any information that may not be immediately apparent. Examples of such annotation include "Images in this study have been flipped, top to bottom" and "Delayed image: 15 minute post contrast injection."

The technologist must understand the difference between image magnification and decreasing the display field of view size and use each function appropriately.

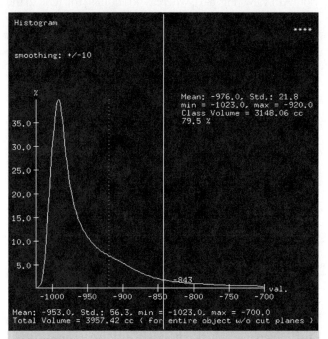

FIGURE 4-12 The appearance and frequency of a range of CT numbers within a region of interest are displayed on a histogram.

REVIEW QUESTIONS

1. Why is a gray scale necessary to display CT images?
2. What does the window width determine?
3. What happens to pixel values that are higher or lower than the range selected by the window width?
4. Provide an example of an area of anatomy that is best imaged with a wide window width. What is an area that is best visualized by a narrow width?
5. What does window level select?
6. When is it helpful to magnify a CT image?
7. What does a high standard deviation indicate?

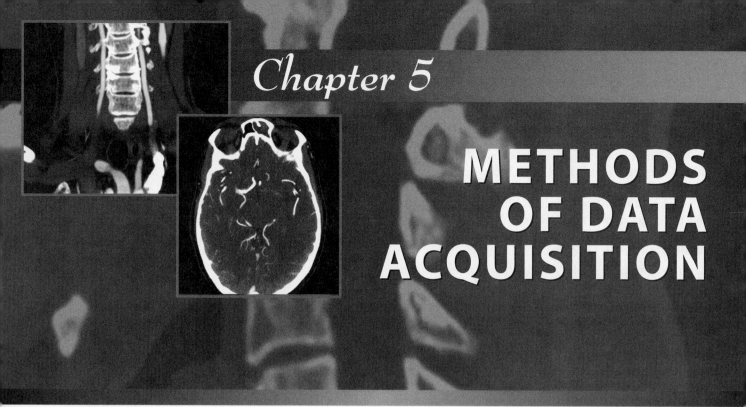

Chapter 5

METHODS OF DATA ACQUISITION

Key Terms: localizer scans • step-and-shoot scanning • axial scanning • clustered scans • slice misregistration • contiguous • single-detector row CT (SDCT) • fan beam • multidetector row CT (MDCT) • cone beam • uniform array • adaptive array • nonuniform arrays • hybrid arrays • helical scanning • spiral scanning • continuous acquisition scanning • helical interpolation methods • 180LI • 360LI • effective slice thickness • slice thickness blooming • slice-sensitivity profile (SSP) • pitch • crosstalk • beam pitch • detector pitch • dual source

Specific options, such as the number of detector channels included in the detector array, are dependent on the model of scanner used. This chapter describes the three general methods in which scanners acquire data: 1) preliminary, or localizer, scanning, 2) axial scanning, and 3) helical (or spiral) scanning.

LOCALIZER SCANS

Most CT studies begin with one or more localizer images. These images are not cross-sectional in nature; rather they are very similar to images acquired with conventional radiographic projection techniques. Because localizer images are not cross sections it is not necessary to rotate the x-ray tube during their acquisition. Localizer scans are digital image acquisitions that are created while the tube is stationary and the table moves through the scan field. The

single projection causes anatomic structures to appear superimposed, like those depicted by conventional radiography. Compared with conventional radiographic images, CT localizer images are of slightly poorer image quality and deliver an approximately equal radiation dose to the patient. The position of the tube determines the orientation of the image. For example, if the tube is positioned above the patient, the resulting localizer scan will be an anterior–posterior (AP) view (Fig. 5-1), whereas positioning the tube to the side of the patient will result in a lateral view (Fig. 5-2).

Localization images are called by various names, depending on the manufacturer. The terms scout, surview, topogram, scanogram, preview, and pilot have all been used to describe these images. In all routine studies, at least one localizer scan is acquired. The optimal scout includes all areas to be scanned and therefore ensures that the anatomy to be imaged has been placed within the range of the system. As an example, a patient may lie out of the scannable range if she is positioned too close to the ends of the scanning table, a problem that can be detected using localizer images. In addition to correct positioning on the table in the head–foot (z axis) direction, the patient must also be centered appropriately in the gantry in both x and y directions. Miscentering a patient in either x or y direction can result in out-of-field artifacts (see Chapter 7). Miscentering in the x direction occurs when the patient lies more to one side of the table. Miscentering in the y direction occurs when the technologist sets the table too low or too high within the gantry. Proper centering is also imperative when automatic exposure control techniques (Chapter 6) are used. Miscentered localizer scans can lead to erroneous calculation of tube current and can affect image quality and the radiation dose to the patient.

40

A

Localizer scan

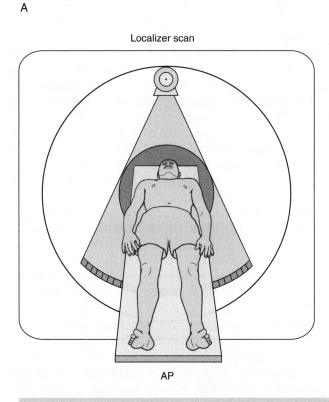

AP

B

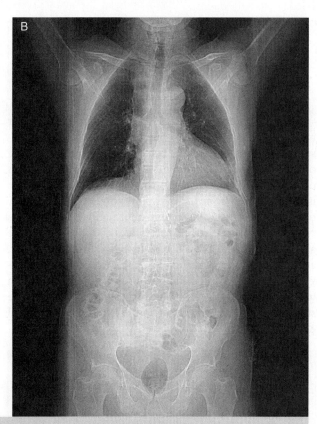

FIGURE 5-1 With the tube positioned above the patient (A), the resulting localizer image will be an anterior–posterior projection, such as the localizer image of the chest and abdomen in (B).

A

Localizer scan

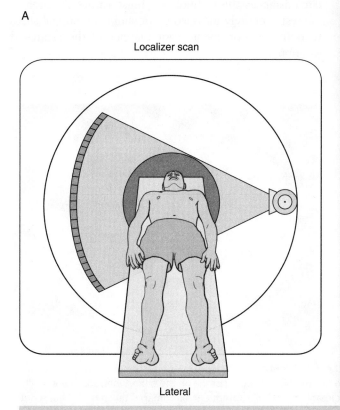

Lateral

B

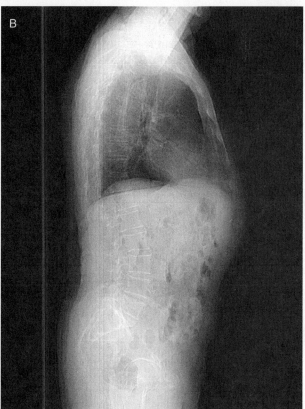

FIGURE 5-2 With the tube positioned at the patient side (A), the resulting localizer image will be a lateral projection, such as the localizer image of the chest and abdomen in (B).

BOX 5–1 Key Concept

All routine CT studies require at least one localizer scan. Proper centering of the localizer scans is particularly important when automatic exposure control options are used.

On all CT systems it is imperative that the operator input the correct directional instructions before data acquisition is initiated. Therefore, before the localizer images are obtained it is necessary to indicate whether the patient is placed head or feet first into the gantry and whether he is lying supine, prone, or in the decubitus position. If the operator accurately enters this information into the system, the software correctly annotates the localizer image and all subsequent cross-sectional images as to left–right, anterior–posterior, and superior–inferior orientation. Conversely, incorrectly inputting any directional instruction will incorrectly annotate all subsequent images in the study and can result in misdiagnosis and serious medical errors (Fig. 5-3).

BOX 5–2 Key Concept

Incorrectly inputting directional instructions into the CT scanner can result in images that have been mislabeled and can result in misdiagnosis and serious medical errors.

As the name implies, localizer images allow the technologist to prescribe the location of cross-sectional slices. The extent of the anatomic area included on localizer images is controlled by the technologist and dependent on the type of study. It is usually selected to extend just beyond the area to be imaged on cross sections. For example, a localizer image for a CT of the chest typically begins at the lower neck and terminates mid-abdomen. A localizer image for a combination chest, abdomen, and pelvis study will also begin at the lower neck but will extend through the pubic bone. Most scan procedures rely on beginning and ending landmarks that can be readily identified on the scout image. For example, an abdomen study typically begins slightly above the level of the right diaphragm and terminates at the level of the iliac crest. Both the diaphragm and the iliac crest are easily identifiable on the localizer image. With some protocols, it is impossible to use readily identifiable landmarks. In these cases, the operator must make an educated guess. If possible, the technologist should take one cross-sectional slice to check the accuracy of the guess before proceeding. For example, this approach is often helpful when scanning the adrenal gland. In this situation, thin slices through the adrenal glands are required. However, from the localizer image, there is no way to precisely predict where the adrenals lie within the abdomen. Obviously, checking the first image before proceeding slows down the examination process, but the delay is justified in that it can reduce the number of unnecessary slices taken and therefore reduce the radiation exposure to the patient. (On multidetector row scanners it may not be possible to obtain just one slice. However, even on these scanners it is possible to limit the scan coverage to 20 mm or less.) There are some situations when such a delay is not feasible, such as when the timing of intravenous contrast material is critical. In these circumstances the technologist must ensure the area of interest is entirely included by obtaining additional slices to both superior and inferior margins of the estimated location.

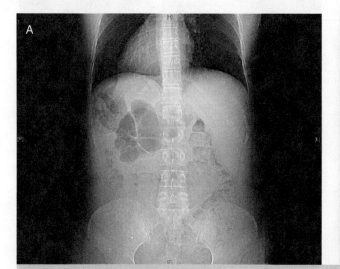
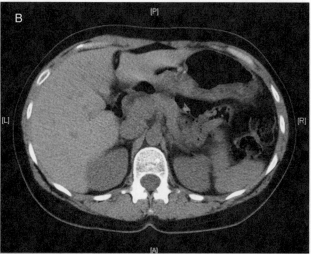

FIGURE 5-3 This is an example of an examination in which the technologist inputted incorrect directional instructions before obtaining the localization scan. Because the patient was incorrectly identified as being prone on the table, when she was actually supine, the right and left labels are reversed, both on the scout image and on all subsequent axial images taken using that scout as a reference. Notice that on the axial image the anterior-posterior annotations are also reversed.

Localizer images also help the technologist select the optimal display field of view (DFOV) and the correct image center. Although both of these parameters can be adjusted after the study is complete by using the raw data (see Chapter 3), department efficiency is improved if they are set correctly from the onset. DFOV and the image center are selected by the careful placement and sizing of lines over the localizer image. The length of the localizer lines demonstrates the DFOV; the center of the line indicates the image center (i.e., *x, y* coordinates). DFOV and image center selection is often improved by including a second localizer scan, taken at 90° from the first (i.e., both AP and lateral views). This process is outlined in Clinical Application Box 5-1.

In addition to using localizer scans to prescribe cross-sectional slices, they are also used once a study is complete. It is standard procedure to include a scout image that is cross-referenced by lines. These lines represent the location of each cross-sectional image (see Chapter 4, Fig. 4-11).

Clinical Application Box 5-1

Selecting a DFOV and Image Center Using Localizer Images

Localizer scans are used to set the extent of anatomic coverage (in the *z* direction) of the subsequent cross-sectional slices. To do this the operator selects the location of the first and last cross-sectional slices. Localizer scans can also be used to determine the appropriate image center and DFOV. To illustrate, assume that a scan of the lumbar spine is needed. The patient is positioned in what the operator estimates to be the center of the gantry. AP and lateral localizer views are acquired, and the operator begins the process of prescribing the cross-sectional slices (the exact command to initiate this process will vary depending on scanner manufacturer). The AP image appears with a line that represents the existing image center in the right–left direction (Fig. 5-4A). This line represents the true right–left center of the gantry. The length of the line represents the DFOV and shows the operator what area (from right to left) that will be included on the cross-sectional images. The line can be adjusted by moving it either to the right or to the left (changing the subsequent image center), or by expanding or shrinking the length (changing the DFOV; Fig. 5-4B). The AP localizer can only be used to adjust the image center in the right–left direction.

In a similar manner, a lateral localizer can be used to adjust the subsequent image center in the top–bottom (or anterior–posterior) direction. In Figure 5-4C the line reflects the true top–bottom center of the gantry. In Figure 5-4D the line is adjusted so that subsequent cross-sectional images will include the lumbar spine.

The lateral localizer can also be used in setting the degree of gantry tilt as illustrated by Figure 5-4E.

STEP-AND-SHOOT SCANNING

Introduced in the first chapter, earlier scanners operated exclusively in the step-and-shoot method. This method is also referred to as axial scanning, conventional scanning, serial scanning, or sequence scanning–all imprecise terms that tend to create confusion in the field. Key aspects of the step-and-shoot method are that the CT table moves to the desired location and remains stationary while the x-ray tube rotates within the gantry, collecting data. Early systems, which contained only a single row of detectors in the *z* axis, obtained data for one slice with each rotation. This method of scanning was used, in much the same fashion, by both third- and fourth-generation scanners (see Chapter 2). A minor difference was that, whereas third-generation systems typically used a 360° rotation for each acquisition, fourth-generation systems most often used a 400° rotation. In all types of scanners using this method there is a slight pause in scanning between data acquisitions, referred to as the interscan delay, as the table moves to the next location. In early scanners the time for a complete cycle (i.e., table movement to correct position, gantry rotation for scan acquisition, table movement to next position) allowed only a single scan to be acquired each time the patient held her breath. Newer scanners shortened the cycle time dramatically, allowing axial scans to be "clustered." This is the practice of grouping more than one scan in a single breath-hold. The number of scans grouped together is dependent on the speed of the specific scanner used and on how long a patient can reasonably be expected to hold her breath. The number of scans per cluster and the breathing time between clusters are programmable features and can be adjusted as specific patient conditions dictate. Grouping scans in this fashion decreases examination time and reduces slice misregistration (discussed later in this chapter).

BOX 5–3   Key Concept

The older, traditional method of scanning is referred to as axial scanning, conventional scanning, serial scanning, sequence scanning, or step-and-shoot scanning. Key to this method is that the CT table moves to the desired location and remains stationary while the x-ray tube rotates within the gantry, collecting data.

Scans produced with the step-and-shoot method result in images that are perpendicular to the *z* axis (or tabletop) and parallel to every other slice, like slices of a sausage (Fig. 5-5).

Advantages

In evaluating image quality using phantoms (that do not breathe or move), step-and-shoot methods result in the highest image quality, superior to that of helical methods.

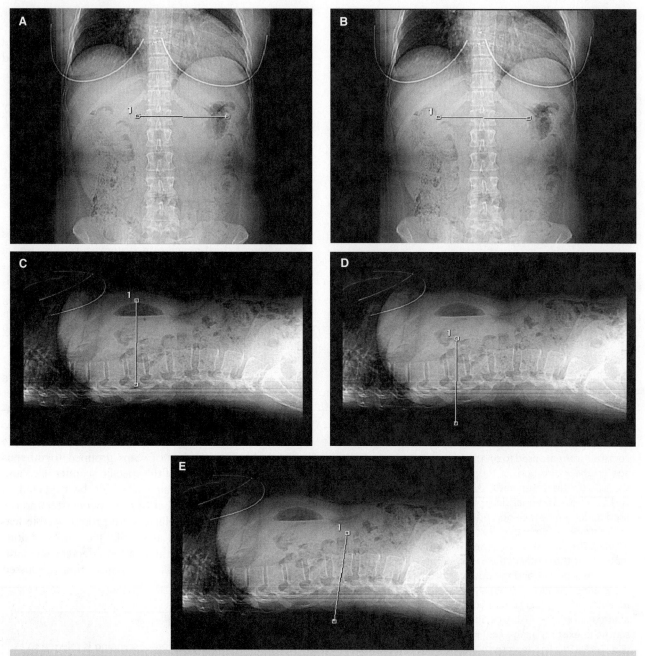

FIGURE 5-4   Selecting a DFOV and image center using localizer images.

This is because of their axial nature (i.e., slices are perpendicular, not slanted) and the fact that the patient table remains stationary during data acquisition.

Axial scans can be programmed to acquire data for contiguous slices (in which one slice abuts the next) or in a noncontiguous fashion, in which some areas of the patient are skipped between slices or slice data overlaps. Scanners can also be programmed to repeat scans at the same slice location (i.e., no table incrementation). Such protocols are often called cine or dynamic methods and are done when how a structure appears over time is of interest. Gapped images are taken when a survey of an area is needed (i.e., representative slices are sufficient, and imaging of every part of the region is not required). Because some areas are not exposed, studies made up of gapped slices will reduce the radiation dose to the patient. Gapped slices are often used for high-resolution chest studies and for the unenhanced portions of chest studies when aortic dissection is suspected. Axial protocols that use overlapping slices are rare because they increase the radiation dose to the patient but typically do not provide additional diagnostic information.

BOX 5–4   Key Concept

Axial slices can be programmed so that the data acquired are contiguous, gapped, or overlapping.

For these reasons, all current scanners offer the option of axial scanning. Although helical scanning has replaced many axial protocols, there are still a number of procedures in which axial methods are preferred.

Disadvantages

The primary disadvantage to the axial method is that the cumulative effect of the pauses between each data acquisition adds to the total examination time. Although the cumulative delay may be less than 30 seconds, even this brief delay is often significant. This is particularly true when blood vessels, which remain contrast-filled for very short periods, are of primary interest or when a patient's breathing will result in motion artifact on the image. In addition, compared with helical data, data acquired in the step-and-shoot method are more limited in how they can be reconstructed.

Misregistration

The delay inherent in axial scan sequences decreases the likelihood that a patient will be able to hold his breath throughout the examination. When a scan sequence is longer than a single breath-hold, scans must be briefly suspended to give the patient time to exhale, take in a new breath, and hold it once again. This can result in slice misregistration, which occurs when a patient breathes differently with each data acquisition.

To better visualize how misregistration can result in error, imagine this scenario: A shallow breath places a group of slices acquired at a specific level of anatomy. The patient is allowed to breathe and the table is moved to the next scan position. The next set of scans is taken, but the patient takes a deep breath instead. This difference in breathing places the second group of scans in an incorrect anatomic position relative to the first set of slices. Valuable information may be missed because of this effect (Fig. 5-6).

Single-Detector Row Systems

Detector elements used in the CT system were introduced in Chapter 2. Until the 1990s all commercial scanners contained many detector elements aligned in a single row (Fig. 5-7). The single-row design was used in both third- and fourth-generation systems. In third-generation systems approximately 700 detector elements were arranged in an arc; fourth-generation systems used as many as 4,800 detectors in a single row arranged in a complete ring. In scanners with a single-detector row, each detector element is quite wide in the z direction

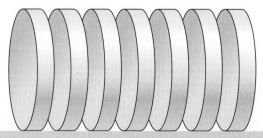

FIGURE 5-5   Axial slices lie parallel to one another. The slice beginning matches exactly the slice end, and perfect circles are formed that are perpendicular to the z axis.

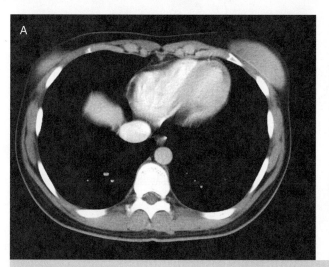
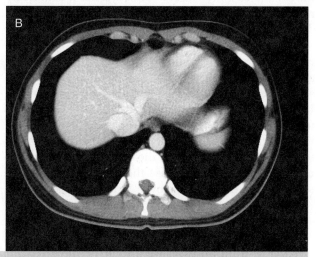

FIGURE 5-6   Slice misregistration caused by patient breathing. These two slices are taken at contiguous table positions; slice (A) is the last slice in the first group of axial slices. The patient was allowed to breathe and then once again asked to hold his breath. Slice (B) was the first slice in the second group of scans. Slice (B) is just 5 mm more inferior, yet it appears dramatically more inferior. It is possible to miss lesions as large as 1 cm as a result of slice misregistration.

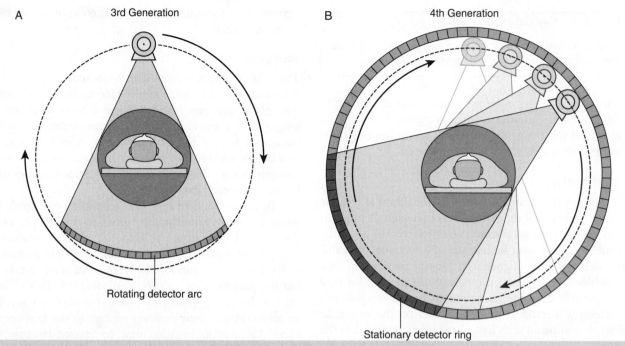

FIGURE 5-7   Single-detector row scanners have many detectors situated in an arc (third-generation) or a ring (fourth-generation).

(approximately 15 mm) and opening or closing the collimator controls the slice thickness by controlling the portion of the detector's width that is exposed to the incoming x-rays (Fig. 5-8). The width of the detectors (in the z axis) in a single-detector array places an upper limit on slice thickness. Opening the collimation beyond this point would do nothing to increase slice thickness, but would increase both the dose to the patient and the amount of scattered radiation. Therefore, in these systems the largest allowable slice thickness is less than the detector width, typically 10 mm. The radiation emitted from the collimated x-ray source in these systems is commonly referred to as a fan beam. Each gantry rotation produces data for a single slice.

Calculating the area of patient anatomy to be covered during an examination with a single-detector row, axial scan method is a simple process of multiplying the slice increment selected by the number of slices acquired. If slices are contiguous the slice increment will be equal to the slice thickness. For example, an examination protocol of the abdomen calls for contiguous, 5-mm slices to be taken from the level of the diaphragms to the level of the iliac crest. In this case the collimator is opened to 5 mm, and the table is moved 5 mm after each gantry rotation. Using an AP localizer image to plan the study, 40 images would be required if the total z distance to be scanned is 200 mm (40 images × 5 mm). For the sake of illustration, if the 40 slices were to be acquired using a 5-mm slice thickness, but a 7-mm slice increment (skipping 2 mm of anatomy between each slice), then the total distance from first slice to last would be 280 mm (40 images × 7 mm).

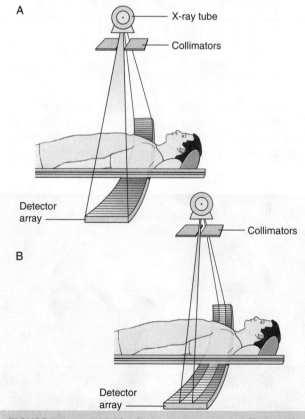

FIGURE 5-8   In a single-detector row system, different slice thicknesses are obtained by means of adjusting prepatient collimation of the x-ray beam. In the figure on the left the collimators are open to their maximum, producing the widest slice width available; on the right the collimators are partially closed, resulting in a thinner slice.

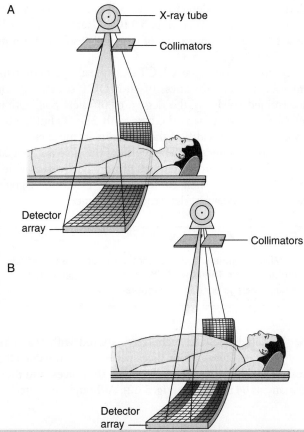

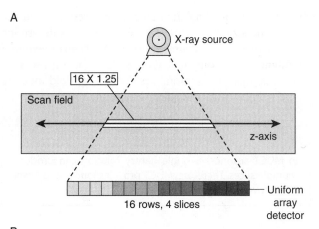

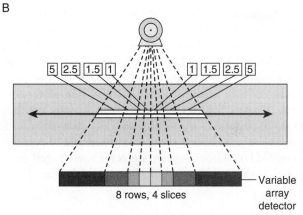

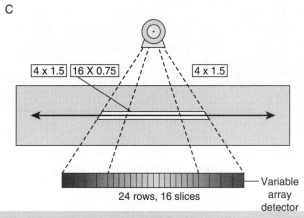

FIGURE 5-10 In some MDCT systems the width of the detector rows are uniform (A). In others, the width of the detector row is variable, with the rows thinner in the center and wider at the periphery (B, C).

FIGURE 5-9 Like third-generation single-detector row scanners, multidetector row scanners contain many detectors situated in an array. However, they have many parallel arrays that are capable of collecting data for multiple slices with a single gantry rotation. Slice thickness is controlled by a combination of prepatient collimation and detector configuration.

Multidetector Row Systems

Newer CT systems continue to use many detector elements situated in a row. However, they may contain from 4 to 64 parallel rows. In multidetector row (MDCT) scanners a single rotation can produce multiple slices. Therefore, MDCT provides longer and faster *z* axis coverage per gantry rotation. Additionally, many MDCT systems have increased the speed of gantry rotation, which further increases volume coverage per unit time. Slice thickness is determined by a combination of the x-ray beam width (controlled by the collimators) and the detector configuration (Fig. 5-9). The radiation emitted from the collimated x-ray source in these systems is commonly referred to as a cone beam. Multiple detector channels can be used for either axial or helical data acquisitions. Depending on the scanner manufacturer and the number of detector rows, the parallel rows may be of equal size, referred to as a uniform array, or they may be variable, with thinner rows centrally and wider rows peripherally (Fig. 5-10). These variable-width detector

rows are also called adaptive arrays, nonuniform arrays, or hybrid arrays.

To understand how MDCT systems change many of the rules established with single-detector row CT (SDCT), we first consider a system capable of acquiring four simultaneous slices. These systems are characterized by multiple parallel rows of detector elements (as thin as 1 mm) that can be combined in various ways to yield four contiguous slices for each gantry rotation. The parallel rows can be thought of as dividing the detector into segments in the z axis. The size and number of segments used determine the slice thickness and number of slices that can be acquired simultaneously. Compared with SDCT, for a given slice thickness, this configuration results in a fourfold increase in the volume of data acquired in a single rotation.

BOX 5–5   Key Concept

In MDCT scanners a single gantry rotation can produce multiple slices. Therefore, MDCT provides longer and faster z axis coverage per gantry rotation.

Scanners with four data acquisition channels have more than four parallel rows of detectors. This allows for scanning with various slice thickness. For example, the General Electric Lightspeed QX/I (GE Healthcare, Milwaukee, WI) scanner system uses 16 detector rows, each 1.25 mm wide, arranged side-by-side along the z axis. These rows can be grouped in various combinations to generate four slices. Using one detector row for each slice will provide slices that are each 1.25 mm thick (Fig. 5-11A). Grouping two detector rows together will provide slices that are each 2.5 mm thick (Fig. 5-11B).

Combining three detector rows will result in slices that are each 3.75 mm thick (Fig. 5-11C). Using all the available 16 detectors in groups of four will result in a 5-mm slice thickness (Fig. 5-11D).

Using the four-slice MDCT example above it is apparent that the slice thickness of an MDCT scanner is not determined solely by the degree of physical collimation of the x-ray beam as is the case with SDCT, but is also impacted by the width of the detectors in the slice thickness (z axis) dimension. The width of the slice is changed by combining different numbers of individual detector elements together. When combined, the electronic signals generated by adjacent detectors are summed.

BOX 5–6   Key Concept

In MDCT scanners a single gantry rotation can produce multiple slices. Therefore, MDCT provides longer and faster z axis coverage per gantry rotation.

Although MDCT technology started with scanners that produced two or four slices per rotation, the detector designs quickly advanced, offering 16 thin slices, and then as many as 64 thin slices (Fig. 5-12). Although the detector

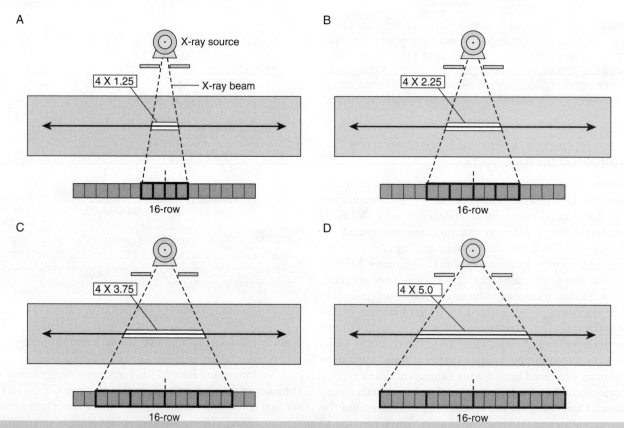

FIGURE 5-11   A–D. The slice thickness of an MDCT scanner is not determined solely by the degree of physical collimation, but also by the width of the detectors in the slice thickness (z axis) dimension. Combining different numbers of individual detector elements together changes the width of the detectors.

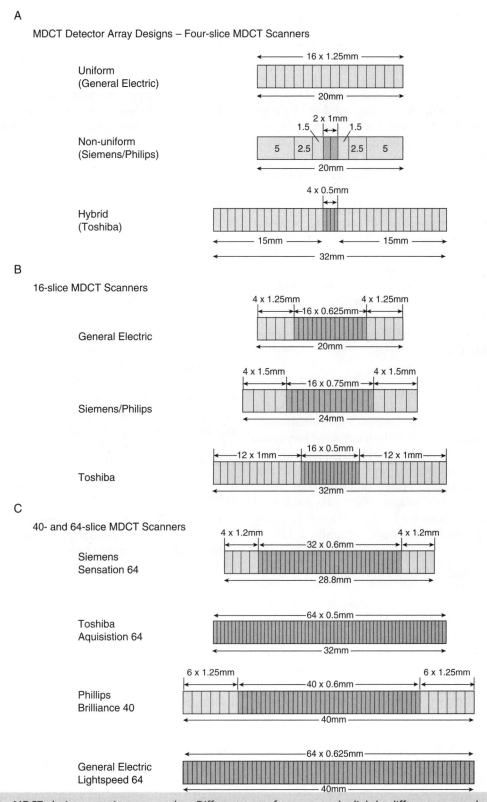

FIGURE 5-12 MDCT designs continue to evolve. Different manufacturers took slightly different approaches to detector configuration.

configuration schemes vary with each permutation, with regards to slice thickness, the concept remains the same as with the earlier 4-slice models. That is, different combinations of detector elements can be combined to vary the slice thickness reconstructed.

It is likely that future technical enhancements will continue this trend of an increasing number of detector channels placed in the z axis. Prototypes for 256-row detectors are currently being tested. The biggest advantage of the 256-row scanners will be their ability to image the heart, brain, and many other organs in a single rotation.

As an interesting side note, MDCT designs were responsible for the demise of fourth-generation scanning systems. Fourth-generation systems contained a complete ring of detectors. To form a complete ring, many separate detector elements were required. As many as 4,800 detectors were necessary to form a single row. Should that design be expanded to a 64-slice MDCT, 307,200 detectors would have to be used. The expense associated with so many detectors made the fourth-generation design unfeasible for MDCT.

Applications

Axial scans are typically used in protocols in which the acquisition speed is not a major concern and optimal resolution is required, such as studies of the internal auditory canal. It is also used for studies in which slices are gapped, or when the exposure will be interrupted, such as the case with prospective electrocardiography-gated cardiac studies. These studies attempt to acquire images only during portions of the cardiac cycle that have the lowest cardiac motion. (See Chapter 20 for a complete explanation of cardiac CT.)

HELICAL SCANNING

Since its introduction in the late 1980s, helical CT has revolutionized clinical imaging. Also called spiral (or continuous acquisition) scanning, helical scanning brought dramatic improvement in scanning speed by eliminating the interscan delay. There are three basic ingredients that define a helical scan process: a continually rotating x-ray tube, constant x-ray output, and uninterrupted table movement.

Increasing the scan speed results in improved image resolution owing to the ability to obtain images with improved iodinated contrast concentration, decreased respiratory and cardiac motion artifact, and superior multiplanar and three-dimensional (3-D) reformation capabilities. In addition to improved diagnostic accuracy, the speed associated with helical scanning is also beneficial in regards to patient comfort and department productivity.

Originally, helical scanners were constructed with a single row of detectors. Since then, MDCT systems with as many as 64 detector rows have been introduced. By further improving scan speed, these systems have made clinical applications, such as CT angiography (CTA) and virtual bronchoscopy, feasible.

This section briefly reviews the technology of helical scanning from its inception to current day. In much the same way that a student must first learn arithmetic before studying algebra, we first review the evolution of single-detector helical systems before moving to the more complicated MDCT systems.

Historical Perspective

Many of the long-standing problems with standard axial CT were overcome with the introduction of helical scanning. Helical scanning offers many advantages, including the ability to optimize iodinated contrast agent administration, the reduction of respiratory misregistration, and the reduction of motion artifacts from organs such as the heart.

Helical scanning is often referred to as volumetric scanning. This refers to the fact that the end result of such a scanning method is a block of data, not separate slices, as occurs in traditional axial scanning. Acquiring information in a volume allows data manipulation possibilities not previously available with the older axial methods. However, it is important to remember that although the end result is a block of data, in the majority of cases the information is acquired in ribbons—and not a block at a time, thus placing certain limitations on data manipulation.

BOX 5-7   Key Concept

There are three basic ingredients that define a helical scan process: a continually rotating x-ray tube, constant x-ray output, and uninterrupted table movement.

To take helical scanning from theory to practice, many obstacles associated with traditional axial CT had to be overcome. The major improvements leading to its development were 1) x-ray gantries with a slip ring design, 2) more-efficient tube cooling, 3) higher x-ray output (i.e., increased mA capability), 4) smoother table movement, 5) software that adjusts for table motion, 6) improved raw data management, and 7) more-efficient detectors.

Slip Rings

Before helical scanning systems, CT gantries moved first in one direction, then stopped as the table moved to the next position. The gantry then reversed direction for the next acquisition. Each 360° rotation produced one image. On these older systems, when the x-ray tube stops to move in the opposite direction, all the momentum is lost, considerably slowing the scan process. In contrast, within newer systems slip rings allow the tube to move continually in the same direction. Slip ring technology eliminates cumbersome electrical cables and makes possible a data-gathering system using a continuous rotation of the x-ray source. The x-ray source can reach much higher speeds, thereby decreasing the time necessary for each data acquisition. Before slip ring technology scanners took from 2 to 5 seconds to complete a single rotation, whereas a slip ring scanner can rotate in 1 second or less.

Also important is the role slip ring technology plays in eliminating the interscan delay. In conventional scanning, this is the time required between each acquisition when the table moves to the next scan position and the scanner readies itself for the next acquisition. On older CT systems, this interscan delay could range from 3 to 15 seconds per slice.

More-Efficient Tube Cooling

There is constant x-ray output throughout a helical scan acquisition. The longer any x-ray tube is on, the more heat is built up within the system. The length of acquisition in helical scanning is selected by the operator and can last more than 60 seconds without a pause for cooling. Because of these extended scan times with no opportunity for tube cooling, helical scanning places tremendous stress on the x-ray tube.

Improvements in tube heat capacity and heat dissipation have helped to rid helical systems of some of the heat generated. Even so, tube heat can still be a significant issue, often limiting the length of the helical acquisition and the milliampere-seconds (mAs) used to scan.

Higher X-ray Output

On older axial systems, scans were often acquired using a scan time of 3 seconds and an mA of 100, resulting in a total of 300 mAs used to produce the image (see Chapter 6 for a full discussion of these and other scan parameters). In a helical scan, the tube makes a complete rotation in 1 second or less. This would drop the overall mAs to one-third (or less) of that of the axial scan if the mA remained the same. However, all other factors being equal, a helical scan will require as much overall mAs as an axial image. One way to compensate for the dramatic decrease in scan time is by increasing the mA options available. To increase the mA choices possible, it is necessary to increase the size of the generator. However, tube heat limits the amount that mAs settings can be increased.

More-Efficient Detectors

Another way manufacturers have compensated for the lower mAs that results from the shortened scan time is to improve the efficiency of the detectors in the helical system. Because systems that have helical scanning capabilities possessed more-efficient detectors than the systems that preceded them, it led to the false belief that helical scans required a lower overall mAs than axial scans. This is not true. The more-efficient detectors allow the total radiation dose to be lower for both helical and axial scans

done on the newer systems. Therefore, on a given CT system, the overall mAs needed to produce an adequate image is approximately equal, whether the slice is produced in an axial or a helical mode.

Smoother Table Movement and Special Software

It is well accepted that motion artifact degrades images. This is particularly true of CT images. Because images are created while the table is in motion, helical scanning requires the table to move very smoothly. A jerky movement will produce an unacceptable amount of motion artifact. In addition, manufacturers created special software that adjusts for the smooth table motion. This correcting software led to another popular helical CT misconception–that patient motion can be eliminated with the helical scanning software. This is not true. The table motion involved in helical CT is relatively predictable compared with the usual sources of patient movement. Because table velocity is smooth and well known, correction can be made for this movement. Other motion artifacts, such as those caused by cardiac pulsations, patient breathing, peristalsis, and gross movement are not significantly reduced by software corrections.

Improved Raw Data Management

The last major development necessary was improved raw data management. Because scanning takes place so quickly, huge amounts of data are generated in a very short time. In addition, helical slices are often taken with much thinner collimation (slice thickness) than that used with older axial scans. Furthermore, because volumetric helical data allow enhanced manipulation possibilities, data must be available until the workload permits the staff to appropriately use the data. Hence, data storage capabilities had to be expanded to make helical scanning feasible.

Fundamentals of Helical Technology

There are fundamental differences between traditional axial images and those acquired in a helical scan process. An axial image is taken so that each slice is parallel to

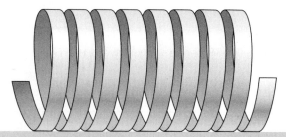

FIGURE 5-13 Helical scans are not precisely axial because the beginning of the slice does not match up with the end of the slice. Therefore, the slices are at a slight angle, similar to a spring.

every slice (Fig. 5-5). In contrast, with helical scanning, the x-ray output is continually on while the table moves through the gantry. What results are slices in which the beginning point and the end point are not in the same z axis plane. Helical CT creates slices that are at a slight tilt, similar to the rungs in a spring (Fig. 5-13).

Helical Interpolation

The computer uses various methods of interpolation to, in effect, take the slant and blur out of the helical image. These complex statistical methods create images that closely resemble those acquired in a traditional axial mode.

Different techniques of interpolating helical scan data have been developed. The specific interpolation technique used depends on the manufacturer and the detector configuration. For SDCT systems the two most common schemes are the 360° and the 180° linear interpolations (abbreviated 360LI and 180LI). These schemes have been expanded on for use in MDCT systems. Evolving methods have improved the quality of the helical image, in most cases making them indistinguishable from axial images. Despite the improvement, the fact remains that any method of interpolation is associated with some, although often quite minimal, loss of image resolution. In addition, interpolation methods can have a negative impact on the effective slice thickness.

In general, the more interpolation required to process an image, the more pronounced these disadvantages become. As the angle of the slice becomes steeper, the interpolation required to adjust the data increases.

Effective Slice Thickness

Interpolation methods can also result in a scan that is wider than that selected by the operator (Fig. 5-14). This is referred to as slice thickness blooming or degradation of the slice-sensitivity profile (SSP; discussed in more detail in Chapter 6). In early helical scanners, slice thickness blooming was quite pronounced. The actual slice thickness could be nearly 20% wider than that selected through the collimator opening. This meant that although a 10-mm slice thickness was being selected, the effective slice was actually closer to 12 mm wide. However, interpolation methods quickly improved from those first introduced, and this effect is not nearly as pronounced on scanners in use today. The various interpolation techniques come with tradeoffs, for example, in SDCT the 180LI interpolation algorithm produces thinner SSP than the 360LI algorithm at the cost of higher noise.

Other factors play a role in the SSP of helical images. In both SDCT and MDCT systems, these include factors such as table speed (pitch), detector width (especially in MDCT), and "crosstalk" between neighboring slices (image noise resulting from the scattering of x-ray photons by adjacent detectors). For SDCT helical, a faster table results in a broader SSP and therefore a larger effective slice thickness. For MDCT systems, the relationship between table speed and SSP is more complex.

Pitch

During a helical scan acquisition, the x-ray tube is continually on while the table moves through the gantry. Pitch is a parameter that is commonly used to describe the CT table movement. It is most commonly defined as the travel distance of the CT scan table per 360° rotation of the x-ray tube, divided by the x-ray beam collimation width. When the table feed and beam collimations are identical, pitch is 1. When the table feed is less than the beam collimation, pitch is less than 1 and scan overlap occurs.

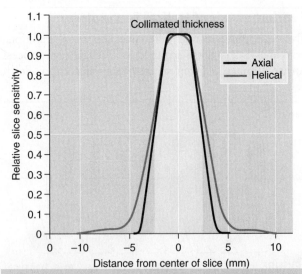

FIGURE 5-14 Axial and helical slice sensitivity profiles from an SDCT system for a collimated slice thickness of 5 mm with a pitch of 1 and a 180° helical interpolation.

> **BOX 5–8 Key Concept**
>
> Pitch is a parameter that is commonly used to describe the CT table movement throughout a helical scan acquisition. It is most commonly defined as the travel distance of the CT scan table per 360 rotation of the x-ray tube, divided by the x-ray beam collimation width.

The concept of pitch is more complicated when discussing MDCT; therefore, our discussion begins with pitch as it relates to SDCT.

Pitch in SDCT

Recall that in SDCT systems the width of the collimator opening is the sole determinant of slice thickness. To understand pitch in an SDCT system let us first consider what happens to the table speed when the pitch is set at 1. To maintain a pitch of 1, the table speed will vary according to the slice thickness selected. For example, assume a 5-mm slice thickness is selected and the table is programmed to move a 5-mm distance for each 360° rotation of the x-ray tube. If the tube makes a full rotation in 1 second, the table must travel 5 mm each second. If a 10-mm slice thickness is selected, the table must move faster; that is, it will move 10 mm per second. Table speed and slice thickness are directly related in a helical scan process.

When the table moves a distance that is equal to the slice thickness during each gantry rotation, the pitch is described as 1. Therefore, pitch describes the relationship of the table speed to the slice thickness.

If the pitch is 1 and the slice thickness (i.e., collimation) is set at 5 mm, the table will move at a speed that allows the gantry to rotate once for every 5 mm of table travel. If the pitch is adjusted to 2, and the slice thickness is kept at 5 mm, the gantry will rotate once for every 10 mm of table motion. This is accomplished by increasing the table speed.

To understand how pitch affects the image, imagine what happens to the data if the spiral is stretched out, like pulling the ends of a spring. The slant becomes more pronounced. Therefore, as the pitch increases, so does the slice angle. More interpolation is required to straighten the image. Consequently, as pitch increases, the effects of interpolation become more pronounced. These effects include image unsharpness and effective slice thickness blooming.

Although it may seem that increasing the pitch would result in data for some anatomic areas being skipped, this is not true. Information is collected for each table position regardless of pitch. However, as pitch increases, fewer data are acquired for each table position.

The operator may select the pitch on a helical scan. Like mA settings, available pitch settings vary, depending on the manufacturer. In SDCT scanners typical pitch settings are 1, 1.2, 1.5, and 2.

Pitch is sometimes expressed as a ratio of table speed to slice thickness. Hence, a pitch of 2:1 indicates that the table will move twice the distance of the slice thickness for each rotation of the gantry. This is the same statement as saying the pitch is 2.

BOX 5–9   Key Concept

Increasing the pitch will result in a scan covering more anatomy lengthwise for a given total acquisition time. It will also reduce the radiation dose to the patient (if other scan parameters are held constant). A decrease in pitch slows down the table speed. A pitch of less than 1 will result in overlapping slices. Therefore, decreasing the pitch will decrease the amount of anatomy covered per unit time and increase the radiation dose to the patient.

Increasing the pitch will result in a scan covering more anatomy lengthwise for a given total acquisition time. It will also reduce the radiation dose to the patient. A decrease in pitch slows down the table speed. A pitch of less than 1 will result in overlapping slices. Therefore, decreasing the pitch will decrease the amount of anatomy

covered per unit time and increase the radiation dose to the patient. A pitch of less than 1 is not commonly used in SDCT. In fact, on some SDCT systems, a pitch of less than 1 is not an available option.

A compromise is necessary when the pitch is extended beyond 1. In exchange for the shortened examination time and the reduced patient radiation dose comes the loss of image sharpness and a decrease in the SSP. These sacrifices are not linear. In fact, these disadvantages are minimal when the pitch does not exceed 1.5. The impact on the image is more significant when pitch is extended beyond this point. This general rule governing pitch is somewhat altered for MDCT systems and is discussed later in this chapter.

Because of the trade-offs necessary when pitch is increased, it is important to accurately assess the advantages and disadvantages in specific scenarios. In many cases, the pitch is increased slightly to allow an entire area to be covered in a single breath-hold. It is also an appropriate option when tube heat limits the length of a helical scan acquisition.

On SDCT systems, increasing the pitch in a helical scan beyond 1.5 is associated with a significant trade-off in the slice profile. Therefore, using a pitch higher than 1.5 is typically reserved for applications in which the few seconds that the increased pitch saves will make a major impact on the outcome. The most prevalent application for using an extended pitch is CT angiography. Because these studies require scanning to take place while vascular structures contain high amounts of an iodinated contrast agent, scan speed is paramount.

Pitch in MDCT Systems   The simultaneous data acquisition from parallel rows of detectors requires rapid table advancement during scanning. MDCT stretches our earlier concept of pitch. Pitch is still defined as the relationship between slice thickness and table travel per rotation. But we must remember that the terms collimation and slice thickness are no longer synonymous (Fig. 5-15). This detail has given rise to more than one definition of pitch as it relates to MDCT systems. The most common definition is referred to as beam pitch, and relates more closely

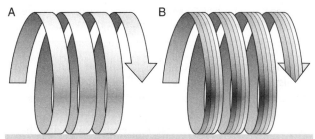

FIGURE 5-15   A. In an SDCT helical scanner the thickness of the x-ray beam equals the thickness of the final slice. **B.** In an MDCT spiral scan the thickness of the x-ray beam is divided over parallel rows of detectors, in this illustration producing four slices with each gantry rotation.

to the definition established in SDCT. Beam pitch can be defined as table movement per rotation divided by beam width. The beam width can be determined by multiplying the number of slices by slice thickness. For example, with a 4-slice MDCT at 4×1.25-mm slice thickness and a table-feed of 6 mm per rotation, the pitch is 1.2.

$$6/(4 \times 1.25) = 6/5 = 1.2$$

This same equation can be used regardless of the number of detector rows in the system. With a 16-slice scanner at 0.5-mm slice thickness and table movement of 12 mm per rotation, the pitch is 1.5.

$$12/(16 \times 0.5) = 12/8 = 1.5$$

Or, with a 64-slice MDCT at 64×0.5-mm slice thickness and a table-feed of 48 mm per rotation, the pitch again is 1.5.

$$48/(64 \times 0.5) = 48/32 = 1.5$$

Less common, the pitch for an MDCT scanner is defined by using the detector aperture, rather than the x-ray beam width. Termed *detector pitch*, it is defined as table movement per rotation time divided by the selected slice thickness of the detector. Physicists do not favor this system because it does not demonstrate clearly the degree of overlap between adjacent scans and is therefore less useful for radiation dose and image quality consideration.

On an SDCT system and a given beam collimation, slice thickness blooming increases with table speed (pitch). With an MDCT system set at a given collimation, there are certain table speeds that produce the best image quality and slice profile. These optimal speeds are when the detector channels interleave at equally spaced intervals after each 180° gantry rotation. This type of interleaving maximizes the number of unique z axis data points necessary for helical interpolation. Most scanners come with recommended pitch values that optimize speed and image quality. In general, a pitch between 1 and 1.5 is most common.

BOX 5-10   Key Concept

In general, in both SDCT and MDCT systems a pitch between 1 and 1.5 is most common.

Changing the pitch will affect the MDCT scan acquisition in the same ways it affects SDCT. To review, increasing the pitch will shorten the total acquisition time for a given distance covered, although there will be some penalty in image noise related to fewer data being acquired (i.e., undersampling). Again, this effect is usually small at pitch levels less than 1.5. Increasing pitch will also decrease radiation dose to the patient provided the technique remains constant. Extended pitch values may result in an increase in streak artifact.

Helical Scan Coverage

The formula for determining how many images are created and how much anatomy (lengthwise) is covered in a helical scan acquisition builds on the formula used to calculate distance covered in an axial scan sequence.

SDCT Scan Coverage

Number of Images Created in a Helical Scan Sequence

Pitch × total acquisition time × 1/rotation time
= number of images

Example 1: When it takes 1 second for each tube rotation, a 30-second helical scan acquisition will produce 30 images when the pitch is set at 1. That is, $1 \times 30 \times 1/1 = 30$.

Distance Covered in an SDCT Helical Scan Sequence

Pitch × total acquisition time × 1/rotation time × slice thickness = amount of anatomy covered

Example 2a: A helical scan with a 30-second total acquisition time, a 1-second rotation time, and a 5-mm slice thickness, with a pitch of 1.

1×30 s $\times 1/1$ s $\times 5$ mm $= 150$ mm of anatomy covered

Example 2b (change in slice thickness): When slice thickness is 10 mm (other factors unchanged from the proceeding example).

1×30 s $\times 1/1$ s $\times 10$ mm $= 300$ mm of anatomy covered

Example 2c (change in gantry speed rotation): When the gantry takes just 0.5 seconds to make a complete rotation (other factors unchanged from example 2a).

1×30 s $\times 1/0.5$ s $\times 5$ mm $= 300$ mm of anatomy covered

---

Clinical Application Box 5-2

Adjusting Pitch to Extend Scan Coverage

A patient will undergo an abdominal CT on an SDCT scanner. Assume the patient's abdomen is 220 mm from diaphragm to iliac crest. A high mA setting is required to accommodate the patient's size. The tube heat limits the scan acquisition to 30 seconds. Using a 5-mm slice thickness and a pitch of 1, only 150 mm will be covered in a single acquisition. However, if the pitch is increased to 1.5, the helical coverage will be extended to 225 mm, which will acquire data for the entire area of interest in a single helical acquisition.

Example 2d (change in pitch): When the pitch is set at 1.5 (other factors unchanged from example 2a).

$$1.5 \times 30\ s \times 1/1\ s \times 5\ mm = 225\ mm \text{ of anatomy covered}$$

MDCT Scan Coverage The formula must only be adjusted slightly to accommodate for MDCT.

Distance Covered in an MDCT Helical Scan Sequence

Pitch × total acquisition time × 1/rotation time
× (slice thickness × slices per rotation) = amount of anatomy covered

Example: A helical scan with a 20-second total acquisition time, a 0.5-second rotation time, a 2.5-mm slice thickness, 4 slices per rotation, with a pitch of 1.2.

$$1.2 \times 20\ s \times 1/0.5\ s \times (2.5\ mm \times 4)$$
$$= 480\ mm \text{ of anatomy covered}$$

Changing Slice Incrementation Retrospectively

Because helical scans result in a block of data, a choice can be made as to where in that block an image is created. This flexibility allows the creation of overlapping slices retrospectively. It does this without increasing the radiation dose to the patient, as is the case when axial images are scanned in an overlapping fashion.

BOX 5–11   Key Concept

Helical data allow the slice incrementation to be changed, retrospectively. This allows the creation of overlapping slices, without increasing the radiation dose. In some situations, changing the slice incrementation can reduce the partial volume effect.

In addition to creating overlapping images, changing slice incrementation offers other advantages. In some cases it may help reduce the partial volume effect. Figure 5-16A represents a volume of helical data taken on an SDCT system with a 10-mm slice thickness. Initially, one image is produced for each 10 mm of data. On images 2 and 3, a lesion is seen. It is suspected that the partial volume effect may be producing an inaccurate representation of this lesion. As Figure 5-16A illustrates, at least 5 mm of normal tissue is being averaged with the lesion.

Because this data are acquired in a helical fashion, we can retrospectively change the portion of data used, which produces a new image. In this example, an image is created from data at table positions 15 through 25. Figure 5-16B demonstrates that image 6 will contain the entire lesion in a single slice, rather than straddling two separate slices. In this way, the partial volume effect can be reduced or eliminated, resulting in a more accurate image. Images can be reconstructed with a very small data incrementation (<1 mm). Continuing with the earlier example and using a

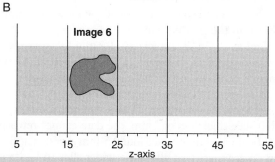

FIGURE 5-16 A. Volume averaging can occur when objects straddle slices. **B.** By changing the slice center, the partial volume effect is reduced.

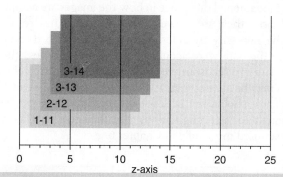

FIGURE 5-17 Data can be reconstructed along the *z* axis with incrementation of as little as 1 mm.

data incrementation of 1 mm, images could be made from the data corresponding to table position 1 through 11, 2 through 12, 3 through 13, and so forth. Figure 5-17 illustrates this concept.

Overlapping images are also an asset to multiplanar and 3-D image reformation (see Chapter 8). Using overlapping images helps reduce the stairstep appearance often seen along the edges of a reformatted image.

Even though the data incrementation can be changed on a single-row detector helical system, slice thickness cannot be altered retrospectively. On these systems, slice thickness is controlled exclusively by the width of the collimator during scanning. Therefore, if a lesion is only 1 mm in size (in our previous example), the partial volume effect cannot be reduced regardless of how the sections are reconstructed, because 9 mm of normal tissue would always be present in the image.

MDCT: Reconstructed Slice Thickness

MDCT systems offer opportunities for retrospectively changing slice thickness that are not available on SDCT systems. However, the choices available for the reconstructed slice thickness are not unlimited, even with the MDCT scanners. It is important to keep in mind that the thinnest images that can be reconstructed for a data set are predetermined by the slice thickness used for the data acquisition. The degree that the acquired slice thickness limits the reconstructed slice thickness varies according to manufacturer and specific model of scanner (information is included in the product literature). On all systems images acquired at a thin slice thickness, 0.5 mm for example, can be added together to created a thicker slice for viewing. Hence, four slices of 0.5 mm each could be combined to create a 2-mm slice for viewing. However, on many systems the reverse is not true. That is, if the data are acquired with a slice thickness of 2 mm, the data cannot retrospectively be divided to produce four 0.5-mm slices. In addition, even on scanners that allow the wider slice to be divided retrospectively, scan parameters (mAs and kVp) that are adequate for the wider slice may be insufficient for good image quality in a narrower slice produced from the same data. It is important to remember with MDCT that there is a fundamental difference in how the images are acquired and how they are viewed. This difference has resulted in the necessity to differentiate between slice thickness (how the data were acquired) and image thickness (how the data are reconstructed). To restate, the image thickness may be greater than the slice thickness, but the image thickness should not be less than the slice thickness. The rationale for selecting various slice thickness options will be explored more fully in Chapter 6.

BOX 5-12   Key Concept

The thinnest image that can be reconstructed for a helical data set is often predetermined by the slice thickness used for the data acquisition. For MDCT acquisitions the image thickness may be greater than the slice thickness, but in many cases the image thickness cannot be less than the slice thickness.

Dual-Source CT

A new CT technology was introduced to U.S. hospitals in 2006. Known as dual-source CT, the new design uses two sets of x-ray tubes and two corresponding detector arrays in a single CT gantry. Figure 5-18 illustrates the theoretical design. In practical application, the second detector array is restricted by the space available in the gantry. Therefore, one detector array covers the entire scan field of view (approximately 50 cm), whereas the second detector is limited to a smaller, central field of view. Figure 5-19 illustrates the actual design. With the two tubes and detectors mounted at right angles, both helical acquisitions run simultaneously.

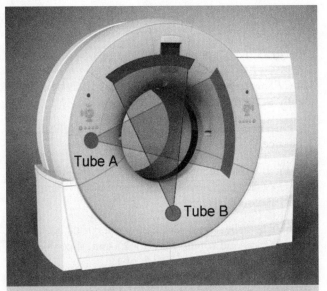

FIGURE 5-18 The dual-source CT design uses two x-ray tubes and two corresponding detectors positioned at 90° from each other. (Reprinted with permission from Flohr TG, Schoept UJ, Ohnesorge BM. Chasing the heart: new developments for cardiac CT. J Thorac Imag 2007;22:4–16.)

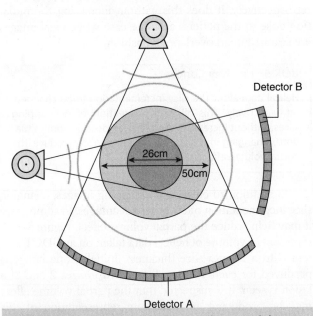

FIGURE 5-19 In practical application, the second detector array is restricted by the size available in the gantry. Therefore, one detector array covers the entire scan field of view (approximately 50 cm), whereas the second detector is limited to a smaller, central field of view. (Reprinted with permission from Flohr TG, Schoept UJ, Ohnesorge BM. Chasing the heart: new developments for cardiac CT. J Thorac Imag 2007;22:4–16.)

The idea of the dual-source CT is not new. The concept was attempted years ago on single-slice scanners, but the early helical scan technology limited its application. Siemens Medical Solutions (Forchheim, Germany) resurrected the idea to produce the Somatom Definition CT scanner.

The primary goal of the dual-source design is increased scan speed. This is particularly valuable in cardiac scanning in which it is hoped that the increased speed will allow clinicians to dispense with the use of β-blockers for slowing heart rates during cardiac CT studies (see Chapter 20). The radiation dose to the patient is no higher when the dual-source CT scanner is used in cardiac scanning.

A second potential advantage of the dual-source CT system arises from the fact that the two x-ray tubes, although working simultaneously, have the ability to produce x-ray photons possessing different energies. That is, for a given scan each x-ray tube can use a different kVp setting. Recall that beam attenuation is caused by absorption and scattering of radiation by the object scanned. The attenuation is dependent not just on the density of the object scanned but also on the energy of the x-ray photons. Thus, additional information can be learned about the object scanned when two x-ray energies are used and the difference in attenuation is analyzed. This works particularly well in materials with high atomic numbers, such as iodine. Theoretically, this strategy can be used to differentiate iodine from other dense materials. Another idea is to use the dual-energy concept to differentiate body tissues without the application of contrast media. However, because soft tissues do not possess high atomic numbers this is likely to be more difficult to achieve.

SUMMARY

Modern scanners offer three basic options for scanning: localization scans, axial scans, and helical scans. Understanding the appropriate application for each option is paramount. Although helical scan methods are now the most widely used, there remain specific situations in which axial methods are preferred. Since its inception, helical technology has been continuously refined with new and improved MDCT systems. Options such as the availability of submillimeter slice thickness continue to open new avenues for clinical application. Understanding the fundamental aspects of a helical scan process is the first step in grasping these complex but exciting developments in the field of CT.

REVIEW QUESTIONS

1. What is the benefit of obtaining both AP and lateral localizer images?
2. List some possible ramifications of incorrectly inputting directional instructions.
3. What are the advantages and disadvantages of axial scan methods? In what situations are axial methods preferable to helical scan methods?
4. Explain how the detectors in MDCT systems can be grouped to produce slices of various thicknesses.
5. What are the three basic ingredients that define a helical scan process?
6. Why are special interpolation methods required for helical data?
7. Explain the term pitch. What trade-offs are necessary when pitch is increased?
8. Explain why it might be beneficial to retrospectively change the slice incrementation of helical data.

RECOMMENDED READING

Bushberg JT, Seibert JA, Leidholdt EM, Boone JM. The Essential Physics of Medical Imaging. 2nd ed. Philadelphia: Lippincott Williams & Wilkins, 2001.

Bae KT, Whiting BR. Basic principles of computed tomography physics and technical considerations. In: Lee JKT, Sagel S, Stanley RT, Heiken JP, eds. Computed Body Tomography With MRI Correlation. 4th ed. Philadelphia: Lippincott Williams & Wilkins, 2005.

Lipson SA. MDCT and 3D Workstations: A Practical Guide and Teaching File. Secaucus, NJ: Springer-Verlag, 2006.

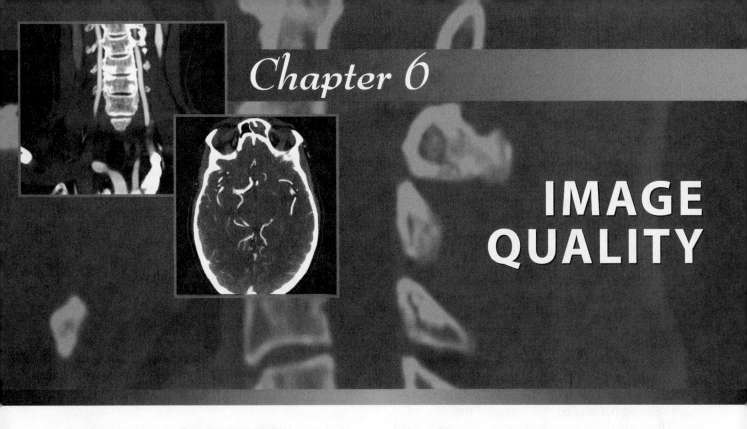

Chapter 6

IMAGE QUALITY

Key Terms: scan parameters

- milliamperes • scan time • slice thickness
- field of view • reconstruction algorithm
- kVp • pitch • milliampere-seconds
- uncoupling effect • convolution filter
- high-contrast resolution • contrast detectability
- low-contrast resolution • spatial resolution
- line pairs phantom • spatial frequency
- modulation transfer function • image fidelity
- MTF graph • limiting resolution • in-plane
resolution • longitudinal resolution • isotropic
- sampling theorem • Nyquist sampling theorem
- focal spot size • receiver operator characteristics
- quantum noise • quantum mottle
- signal-to-noise ratio • standard deviation • subject
contrast • contrast-detail response • contrast-detail
curve • displayed contrast • temporal resolution

In this chapter we consider factors that influence the quality of the CT image, the various aspects of image quality, and the methods available for assessing image quality.

SCANNING PARAMETERS

Many factors affect the quality of the image produced. Some of these variables can be regulated by the operator, whereas others, such as patient size, cannot.

Among the factors that the operator can control are milliampere (mA) level, scan time, slice thickness, field of view, reconstruction algorithm, and kilovolt-peak (kVp). When using helical scan methods, the operator also has a choice of pitch. As a group, these factors are usually referred to as scanning parameters. We begin our discussion of image quality with a brief definition of each parameter. We then look at how each of the factors affects the various aspects of image quality.

BOX 6–1   Key Concept

The total x-ray beam exposure in CT is dependent on a combination of mA setting, scan time, and kVp setting.

mA and scan time together are referred to as mAs and defines the quantity of the x-ray energy.

kVp setting defines the quality (average energy) of the x-ray beam.

As in standard radiography, the total x-ray beam exposure in CT is dependent on a combination of mA setting, scan time, and kVp setting. Milliampere level and scan time together define the quantity of the x-ray energy, whereas kVp setting defines the quality, or average energy, of the beam. These factors are roughly analogous to water flowing through a hose. The intensity, or force, with which the water flows through the hose can be compared to the kVp level. The quantity of water that flows through the hose is similar to the milliampere level. The length of time the water flows can be compared to scan time. The product of milliampere setting and scan time is known as milliampere-seconds (mAs) and is the quantitative measure of the x-ray beam. It is also referred to as tube current.

Milliampere-Second Setting

Within the x-ray tube are filaments, and a cathode and anode. The filament provides the electrons that create the x-ray beam. The system heats the filament until electrons start to "boil off" and break away from the filament. These electrons are then pulled across to strike the anode. This current of electrons that flow from the filament to the anode is measured in mA. Increasing the mA increases the number of electrons that will produce x-ray photons. Use of a small filament size concentrates the focal spot, reducing the penumbra (i.e., geometric unsharpness), which, in turn, positively affects image quality. Unfortunately, small filaments cannot tolerate high mA. Therefore, systems typically provide two separate filaments. A small filament is provided for lower mA settings (typically less than 350 mA) and a large filament for higher settings. In reality, the loss of resolution caused by a larger filament is slight and difficult to see on a standard CT image.

In SDCT, scan time is the time the x-ray beam is on for the collection of data for each slice. Most often it is the time it takes for the gantry to make a complete 360° rotation, although with overscanning and partial scanning options, there may be some mild variation. In most situations a full scan reconstruction algorithm is also used in MDCT. Therefore, in most cases the scan time in MDCT is the time it takes for the x-ray tube to make a 360° rotation, even though many slices may be produced. Typical choices of scan time for a full rotation range from 0.5 to 2 seconds. In cardiac applications, images may be created from data acquired from less than a 360° rotation, hence the scan time for these protocols are shorter, in the range of 0.35 to 0.45 seconds.

The quantity of x-ray photons produced is a product of mA and scan time. An example illustrates this relationship. If a 320 mAs setting is required for a specific study of the abdomen, this number can be obtained from a variety of combinations, based on the mA settings and scan times available with a specific system. For example, the selection of 160 mA and a 2-second scan time provides the same quantity of x-ray energy as 640 mA and a 0.5-second scan time.

BOX 6–2   Key Concept

Higher mA settings allow shorter scan times to be used. A short scan time is critical in avoiding image degradation as a result of patient motion.

Scanners vary in the mAs settings that they offer. The previous example shows how higher mA settings allow shorter scan times to be used. This practice is critical in avoiding image degradation as a result of patient motion. Even with a cooperative patient who remains still

and suspends respirations on command, motion can be a factor because of involuntary movement such as peristalsis and cardiac motion. Shorter scan times reduce, but do not eliminate, artifacts caused by motion. The degree to which involuntary motion affects an image is largely dependent on the area scanned. For example, it is a great concern when the purpose of the scan is to evaluate the patency of the small, pulsatile, coronary arteries but much less important in routine abdominal studies and virtually nonexistent in routine head studies. As a general rule, if the total mAs level can be maintained, it is preferable to use the shortest scan time available. However, there are exceptions to this rule. Slower scan speeds are favored for use in radiation therapy planning when evaluating organ movement during respiration.

As the mAs level increases, so does the amount of heat being generated within the x-ray tube. This heat is a limiting factor in all scanners. On most systems, there is a direct correlation between mAs level and interscan delay time. The higher the mAs setting, the longer the time between scans while the tube cools off enough to allow another scan sequence.

In the last decade, x-ray tubes have improved dramatically in their heat tolerances. Improvements in scanner design have allowed scans to be performed with higher mA settings and much shorter scan times. This capacity has opened the door for new applications, such as cardiac imaging, that demand very thin slices be acquired rapidly. Such new uses push the limits of even the improved technology. Hence, maximum mAs capabilities, minimum interscan delays, and corresponding heat dissipation rates remain significant factors that distinguish scanners in various price ranges.

A number of factors affect which mAs level is selected. These factors are basically the same as in conventional radiography. Specifically, the thicker and denser the part being examined, the more mAs required to produce an adequate image. For example, a CT study of the lungs will require less mAs than that of the abdomen because the chest is composed primarily of the lungs, which contain air and are less dense than the organs of the abdomen.

BOX 6–3   Key Concept

The factors affecting the mAs selected for a CT study are basically the same as in conventional radiography: the thicker and denser the part being examined, the more mAs that is required to produce and adequate image.

Determining the optimal mAs setting is often a matter of trial and error. Manufacturers often make general recommendations for the setting required for various examinations. Differences in mAs of less than 20% may not result in a visible change on the image. This allows for a bit of latitude in selecting mA and scan time.

The mAs can be obtained from various combinations of mA and scan time settings. For example, assume the recommended setting for a specific study of the abdomen is 280 mAs. Further, assume that the scanner allows mA choices in 20-mA increments from 20 to 700, and offers a choice of scan times from 0.4, 0.6, 0.8, 1.0, and 2.0 seconds. Many different combinations of mA and scan time will produce mAs close to 280. Some choices: 0.4 seconds and 700 mA (280 mAs), 0.6 seconds and 460 mA (276 mAs), 0.8 seconds and 340 mA (272 mAs), 1.0 second and 280 mA (280 mAs), and 2.0 seconds and 140 mA (280 mAs).

Tube Voltage or Kilovolt Peak

Most CT systems allow the operator to adjust the tube voltage. These are referred to as kilovolt peak, or kVp, settings. In CT, kVp does not change contrast as directly as it does in film-screen radiography. Compared with mA selection, choices of kVp are more limited. On some systems, the kVp setting is fixed, typically at 120 kVp. Increasing the kVp setting increases the intensity of the x-ray beam and the beam's ability to penetrate a thick, dense anatomic part. Routine body CT for adult patients is performed with 120 to 140 kVP. Because of their smaller size, pediatric patients are often scanned with 80 kVp.

Impact of mAs and kVp Settings on Radiation Dose

The appropriate selection of mAs and kVp is critical to optimize radiation dose and image quality. Reducing the mAs while holding the kVp constant reduces the radiation dose to the patient. Dose is also reduced if the kVp is reduced while the mAs is held constant. However, excessively lowering the kVp may result in a dramatic increase in the amount of x-ray attenuated by patient tissue, because the x-ray beam will be too weak to penetrate the patient. This is particularly true for large patients.

BOX 6-4   Key Concept

The appropriate selection of mAs and kVp is critical to optimize radiation dose to the patient and image quality.

It is a more common practice to manipulate the mAs, rather than the kVp, when modifying the radiation dose. This is true for two reasons. First, the choice of mA is more flexible, with available settings typically ranging from 20 to 800 mA. Another practical advantage of adjusting the mA instead of kVp is that its effect on image quality is more straightforward and predictable.

The Uncoupling Effect

The relationship between radiation dose and CT image quality is complex, particularly because of the uncoupling effect. This effect makes CT physics somewhat different from that of film-screen radiography, in which the relationship between dose and image quality is clear and well understood by technologists. In film-screen radiography,

when the radiation dose is too high, the film is overexposed and the image obtained is too dark; therefore, the technique (mA or kVp) is adjusted. With digital technology, whether it be in CT or computed radiography (CR), the image is uncoupled from the dose, so even when an mA or kVp setting that is too high is used, a good image results. This effect can make it difficult to identify when a dose that is higher than necessary is used. The uncoupling effect does not play a role when the mA or kVp setting is too low, because quantum noise (discussed later in this chapter) will result and provide evidence of the inadequate exposure settings. Digital radiography, which is also affected by the uncoupling effect, is rapidly replacing the older film-screen method. However, many current CT technologists began their careers as radiologic technologists and were trained when film-screen methods were the norm. Consequently, CT technologists are sometimes unfamiliar with the physical characteristics of the newer digital imaging methods.

BOX 6-5   Key Concept

Uncoupling Effect—using digital technology, the image quality is not directly linked to the dose, so even when an mA or kVp setting that is too high is used, a good image results.

Automatic Tube Current Modulation

Adapting the mAs to the patient's size and weight is a key factor in reducing radiation exposure from CT examinations (also see Chapter 14). Software that automatically adjusts the tube current (mAs) to fit specific anatomic regions is increasingly used in clinical practice. This software adjusts mAs during each gantry rotation to compensate for large variations in x-ray attenuation, such as when scans move from the shoulders to the rest of the thorax. In some software designs the variation of tube output is predefined by means of an analysis of the AP and lateral localizer scans. Other designs adjust the mAs in near real-time by evaluating the signal from the detector row. Still other designs combine these two approaches. These automatic exposure control techniques report a 15% to 40% reduction in dose, without degrading image quality. Software currently available adjusts only the tube current (mAs); however, future designs may also incorporate tube voltage (kVp) adjustments.

Slice Thickness

Slice thickness is important in CT and has a significant impact on image quality. In discussions of image quality we are primarily interested in the slice thickness (how the data were acquired) rather than image thickness (how the data are reconstructed).

Field of View

Scan field of view (SFOV) determines the area, within the gantry, for which raw data are acquired. Scan data are always acquired around the gantry's isocenter. The display field of view (DFOV) determines how much, and what section, of the collected raw data are used to create an image (see Chapter 3).

Reconstruction Algorithms

Depending on the manufacturer, this feature may be called algorithm, convolution filter, FC filter, or simply filter. Current scanners offer several algorithm choices that are designed to reconstruct optimal images depending on tissue type. By choosing a specific algorithm, the operator selects how the data are filtered in the reconstruction process. Filter functions can only be applied to raw data (not image data). Therefore, to reconstruct an image using a different filter function, the raw data must be available for that image. It is important to differentiate reconstruction algorithms from merely setting a window width and level. Changing the window setting (see Chapter 4) merely changes the way the image is viewed. Changing the reconstruction algorithm will change the way the raw data are manipulated to reconstruct the image.

Pitch

Pitch is the relationship between slice thickness and table travel per rotation during a helical scan acquisition (see Chapter 5). Specific pitch settings available vary and depend on manufacturer and detector row number and configuration.

SCAN GEOMETRY

Another factor is tube arc. Traditionally, a CT image is thought to comprise data collected from one 360° rotation of the x-ray tube. In this case, two matching (or, in some sense, mirror) samples are taken 180° apart. These samples contribute similar information to the reconstructed image. By averaging the information from two similar views, the image is usually improved.

Although a 360° tube rotation per scan is the most common selection, it is not the only choice. It is possible to obtain a partial scan, which is acquired from 180° plus the degree of arc of the fan angle. Although this scan is slightly more than a half circle, these scans are often referred to as half-scans. Only half of the otherwise available data are available to reconstruct the image with partial scans; therefore, they are inferior to standard 360° scans. However these scans do have a limited application in studies that require short scan times.

Another tube arc option is the 400° scan, known as an overscan. The overscan adds approximately the width of the field of view to the full scan [360° (full scan) + 40 (typical field of view) = 400° scan]. These were more commonly used in fourth-generation scanner designs. In a stationary detector design, the views are not recorded instantaneously, but are taken over approximately one-fifth of the scan time. Because this timing increased the inconsistency of data within views, motion was more of a problem. This disadvantage was minimized by using overscans. By allowing some overlap of data from the first and last tube positions, overscans reduced motion artifacts.

IMAGE QUALITY DEFINED

Image quality is a basic concept that applies to all types of images including photographic and video images as well as a wide variety of images produced for medical purposes. At the most fundamental level, image quality is a comparison of the image to the actual object. In many regards "quality" is a subjective notion and is dependent on the purpose for which the image was acquired. In CT, image quality is directly related to its usefulness in providing an accurate diagnosis. For example, an image of an infant using a very low technique may appear quite noisy, but it may still be adequate if the image is taken to follow up a large abnormality, such as an abscess. Clearly, the usefulness of an image can only be assessed on a case-by-case basis. This chapter deals primarily with the more objective measures of image quality. These tools help make possible comparisons of one imaging system to another, or the same system over time. Analytic methods attempt to assess the degree to which a system reliably detects and accurately depicts subtle abnormalities. However, it is important to keep in mind that the true test of the quality of a specific image is whether it serves the purpose for which it was acquired.

BOX 6-6   Key Concept

Image quality relates to how well the image represents the object scanned. However, the true test of the quality of a specific image is whether it serves the purpose for which it was acquired.

Just as a variety of factors influence a photograph's portrayal of reality, many factors influence how well a CT image represents the actual object scanned. Image accuracy may also be referred to as image fidelity. To assess how well the image represents real anatomy, we are concerned with two main features: detail (or high-contrast) resolution and contrast detectability (or low-contrast resolution). High-contrast resolution is the level of detail that is visible on the image. For example, if two thin wires lie close together in an object, will they be seen as two separate lines on the image? Low-contrast resolution is the ability of the system to differentiate between objects with similar densities. For example, consider an object that is nearly the same density as its background. Will this object be distinguishable on the CT image?

SPATIAL RESOLUTION

Spatial resolution is another term used for detail resolution. Spatial resolution is the system's ability to resolve, as separate forms, small objects that are very close together. Examples of imaging challenges that depend on spatial resolution are two 1-mm-diameter iodinated contrast-filled arteries that are just 1 mm apart, and small bone fragments in a crushed ankle.

Spatial resolution can be measured using two methods. It can be measured directly, or it can be calculated from analyzing the spread of information within the system. This latter data analysis is known as the modulation transfer function (MTF). By quantifying spatial resolution in one of these ways, it is possible to compare a system's performance with another CT system or the same system on a different day.

Direct Measurement of Spatial Resolution

To measure spatial resolution directly, a line pairs phantom is used. This type of phantom is made of acrylic and has closely spaced metal strips imbedded in it (Fig. 6-1).

The phantom is scanned, and the number of strips that are visible are counted. A line pair is *not* a set of two lines, but rather, a line and the space between lines. This is the conventional definition because it would be impossible to differentiate neighboring strips if there was no space between the lines. With this in mind, if 20 lines can be seen in a 1-cm section in an image of the phantom, the spatial resolution is reported as 20 line pairs per centimeter (lp/cm).

Spatial Frequency

The number of line pairs visible per unit length is also called spatial frequency. This is a characteristic of any structure that is periodic across a position in space and is a measure of how often the structure repeats per unit of distance. If objects are large, not many will fit in a given length. If the objects are smaller, many more will fit into the same length. How *frequently* an object will fit into a given *space* is its spatial frequency. Therefore, a large object will have a low spatial frequency, and small objects will have a high spatial frequency (Fig. 6-2).

Evaluating Spatial Resolution Using the MTF

Spatial resolution can also be calculated using the modulation transfer function (MTF). The MTF is the most commonly used method of describing spatial resolution ability, not only in CT, but also in conventional radiography. It is often used to graphically represent a system's capability of passing information to the observer.

Although it is not essential for the technologist to understand the mathematics associated with the MTF, it is important to understand what MTF indicates.

The ability of the system to accurately portray an object varies according to the size of the object (spatial frequency). As objects become smaller (higher spatial

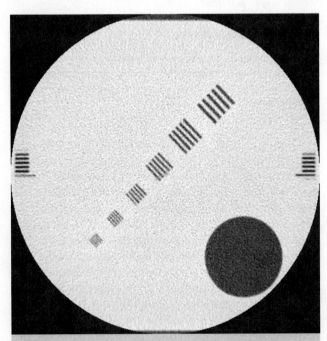

FIGURE 6-1 Spatial resolution can be measured using a phantom made of Lucite. Imbedded in the Lucite are closely spaced metal strips.

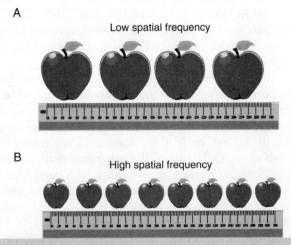

A

Low spatial frequency

B

High spatial frequency

FIGURE 6-2 A simplified illustration of spatial frequency. **A.** If objects are large, not many will fit in a given length and they are said to have low spatial frequency. **B.** If the objects are smaller, many more will fit into the same length. These are said to have high spatial frequency.

frequency), they will not be as accurately depicted on the CT image (i.e., all other things being equal, smaller objects are harder to see). The MTF is the ratio of the accuracy of the image compared with the actual object scanned. Therefore, MTF indicates image fidelity. The MTF scale is from 0 to 1. If the image reproduced the object exactly, the MTF of the system would have a value of 1. If the image were blank and contained no information about the object, the MTF would be 0. Because the actual MTF calculated from most objects is between these two extremes, it will have a value between 0 and 1.

In graphic form, MTF is charted against the spatial frequency (object size). These charts are typically referred to as MTF graphs and depict spatial frequency on the x axis and MTF along the y axis (Fig. 6-3). As expected, this graph shows that as the size of the object increases, the MTF also increases. This finding correlates with the common sense observation that as the size of the object increases, it can be more accurately portrayed on the image. The ability of a specific system to portray objects of varying sizes can be evaluated by examining a graph of its MTF. By charting the MTF of two separate CT systems, we can compare their ability to accurately resolve objects in the image (Fig. 6-4). An MTF curve that extends farther to the right indicates higher spatial resolution, which means the imaging system is better able to reproduce small objects. In Figure 6-4, scanner B will produce images of higher spatial resolution than scanner A. The relationship between the size of the object and its portrayal on the image is a complicated one. The relationship is not linear; hence an object twice the size of another object may not necessarily possess twice the image fidelity.

Limiting resolution is the spatial frequency possible on a given CT system at an MTF equal to 0.1. Figure 6-5

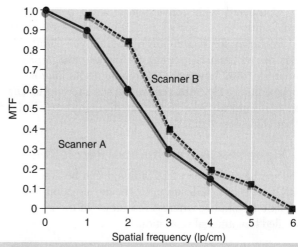

FIGURE 6-4 By graphing the MTF of two separate CT systems, we can compare their ability to accurately resolve objects in the image. An MTF curve extending to the right indicates a system with higher spatial resolution capabilities.

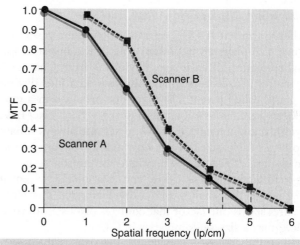

FIGURE 6-5 The limiting resolution is the spatial frequency possible on a given CT system, at an MTF equal to 0.1. In this example, the limiting resolution of scanner A is 4.3 and scanner B is 5.0.

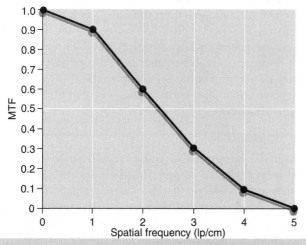

FIGURE 6-3 The ability of a CT system to accurately portray an object varies according to the size (spatial frequency) of the object. In a typical MTF graph the x axis corresponds to the spatial frequency of the object.

illustrates the concept of limiting resolution. First, identify the number 0.1 on the y axis. This is considered the lowest MTF possible that will still result in a (barely) visible object. Follow this line across until it intersects the MTF curve of scanner A. We can see that at an MTF of 0.1, scanner A will have a spatial frequency of 4.3, whereas at the same MTF, scanner B will have a spatial frequency of 5.0. These numbers reflect the limiting resolutions of scanners A and B, respectively. Although CT scan resolution is often stated in these numerical terms, it is often easier to think in terms of the object size that can be reproduced in the image. In our example, scanner B will be better able to reproduce small objects than will scanner A.

Compared with conventional radiography, CT has significantly worse spatial resolution. The limiting spatial frequency for screen-film radiography is about 7 line pairs per millimeter (lp/mm), for digital radiography it is about 5 lp/mm; however, the limiting resolution for CT is approximately 1 lp/mm. As we will see later in this chapter, it is contrast resolution that distinguishes CT from other clinical modalities.

In-Plane Versus Longitudinal Resolution

The spatial resolution of a CT image can be described in two dimensions. Resolution in the xy direction is called in-plane resolution, whereas resolution in the z direction is called longitudinal resolution.

Factors Affecting Spatial Resolution

The spatial resolution of a CT imaging system depends on the quality of raw data and the reconstruction method. In turn, the quality of the raw data is affected by several factors, many of which can be adjusted by the operator.

Matrix Size, Display Field of View, Pixel Size

Matrix size and DFOV selection determine pixel size. Pixel size plays an important role in the in-plane spatial resolution of an image. Reviewing from Chapter 1, a matrix is used to segment the raw data into distinct squares called pixels. The pixels are arranged in a grid-like arrangement of columns and rows. Each pixel has a width x, and a length y. In CT, pixels are always square, so $x = y$. Matrix size refers to how many pixels are present in the grid. Because the perimeter of the square matrix is held constant, the greater the total pixels present in the image, the smaller each individual pixel. Therefore, matrix size is one factor that controls pixel size. In practice, matrix size seldom varies in CT.

DFOV determines how much raw data will be used to reconstruct the image. Changing the DFOV will also alter the size of the image on the screen. Recall from Chapter 3 that DFOV works like the zoom on a camera and can be used to show the entire area, or to display a specific region of interest in greater detail. Increasing the DFOV increases the size of each pixel in the image. The pixel size reflects how much patient data is contained within each square. A larger pixel will include more patient data. The relationship between pixel size, matrix size, and DFOV is apparent in the equation:

$$\text{pixel size} = \text{DFOV}/\text{matrix size}$$

How does a change in pixel size affect spatial resolution? Recall that the information contained in each pixel is averaged, so that one density number, or Hounsfield unit (HU), is assigned to each pixel. If an object is smaller than a pixel, its density will be averaged with the density of other tissues contained in the pixel, creating a less accurate image.

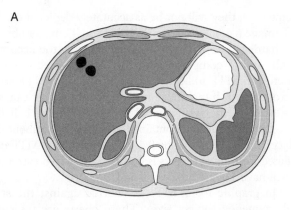

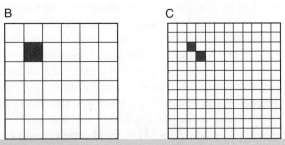

FIGURE 6-6 **A.** Two small objects in the patient. **B.** When reconstructed to lie within a single pixel, they will be represented on the image as a single object. **C.** If a smaller pixel is used, the objects can be displayed as two distinct shapes.

A large pixel size will make it more likely that multiple objects are contained within a pixel. When pixels are smaller, it is less likely that they will contain different densities, therefore decreasing the likelihood of volume averaging. Hence smaller pixel size will improve spatial resolution.

To illustrate, Figure 6-6A represents a section of patient data containing two, closely spaced, high-density objects. If these two small objects are reconstructed so that they are contained in a single pixel, such as in Figure 6-6B, they will be represented on the image as a single object. However, if a smaller pixel size is used, the objects can be displayed as two distinct shapes (Fig. 6-6C).

Because no object smaller than a pixel can be accurately displayed and the matrix size and DFOV influence the pixel size, it follows that matrix size and DFOV affect spatial resolution.

Slice Thickness

Chapter 1 introduced the concept of volume averaging and its relationship to slice thickness. In this section we review and expand on that association. In general, thinner slices produce sharper images because to create an image the system must flatten the scan thickness (a volume) into two dimensions (a flat image). The thicker the slice, the more flattening is necessary.

The raw data are segmented in the longitudinal (head/foot) direction by the slice thickness, representing a volume (a physical cross section) in the patient. Each segmented

Calculating Pixel Size When DFOV or Matrix Size Is Changed

DFOV may be given in either millimeters or centimeters. Regardless of what units are given, they must be consistent to solve the equation.

Problem 1: The DFOV used for an abdominal study is 42 cm and a 512 matrix is used. What is the pixel size in mm?

Step 1 (Lay out the equation):

42 cm/512 = pixel size

Step 2 (Convert DFOV units from cm to mm and solve the equation):

420 mm/512 = 0.82 mm

Problem 2: The DFOV used for a head study is 25 cm and a 512 matrix is used. What is the pixel size in mm?

Step 1 (Lay out the equation):

25 cm/512 = pixel size

Step 2 (Convert DFOV units from cm to mm and solve the equation):

250 mm/512 = 0.49 mm

In the above examples we see that with the matrix held constant, a 42 DFOV will result in a larger pixel than a 25 DFOV. More raw data are crammed into each of the larger pixels. This reduces the spatial resolution in the image.

Problem 3: The DFOV used for a head study is 25 cm and a 256 matrix is used. What is the pixel size in mm?

Step 1 (Lay out the equation):

25 cm/256 = pixel size

Step 2 (Convert DFOV units from cm to mm and solve the equation):

250 mm/256 = 0.98 mm

Compared with problem 2, this shows that a smaller matrix for a constant DFOV results in larger pixels and therefore less spatial resolution.

BOX 6–8   Key Concept

Slice thickness plays an important role in volume averaging, thereby affecting spatial resolution in the image.

New CT scanners allow for very thin slice thickness; often the goal is to produce isotropic voxels.

Historically, the impact of slice thickness on image quality is substantially more pronounced than pixel size. When comparing the x, y, and z dimensions, using the typical matrix and DFOV, the z axis tended to be considerably longer than either the x or y dimensions (Fig. 6-8). Recall from the practice equations that the pixel size for an abdominal image taken with a 42-cm DFOV is 0.82 mm. Compare this to a typical slice thickness of 5 mm used before the newer MDCT scanners. In such a situation, the z axis is six times longer than the x or y directions.

The advent of scanners capable of acquiring 16 or more slices simultaneously has changed this well-established premise. These newer systems allow a slice thickness of between 0.5 mm and 1 mm. Although these thin slices are often summed for a wider display slice, the spatial resolution is dependent on the way they were scanned. Hence, two 1-mm slices added together to display a single 2-mm slice will retain the spatial resolution of the original 1-mm slices. MDCT scanning results in isotropic

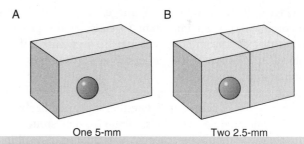

One 5-mm   Two 2.5-mm

FIGURE 6-7   A. A 2-mm object is contained in a 5-mm slice, resulting in significant volume averaging on the image. **B.** Slice thickness is decreased to 2.5 mm and volume averaging is significantly decreased.

portion of data is called a voxel (see Chapter 1). The voxel size also plays a role in volume averaging, and hence affects spatial resolution. The matrix divides data into squares with an x and y dimension. The operator's selection of slice thickness accounts for the z axis segmentation and results in a rectangular solid; however, if the slice thickness is set equal to the pixel width, the voxel can have equal lengths on all sides (i.e., be a cube). All of the tissue within the voxel is averaged together to produce one CT number.

Figure 6-7 illustrates how slice thickness affects the amount of volume averaging in the image. In Figure 6-7A, a 2-mm object is contained in a 5-mm slice. This results in image data that averages 3 mm of normal tissue with the 2-mm abnormality. In Figure 6-7B the slice thickness is decreased to 2.5 mm. The resulting image data now averages just 0.5 mm of normal tissue with the 2-mm abnormality. In doing so an image is created that more closely represents the actual object scanned. Therefore, narrowing the slice improves the images' longitudinal resolution.

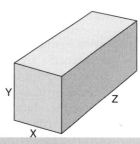

FIGURE 6-8   Before the newer MDCT scanner that can routinely scan with very thin slices, the z axis was considerably longer than either the x or y axes.

(or near-isotropic) voxels. An isotropic voxel is a cube, measuring the same in the $x, y,$ and z directions. When the imaging voxel is equal in size in all dimensions there is no loss of information when data are reformatted in a different plane. This is particularly important for imaging small vascular structures. For example, the coronary, peripheral, and carotid arteries frequently follow a twisting path and often run perpendicular to the image plane. Because each slice only encompasses a small amount of data, to follow these arteries multiple slices must be assembled in the z axis. An isotropic voxel ensures that there is no data loss with either multiplanar reformation (MPR) or volume rendering (VR).

Sampling Theorem   Patients are not composed of uniform density squares that can be trusted to fall neatly into separate pixels. Instead, an actual object may not lie entirely within a pixel. Sampling theorem (also called the Nyquist Sampling Theorem), used in telecommunication and many types of signal-processing applications, provides insight into the parameters necessary to accurately depict an object in a reconstructed image. As applied to CT image reconstruction, sampling theorem can be roughly summarized by the following statement: because an object may not lie entirely within a pixel, the pixel dimension should be half the size of the object to increase the likelihood of that object being resolved.

This theorem accounts for the element of random chance in the creation of a CT image. To understand this theorem, it is again important to consider the possible ways that data from an object may be segmented. If the object in question is the same size as a pixel, it is possible that by chance the object may fall entirely within a single pixel. Figure 6-9A represents this possibility. However, random chance will dictate that it is more likely the object will straddle two pixels. Figure 6-9B illustrates this possibility. It should be apparent that the image resulting from the case portrayed by Figure 6-9B would be inferior to that of the image resulting from Figure 6-9A. A third possibility could also arise. In Figure 6-9C the object falls at the junction of four separate pixels. Therefore, only a fourth of the object will be averaged with three-fourths of a pixel of normal tissue. This would be the worst-case scenario and would result in an image with the poorest spatial resolution.

Sampling theorem states that we reduce the likelihood of our worst-case scenario occurring by reducing the size of the pixel. We can see that in Figure 6-9D, the smaller pixel size will improve spatial resolution by allowing four pixels to represent the object, with no normal tissue included. However, even with the smaller pixel size, cases such as that depicted by Figure 6-9E will still arise. In this case, the object will fall so that only two of the pixels accurately represent the object, whereas the four surrounding will have some degree of volume averaging.

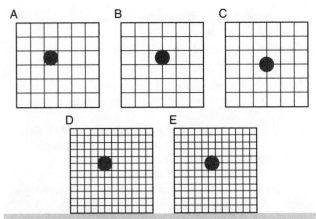

FIGURE 6-9   Random chance plays a role in whether a small object will be seen on the reconstructed image. In (A), (B), and (C) the object to be displayed is the same size as the pixel. The three figures show different scenarios as to how the object could be reconstructed, each resulting in a different level of volume averaging. In (D) and (E), a smaller pixel size is used, and the scenarios regarding the likelihood of volume averaging improve.

However, we can see from our illustrations that the situation depicted in Figure 6-9E is preferable to that of Figure 6-9C. To review, by reducing the size of the pixel we can increase our chance of accurately representing a small object. The theorem further states that by making the pixel size half the size of the object we will increase the likelihood that the object is accurately resolved on the image.

Reconstruction Algorithm

All CT systems offer a choice of different reconstruction algorithms that are chosen by the operator (or built into the scan protocols). The appropriate reconstruction algorithm depends on which parts of the data should be enhanced or suppressed to optimize the image for diagnosis. Some will "smooth" the data more heavily, by reducing the difference between adjacent pixels. This can help to reduce the appearance of artifacts (such as those that result from dental fillings) but do so at the cost of reduced spatial resolution. Conversely, some filters accentuate the difference between neighboring pixels to optimize spatial resolution, but must make sacrifices in low-contrast resolution. These latter filters are most often used when there are great extremes of tissue density and when optimal low-contrast resolution is not necessary. An example is images of the internal auditory canal in which the tiny bones of the inner ear are displayed; the tissue densities of interest are limited to bone or air, with high inherent tissue contrast so the image can be reconstructed for spatial rather than contrast fidelity (Fig. 6-10). These types of high-contrast reconstruction algorithms are often called bone or detail filters. The advantage of these types of filters is gained at

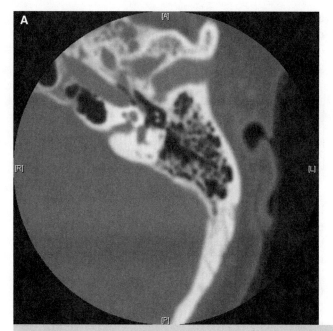 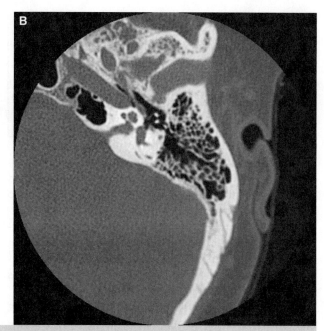

FIGURE 6-10 Image (A) was reconstructed using a standard filter. The same data were reconstructed with a bone filter in image (B). Notice the increased spatial resolution. Images courtesy of the University of Michigan Health Systems.

the cost of reduced visibility of the soft tissue structures, for which the high-contrast filter produces a noisy effect. For this reason, certain studies require the data to be reconstructed with two separate algorithms. One optimizes low-contrast detectability in the soft tissue. The second provides optimal high spatial resolution and is preferable for bone.

Focal Spot Size

As mentioned earlier, the focal spot size affects image quality, but the effect is minimal. As in any x-ray imaging procedure, larger focal spots cause more geometric unsharpness in the image and reduce spatial resolution.

Pitch

The pitch used in helical scanning can affect spatial resolution. In general, increasing the pitch reduces resolution. However, the impact of increased pitch is more pronounced in SDCT than in MDCT systems. This is related primarily to the fact that in SDCT as pitch increases so does the slice sensitivity profile (i.e., effective slice thickness; see Chapter 5). Optimal choice of pitch depends on the detector configuration and the CT projection data interpolation scheme used. In practice, pitch values from 1 to 2 are commonly used in both SDCT and MDCT.

BOX 6–9   Key Concept

In general, increasing the pitch reduces resolution in the image.

Patient Motion

Motion creates blurring in the image and degrades spatial resolution. Hence, shortened scan times may help improve spatial resolution to the extent that they may reduce the effects of both involuntary motion (e.g., heart) and overt patient motion.

CONTRAST RESOLUTION

The second major aspect of image quality is that of contrast resolution (or low-contrast resolution). It is the ability to differentiate a structure that varies only slightly in density from its surrounding. An example of an imaging challenge that is dependent on contrast resolution is that of a liver lesion surrounded by healthy liver tissue. Recall that in order to see a difference on an image there must be a density difference between the object and its background. The ability to distinguish an object that is nearly the same density as its background is referred to as low-contrast detectability. Contrast resolution may also be referred to as the sensitivity of the system; hence the term low-contrast sensitivity is also used.

CT is superior to all other clinical modalities in its contrast resolution. It is generally accepted that for an object to be visible on an image produced from screen-film radiography the object must have at least a 5% difference in contrast from its background material, whereas CT is an excellent low-contrast discriminator and can differentiate an object with a 0.5% contrast variation. In CT, the contrast difference between objects is typically characterized by the percentage linear attenuation coefficient: 1% contrast difference corresponds to a difference of 10 HU.

Contrast resolution is measured using phantoms that contain objects, typically cylindrical, of varying sizes and with a small difference in density (typically from 4 to 10 HU) from the background (Fig. 6-11). The most common method requires an observer to detect objects as distinct. To some degree this is subjective, because different observers will often look at the same image and evaluate it differently. This subjectivity is broadly referred to as receiver operator characteristics.

By definition, contrast resolution involves differentiating an object from its very similar density background. Because the difference between object and background is small, noise plays an important role in low-contrast resolution.

Noise

Simply defined, image noise is the undesirable fluctuation of pixel values in an image of a homogeneous material. We can recognize noise as the grainy appearance or "salt-and-pepper" look on an underexposed image. Noise is caused by the combination of many factors, the most prevalent being quantum noise, or quantum mottle. Quantum mottle occurs when there are an insufficient number of photons detected. It is inversely related to the number of photons used to form the image. Hence, as the number of x-ray photons used to create an image decreases, noise increases. In CT, the number of x-ray photons detected per pixel is also often referred to as signal-to-noise ratio (SNR), although this is not the technical definition of that term. In addition to image processing, SNR is used in many other

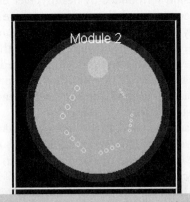

FIGURE 6-11 A scanner's low-contrast resolution can be measured using a phantom that contains objects of varying sizes and with a small difference in density from the background. The more objects visible, the better the system's low-contrast resolution capability.

applications including acoustics. SNR compares the level of desired signal (such as music) to the level of background noise. The higher the ratio, the less obtrusive the background noise is.

If an image is created of an object that is known to be uniform in density, such as a water phantom, then all measured points within that image should in theory be the same, but in practice they are not. Fluctuations of CT numbers at adjacent points indicate noise in the image. The standard deviation (SD) measurement is an indication of the amount of variance among pixel values in a designated region of interest (ROI) (Chapter 4). The SD measurement of an ROI of a known uniform phantom will indicate the degree of noise in an image. The smaller the SD, the less the noise and the better the contrast resolution capability. It follows that factors that influence the noise levels will also affect contrast resolution.

Factors Affecting Contrast Resolution

Many factors affect contrast resolution. Many of these factors influence contrast through their relationship to image noise.

mAs/Dose

The mAs selected for scanning directly influences the number of x-ray photons used to produce the CT image, thereby affecting the SNR and the contrast resolution. Doubling the mAs of the study increases the SNR by 40%. Therefore, if the initial image was degraded by quantum noise then doubling the mAs will improve the contrast resolution of repeat scans.

The dose increases linearly with mAs per scan. It follows that increasing mAs, will improve contrast resolution, but at the cost of a higher radiation dose to the patient. Determining the appropriate mAs for a scan must be made in the context of the clinical task at hand. A relatively high amount of noise may be tolerable if the clinical task is primarily dependent on the image's spatial resolution. Examples of indications in which a lower mAs might be acceptable are solid nodule detection in the lung, coronary artery calcium detection, or the identification of emphysema in the lung. Conversely, abdominal studies (for liver or kidney lesion detection) are examples of examinations that depend on the images' low-contrast resolution, and therefore require that mAs be set to a level that reduces noise.

Pixel Size

Keeping all other scan parameters the same, as pixel size decreases, the number of detected x-ray photons per pixel will decrease. Fewer photons per pixel results in an increase in noise and a subsequent decrease in contrast resolution.

Slice Thickness

The slice thickness has a linear effect on the number of x-ray photons available to produce the image–a 5-mm slice will have twice the number of photons as a 2.5-mm slice. Because thicker slices allow more photons to reach the detectors they have a better SNR and appear less noisy. However, this improvement comes at the cost of spatial resolution in the z axis.

Reconstruction Algorithm

As mentioned earlier, bone algorithms produce lower contrast resolution (but better spatial resolution), whereas soft tissue algorithms improve contrast resolution at the expense of spatial resolution.

Patient Size

For the same x-ray technique, larger patients attenuate more x-rays photons, leaving fewer to reach the detectors. This reduces SNR, increases noise, and results in lower contrast resolution.

Other Contrast Resolution Considerations

Although the level of image noise is paramount in discussions of contrast resolution, other factors play a role in whether an object will be discernible from its surroundings. Subject contrast relates to the inherent properties of the object scanned. For a given technique, the level of contrast that is visible will decrease as the object size decreases. Stated more simply, if everything else is held constant, small objects are more difficult to see than larger objects. The relationship between object size and visibility is called the contrast-detail response. Measuring and charting this relationship results in what is known as a contrast-detail curve.

The inherent contrast of an organ relates to its physical properties. For example, the lung is said to possess high inherent contrast because it is primarily air-filled. The low-attenuation lungs provide a background that makes nearly any other object discernible because of its dramatic difference in density. For example, consider a calcified nodule. It is easily discernible in the lung, in which the surrounding air provides a substantial amount of natural contrast. Imagine the difficulty in recognizing the nodule if it were to lie against the iliac crest.

The displayed contrast of an image is dependent on the window settings used for its display. For low-contrast objects to be visible, the window level must be set near the average density of the object and the window width must be narrow enough so that only small groups of HU are represented in each shade of gray displayed (see Chapter 4). The images in Figure 6-12 illustrate this concept.

TEMPORAL RESOLUTION

The word temporal has two distinct definitions–in medicine the word typically refers to being near the temple of the head (i.e., temporal bone). However, in discussions of image quality, temporal (from the root "tempo")

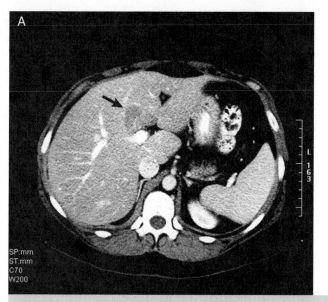
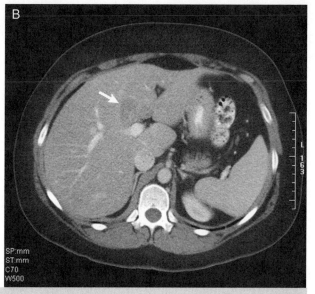

FIGURE 6-12 The effect of window settings on low-contrast resolution. An oblong, hypoattenuating mass is seen in the medial segment of the left hepatic lobe (arrow). The liver lesion is more easily discernible when the image is displayed with a narrow window width (A). The same image, displayed with a wider window width—the liver lesion is nearly indistinguishable (B). Images courtesy of the University of Michigan Health Systems.

refers to the characteristic of being limited by time. The temporal resolution of a system refers to how rapidly data are acquired. Temporal resolution is controlled by gantry rotation speed, the number of detector channels in the system, and the speed with which the system can record changing signals. The temporal resolution of a system is typically reported in milliseconds (ms), which are thousandths of a second. For example, a specific 64-slice detector (Somatom Sensation 64, Siemens Medical Solutions, Forchheim, Germany), with a gantry rotation speed of 330 ms, reports the temporal resolution as 83 to 165 ms. High temporal resolution is of particular importance when imaging moving structures (e.g., heart) and for studies dependent on the dynamic flow of iodinated contrast media (e.g., CT angiography, perfusion studies).

BOX 6–12   Key Concept

Temporal resolution refers to how rapidly data are acquired. It is controlled by gantry rotation speed, the number of detector channels in the system, and the speed with which the system can record changing signals.

SUMMARY

It should be clear that there is a compromise between spatial resolution and contrast resolution. In addition, image quality is closely linked to radiation dose. Improvement in image quality most often comes at a cost of increased radiation dose. In fact, in CT there is a well-established relationship among SNR, pixel dimensions, slice thickness, and radiation dose. Manipulating scan parameters may improve one aspect of image quality while decreasing another aspect. Technologists must be aware of these tradeoffs. The clinical task at hand must be the overarching consideration in making specific decisions regarding scan protocols.

REVIEW QUESTIONS

1. What factors are referred to as scanning parameters?
2. What factors define the quantity of x-ray energy produced?
3. What factor defines the intensity of the x-ray beam?
4. Define partial scan and overscan.
5. Define spatial resolution.
6. How is the CT image affected by too low an mAs setting? How is it affected if the mAs setting is too high?
7. Give examples of examinations in which images may need to be reconstructed twice, using different algorithms.
8. How does a change in slice thickness affect the spatial resolution? How does it affect contrast resolution? What effect will it have on patient dose?
9. List the factors that affect spatial resolution. List the factors that affect contrast resolution.

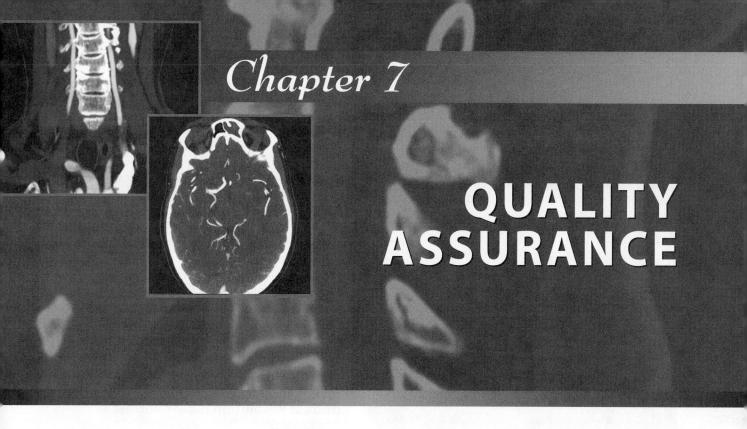

QUALITY ASSURANCE

control tests must be documented in a consistent format, and 3) the quality control test should indicate whether the tested parameter is within specified guidelines.

BOX 7–1   Key Concept
Quality assurance programs should be designed around three basic concepts: 1.   The tests that make up the program must be performed on a regular basis 2.   The results from all tests must be recorded using a consistent format 3.   Documentation should indicate whether the tested parameter is within specified guidelines

QUALITY ASSURANCE METHODS

Quality control programs are designed to ensure that the CT system is producing the best possible image quality using the minimal radiation dose to the patient. An effective program provides a method for the systematic monitoring of the system's performance allowing the identification of specific problems or malfunctions. Responsibility for performing and documenting quality control tests is often shared between CT technologists and medical physicists. Technologists typically perform and record routine quality control tests; testing done by physicists is typically annual or semiannual. A medical physicist is required to obtain necessary dosimetric data.

Quality assurance programs should adhere to three basic rules: 1) the tests that make up the program must be performed on a regular basis, 2) the results from all quality

As described in Chapter 6, phantoms can be used to evaluate both spatial and contrast resolution. Many other aspects of image quality can be evaluated using phantoms. Many manufacturers produce phantoms for CT quality control purposes. Most phantoms are designed with many components so that a single phantom can be used to examine a broad range of scanner parameters. For example, the American College of Radiology (ACR) CT accreditation phantom is a solid phantom that contains four modules, and is constructed primarily from a water-equivalent material. Each module is 4 cm deep and 20 cm in diameter, with external alignment markings to allow centering of the phantom in the *x, y,* and *z* axes. Module 1 is used to assess positioning and alignment, CT accuracy and slice thickness. Module 2 is used to assess low-contrast resolution. Module 3 is used to assess CT number uniformity and the accuracy of in-plane distance measurements. Module 4 is used to assess spatial resolution (Fig. 7-1). Below is a summary of the various features that can be evaluated and the types of phantoms that are used.

BOX 7–2   Key Concept

Many aspects of image quality can be evaluated using phantoms. Most phantoms are designed with many components so that a single phantom can be used to examine a broad range of scanner parameters.

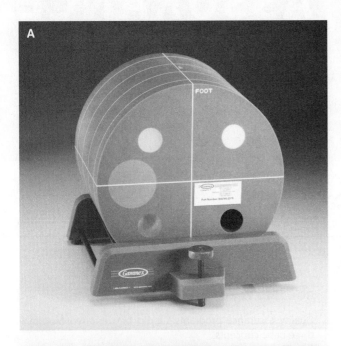

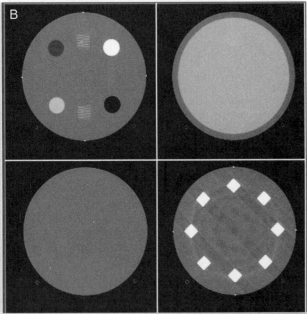

FIGURE 7-1   ACR CT accreditation phantom (A) consists of four modules that can be used to examine a broad range of scanner parameters. Cross-sectional image from each of the modules are shown in (B). Images courtesy of Gammex, Inc.

Spatial Resolution (High-Contrast Resolution)

Spatial resolution can be calculated from the analysis of the spread of information within the system using the MTF. This process is cumbersome and, when performed, is typically done by a physicist. Measuring the spatial resolution directly, using a line pairs phantom, is a simpler method and is often performed by a technologist. A typical line pairs phantom contains groups of lead strips having different strip width and spacing. In each group, the lead width is equal to the lead spacing. The spatial resolution is given as the maximum number of visible line pairs (lead strip and space) per millimeter.

At a minimum, the spatial resolution measured should be equal to the manufacturer's specifications for that scanner. The spatial resolution of current scanners when images are reconstructed in a high-resolution algorithm is in the range of 10 to 20 lp/cm. This test is performed monthly in most quality assurance programs.

Contrast Resolution (Low-Contrast Resolution)

To evaluate contrast resolution a phantom is used that contains objects of varying sizes. These objects have only a small difference in density from their background. The phantoms are scanned at different mAs settings. The most common method requires an observer to detect objects as distinct. At the minimum, contrast resolution should be such that with a density difference of 0.5% a 5-mm object can be displayed. This test is performed monthly in most quality assurance programs.

Slice Thickness Accuracy

Measurements of selected slice thickness are determined using a phantom that includes a ramp, spiral, or step-wedge. The phantom contains objects with known measurements and provides a standard to compare with the scanner. For a slice thickness of 5 mm or greater, the slice thickness should not vary more than ±1 mm from the intended slice thickness. For a slice thickness of less than 5 mm, the slice thickness should not vary more than ±0.5 mm. This test is usually performed semiannually.

Laser Light Accuracy

Laser lights located both inside and outside the gantry are used extensively for patient positioning and alignment. Accurate laser light performance is critical and can be measured, most often using a specific phantom designed for the purpose and provided by the scanner manufacturer. The light field should coincide with the radiation field to within 2 mm. This test is usually performed semiannually.

Noise and Uniformity

A water phantom (or any phantom known to be uniform in density) is scanned. Noise is measured by obtaining the standard deviation (SD) of the CT numbers within a region of interest (ROI).

Uniformity refers to the ability of the scanner to yield the same CT number regardless of the location of an ROI within a homogeneous object. Like noise, uniformity is most commonly measured using a water phantom. Placing several ROIs within the phantom, it is hoped that each will possess the same measurement. If fluctuations exist at different regions within the phantom (e.g., if a ring around the perimeter measures differently from the center), then a problem with the system's cross-field uniformity can be diagnosed (Fig. 7-2).

For noise measurements, the standard deviation of an ROI in a water phantom should not exceed 10. For uniformity measurements, there should be no more than a ±2 HU variation from an ROI placed at the center of the water phantom to those placed at the periphery. These tests should be performed on a weekly basis.

Linearity

This refers to the relationship between CT numbers and the linear attenuation values (Chapter 1) of the scanned object at a designated kVp value. Over time these values can vary as a result of minute changes in detector channel variations and responses. Daily calibrations help to avoid fluctuations in linearity by compensating for these tiny changes. To assess linearity a phantom containing a variety of objects with known densities is scanned and the objects measured (Fig. 7-3). The plotted values should demonstrate a straight line between the average CT number and the linear attenuation coefficients. Any deviation from the straight line indicates scanner malfunction. Linearity is typically measured semiannually.

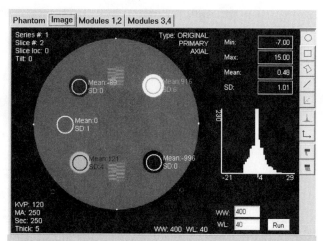

FIGURE 7-3 Linearity refers to the relationship between CT numbers and the linear attenuation values of the scanned object at a designated kVp value. To assess linearity a phantom containing a variety of objects with known densities is scanned and the objects measured. Image courtesy of Gammex, Inc.

Examples of quality control reports generated from tests performed on the ACR CT accreditation phantom are provided in Figure 7-4.

Radiation Dose

It is important to monitor the amount of radiation to which patients and staff are exposed. Technologists must be well acquainted with the factors (e.g., slice thickness, mAs, kVp) that affect the radiation dose to the patient. Technologists should also be able to provide safety instructions to anyone (e.g., patient's family members) who must remain in the scan room. Advice should include donning protective apparel (e.g., lead aprons, thyroid shields) and directing them to areas within the room with the least exposure.

Dose measurements are required for each of a facility's CT scanners. These measurements are performed by a medical physicist who follows very detailed specifications to report parameters such as effective dose and dose length product. Measurements are made using standard head and body CT dose index (CTDI) phantoms and a pencil ionization chamber. Using the CTDI measurement, the physicist must calculate several descriptors of dose for an adult head, pediatric abdomen, and adult abdomen examination. These measurements are compared with reference dose values. For example, ACR reference CTDI$_{vol}$ (effective January 1, 2008) are as follows: adult head, 75 mGy; adult abdomen, 25 mGy; pediatric abdomen (5 years old), 20 mGy. If a dose for any of the three examinations exceeds the respective reference value, the site is expected to submit documentation detailing their investigation, corrective action if necessary, or justification of the higher dose level.

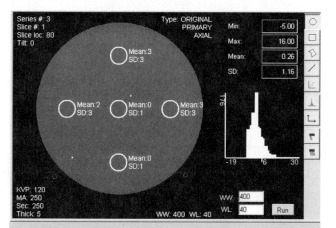

FIGURE 7-2 Uniformity refers to the ability of the scanner to yield the same CT number regardless of the location of an ROI within a homogeneous object. Uniformity is most commonly measured using a water phantom. Placing several ROIs within the phantom, it is hoped that each will possess the same measurement. Image courtesy of Gammex, Inc.

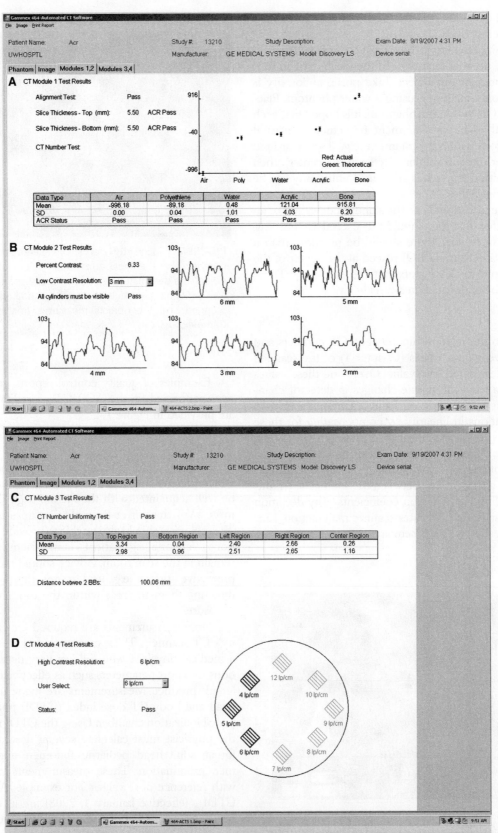

FIGURE 7-4 Examples of quality control reports generated from tests performed on the ACR CT accreditation phantom. A report of alignment, slice thickness, and linearity results is created from module 1 (A). A report of low-contrast resolution results is created from module 2 (B). A report of CT number uniformity and in-plane distance accuracy results is created from module 3 (C). A report of high-contrast resolution results is created from module 4 (D). Images courtesy of Gammex, Inc.

IMAGE ARTIFACTS

Artifacts are defined as anything appearing on the image that is not present in the object scanned. Artifacts have many different presentations and can be attributed to many causes. They can be broadly classified as physics-based (resulting from the physical processes associated with data acquisition), patient-based, or equipment-induced. Artifacts can seriously degrade the quality of CT images, sometimes to the point of rendering them diagnostically unusable. Recognizing various artifacts and understanding why they occur and how they can be prevented or reduced is an important aspect of image quality assurance. Recognizing the possible causes of artifacts can save a significant amount of time and money. Ideally, better identification of artifacts can permit them to be corrected without a service call; or, if the severity of the artifact requires a service engineer, the call can be placed promptly.

BOX 7–3   Key Concept

Any object seen on the image that is not present in the object scanned is considered an artifact. A variety of sources cause artifacts.

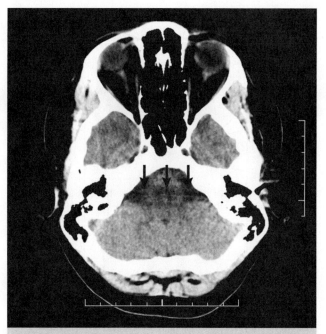

FIGURE 7-5 Beam hardening from the dense petrous bones creates low attenuation streaks in the image (arrows).

Beam Hardening

The polychromatic nature of the x-ray beam used in CT and its effect on the creation of beam-hardening artifacts was discussed in Chapter 1. To summarize here, as an x-ray beam passes through an object, lower-energy photons are preferentially absorbed, creating a "harder" beam. Individual rays are hardened to differing degrees, and this variation cannot be adjusted for by the reconstruction algorithm. A common clinical example of beam hardening occurs between the petrous bones in the head, where streak artifacts appear between the two bones on the image. The degree of beam hardening is dependent on the composition of the part examined and the extent the beam must travel through various tissues. The beam is hardened more by dense objects (e.g., more by bone and less by fat). Two types of artifact can result from this effect, cupping artifacts (the periphery of the image is lighter) and the appearance of dark bands or streaks between dense objects in the image (Fig. 7-5).

CT systems use three features to minimize beam hardening: filtration, calibration correction, and beam-hardening correction software. Filtering the beam by a metallic material such as aluminum filters out the lower-energy components of the beam before they pass through the patient. An additional filter shaped like a bow tie is used for body studies to further harden the edges of the beam, which will pass through the thinner parts of the patient (Chapter 2). Scanners are calibrated in a range of sizes so that beam-hardening compensation can be tailored to different parts of the patient. For example, a head scan field of view (SFOV) typically uses correction to reduce cupping artifacts often seen in the posterior fossa.

Correction software that reduces beam-hardening artifacts can also be included in bone or detail reconstruction algorithms. Raising the kVp will increase the average photon energy of the beam, therefore reducing beam hardening to some extent.

The best strategy available to the operator to avoid beam hardening is to select the appropriate SFOV to ensure the correct filtration, calibration, and beam-hardening correction software is used.

Partial Volume Artifact

There are a number of ways in which the partial volume effect can reduce image quality (Chapter 6). Recall that the partial volume effect occurs when more than one type of tissue is contained within a voxel. Although related, partial volume artifacts are a separate problem from that of partial volume averaging. One type of partial volume artifact occurs when a dense object lies to the edge of the FOV. This can result in the object showing up in only a small number of views collected from the tube's 360° path. To illustrate, Figure 7-6 exaggerates the geometry of the x-ray beam to demonstrate how an object that lies to the periphery may not appear on all views. The inconsistencies between the views cause shading artifacts to appear in the image. The best method of reducing partial volume artifacts is to use thinner slices.

Aliasing

An adequate number of projections, as well as an adequate amount of data within each projection, must be available to reconstruct a CT image of optimal quality. Insufficient

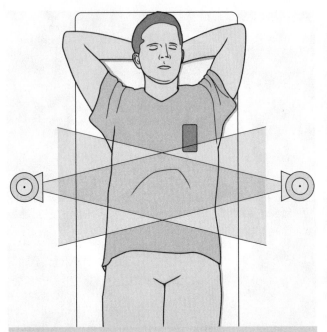

FIGURE 7-6 Partial volume artifacts can occur when dense objects lie to the edge of the SFOV and are only present in some of the views used to create the image.

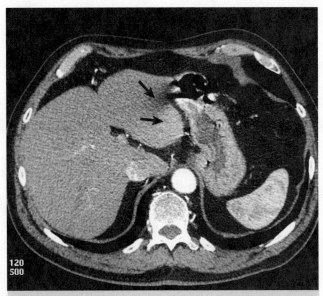

FIGURE 7-7 The irregular shading in the left lobe of the liver (indicated by arrows) in this image is caused by a combination of edge gradient effect and beam hardening. The artifacts arise from the pronounced difference in density between the air and barium in the stomach.

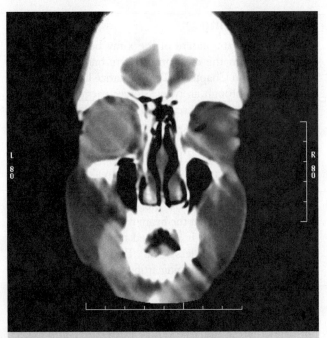

FIGURE 7-8 The diagonal shading degrading this image is caused from patient movement during the scan.

projection data (for instance, when the helical pitch is greatly extended) is known as undersampling. Undersampling causes inaccuracies related to reproducing sharp edges and small objects and results in an artifact known as aliasing, in which fine stripes appear to be radiating from a dense structure. Because aliasing artifacts consist of evenly spaced lines they are easy to distinguish from anatomic structures and, therefore, seldom do they render an image undiagnostic. However, when resolution of fine detail is important, aliasing artifacts should be avoided to the degree possible. Aliasing artifacts can be combated by slowing gantry rotation speed (i.e., increasing scan time) or by reducing the helical pitch.

Edge Gradient Effect

The edge gradient effect results in streak artifact or shading (both light and dark) arising from irregularly shaped objects that have a pronounced difference in density from surrounding structures. A common clinical example is artifacts that result when barium and air lie adjacent to each other in the stomach (Fig. 7-7). Artifacts from the edge gradient effect are largely unavoidable, but are somewhat reduced by thinner slices. Using a low HU-value oral contrast, such as Volumen, or water (a neutral HU contrast agent) in place of a barium suspension can eliminate the streak artifacts from the gastrointestinal tract.

Motion

Artifacts from patient motion typically appear as shading, ghosting (objects appear to have a shadow), streaking or blurring (Fig. 7-8). Manufacturers have built features into the CT systems to reduce motion artifacts such as overscan and partial scan modes, software correction, and cardiac gating.

Voluntary motion can be reduced or eliminated by adequately preparing the patient for the examination. Time is well invested in explaining the procedure to the patient, reinforcing the importance of remaining still, and confirming that the patient understands any breathing requirements. Positioning aids such as an angle sponge placed beneath the patient's knees will also reduce motion by ensuring the patient is more comfortable during the examination. In some situations, immobilization devices such as straps and wedge sponges can provide the patient additional stability. In some situations, particularly with pediatric patients, it may be necessary to immobilize the patient by means of sedation. Scanning the chest and abdomen using the shortest scan time possible also helps to minimize artifact from involuntary motion. Cardiac protocols often include pharmacologic methods to lower the patient's heart rate in an effort to reduce motion artifact on the images (see Chapter 20).

Metallic Artifacts

Metal objects in the SFOV will create streak artifacts (Fig. 7-9). They occur, in part, because the density of the metal is beyond the range of HU values that the system is designed to handle. The range of x-ray intensity values to which the scanner can accurately respond is called the *dynamic range*. The upper limit on older CT systems was often 1,000 HU (that of dense cortical bone). Metal objects have attenuation values higher than 1,000. Newer systems have expanded the HU scale and can include values as high as 4,000, thereby reducing the impact of metallic streak artifacts. However, beam hardening, partial volume, edge gradient, and aliasing all contribute to the streaks that result from metal in the SFOV.

The best way to reduce metallic artifact is to minimize the metal present in the SFOV. Patients are asked to take off any removable metal objects such as jewelry before scanning begins. For body scans, patients should change into a hospital gown to avoid scanning zippers, safety pins, etc. For nonremovable items, such as dental fillings, prosthetic devices, and surgical clips, it is sometimes possible to angle the gantry to exclude the metal objects. When it is impossible to scan the required anatomy without including metal objects, increasing technique, especially kVp, may help penetrate some objects, and using thin sections will reduce the contribution caused by partial volume artifact.

Out-of-Field Artifacts

Out-of-field artifacts are caused by anatomy that extends outside of the selected SFOV. These artifacts occur because the anatomy outside the SFOV attenuates and hardens the x-ray beam, but is ignored in the image reconstruction process. A common clinical example is when imaging of the body must be done with the patient's arms down by their side, rather than raised out of the way of the scan (Fig. 7-10). If the

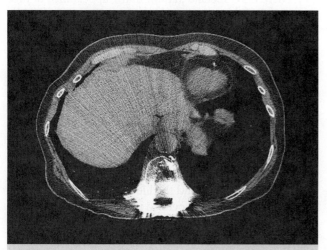

FIGURE 7-9 Metallic hardware in the patient's spine resulted in streak artifacts.

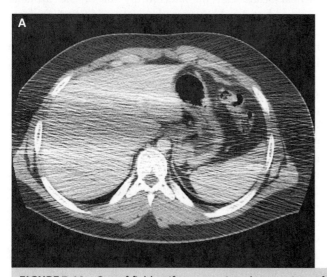
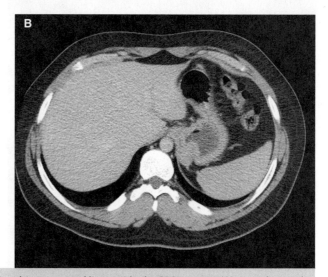

FIGURE 7-10 Out-of-field artifacts can arise when portions of the object scanned lie outside the SFOV. Image (A) was taken with the patient's arms down by his side, resulting in pronounced artifacts. The scan was repeated, and image (B) was taken after the patient's arms were raised to lie outside of the scan field.

arms are outside the scan field they will not be seen on the image, but their presence can lead to severe artifacts in the image. In addition, obese patients may obstruct the reference detectors, further contributing to image artifacts. Out-of-field artifacts appear as streaks and shading on the image.

Out-of-field artifacts can be avoided when an SFOV can be selected that is larger than the patient. For exceptionally large patients who exceed even the largest SFOV, out-of-field artifacts are inevitable. Encouraging patients to raise their arms out of the way of the SFOV will also avoid artifact.

Ring Artifacts

Ring artifacts occur with third-generation scanners and appear on the image as a ring or concentric rings centered on the rotational axis (Fig. 7-11). They are caused by imperfect detector elements–either faulty or simply out of calibration. In some instances technologists may eliminate circular artifacts by recalibrating the scanner. Should that fail, the problem must be reported to a service engineer for repair.

Tube Arcing

A common cause of equipment-induced artifact occurs when there is an undesired surge of electrical current (i.e., a short-circuit) within the x-ray tube. This is referred to as either high-voltage arcing or tube arcing. Arcing tends to occur whenever there is a large difference in electrical potential, such as the case between the anode and cathode in an x-ray tube. In an x-ray tube, arcing can occur

through residual gas molecules present within the evacuated envelope of the x-ray tube. As an x-ray tube ages, the tendency to arc often increases owing to such factors as degradation of the vacuum within the tube, which results in increased gas pressure. Arcing can also occur through the oil in the x-ray tube housing. Once an x-ray tube starts to arc, a cascade-type effect may occur that sets events in motion that contribute to yet more frequent arcing. The arcing causes a momentary loss of x-ray output, which contaminates the x-ray signal collected at the detectors, affecting proper image reconstruction and hence producing artifacts. In the early stages the arcing may be infrequent, and small artifacts begin to appear in the images. However, as the tube ages further, the frequency and severity of the arc often increase, resulting in images with more pronounced artifacts.

There is no specific pattern in the appearance of tube arc artifacts. Their effect on the image will vary depending on the severity and frequency of arching. Artifacts from tube arcing can range from a single slight streak to multiple streaks that combine to render the image diagnostically useless. In most cases of tube arcing the CT system will produce an error message that can help the technologist identify the problem. A service engineer should be called when tube arcing occurs. In addition to the error message, the technologist should describe the arcing pattern to the service engineer and report on the frequency of the error. The engineer may be able to remove residual gasses and thereby extend the life of the x-ray tube. Given the considerable cost associated with installing a new tube and the length of time the system is inoperable while it is being serviced, it is desirable to extend the service life of the x-ray tube.

Helical and Cone Beam Effect

Helical scans can be affected by all of the artifacts explained so far. However, there are additional artifacts that can occur in helical scanning attributable to the helical interpolation and reconstruction process. The introduction of helical scanning necessitated new image reconstruction methods because now the table moved continuously during data collection and the views needed to reconstruct the images were not all in the same plane. To address these problems, interpolation methods used measurements from either side of the image plane to create each image (see Chapter 5). This interpolation can result in artifacts, particularly when anatomic structures change rapidly in the z direction. Higher pitches require more interpolated data, and result in more artifacts. Helical interpolation artifacts result in subtle inaccuracies in CT number and can be easily misinterpreted as disease. These artifacts can best be avoided by using a low pitch whenever possible.

The interpolation process becomes even more complicated as the number of detector rows increase. Windmill artifacts (Fig. 7-12) appear only on MDCT helical systems.

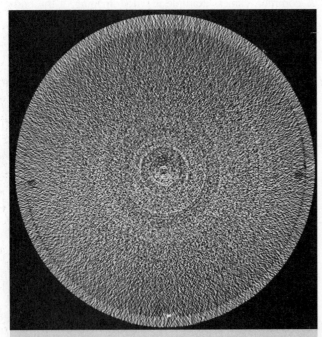

FIGURE 7-11   Ring artifacts appear from a malfunctioning or miscalibrated detector element in a third-generation scanner.

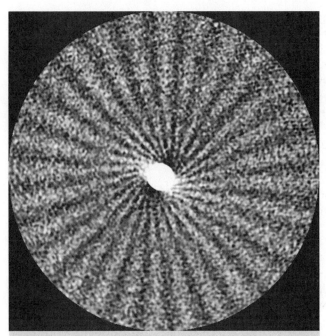

FIGURE 7-12 CT image of a phantom shows windmill artifact.

As the number of detector channels increases, a wider collimation is required and the x-ray beam becomes cone-shaped rather than fan-shaped. The data collected in each acquisition does not correspond to a flat plane, but rather to a cone shape. This can result in artifacts from the so-called cone beam effect. These are similar to partial volume artifacts if they occur from objects located to the edge of the FOV. They appear as either streaks or as bright and dark shading near areas of large density differences (e.g., bone and muscle). Cone beam artifacts are more pronounced for the outer detector rows. The larger the cone beam (i.e., more detector channels), the more pronounced the effect. This is why certain protocols for 64-detector row scanners do not use all of the available detector rows for data acquisition. In protocols in which high image resolution is paramount and the speed of the scan acquisition is not as important, protocols may be designed so that only the 32 center rows of the detector array are used. In addition, manufacturers have addressed the problem with new and innovative cone beam reconstruction algorithms that replace the standard reconstruction techniques used on SDCT systems.

TABLE 7-1 Troubleshooting Artifacts on the CT Image

Manifestation	Possible Cause	Corrective Steps
Beam-hardening artifact (broad streaks, cupping, vague areas of low density)	X-ray beams are composed of different energies	Use appropriate filtration, calibration, and correction software. Increase kVp setting.
Aliasing effect (fine lines)	Too few samples	If a partial scan was used, rescan using a complete arc. Increase scan time. Reduce pitch.
Edge gradient effect (straight line radiating from high-contrast areas, such as barium adjacent to air)	Angle of x-ray beam varies between two similar views	Largely unavoidable. Somewhat reduced by thinner slices. Use low or neutral HU-value oral contrast in place of barium.
Motion (shading, streaking, blurring, or ghosting)	Voluntary or involuntary patient motion	Give clear breathing instructions to the patient and reinforce the importance of holding still. Use positioning aids or immobilization devices. Consider sedation, particularly for pediatric patients. Use shortest scan time possible. For cardiac protocols, consider β-blockers.
Metallic (streaks)	Objects present that are beyond the dynamic range of the scanner	Whenever possible, remove metallic objects from SFOV. Angle gantry. Increase technique, particularly kVp. Use thin slices.
Ring (a single ring or concentric rings)	Detector problem	Recalibrate; if rings persist, call service
Tube arcing (no specific pattern; can range from a single streak to severe mottling)	Electrical surge within the x-ray tube	Call service
Spiral interpolation artifacts (subtle inaccuracies in CT number)	Images are created from views that are not all in the same plane	Lower pitch
Cone beam effect (lines appear in a windmill formation)	Only on MDCT, from the cone-shaped x-ray beam	Use pitch selections recommended by manufacturer

Artifacts Arising From Multiplanar or 3D Reformations

A variety of artifacts can occur when image data are reformatted to produce three-dimensional (3D) images or images in planes other than that in which the patient was scanned. These artifacts will be discussed in Chapter 8.

SUMMARY

A CT quality assurance program is a planned and systematic approach to ensure that CT equipment conforms to established standards. An effective program identifies variances in system performance that can uncover specific problems or malfunctions. A well-designed and implemented quality assurance program can provide confidence that a CT system will perform patient examinations satisfactorily.

Many types of artifacts exist in CT. More than one type of artifact may play a role in a specific image. All artifacts degrade the image. It is helpful to be able to identify the types and causes of artifacts. Table 7-1 lists the most common artifacts, their typical causes, and steps that can be taken to resolve them.

REVIEW QUESTIONS

1. List the three basic tenets of a quality assurance program.
2. What type of phantom is used for measuring spatial resolution?
3. Why is low-contrast resolution evaluated at different mAs settings?
4. Explain how noise is measured using a water phantom.
5. What tools do medical physicists use to measure radiation dose?
6. What are the three general classifications of artifacts?
7. What factors affect beam-hardening artifacts?
8. List strategies to reduce or eliminate motion artifacts.
9. What steps can be taken to avoid out-of-field artifacts? When are these artifacts unavoidable?

RECOMMENDED READING

Papp J. Quality management in the imaging sciences. 1st Ed. Chapter 12: Quality Control in Computed Tomography (Lorrie Kelly). St. Louis: Mosby, 1998.

Bushong SC. Radiologic Science for Technologists–Physics, Biology and Protection. 6th Ed. St. Louis: Mosby, 1997.

Bushberg JT, Seibert JA, Leidholdt EM Jr, Boon JM. The Essential Physics of Medical Imaging. 2nd Ed.

Barrett JF, Keat N. Artifacts in CT: recognition and avoidance. RadioGraphics 2004;24:1679–91.

New CT Accreditation Dose Requirements Effective January 1, 2008. Available at http://www.acr.org/accreditation/FeaturedCategories/ArticlesAnnouncements/NewDoseReq.aspx. Accessed September 14, 2007.

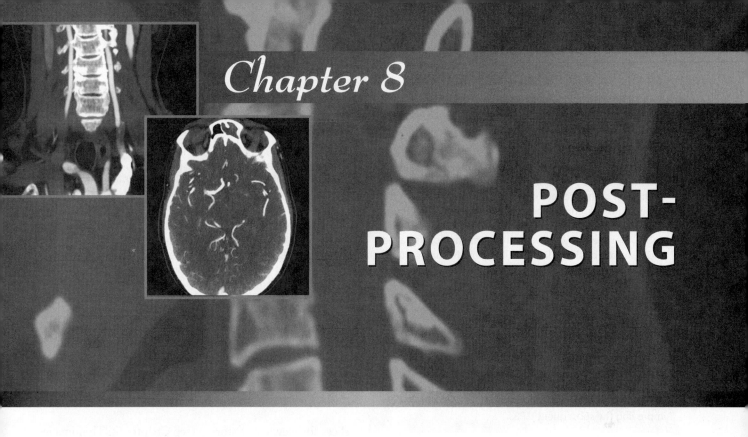

Chapter 8

POST-PROCESSING

Key Terms: prospective reconstruction
• retrospective reconstruction • overlapping
reconstruction • image reformation • image
rendering • multiplanar reformation • manual MPR
• real-time MPR • scanner-created MPR
• workstation-created MPR • three-dimensional
reformation • surface rendering • shaded-surface
display • threshold CT values • projection displays
• maximum-intensity projection • minimum-
intensity projection • volume rendering • opacity
value • endoluminal imaging • virtual
endoscopy • virtual bronchoscopy • virtual
colonoscopy • region-of-interest editing
• manual segmentation • fully automated
segmentation • semiautomatic segmentation
• segmentation errors • stair-step artifacts

Previous chapters have focused on the steps involved in acquiring raw data and in manipulating those data so that an initial image can be formed. These images, planned before actual scanning begins, are most often called prospective reconstructions. Modern scanners allow many opportunities to manipulate both raw data and image data after scanning has taken place. Collectively, these techniques are referred to as post-processing.

Although throughout the CT literature the terms are often used interchangeably, in this text, the term "reconstruction" is used when raw data are manipulated to create pixels that are then used to create an image. The term "reformation" is used when image data are assembled to produce images in different planes, or to produce three-dimensional (3D) images.

BOX 8–1   Key Concept

In this text, the term reconstruction is used when raw data are manipulated to create pixels that are then used to create an image.
The term reformation is used when image data are assembled to produce images in different planes, or to produce 3D images.

RETROSPECTIVE RECONSTRUCTION

Reconstructing raw data to create new images can only be done from the operator's console. Even though many parameters can be changed retrospectively, the images that result are always in the same plane (i.e., coronal, axial) and the same orientation as were the original images.

Provided the raw data are available they can be reused to create new images. Some parameters can be modified retrospectively. Display field of view (DFOV), image center, and reconstruction algorithm can be changed on both axial and helical data. Previous chapters provided examples of why these parameters might be changed retrospectively. In addition, parameters are sometimes changed retrospectively to make them consistent throughout the study. This could occur when one parameter (such as DFOV) varied among the prospective images in a study, preventing their reformation into a single image.

Clinical Application Box 8-1

Retrospective Reconstruction

Assume a scan of the chest, abdomen, and pelvis is performed with 5-mm contiguous slices. Because the patient's abdomen is much larger in diameter than either the chest or the pelvis, the technologist selects a 34 DFOV from the apices to just superior to the diaphragm, a 45 DFOV through the abdomen, and a 36 DFOV from the iliac crest to the pubis. After the images have been reconstructed, displayed, and reviewed by the radiologist, it is thought that multiplanar reformation (MPR) may aid diagnosis. Because of the differing DFOVs, the prospective images will not allow the generation of MPRs that include the chest, abdomen, and pelvis together (separate MPR images of the chest, abdomen, and pelvis could be created). However, assuming the raw data are still available, retrospective reconstructions can be created in which the DFOV is consistent among all slices. In this example, it would also be beneficial to change the slice incrementation so that the new images are created every 2.5 mm, thus creating overlapping images and improving the subsequent MPRs.

Clinical Application Box 8-2

Are Overlapping Reconstructions Needed?

Overlapping reconstructions of data for use as source images in MPR or 3D reformation are particularly useful when the slice thickness substantially exceeds pixel size. They are less beneficial when the voxel size is isotropic. For example:

A scan protocol that focuses on the circle of Willis uses a 0.5-mm slice thickness and a 24-cm FOV. Pixel size = 240 mm/512 = 0.46 mm. Because the slice thickness is nearly equal to the pixel size, overlapping reconstructions are probably not necessary.

A scan protocol that focuses on the thoracic aorta uses a 2-mm slice thickness and a 30-cm FOV. Pixel size = 300 mm/512 = 0.58 mm. Because the slice thickness is significantly greater than the pixel size, overlapping reconstructions are indicated.

Overlapping Reconstructions

On helical data from either SDCT or MDCT systems, image incrementation can be changed. This is often done to produce overlapping images that are then used in multiplanar or 3D reformations. When the slice thickness is wider or the FOV is larger, it is common practice to reconstruct images with an overlap of approximately 50% whenever multiplanar or 3D post-processing is expected to occur. For example, a case scanned with a slice thickness of 3.0 mm would be reconstructed every 1.5 mm. The decision as to whether overlapping slices may be beneficial depends on the voxel size in the specific study. When scans are generated with isotropic (or near isotropic) voxels, not much is gained from overlapping reconstructions. Reviewing from Chapter 6, a voxel is isotropic when the *xy* direction is equal to the slice thickness. Therefore, as a general rule, when slice thickness is very thin (0.5 mm) and FOV is small (<25 cm), overlapping reconstructions are generally not worth the inconvenience associated with storing the larger data set. In a specific circumstance the benefit of creating overlapping reconstructions can be assessed by calculating the pixel size and comparing it with the slice thickness. The more the slice thickness exceeds pixel size (i.e., the voxel is a rectangular solid rather than a cube), the greater the benefit of overlapping reconstructions for source data in multiplanar reformation (MPR) and 3D reformation.

Retrospectively Changing Image Thickness

On MDCT systems, data from the parallel rows of detectors can be combined in different ways to create thicker slices for viewing or storing (see Chapter 5). Thin images are wonderful when used as source images for generating reformations, but can be cumbersome for primary image review. The goal of using a thin slice for scanning and reconstructing thicker slices for viewing and storing is to maintain the advantage of high-resolution imaging but also create image files that are manageable and more easily reviewed by radiologists.

BOX 8–2   Key Concept

The goal of using a thin slice for scanning and reconstructing thicker slices for viewing and storing is to maintain the advantage of high-resolution imaging but also create image files that are manageable and more easily reviewed by radiologists.

IMAGE REFORMATION

Image reformation is also called image rendering. Once again, the slice of bread analogy is helpful for clarification of the process. If the slices of bread are stacked so that they resemble an intact loaf and the loaf is cut in a different fashion (e.g., diagonally), the slices of bread can be seen from a new perspective. Using this example it is clear that all of the original slices of bread must have some common features to facilitate stacking them into a loaf. For example, they must be the same size, their edges must all match up, they must have the same original slice angle, and there must be no missing slices. Similarly, to successfully reformat a CT study all the source images must have an identical DFOV, image center (i.e., the *xy* coordinates must be the same), and gantry tilt, and they must be contiguous (i.e., no nonimaged spaces between slices). Because lining up the images exactly is vital in reformation, even a small amount of patient motion seriously degrades the end product. When a patient moves during the scan process, the images themselves may technically "line up," but the structures represented by the images may have moved between slices.

The direct scan plane in CT is primarily limited to the transverse plane. Only for the head and some extremities can scans be obtained directly in a coronal orientation by means of patient positioning. In many clinical situations the scanned plane is not optimal for diagnosis. In these situations image reformation can be a valuable adjunct.

Image reformation uses only image data (not raw data) to generate images in a plane or orientation different from the prospective image. These reformatted images are used to better display anatomic relationships (Fig. 8-1). Reformatted images can be of either a 2D or 3D

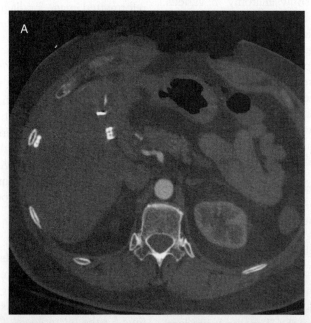

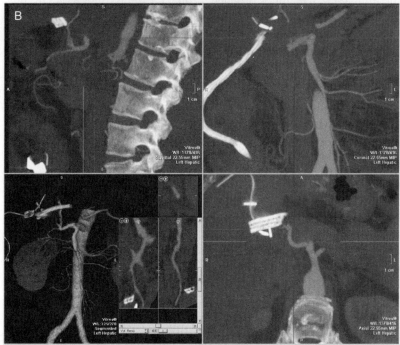

FIGURE 8-1   Reformatted images are used to better display anatomic relationships. Image (A) is a standard axial. The reformatted images in (B) demonstrate the origin of the replaced right hepatic artery arising from the superior mesenteric artery.

nature. In general, the thinner the original slice, the better the reformatted image.

Multiplanar Reformation

Reformation that is done to show anatomy in various planes is referred to as multiplanar reformation (MPR). MPRs are 2D in nature. Unlike 3D displays, 2D image displays always represent the original CT attenuation values (Fig. 8-2). MPRs can typically be created either at the operator's console or at a separate workstation. They can be created in transverse, coronal, sagittal, or oblique planes (Fig. 8-3). Curved planar reformation (CPR) allows images to be created along the centerline of tubular organs (e.g., vascular structures, common bile duct, ureters; Fig. 8-4).

The advent of MDCT has expanded the use of multiplanar images in diagnosis. This is because the volumetric image data sets that result from MDCT methods produce very high quality multiplanar images, and modern software allows the reformations to be generated quickly and easily. In addition, when voxels are isotropic, any oblique plane can be created with virtually no loss of image quality. The reformatted image is virtually identical in quality to the original axial reconstruction. If the voxels are not isotropic, image quality can be improved by using overlapping source images. Although MPRs were available before MDCT, there was often substantial image quality degradation between the axial and reformatted images, undermining the radiologists' confidence in relying on the reformatted image for diagnosis. MDCT has changed this; radiologists are now free to interpret images in whatever plane is most appropriate for a given clinical situation.

Manual and Real-Time MPR

Manual methods of MPR require that the operator input the criteria, such as the thickness of the MPR, the plane desired, and the number or incrementation of the resulting planar images. Real-time (or interactive) reformation refers to the feature that allows the operator to manually change (typically by moving a mouse) the image plane while the software continually updates the image. This feature permits the operator to use trial and error to obtain the ideal image plane.

Scanner-Created MPR

Most current scanners also allow protocols to be programmed so that MPRs are automatically generated by the scanner software. Advantages of scanner-created MPRs are that they ensure the MPRs are always done and they save time for the technologist. On most scanners, only straight

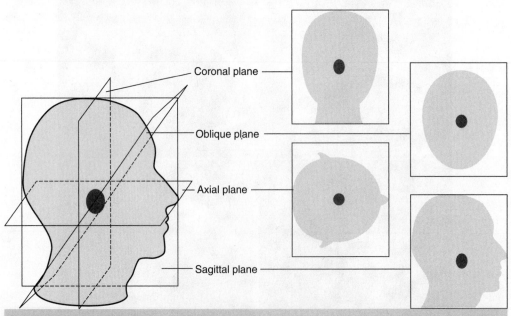

FIGURE 8-2 Unlike 3D displays, the 2D image process always retains the original CT attenuation values. In this example, axial source images of the head are stacked, and a reformatted image is created in the coronal plane. Pixels (highlighted) in the axial slice will retain their attenuation values in the corresponding pixels in coronal reformation.

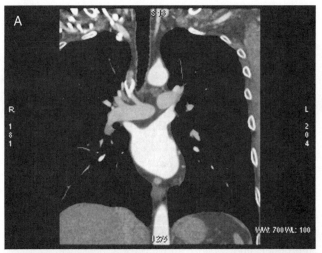

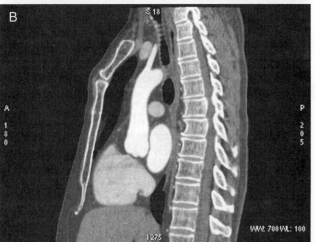

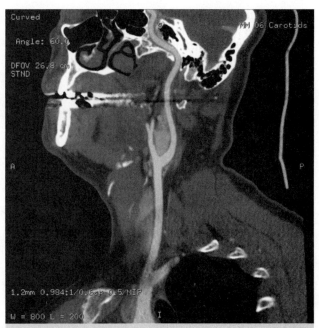

FIGURE 8-4 Curved reformations can be created to follow vascular structures, just as in this reformatted image of the carotid artery. Image courtesy of the University of Michigan.

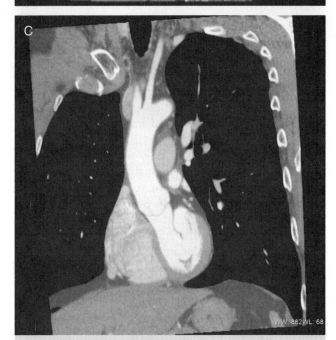

FIGURE 8-3 **A.** MPR in the coronal plane. **B.** MPR in the sagittal plane. **C.** MPR in the oblique plane. Images courtesy of the University of Michigan.

sagittal and coronal planes can be automatically generated with the criteria set in advance. If oblique or curved images are needed, the technologist must create them manually.

Workstation-Created MPR

Current picture archive and communication systems (PACS) or specialized independent workstations allow users to generate MPRs directly on the monitor. This allows radiologists the flexibility and interactivity to create images that are suited to the specific clinical situation. However, to create the highest quality reformations, the thinnest possible slice must be available. This means that all of the slices must be sent to the workstation, rather than just the thicker slices often reconstructed for viewing purposes. Data sets are frequently huge, containing hundreds (sometimes thousands) of images, potentially slowing down the PACS network.

Three-Dimensional Reformation

The addition of special software allows another class of reformat to be performed. 3D reformation seeks to represent the entire scan volume in only one image. Unlike 2D displays, 3D techniques manipulate or combine CT values to display an image; the original CT value information is not included. For example, the technique known as surface rendering (SR) includes only information from the surface of an object. Because the 3D rendering process can be time-consuming, 3D software is generally available only on independent workstations so as to not tie up the operator's console.

All 3D techniques use a process that draws an imaginary line from the viewer through the data volume. Displays are generated by taking into account some or all (depending on the technique used) of the CT values along each line and appropriately weighting each point. The process is complex. Fortunately, understanding the intricacies of the method is not essential to effectively generating 3D displays.

The principles of MPR apply to 3D reformats, especially the axiom that the thinner the original CT slices, the better the final 3D image. Like MPRs, 3D software programs allow for different combinations of slice thickness within a single 3D model. Consequently, a scanning protocol of thin slices through the area of primary interest (e.g., fracture or tumor site) could be followed by thicker slices through the remaining structures. Again, all slices must be contiguous, with no change in gantry tilt, table height, and DFOV. Patient motion during the data acquisition sequence does not prevent 3D reformats from being produced, but will degrade the image quality.

A variety of 3D techniques exist that display data aggregated from the scan volume in different ways. Techniques such as surface rendering and volume rendering (VR) produce images immediately recognizable as 3D. That is, the sliced loaf of bread from our earlier analogy is reassembled to appear whole. Other 3D techniques, such as maximum-intensity projections (MIP) assemble data from a volume but display the data in images that appear flat.

Surface Rendering

Surface rendering (SR), also known as shaded-surface display (SSD), is similar to taking a photograph of the surface of the structure in that the voxels located on the edge of a structure are used to show the outline or outside shell of the structure (Fig. 8-5). In most forms of SR the images are created by comparing the intensity of each voxel in the data set to some predetermined threshold CT value. The software will include or exclude the voxel depending on whether its CT number is above or below the threshold and use this information to create a surface

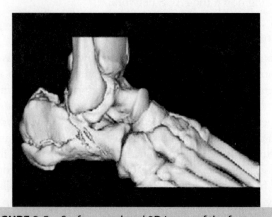

FIGURE 8-5   Surface-rendered 3D image of the foot.

of an object. The remaining voxels in the image are usually invisible. SR is useful for examining tubular structures, such as the inside surfaces of airways, the colon, and blood vessels.

Selecting the appropriate threshold CT values of the voxels that will be displayed is critical. Unfortunately, it is difficult to define clear guidelines for threshold assignment. If the threshold is too narrow, actual protruding structures can be imperceptible. If the threshold is too inclusive, nontissue materials (e.g., fluids) can be displayed as if they were tissue and can obscure protruding structures. Manipulating the predefined threshold value can dramatically change the appearance of displayed structures. For example, lowering or raising the threshold value can change the included wall thickness of bony structures and hence alter the size and surface appearance.

BOX 8-6   Key Concept

Setting the appropriate threshold CT values for surface rendering is critical.

An advantage to SR is that because it only uses a small portion (approximately 10%) of the data available, images can be created quickly even on less powerful computers. However, in recent years computer capacity has expanded dramatically, making this less important. Most uses of SR have been replaced by VR. SR remains a useful technique for orthopedic imaging as it excels at showing bone surfaces. Images can be rotated and viewed from any angle. Editing the data set (discussed later) can improve the SR display by removing obscuring structures.

Projection Displays

Two common 3D techniques are the MIP (Fig. 8-6) and the minimum-intensity projection (MinIP; Fig. 8-7). The MIP examines each voxel along a line from the viewer's eye through the data set and selects only the voxel with the highest value for inclusion in the displayed image. The rest of the voxels are ignored. This method tends to display bone and contrast-filled structures; lower-attenuation structures are not well visualized. In a similar fashion, MinIP involves selecting the voxel with the minimum value from the line for display. Such images can be useful to display the bronchial tree. MIP and MinIP images can be generated from the entire data set or from only a selected portion of it. Limiting the data set is useful when other structures are present that may obscure the area of interest. For example, an MIP image of the blood vessels can be obscured when other high-density structures such as bone, enhancing organs, or calcifications are present and overlying the vessels. Creating an MIP from only a portion of the data set is called the variable sliding slab method. Editing the data set can also minimize superimposition effects by deleting structures that are not of clinical interest.

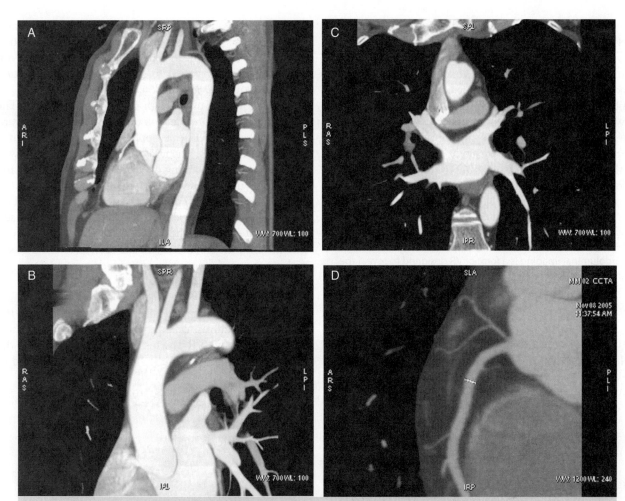

FIGURE 8-6 Examples of MIP images. **A.** Aortic arch. **B.** Ascending aorta and branches. **C.** Left atrium demonstrating pulmonary veins. **D.** Right coronary artery. Images courtesy of the University of Michigan.

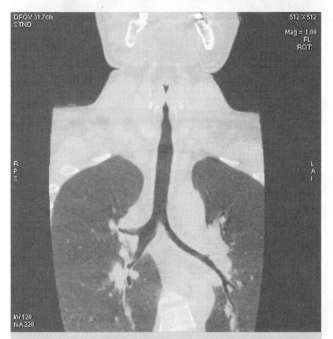

FIGURE 8-7 MinIP image of the trachea. Image courtesy of the University of Michigan.

BOX 8–7   Key Concept

Two common 3D techniques are the MIP and the MinIP. The former selects voxels with the highest value to display; the latter selects voxels with the lowest value.

Volume Rendering

VR is a 3D semitransparent representation of the imaged structure. It has become the favored 3D imaging technique with applications in every type of examination performed with CT. An advantage of VR compared with other 3D techniques is that all voxels contribute to the image. This allows VR images to display multiple tissues and show their relationships to one another.

BOX 8–8   Key Concept

VR has become the favored 3D imaging technique. An advantage of VR is that all voxels contribute to the image, allowing the image to display multiple tissues and show their relationship to one another.

Like other 3D methods, VR displays are built by collecting and manipulating data along a line from the viewer's eye through the data set. However, VR techniques sum the contributions of each voxel along the line. Each voxel is assigned an opacity value based on its Hounsfield units. This opacity value determines the degree to which it will contribute, along with other voxels along the same line, to the final image. The process is repeated for the voxels along each line, with each line producing one voxel in the VR image. Unlike other 3D techniques, with VR no information is ignored or discarded; every voxel contributes to the final image.

BOX 8–9   Key Concept

Endoluminal imaging is a form of VR designed to reveal the inside of the lumen of a structure. The technique is also called virtual endoscopy, virtual bronchoscopy, and virtual colonoscopy.

The pixels in the final VR image can be assigned a color, brightness, and degree of opacity. For example, normal soft tissue can be assigned high transparency, contrasted vessels slight opaqueness, and bone strong opaqueness (Fig. 8-8). In many cases color is used, with the color intensity varied to generate depth information for a traditional 3D impression.

VR allows the user a high degree of interactivity. The user can easily change the look of the VR by changing variables such as the color scale, applied lighting, opacity values, and window settings. The image can be rotated and viewed from any angle. By varying opacity and window width and level functions, anatomy can be displayed or made invisible. This allows the user to quickly classify structures based on their attenuation. For example, adjusting the window settings can often remove the soft tissue from the VR display so that the contrast-enhanced vascular structures can be seen, without the need for time-consuming data set editing.

Endoluminal Imaging

A form of VR that is specifically designed to look inside the lumen of a structure is called endoluminal imaging, or alternately, perspective VR The technique aims to simulate the view of an endoscopist, hence it is commonly referred to

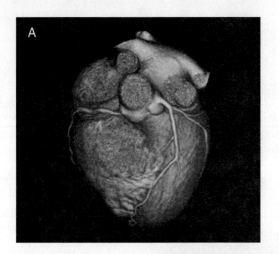
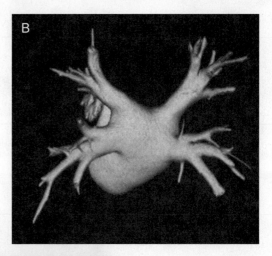
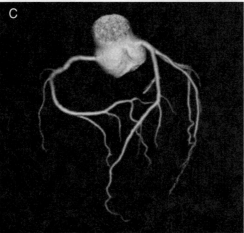

FIGURE 8-8   Examples of VR images of the heart (A), the left atrium and pulmonary veins (B), and the coronary artery tree (C). Images courtesy of the University of Michigan.

as virtual endoscopy. The technique can be used to image areas that are amenable to endoscopic evaluation, such as the lumen of the bronchial tree (virtual bronchoscopy), lumina of the larger blood vessels, the inside surface of the colon (virtual colonoscopy or CT colonography), and the mucosa of the paranasal sinuses. Endoluminal imaging visualizes a structure as if it were hollow and the viewer were inside of it (Fig. 8-9). Once inside, a viewer can "fly through," which provides the impression of a virtual flight through the selected body region equivalent to directing an endoscope into the lumen. For easy navigation a path through the lumen is needed. Because manually tracking such a path is time-consuming, some software programs automatically calculate a centerline path through the air- or contrast-containing structure. Users may also change their virtual field of view. That is they may look forward, backward, or to the sides and get closer to the luminal wall or further away. Software can also correlate findings on the 3D endoluminal imaging with the 2D cross-sectional source images to allow better characterization and localization of abnormalities.

Region-of-Interest Editing

The process of selectively removing or isolating information from the data set is referred to as region-of-interest editing or segmentation. The purpose is to better demonstrate the areas of interest by removing obscuring structures. Current 3D software offers choices of manual, automatic, and semiautomatic segmentation techniques.

BOX 8-10   Key Concept

Region-of-interest editing is done to remove obscuring structures from the 3D image. 3D software allows this editing to be in a manual, automatic, or semiautomatic fashion.

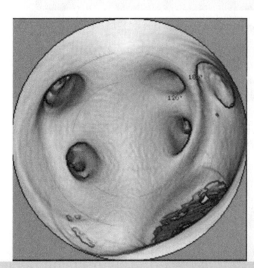

FIGURE 8-9 An endoluminal image of the left atrium and lumens of the pulmonary veins. Image courtesy of the University of Michigan.

Manual Segmentation

Manual segmentation refers to the process by which a user identifies and selects data to be saved or removed. Manual segmentation can be done on either 2D or 3D images. The user traces an outline around anatomy to be saved or discarded on a series of axial or MPR images, or a 3D model. In some situations, manual segmentation can be a fast and simple process, such as editing the head holder out of the data set (Fig. 8-10). In other situations it is very hard to separate the object from the image background and the task can become tedious and time-consuming, particularly when significantly changing anatomy necessitates the editing be performed in a slice-by slice fashion.

Fully Automated Segmentation

Manufacturers have developed software that can automate the process of segmenting. However, fully automatic segmentation methods are usually impractical because of image complexity and the variety of image types and clinical indications. In addition, low contrast between structures can cause otherwise robust automatic algorithms to fail.

Semiautomatic Segmentation

Semiautomatic segmentations methods combine many of the benefits of manual and automatic segmentation

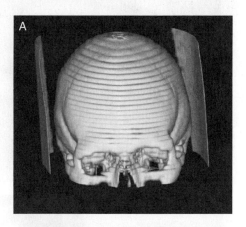

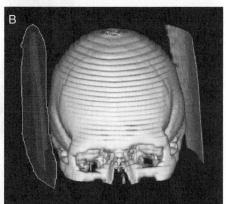

FIGURE 8-10 Manual segmentation technique. Image (A) shows the CT head holder. In image (B), the technologist traced the right side of the head holder for removal.

techniques. By supplying initial information about the region of interest, the user may guide an otherwise automatic segmentation process. For example, the user may pick a point on a bone and the software automatically adds adjacent points until the bone is completely selected and may then be edited out. Or the user may draw a line around a structure and the software then moves the line to more accurately reflect the interface between the structure and adjacent tissues. When completed, the user must carefully examine the finished product for any errors introduced by the automated methods. Such errors can be corrected by manual editing.

Factors That Degrade Reformatted Images

A number of factors can degrade the post-processed images, reducing their usefulness in diagnosis. Even worse, some factors can result in inaccurate or misleading images that could lead to incorrect diagnosis. Anyone who generates reformatted images (i.e., radiologist or

technologist) must pay careful attention so that post-processing pitfalls are avoided. In addition, the radiologist interpreting these images must understand the type of images being viewed, and the various limitations and strengths of different rendering and segmentation techniques.

Segmentation Errors

Errors in the reformatted image can be introduced when important vessels or other structures are inadvertently edited out of the data set. In some instances segmentation errors are quite obvious, because an expected structure is absent (Fig. 8-11). Unfortunately, many segmentation errors can be quite subtle, even impossible to identify from a single reformatted image. This is particularly true when the missing structure is unexpected, such as an accessory artery. Segmentation errors include those that exclude small arteries and arteries that are stenotic, and the creation of false areas of narrowing that can mimic true stenosis

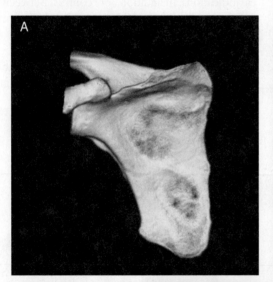
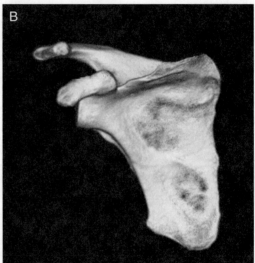
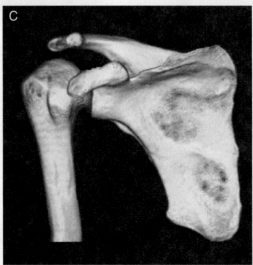

FIGURE 8-11   This series of three images illustrates obvious segmentation errors. In images (A) and (B) the user mistakenly removed portions of the shoulder girdle when editing out items on the surface of the patient's skin. Image (C) shows the 3D image without segmentation errors.

on the 3D reformation. Errors are more common when automatic segmentation and vessel-tracking techniques are used. However, segmentation errors can occur even when a veteran user guides the process. For this reason, radiologists are cautioned against depending exclusively on segmented images. By also reviewing unsegmented volumes, MIPs, and the source data, radiologists minimize the risk that an important finding is overlooked.

Image Noise

Excessive image noise in the source images will significantly limit the quality and utility of 3D rendered images. Excessive noise diminishes image quality, particularly its low-contrast resolution, making it difficult to distinguish between tissue types. This is particularly problematic for vascular studies because the contrast between soft tissue and iodine-enhanced vessels is reduced. MPR images are not as degraded by image noise.

In many situations noisy images can be avoided by using appropriate scan parameters (i.e., high mAs, lower pitch setting, slower rotation speed) for the patient's size. In obese patients, a larger DFOV and thicker slices will also help to reduce image noise. In these patients it is also helpful to reconstruct thicker slices to use as source data for reformation and for review. For example, if the data were acquired at 2.5 mm, summing data to reconstruct 5-mm slices will reduce noise.

Artifact

Artifacts on the source data will also degrade the reformatted images. The most common artifacts are a result of motion or from high-density material (e.g., surgical clips) that produce streaks. Stair-step artifacts can occur when voxels are not isotropic.

Motion artifacts result from patient movement, breathing, pulsation, or peristalsis (Fig. 8-12). In many cases motion artifacts are easily recognized and therefore not confused with abnormality. Occasionally motion

artifacts are subtle and carry the potential for misinterpretation. Subtle motion artifacts are of greater concern on MPRs on which they can mimic a fracture or a vascular lesion. A careful review of the source images (in which motion artifacts can be more easily identified) is recommended when doubt exists. Pulsation artifacts can be misleading and are particularly hard to identify, both on the source images and on the reformatted images. Motion artifacts in cardiac CT that are related to heart rate irregularities are called banding artifacts. Pulsation artifacts can be reduced by using electrocardiogram-gating techniques (see Chapter 20).

Streak artifacts can be traced to many sources (see Chapter 7), but most often are caused by metallic objects or very dense iodinated contrast in a vessel (such as the brachiocephalic vein). Streak artifacts have a characteristic appearance on both the source images and MPRs and are typically not problematic. They can be more troubling on VR or SR images on which they leave gaps in the model. This is because the streaks have widely different CT numbers from the background and are filtered out by the threshold set. In orthopedic cases, adjusting the window setting may be useful in reducing the artifacts while still demonstrating relevant anatomy. In vascular cases in which streak artifact appears on source images, VR or SR is abandoned.

As mentioned earlier, the best reformations are generated from voxels that are isotropic (or near isotropic). When the slice thickness exceeds the pixel dimensions in the source data, artifacts appear on the reformatted images. So-called stair-step artifacts are present when smooth objects, such as the aorta, appear to have edges that resemble a flight of stairs (Fig. 8-13).

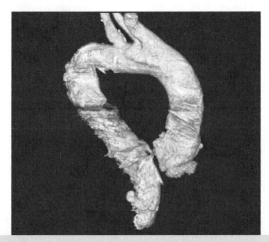

FIGURE 8-12 This 3D reformation of the aortic arch is seriously degraded by motion artifact from the source images. In this case the motion was a result of overt patient movement.

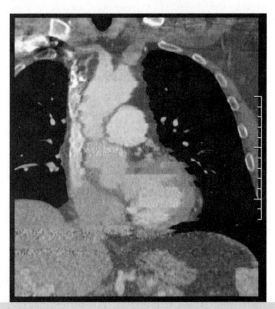

FIGURE 8-13 Stair-step artifacts result when wide slices are used as source images for the MRP. In this case, patient motion further degrades the reformatted image and makes the stair-step artifacts more pronounced.

SUMMARY

Several post-processing techniques are common to clinical radiology departments. Advances in CT design, particularly MDCT with its ability to obtain very thin slices very rapidly, has resulted in an explosion of new post-processing applications. Technologists should make the distinction between image reconstruction, which uses raw data to create new images, and that of image reformation, which uses image data to view anatomic information from different perspectives.

REVIEW QUESTIONS

1. Explain the difference between the terms reconstruction and reformation. Give an example of a clinical application for each.
2. What is a disadvantage to the many thin slices produced by MDCT systems? How can this disadvantage be overcome?
3. Which parameters must be consistent in the source images to create reformations?
4. Explain what is meant by manual MPR, real-time MPR, scanner-created MPR, and workstation-created MPR.
5. What is the primary difference between 2D and 3D reformation techniques?
6. Define the following 3D techniques: surface rendering, MIP, MinIP, VR, and endoluminal imaging.
7. Describe the three types of segmentation methods available.

RECOMMENDED READING

Lipson S. MDCT and 3D Workstations: A Practical Guide and Teaching File. New York: Springer, 2006.

Kalender WA. Computed Tomography: Fundamentals, System Technology, Image Quality, Applications. 2nd Ed. Erlangen, Germany: Publicis Corporate Publishing, 2005.

Cody DD. Image processing in CT. AAPM/RSNA physics tutorial for residents: topics in CT. RadioGraphics 2002;22:1255–68.

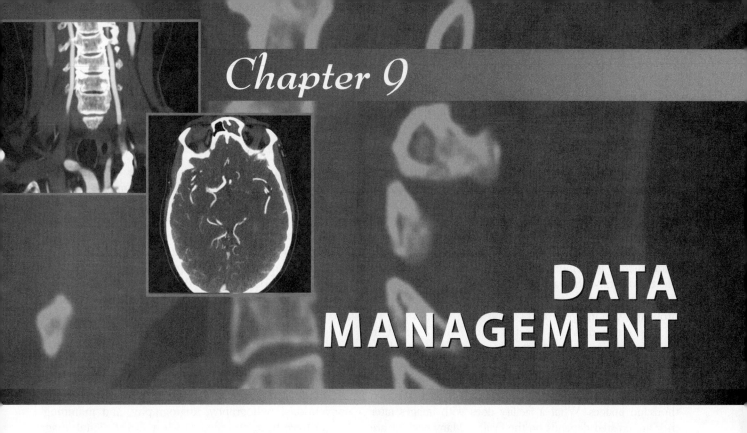

Chapter 9

DATA MANAGEMENT

Key Terms: informatics • imaging informatics • hospital information systems (HIS) • clinical information systems (CIS) • computerized physician order entry (CPOE) • electronic health record (EHR) • electronic medical record (EMR) • radiology information system (RIS) • picture archive and communication system (PACS) • information technology (IT) • local area network (LAN) • wide area network (WAN) • wired • wireless • topology • Ethernet, peer-to-peer (P2P) network • client-server network • core servers • bandwidth • bits • bytes • lossy compression • lossless compression • protocol • redundancy • DICOM • Health Level Seven • direct digital capture • frame grabbing • CRT • LCD • luminance • online archiving • near-line archiving • off-line archiving • redundant array of inexpensive disks (RAID) • compact discs • digital versatile discs • Blu-ray discs • optical jukebox • optical disc libraries • robotic drives • autochangers • magnetic tape • enterprise-wide distribution • virtual private networks (VPN)

INTRODUCTION TO INFORMATICS

The collection, classification, storage, retrieval, and dissemination of recorded information are known as informatics. Imaging informatics is a subspecialty that is vital to radiology and is devoted to how information about medical images is exchanged within the radiology departments and throughout the medical enterprise. Although it is often thought of as how images get from one place to another, imaging informatics is actually much broader in scope.

Radiology professionals are exposed to a myriad of medical information systems from both outside the radiology department and within it. Hospital information systems (HIS) focus on administrative issues, such as patient demographic data, financial data, and patient locations within the hospital. Clinical information systems (CIS) may be integrated into the HIS, but are often separate systems that keep track of clinical data. Individual facilities may also have a computerized physician (or provider) order entry (CPOE) system that electronically transmits clinician orders to radiology and other departments. A generic term for a digital patient record is electronic health record, or EHR. These are often composed of electronic medical records (EMR) from a variety of sources, including radiology. However, in general usage, EHR and EMR are used synonymously.

Within the radiology department there are two key elements that form the information infrastructure. First is the radiology information system (RIS). The RIS is most often designed for scheduling patients, storing reports, patient tracking, protocoling examinations, and billing. The RIS should have two-way communication with both the HIS and the CIS. Ideally, the RIS ties together all the computer systems within the radiology department. The second key element is the imaging network, most often called the picture archive and communication system (PACS). The term PACS encompasses a broad range of technologies necessary for the storage, retrieval, distribution, and display of images. PACS networks are the primary focus of this chapter. Using the informatics infrastructure is an integral part a technologist's job. They must understand the various communication tools to perform their jobs efficiently and effectively and to correct problems with image quality.

The large data sets created from MDCT result in higher-resolution images that aid in more accurate diagnosis, but present significant challenges in how the images are handled after they are acquired. For example, it is not uncommon for a coronary study to produce well over two thousand images. What a facility does with images after they are created depends on the facility. Many options are available.

Hardcopy Versus Electronic Archiving

The exclusive use of film or other hardcopy media for documentation and subsequent interpretation is no longer practical, for both financial and quality reasons. The total cost of film-based systems include the cost of film, film storage, lost examinations (including the cost of repeating examinations when they are lost), and time spent for clerical staff and clinicians to handle the film and accompanying jackets. Even considering just one component, the cost of film, a case can be made against hardcopy archiving. For example, a single sheet of film costs more than a compact disc (CD). For documentation of one of the cardiac studies mentioned above approximately 100 films would be required, whereas a single CD can easily hold this volume of data. Another significant disadvantage of hardcopy is that it limits the viewer to only that information captured on the film, whereas reading cases from a monitor allows the option of interactive adjustment to suit the particular clinical need. In addition, obtaining an older examination for comparison can be time-consuming when one must wait for the hardcopy file to be found and pulled, whereas electronic systems can provide near instant access to prior studies.

The conversion from a primarily film-based system to an electronic system can be gradual, starting with a select set of modalities or with limited functionality and becoming more inclusive over time; or it can be dramatic, allowing complete conversion to digital acquisition, transfer, interpretation, storage, and transmission. It should be mentioned that the radiology industry as a whole is not likely to achieve a true filmless system for some time. Even when institutions move away from film-based systems, it is common that they still use printed media for patients to take studies to referring physicians.

PACS FUNDAMENTALS

PACS is used to refer to a broad range of technologies that enable digital radiology. Using a computer network the PACS technology allows the integration of image acquisition devices, display workstations, and storage systems. This technology has a huge influence on the workflow of radiologists and technologists. It can also have a tremendous impact on referring physicians, in that it can allow easy remote access to the images of their patients, improving turnaround times and patient care. PACS can also provide an excellent resource for education, statistical analysis, and research.

To be included in a PACS, images must be in a digital form. CT, like magnetic resonance imaging (MRI) and positron emission tomography (PET), is intrinsically digital. All other modalities (i.e., nuclear medicine, ultrasound, conventional radiography, angiography, and mammography) have been modified to allow direct digital image capture.

A PACS requires many complex components that must function collaboratively. Vast amounts of data pass through any PACS, and there is near-constant demand for access to these data from technologists, radiologists, and referring clinicians. Along with an investment in hardware and software, a necessary component of any PACS is a skilled team of information technology (IT) personnel to keep the PACS running smoothly. These individuals must possess a thorough understanding of the technology so that they can be relied on to troubleshoot most problems. However, to ensure optimal workflow and image quality, technologists should become familiar with the basic elements of the PACS: networking, digital image format standards, image acquisition, workstations, data storage, and image distribution. It is not unusual for technologists to transition to become PACS administrators.

Networking

A group of two or more computers linked together is a network. Although the network and the PACS are two distinct environments, they converge in such a way that makes the success of the latter dependent on the strength of the former. Even the most state-of-the-art PACS will be a disappointment if the network it is paired with is poorly designed. The network is fundamental to the success of a PACS because it regulates the movement of data and directly affects all users. Network problems can mean that technologists are unable to send images, radiologists are unable to interpret studies, and referring clinicians are unable to access images or reports.

There are many different types and configurations of computer networks. Linked computers that are

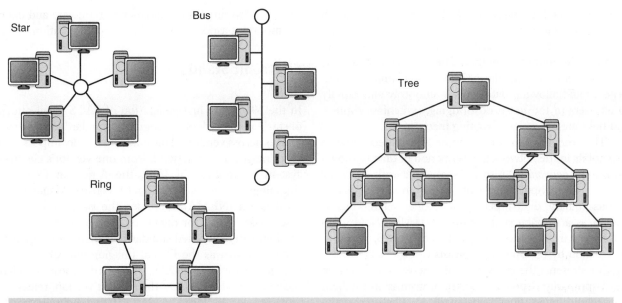

FIGURE 9-1 The geometric arrangement of a computer system is referred to as its topology. Common topologies include bus, star, ring, and tree.

geographically close together (i.e., in the same building) are often called local area networks, or LANs. Computers that are farther apart and must be connected by telephone lines, cables, or radio waves are called wide area networks, or WANs. Networks that are linked by a physical connection (e.g., telephone lines, copper or fiberoptic cables) are referred to as "wired." Networks that use radio waves to transmit data between computers are referred to as "wireless." The geometric arrangement of a computer system is referred to as its topology. Common topologies include bus, star, ring, and tree (Fig. 9-1). A LAN can be a combination of these types of topologies. LANs typically use Ethernet connections to attach computers to the network. Ethernet cables are made up of twisted pairs of copper wire.

Networks can be broadly classified as using either a peer-to-peer or a client-server architecture. In peer-to-peer (or P2P) networks, each party has the same capabilities and any party can initiate communication (Fig. 9-2). P2P networks exploit the diverse connectivity and the cumulative data capacity of network participants, rather than using a centralized resource. Far more common in the PACS setting is the client-server network architecture. Computers in this model are either classified as servers or clients. A server is a computer that facilitates communication between and delivers information to other computers. The server acts on requests from other networked computers, rather than from a person inputting directly into it. Servers are passive, that is, they wait for requests from clients. A server typically accepts connections from a large number of clients. End-users interact directly with client computers to send data requests to one or more connected servers. The servers then accept the requests,

Peer-to-peer network

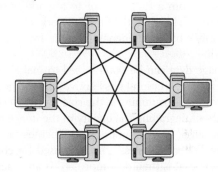

Client-server network

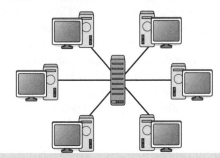

FIGURE 9-2 Networks can be broadly classified as using either a peer-to-peer or a client-server architecture.

process them, and supply the requested information to the client. Clients usually connect to a small number of servers at one time. Each client or server in the network may also be referred to as a node.

Depending on the specific PACS configuration and software there may be one or more servers. The server computers that are integral to the functioning of the PACS are referred to as *core servers*.

Networks can use a variety of strategies to route data from one computer to another. The specific mechanisms selected will have a significant impact on eliminating bottlenecks and allowing data to flow smoothly and rapidly to all users in the network. Bridging, switching, routers, and hubs are examples of routing mechanisms.

The amount of data that can be transmitted between two points in the network in a set period of time is known as *network bandwidth*. Also known as network speed or network throughput, bandwidth is commonly expressed in bits (binary digits) per second; one million bits is known as a megabit and denoted as 1 Mb. [Note: This is different from a megabyte, denoted by MB, which is one million bytes. One byte consists of eight bits.] Bandwidth represents the capacity of the network connection and is primarily dependent on the transmission medium (e.g., copper wires, fiberoptics, wireless). The greater the capacity, the more likely that greater performance will follow, although overall network performance also depends on other factors, such as the number of computers sharing the same bandwidth. The time required for an image to be sent from a PACS server to a workstation depends greatly on the bandwidth of the network infrastructure and the number of simultaneous requests from users on the network.

Image data can be compressed to make transmission more efficient, requiring less bandwidth. The goal of image compression is to minimize the size (in bytes) of an image file without degrading the quality of the image to an unacceptable level. Image compression schemes can be lossless or lossy. When a lossless scheme is used for compression, the image that is then decompressed is an exact replica of the original. Lossy compression methods introduce compression artifacts because not all data are restored. It is difficult to know for certain the level of lossy compression that can be applied to an image without decreasing diagnostic accuracy. Therefore, many PACS use only lossless compression methods. Lossy compression can be used to transmit images that do not need to be of diagnostic quality. This is sometimes referred to as "conversational" quality.

To communication effectively, humans must speak a common language. In a similar fashion, computers communicate by using a specific language, or *protocol*. A protocol defines a common set of rules and signals that computers on the network use to communicate. A common set of protocols used extensively on the Internet is TCP/IP. Protocols are not related to the specific data that are being exchanged, but rather how the data are exchanged between computers.

In the computing world, redundancy is used to describe an arrangement in which two or more components perform the same task–if one element fails the duplication keeps the system functioning while the failed component is repaired. It can also refer to the duplication of data to provide an alternative in case of failure of one part of the process. Planning for redundancy in hardware and data is an important aspect of any PACS implementation.

Electronic Standards

DICOM

In the 1980s, the first generation of PACS faced a major obstacle in the lack of a recognized standard for electronic images across vendors. This made it virtually impossible to send images over a network from one vendor's electronic system to another. In 1985, the American College of Radiology (ACR) and National Electrical Manufacturers Association (NEMA) addressed the issue by publishing a set of standards for digital medical images. The result is a universally adopted standard for medical image interchange known as the Digital Imaging and Communication in Medicine (DICOM) standard. These standards have been updated twice; the current version, released in 1992, is referred to as DICOM v3.0 and includes specifics related to networked environments. The standard are continually updated, so instead of using the version number the standard is often identified using the release year, such as "the 2007 version of DICOM." The scope of DICOM now extends well beyond radiology, having been adopted by vendors in other medical specialties including cardiology, dentistry, and pathology. Although the DICOM standard is used by all imaging system vendors, each vendor will have additional, often proprietary, information that may or may not be used by other vendors.

Health Level Seven

In a similar fashion, the Health Level Seven (HL7) organization works to develop universal standards for clinical and administrative data throughout the healthcare arena. HL7 is also used to refer to some of the specific standards created by the organization. HL7 standards are applied to HIS and RIS systems. Unfortunately, specifications in HL7 and DICOM standard vary widely; therefore, HIS-RIS may not adequately support DICOM, making integration between the RIS and the PACS difficult. Efforts are being made to better improve connectivity between different electronic systems as well as between the electronic systems of different medical facilities.

Image Acquisition

Because CT is inherently a digital modality, the image acquisition from the CT scanner to the PACS should be a direct digital DICOM capture. Transferring the CT data in this way allows the full spatial resolution and image manipulation capabilities (such as adjusting window width and level). Although transferring all of the data through direct digital interfaces is the preferred method, an analog method exists. The analog method is called frame grabbing, in which an image on the monitor is converted to a digital format, somewhat similar to a screen capture. Converting CT data in this way loses the original pixel's metrics. The primary advantage of the frame-grabber method is that it does not require image format compatibility. Any image that is displayed on the monitor, whether or not it complies with DICOM standards, can be captured and transmitted to the PACS. However, although this can be an important advantage in other areas of radiology it is unnecessary in CT because all modern scanners produce images that comply with DICOM standards.

Workstation Monitors

Until the 1990s, the monitors used in radiology departments were all adaptations of the cathode-ray tube (CRT) technology that had been used in televisions for decades. To suit the needs of radiology, typical color CRT monitors were modified and monochrome CRTs were created with special phosphors that could produce the required brightness (luminance), reduce distortion, and display images with higher spatial resolution. Newer liquid crystal display (LCD) and plasma display technologies have been introduced to the medical display device arena and are vying to overtake the role of the CRT monitor in PACS.

The purchase price of the LCD and plasma monitors is approximately two to three times higher than the price of CRT monitors of equal spatial resolution. However, this cost is offset by the longer life span of the newer monitors. The newer technologies are a type of flat-panel monitor, so the amount of desk space required is substantially less than that for CRTs. Quality assurance is simpler, as LCD and plasma technologies do not have many of the physical characteristics that tend to drift in CRT systems (e.g., geometric distortion, focus, raster size). Additionally, the luminance levels of CRT monitors degrade relatively quickly whereas LCD and plasma monitors better maintain their luminosity. Brightness is an important characteristic because subtle findings tend to be more conspicuous on brighter displays and may allow radiologists to interpret images more accurately.

Historically, monitors used for medical image display have been primarily gray scale, rather than color. The main reasons are that a monochrome display is brighter and sharper than its color counterpart. Therefore, gray-scale monitors are best suited for many radiology applications. Because applications such as PET/CT and Doppler ultrasound require a color display, an additional color monitor is often included at PACS workstations.

Data Storage

Imaging departments generate a tremendous amount of data. Innovations like 64-slice CT technology ensure that the growth of information in digital forms will continue. The process of saving image data from the originating modality to an electronic medium is called archiving. These archived images can later be retrieved and displayed on the monitor. If requested by the patient, the archived data can be copied onto a disk or filmed so that a study can be taken to an outside physician. Only image data (not raw data) are stored.

Several devices are available for archiving; these can be broadly classified as online, near-line, or offline, depending on the time and method required for data retrieved. Devices such as hard drives are considered online because they are instantly accessible to the user. Data from near-line devices are readily, although not immediately, available. Data from near-line devices are automatically retrieved from a storage system such as an optical jukebox or tape library, which typically takes 10 to 30 seconds. Offline storage refers to data that are kept in a less accessible location, requiring manual intervention to use. Offline storage can be time-consuming because it requires personnel to locate the appropriate device (usually optical media or tape), then load the media into the reader. Offline storage also carries with it risks of lost data through mislabeled, misplaced, or damaged media.

Redundant Array of Inexpensive Disks

Accessing data stored on hard disks is fast and reliable. A system known as redundant array of inexpensive disks (or drives; RAID) is a storage solution that capitalizes on these facts. RAID schemes divide or replicate data among multiple hard drives. These drives are designed to work together and appear to the computer as a single storage device. There are a number of standard RAID configurations available. These are referred to as levels, nested-levels, and nonstandard levels. The specifics of each configuration are beyond the scope of this text; suffice it to say that RAID 5 is the design most frequently used for PACS archives.

Optical Storage

Optical storage devices, such as compact discs (CD) and digital versatile discs (DVD), can be used for long-term data storage. Although the technology is very similar, a single-sided DVD can store about 7 times the data as a CD. DVDs can be written on both sides, doubling the capacity. Newer DVD technology (double-sided/double-layer DVDs) further increases the capacity to 15.9 GB, more than 25 times that of a CD. Newer yet is the Blu-ray disc (a shortened version of blue array, also called BD), a high-density optical disc that has even greater data storage capacity than a DVD. A dual-layer Blu-ray disc can store 50 GB, more than 3 times that of a double-sided/double-layer DVD.

Optical media are often used in a device called an optical jukebox. These are robotic storage systems that automatically load and unload the optical discs. The devices are also called optical disc libraries, robotic drives, or autochangers.

Tape

Magnetic tape is one of the oldest data storage options, first used to record computer data in 1951. Magnetic tape consists of a long narrow strip of plastic with a magnetizable coating, most often packaged in cartridges and cassettes. The device that performs the actual writing or reading of data is known as a tape drive. Like optical discs, autochangers and tape libraries are often used to automate cartridge loading and unloading. Tapes do not allow random access (see Chapter 3), instead they must wind to the appropriate location on the tape (i.e., sequential access), and therefore retrieval of data is somewhat slower than with optical storage media. Many improvements have been made since magnetic tape was first introduced that have increased tape capacity and reduced retrieval time. When storing large amounts of data, tape can be substantially less expensive than other data storage options. This may not be as true in the future as the cost of optical storage methods continues to decline.

Image Distribution

A vital function of any PACS is getting the correct images to the correct locations in the shortest time possible. Distribution channels can be department-wide (e.g., from the CT scanner to the radiologist's workstation), hospital-wide (e.g., at the request of referring clinicians), and, more recently, enterprise-wide (e.g., at off-site outpatient clinics or for on-call radiologists who wish to review studies from home). The Internet is increasingly being used as a key element in meeting image distribution requirements. Clearly, any image distribution system, whether or not it is web-based, must carefully consider issues of data security. Many security strategies exist that can be used separately or in combination, including firewalls, passwords and usernames, and secure socket layers (Table 9-1). Virtual private networks, or VPNs, are also being used to make the Internet a safe medium for the secure transmission of clinical data. By definition, VPNs overlay another network to provide a particular functionality. In the medical computing world the desired function is to enhance

TABLE 9-1   Glossary of Common Imaging Informatics Acronyms and Terms

Acronym	Term	Meaning
	Bandwidth	The amount of data that can be transmitted between two points in the network in a set period of time.
CIS	Clinical Information System	
CPOE	Computerized Physician Order Entry System (also, computerized provider order entry)	A system that allows referring clinicians to place patient orders, such as radiologic tests, on a computer (rather than by writing prescriptions); the orders will be electronically transmitted to the order-receiving department (e.g., radiology, laboratory).
	Core Servers	Server computers that are integral to the functioning of the PACS.
DICOM	Digital Imaging and Communication in Medicine	A set of universally adopted standards for medical image interchange.
EHR	Electronic Health Record	A health record in a digital form. Often used as a synonym for EMR.
EMR	Electronic Medical Record	A medical record in digital form. Often used as a synonym for EHR.
	Firewalls	Similar to a fire door in a building construction, a firewall is an electronic device used to regulate access to private network resources.
HIS	Hospital Information System	An electronic system designed to manage the administrative, financial, and clinical aspects of a hospital.
HL7	Health Level Seven	An organization that works to develop universal standards for clinical and administrative data.
LAN	Local Area Network	Linked computers that are geographically close together.
PACS	Picture Archive and Communication System	A computer network dedicated to the storage, retrieval, distribution, and display of images.
RIS	Radiology Information System	A system designed for radiology departments that includes functions such as scheduling patients, storing reports, patient tracking, protocoling examinations, and billing.
SSL	Secure Sockets Layer	Originally developed by Netscape, SSL is a protocol for transmitting private documents via the Internet. SSL uses two keys to encrypt data. One key is public (known to all); the other is private and known only to the recipient of the message.
VPN	Virtual Private Network	Technology designed to make the exchange of private information over the Internet more secure by encrypting the information at the source and decrypting it at the destination.
WAN	Wide Area Network	A computer network that covers a broad area and must be linked via telephone lines, cables, or radio waves.
	Wired	Networks linked by a physical connection.
	Wireless	Networks that use radio waves to transmit data between computers.

security by encrypting the information at the source and decrypting it at the destination. A detailed discussion of image distribution strategies is beyond the scope of this text. Many excellent texts on the subject exist for the interested reader.

SUMMARY

As CT technology advances to capture more slices and higher-resolution images, the amount of data collected grows, too. This explosion in the quantity of data acquired poses considerable challenges in how those images can be managed so as to be readily viewable. Radiology departments everywhere are becoming increasingly digital as more-efficient computer-based processes replace slow, inefficient film and paper ones. Every technologist in every clinical setting will be affected by this conversion to new electronic methods of managing patient data.

REVIEW QUESTIONS

1. List the reasons why the exclusive use of film for documentation, interpretation, and archiving is becoming obsolete.
2. In computing terms, what is a network? Explain how radiology workflow can be impacted by the network's performance.
3. In the computing world, what does the term redundancy refer to?
4. What benefits were realized by the implementation of an electronic standard such as DICOM and HL7?
5. List the data storage options for archiving image data.

RECOMMENDED READING

Dreyer KJ, Hirschorn DS, Thrall JH, Mehta A. PACS: A Guide to the Digital Revolution. 2nd Ed. New York: Springer, 2006.

Branstetter BF. Basics of imaging informatics: part 1. Radiology 2007;243:656–67.

Branstetter BF. Basics of imaging informatics: part 2. Radiology 2007;244:78–84.

Section II

PATIENT CARE

CHAPTER 10 • Patient Communication

CHAPTER 11 • Patient Preparation

CHAPTER 12 • Contrast Agents

CHAPTER 13 • Injection Techniques

CHAPTER 14 • Radiation Dosimetry in CT

INTRODUCTION

As technical advances result in ever-increasing scan speed, CT technologists find that a greater percentage of their work time is spent in direct patient care duties. As respected members of the healthcare team, technologists are expected to provide quality care with medical expertise. Although mastery of the technical components of CT are essential, so too are a great number of other skills necessary to competently and compassionately care for patients.

Providing excellent care begins with an understanding of the patient as a human being who brings his or her emotional as well as physical problems with him or her to the CT department. Imaging professionals are responsible for the patient's safety while under their care. As such, a number of steps must be taken in preparation for the examination. Technologists must understand the factors that affect radiation dose and apply that knowledge to provide quality examinations with the lowest possible patient exposure. In addition, technologists must recognize symptoms of emergency situations, such as an adverse reaction to contrast media, and know what action to take when they occur. This section covers these important topics.

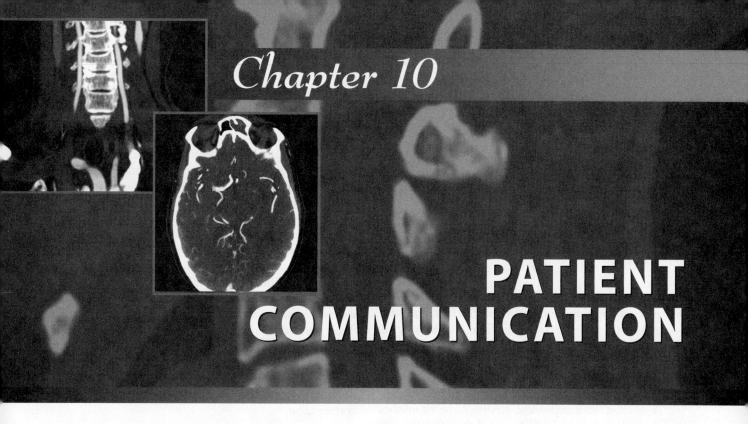

Chapter 10

PATIENT COMMUNICATION

PATIENT COMMUNICATION

Technologists understand the importance of providing their patients with quality care and up-to-date medical expertise. What is often overlooked, however, is the fact that in order to provide this care, technologists must adopt an attentive, personal, interactive style that ensures that patients leave feeling valued and cared for as individuals. Obtaining an accurate medical history and ensuring that the patient understands what is expected of him during a CT examination are critical steps to performing a safe, diagnostically useful study. Only through effective communication can this vital information be gathered and imparted. Therefore, we begin this patient care section with a review of why communication skills are important, basic aspects of the communication process, and practical tips to improve patient interactions.

DO COMMUNICATION SKILLS REALLY MATTER?

When surveyed, healthcare professionals (physicians, nurses, technologists) cite "lack of time" as the chief reason for not talking more to patients. However, researchers have found that professionals who communicate effectively with their patients spend no more time, per patient, than those professionals who report feeling "too rushed to spend time talking."[1] In fact, some studies have shown that total examination time actually *decreased* as communication increased.[2]

Patient concerns are limited to the specific medical care they receive per visit. They expect quality service throughout the entire healthcare experience, including:

- How healthcare workers communicate with patients, from the registration desk to the billing department
- How they and their families are treated by the staff
- The type of information they are given

Technologists must understand that providing patients with the quality service they expect is not only worthwhile and important medically, it also makes good business sense. Improved communication between patient and healthcare providers results in patients who are happier with their overall healthcare experience.[3-7] Increased patient satisfaction has a domino effect and has been linked to many other benefits (Table 10-1).

A number of independent studies have established a link between effective communication and a reduction in malpractice claims.[8-17] These studies confirm that patients feel most satisfied when they feel fully informed. They need to have their questions answered. Patients also express a desire to have interactions that feel personal, caring, and respectful. They want technologists to relate to them as people. Dissatisfied patients have reported feeling that the provider focuses on them only as a disease process (e.g., "the diabetic") or as an organ to be examined (e.g., "the abdomen").[17]

Patients don't care how much you know until they know how much you care.

SIR WILLIAM OSLER

Although the intent of most healthcare professionals is to provide adequate information and intervention, there are a number of ways communication can inadvertently go awry. Physicians, nurses, or technologists often

TABLE 10-1   Benefits of Effective Communication[3-17]

Improved patient safety	Improved examination quality
Improved patient retention	Better staff morale
Increased referral	Reduced staff turnover
Improved patient compliance	Improved collections
Greater profitability	Greater efficiency
Reduced risk of malpractice suits	Increased personal and professional fulfillment of healthcare staff

feel pressed for time and consequently rush the visit. Sometimes they use excessive medical terminology, or they can underestimate the patient's desire for information. These problems may result in the patient's perception that the health professional did not provide enough information or adequately explain the test or procedures.

A number of independent studies have established that patients are more likely to sue if they feel that the healthcare provider didn't care or didn't inform them adequately.[7,9-15] The same communication skills that reduce malpractice risk lead to patient satisfaction and improved quality of care. Caring, concerned technologists who communicate well with their patients are likely to provide the best quality of care. Collaborative relationships with patients provide opportunities for technologists to derive the professional and personal rewards of truly meaningful connections with patients. Although preventing malpractice claims is important, providing high-quality, humanistic care is the best reason to communicate effectively.

THE COMMUNICATION PROCESS

But how can communication be improved? Global suggestions to improve information giving are unlikely to be helpful. After the importance of effective communication is recognized, the next step to improvement is to understand the communication process.

Communication can be defined as the "process of creating meaning." Two words in this sentence are critical: *create* and *meaning*. Messages may be generated from the outside by a radio speaker, television screen, or parent. But meanings are generated from within. Communication does not consist of the transmission of meaning, because meanings are not entirely transmittable or transferable. Only messages are transmittable. Meanings are not entirely contained in the message; they are interpreted by the message receivers.

Many times the sender thinks the message is clear. But the receiver, who must interpret the message through his or her own specific frame of reference, may hear something entirely different. Communication is so difficult because at each step in the process there is a potential

for breakdown. Therefore, it is no surprise that social psychologists estimate that there is usually a 40% to 60% loss of meaning in the transmission of messages from sender to receiver.[2]

Here is a fictitious example of a multipart exchange between a patient in the computed tomography (CT) department and a radiology nurse. The patient asks, "When is the last time I had my painkiller?" (He winces and holds his abdomen.) His direct request is for information on the time he was last administrated an analgesic. His indirect request is for information about when he can have more. He is anticipating action (the nurse giving him the medication) so that he will be comforted. This exchange illustrates that communication consists of much more than the words that are spoken. If the nurse responds only to his direct request and replies, "About 4 hours ago," the patient is likely to feel that she is indifferent to his pain.

It is critical to understand and be aware of the potential pitfalls and to make a conscientious effort to minimize those areas in which there may be loss of meaning in your conversation.

Barriers to Communication

There are many potential barriers to communications. Some examples are as follows:

- Language. The choice of words a sender selects will influence the quality of the communication. It is important to remember that no two people will attribute the exact same meaning to the same words.
- Power struggles. Defensiveness, distorted perceptions, guilt, transference, past transgression. These issues crop up when either the sender or the receiver suffers from low self-esteem or insecurity.
- Misreading of body language, tone, and other nonverbal forms of communication. It also very important to understand that a majority of communication is nonverbal. This means that when we attribute meaning to what someone else is saying, the verbal part of the message actually means less than the nonverbal part. The nonverbal part includes such aspects as body language and tone. For example, when a person crosses her arms, it is typically interpreted as a sign of resistance or lack of cooperation. But occasionally crossed arms simply indicate that the air conditioning is turned up too high and the person is cold.
- Fuzzy transmission. Unreliable or inconsistent messages.
- Receiver distortion. Selective hearing, ignoring nonverbal cues. This often happens if the receiver doesn't like portions of the sender's message. By simply ignoring pieces of the message, the receiver gets a message more to his liking. In the healthcare setting this can sometimes be used to the technologist's

advantage. Assume a patient enters the department and angrily questions, "Fill out another medical history?" The technologist may choose to ignore the tone of voice and just respond to the question, "Yes, we do like to be very thorough–giving you the best care possible is important to us and we want to make sure we don't overlook anything."

- Assumptions. Assuming others see situations the same as you, or have the same feelings as you. Healthcare workers become so accustomed to the hospital environment that they sometimes forget how frightening and strange it can be to someone with no medical background. Also, sometimes by making an assumption, even an incorrect one, we help to make the assumption come true. We think, "Mrs. Jones is always so grumpy," and it colors our communication, which, in turn, annoys Mrs. Jones, who responds by being curt.
- Preconceptions. In the process of communicating, our prejudices often slip through. For example, when a 79-year-old woman being treated in the emergency room repeatedly asked whether her father had arrived yet, the staff automatically assumed her to be suffering from dementia. Imagine their surprise when a 98-year-old man hobbled up to the desk and inquired about the status of his daughter.
- Past experiences. How we perceive communication is affected by past experiences with the individual.
- Cultural differences. Effective communication requires deciphering the basic values, motives, aspirations, and assumptions that operate across geographical lines. Given some dramatic differences across cultures in approaches to such areas as time, space, and privacy, the opportunities for miscommunication while we are in cross-cultural situations are plentiful.

Nonverbal Communication

Studies have shown that as much as 90% of the meaning we derive from communication comes from the nonverbal cues that the other person gives. Often, a person may say one thing but communicates something totally different through vocal intonation and body language. These mixed signals force the receiver to choose between the verbal and nonverbal parts of the message. Most often, the receiver chooses the nonverbal aspects. Mixed messages create tension and distrust because the receiver senses that the communicator is being less than candid.

Nonverbal communication can be categorized five ways: 1) visual, 2) tactile, 3) vocal, 4) use of time, space, and images, and 5) objects or values.

Visual Communication

Visual communication is often called body language and can include facial expression, eye contact, posture, and gestures. The face plays the biggest role in body language. All of us "read" people's faces for insight into what they say and feel. Visual cues can easily be misread, especially when communicating across cultures in which gestures can mean something very different. For example, in American culture, agreement is often indicated by moving the head up and down. In India, however, a side-to-side head movement is the gesture for agreement.

Eye contact is an important aspect of nonverbal communication. There are certain unstated rules in each society. For example, proper street behavior among Americans permits passersby to look at each other until they are approximately 8 feet apart. At this point, both parties cast their eyes away so that they will not appear to be staring. Research psychologists have summed up several of these rules about eye contact. Two that are particularly important when interacting with patients are:

- Persons who seek eye contact while speaking are more believable and truthful.
- If gazes of longer duration replace the usual short, intermittent glances during normal conversation, the target interprets this change as meaning the task is less important than the personal relationship between the two persons.

Think about how these facts may be integrated into interactions with patients. For example, pausing to make eye contact while taking a patient's medical history may convey to the patient that his or her care is more important to the technologist than completing paperwork.

Posture also provides cues about the communicator by indicating self-confidence, aggressiveness, fear, guilt, or anxiety.

Tactile

In this respect, tactile communication cues involve the use of touch to impart meaning. Common examples are a handshake, a pat on the back, an arm around the shoulder, or a hug. The use of touch is a powerful tool to convey caring, but must be used cautiously lest the receiver misinterpret the touch as sexually charged.

Vocal

Vocal cues refer to the intonation of a person's voice. The meaning of words can be altered significantly according to the intonation. Think of the many ways to say "No." With one word you could express mild doubt, terror, amazement, or anger.

Time, Space, and Images

Time may be a form of communication, especially when we view our own status and power in relation to others. Imagine how a subordinate and his boss would view arriving at a designated place for an agreed-upon meeting. If the subordinate shows up late, this action is viewed quite differently than if the boss were late.

Now, consider the long wait common in many doctors' offices. Viewing time in this way may give a patient the impression that the doctor sees her own time as being much more important than that of the patient's.

For most of us, someone standing very close makes us uncomfortable. We feel our space has been invaded. In the context of communication, there are four types of distance: intimate, personal, social, and public. In general, for North Americans these spaces can be defined as follows:[18]

- Intimate distance–18 inches or less; used to discuss confidential matters
- Personal distance–1.5 to 4 feet; which is analogous to a small protective sphere or bubble that a person maintains between themselves and others
- Social distance–4 to 12 feet; described as a psychological distance, people begin to feel anxious when these boundaries are not maintained. This distance can be thought of as a hidden band that contains the group. Social distance is suitable for business discussions and conversations at social gatherings. It is typically the most comfortable distance when working with patients.
- Public distance–12 feet or more; requires a more formal style of language and a louder voice.
- Ethnic, Age, and Sex Differences.
  - There are significant differences in how members of different ethnic groups within a single culture interact.[18] Research has found that Mexican-Americans stand closest to one another, Anglo-Americans stand at an intermediate distance, and Afro-Americans stand at the farthest distance from each other.
  - Age also makes a difference in how close people stand to each other. Children interact at a close distance, whereas adults interact at a farther distance. Adolescents interact at an intermediate distance.
  - Male–female interactions are closest, whereas male–male interactions are farthest and female–female interactions occur at an intermediate range.

Objects

Similarly, we use "objects" to communicate. Objects can be cheap or expensive, neat or messy, interesting or boring, and so forth. For example, if a patient shows up for an appointment to a waiting room in which there are overflowing trash receptacles, newspapers on the floor, and 5-year-old magazines, she will make assumptions about the quality of care she will receive even before her first contact with staff members.

PRACTICAL ADVICE

Because communication is a two-way process, the first step in improving communication skills is to recognize that each of us has responsibilities both as a speaker and a listener.

The Speaker's Responsibilities

- Be audible. Speak loudly enough so that your listener can hear you without undue strain. Be clear.
- Be aware that your listener may not have understood you. In other words, acknowledge the many possibilities for misunderstanding as a normal part of every communication.
- Be willing to ask questions of your listener to see whether he or she understands you. Offer the listener an opportunity to ask for clarification. Be willing to restate and clarify your message. Sometimes when questioned, we repeat what we have just said, using the identical words and a louder, angrier tone of voice. Realize that this behavior ridicules the listener and makes it less likely that he or she will even acknowledge any future misunderstandings.

The Listener's Responsibilities

- Let the speaker know whether he or she is inaudible. Don't just sit there straining to hear; ask the speaker to talk louder, and, if necessary, to repeat the information you have missed.
- Let the speaker know that you are attentive. Look at the speaker. Nod or shake your head. Your response does not have to be verbal, but you should react in some way that demonstrates that you are listening.
- If the speaker's message is unclear, let him or her know that you need a point clarified. However, be tactful and also be willing to accept some of the responsibility for not understanding. "The machinery running makes it very noisy in here and I'm having a hard time understanding you. Did you say you just had a barium examination yesterday?" Be aware that you may not have understood the speaker. Don't be impatient if you occasionally do not understand everything. Misunderstandings and their subsequent clarification are a normal part of the communication process. Try to keep from getting angry. Be willing to paraphrase what you think the speaker means. This is the best way to check whether the message received matches the intended message.

Communication Habits to Avoid

A discussion of strategies to improve communication skills would not be complete without considering those communication habits that should be avoided in the healthcare setting.

- Don't use false reassurance. For example, if a patient admits to being fearful that the biopsy examination being performed will result in the discovery of a terminal cancer, avoid responses such as, "I'm sure you'll be fine," or "Everything is going to be okay." It is entirely possible, maybe even likely, that the patient's condition *will not* be fine. It is better to say nothing rather than to use such hollow statements. A better way might be to use an empathic response, such as "I understand how stressful all these tests are," or "Yes, the uncertainty and waiting can sometimes be the hardest part." Often, there may not be words that can offer comfort. In these situations, a gentle touch on the hand or shoulder can be very reassuring and may succeed in demonstrating that the patient is cared for.

- Don't ignore a patient's wishes. If a patient states that his right arm is the best place for starting an intravenous (IV) line, the technologist has two options. She can use the patient's right arm (or at least look to see whether there is an adequate vein there), or she can explain why the left arm is a better choice, i.e., "Because of the design of the human circulatory system and the specific structures we are looking for in this examination, the doctor prefers we start the IV in the left arm. May I take a look?" In a similar manner, if a patient complains that he can't drink the oral contrast medium, it is not effective for the technologist to simply demand compliance. A better approach is to first show sympathy, explain why the request is legitimate, and then politely repeat the request: "I know that barium isn't the most wonderful tasting cocktail, but it is very important in helping us to see your pancreas. Please try your hardest to get it down so that we can perform the best possible test for you."

- Don't speak like you are talking to a child. Be careful of your inflection. No one likes to be treated like a child. Many technologists fall into the habit of talking to the elderly in a singsong voice as if they were small children or senile. This can be perceived as insulting and disrespectful.

- Don't assume that a nonresponsive patient can't hear. A number of studies have demonstrated that the sense of hearing is quite complex, with much hearing occurring at the subconscious level.[19-21] The lesson to be drawn from such research is that healthcare staff working with the seriously ill must always explain what is being done, at least in simple terms, even if that patient does not appear able to understand.

- Don't carry on a separate conversation with a coworker while a patient is present. This can make the patient feel like you view her as an object or anatomic part rather than as an individual. In most instances, it is fine to carry on a conversation–even one that is totally unrelated to the examination to be performed–if the patient is included in the conversation. To make a patient feel comfortable in sharing in the dialogue, the technologist should explicitly invite the patient to participate. To illustrate, consider the following interchange:

Technologist 1 (comes into the CT room as another technologist is preparing Mrs. Smith for her examination by starting her IV): "Hey, Sue, did you ever find that cow fabric you were looking for?"

Technologist 2: "As a matter a fact, I did. I had to look in three different stores, though. (Looking directly at Mrs. Smith) I'm making a cow costume for my 6-year-old's school Halloween party. I had a heck of a time finding the fabric I wanted. Do you sew?"

By actively involving the patient in the conversation, you show her that her opinion is valued. She is not just a body part to be examined, but also an individual with opinions and feelings.

- Don't think being professional means being cold. As technology improves, technologists have been forced to spend much of their time and energy staying current. Many healthcare professionals, knowing that patients feel comforted when they recognize the staff is competent, try to portray competency by behaving in a very cold, robotic way. Seldom does this bring the desired results. It's important to remember: "Patients don't care how much you know, until they know how much you care." Warm, friendly technologists who are willing to share a little of their personalities with patients are the professionals that will be viewed as most caring by their patients.

- Don't blame the patient. Blame decreases the patient's level of self-confidence and, most often, results in the patient responding with anger or defensiveness. Thus, blame is not an effective communication style. There is a subtle but important distinction between placing blame and requiring the patient to accept responsibility for their actions. Instead of saying, "Why did you miss your last appointment?" try, "I see that you missed your last appointment. What happened?" Rather than saying, "If you had taken the barium as you were instructed to, you wouldn't have to wait so long," try, "We get the best results when we perform the test 2 hours after the patient drinks the barium. I know it's a long time to wait, but it is important to get the best possible results."

- Don't use abbreviations or medical lingo. The use of medical jargon can confuse patients. Worse, if the patient nods knowingly, too embarrassed to admit he or she is baffled, you could risk getting an inaccurate medical history, or at the least, of having an unhappy, noncompliant patient. Use language that patients will understand, with words that create mental pictures, common terms, and analogies.

An example of such imagery includes, "CT pictures are cross-sectional; imagine you're a loaf of bread, each CT picture is like looking at a slice of bread; your skin is like the crust, and your internal organs are like the white part of the bread."

Communication Habits to Adopt

Finally, consider the following list of habits that *do* work well in the healthcare setting.

- Be a good listener. When surveyed, doctors interrupt a patient after just 18 seconds of the patient's description of symptoms.[22] In addition, it is common for healthcare professionals to ask a patient a question, and then, instead of actively listening to the patient, focus their attention on the form, or chart, in front of them. Concerned about time, technologists may be reluctant to use open-ended questions or statements, such as, "Tell me why you think your doctor wanted you to have this examination." However, an uninterrupted narrative usually takes approximately 1 or 2 minutes on average.[23] During this narrative, the technologist's role should be to listen actively. If the patient gives information that must be recorded, politely ask the patient to pause in speaking for a moment while you write down important information. When you are done writing, restart the narrative with a comment like, "Please continue, Mr. Jones, you were telling me about when the pain in your abdomen started."

- Use focused questions. Focused questions allow you to get directly to the relevant points and reduce rambling explanations from the patient. For example, "Tell me about the pain in your arm," or "It says here that you're allergic to iodine. Could you describe your experience the last time you received iodine for an examination?"

- Use the patient's name. It's been said that the most beautiful word in any language is a person's name. By using their name, you assure the patient that he or she is now the focus of your attention. Unless they are much younger, it is best to use a title, such as Mr., Mrs., or Ms., when addressing a patient.

- Use touch to comfort and be aware of nonverbal messages. Patients often judge the quality of communication by both words and nonverbals such as a handshake, eye contact, and the "white spaces" when no words are spoken but an emotional or personal connection is made. This connection must be sincere and honest; a caring attitude can't be simulated.

- Develop a rapport with the patient. Asking questions that have nothing to do with the examination at hand can show the patient that you that are interested in him or her as an individual. "Are you retired? What type of work did you do before you retired?" Or "That's an interesting last name. What nationality is it?" In addition to creating a connection with the patient, communicating in this way often enhances the technologist's job by allowing her to continually learn from her patients.

- Explain before acting. Never attempt to provide care until the patient understands exactly what will happen. Sometimes, in a rush to keep on schedule, technologists will just start a procedure (i.e., putting a tourniquet on a patient's arm). It is important to remember that delivering personal care without explanation and, therefore, a patient's consent has a name other than aid; it is called assault.

- Give the patient an opportunity to ask questions. After you have explained the procedure, give the patient the chance to clarify any points that may be confusing. "Well, that about does it for the explanation. Do you have any questions for me before we get started?"

- Use reflective speech. This technique is great for clarification of a patient's message. "All this medical stuff is like Greek to me," could be answered by you with, "It sounds like you find many of the issues related to your condition to be confusing." Or, in response to "Maybe I had that iodine stuff before," you could ask, "So you're unsure whether you've ever had the contrast before?"

- Give consistent messages. Quality of care must be consistent—across the entire staff and practice, not some of the time, but all of the time. For example, a patient has a CT examination in August, at which time a staff member tells her one thing. Then in December that same patient has a follow-up examination, and she is told something entirely different by another staff member. This type of inconsistency can be disturbing. Patients need to get a unified message. Printed material, videos, and other forms of adjunctive patient education material provide a consistent message that also serves as documentation. However, it is vital that staff members give consistent messages to patients about clinical policies and procedures.

SUMMARY

Technologists provide quality care with medical expertise. However, quality care is also dependent on attentive, personal interaction. Ensuring that patients are satisfied so that they leave the department feeling valued and cared for as individuals is the role and responsibility of everyone involved in health care. For a practice to be successful, technologists and other staff members must honestly and effectively communicate and stay connected to people.

REVIEW QUESTIONS

1. List the benefits of effective communication in the healthcare environment.
2. Identify at least 5 communication habits that healthcare workers should avoid.
3. Describe at least 5 communication habits that healthcare workers should adopt.

REFERENCES

1. Bradley EM. Communication in the Nursing Context. Norwalk, CT: Appleton & Lange, 1990.
2. Davis A. Listening and Responding. St Louis: Mosby, 1984.
3. Dugdale DC, Epstein R, Patilat SZ. Time and the patient-physician relationship. J Gen Intern Med 1999; 14(Suppl):S34–40.
4. Brown SW, Bronkesh SJ, Nelson AM, Wood SD. Patient Satisfaction Pays. Gaithersburg, MD: Aspen Publishers, 1993:9.
5. Gearson R. Beyond Customer Service. Menlo Park, CA: Crisp Publications, 1992:3, 11.
6. Macharia WM, Leon G, Rowe BH, Stephenson BJ, Haynes RB. An overview of interventions to improve compliance with appointment keeping for medical services. JAMA 1992; 267:1813–7.
7. Entman SS, Glass CA, Hickson GB, Githens PB, Whetten-Goldstein K, Sloan FA. The relationship between malpractice claims history and subsequent obstetric care. JAMA 1994;272:1588–91.
8. Beckman HB, Markakis KM, Suchman AL, Frankel RM. The doctor-patient relationship and malpractice. Lessons from plaintiff depositions. Arch Intern Med 1994;154:1365–70.
9. Medical Malpractice: Report. Washington, DC: US Dept of Health, Education and Welfare; DHEW Publication No. OS 73-89, 1973.
10. Leape LL, Brennan TA, Laird NM, et al. The nature of adverse events in hospitalized patients. Results of the Harvard Medical Practice Study II. N Engl J Med 1991;324:377–84.
11. Brennan TA, Leape LL, Laird NM, et al. Incidence of adverse events and negligence in hospitalized patients. Results of the Harvard Medical Practice Study I. N Engl J Med 1991;324:370–6.
12. Hickson GB, Clayton EW, Entman SS, et al. Obstetricians' prior malpractice experience and patients' satisfaction with care. JAMA 1994;272:1583–7.
13. Levinson W, Roter DL, Mullooly JP, Dull VT, Frankel RM. Physician-patient communication. The relationship with malpractice claims among primary care physicians and surgeons. JAMA 1997;277:553–9.
14. Adamson TE, Tschann JM, Gullion DS, Oppenber AA. Physician communication skills and malpractice claims. A complex relationship. West J Med 1989;150:356–60.
15. Sloan FA, Mergenhagen PM, Burfield WB, Bovbjerg RR, Hassan M. Medical malpractice experience of physicians. Predictable or haphazard? JAMA 1989;262:3291–7.
16. Avery JK. Lawyers tell what turns some patients litigious. Med Malpractice Rev 1985;2:35–7.
17. Hall JA, Roter DL, Katz NR. Meta-analysis of correlates of provider behavior in medical encounters. Med Care 1988; 26:657–75.
18. Vangelisti A, Daly JA, Friedrich GW. Teaching Communication: Theory, Research, and Methods. Mahway, NJ: Erbaum Associates, 1999.
19. Ott R, Curio I, Scholz OB. Implicit memory for auditorily presented threatening stimuli: a process-dissociation approach. Percept Mot Skills 2000;90:131–46.
20. Tsunoda T. Human cerebral dominance and significance of a subconscious sensor for detecting auditory signals. Int J Neurosci 1989;47:149–58.
21. Makari G, Shapiro T. On psychoanalytic listening: language and unconscious communication. J Am Psychoanal Assoc 1993;41:991–1020.
22. Gibbs N. Sick and tired. Uneasy patients may be surprised to find their doctors are worried too. Time 1989;134:48–53.
23. Brown SW, Bronkesh SJ, Nelson AM, Wood SD. Patient Satisfaction Pays. Gaithersburg, MD: Aspen Publishers, 1993: 258–9.

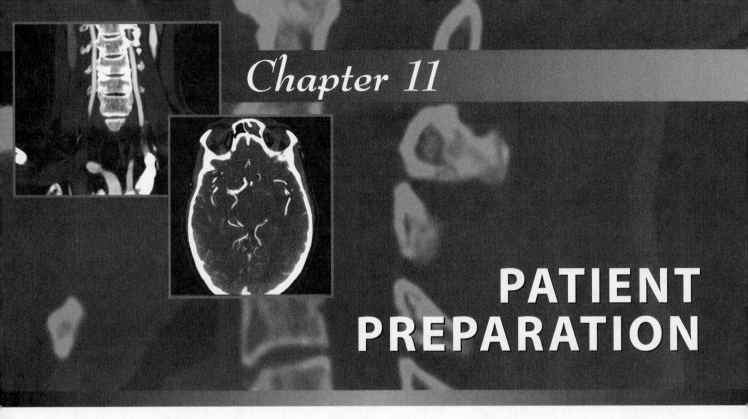

Chapter 11

PATIENT PREPARATION

Many steps are taken before the patient ever sets foot at the imaging facility. Tasks such as scheduling the examination, selecting the appropriate examination protocol, obtaining pertinent medical history, and preparing the CT examination room are often done in collaboration with technologists, clerical staff, and radiologists. The exact order of the steps and what staff member will perform what task varies widely from facility to facility. This chapter considers the tasks that must occur before scanning a patient.

EXAMINATION INITIATION

All CT examinations must be initiated by a clinician with appropriate credentials. In addition to physicians, clinicians who may order diagnostic tests include nurse practitioners (NP) and physician assistants (PA). In outpatient settings, the order is often written by the clinician in his or her private office, and the clerical staff will then phone the scheduling division of the imaging facility to arrange an appointment. Scheduling staff then transmit the appointment to the CT department. This process introduces the potential for transcription errors at several points; therefore, it is recommended that the original requisition written by the ordering clinician be faxed or electronically transmitted to the imaging facility. In any case, it is essential that before any CT examination is performed, a copy of the original order requisition is available to the technologist so that she can verify that the appropriate examination has been planned. Ideally, some patient screening should occur at the time the examination is scheduled. This will help to schedule patients more efficiently by adequately planning for issues such as contrast media allergies and claustrophobia.

110

> **BOX 11-1   Key Concept**
>
> Before the CT examination begins the technologist must review the physician's order and read all clinical data provided. Any discrepancies between the written order, the examination scheduled, or the examination the patient thinks was ordered must be reconciled.

The process for initiating inpatient examinations is different than that for outpatients but may also include opportunities for transcription errors. The most accurate method for transmitting orders to the radiology department is via an electronic system in which the ordering clinician places the electronic order herself. Generically called computerized physician order entry (CPOE), these systems eliminate the transcription errors that can arise when an intermediary (e.g., clerk or nurse) must read a hand-written order and translate it into an electronic order. They also ensure that the order is legible. However, in many institutions CPOE is not available. Whenever the original order is transcribed by someone other than the ordering clinician, the process must include, as a final step, the technologist verifying the original clinician's order against that of the scheduled examination. This is often accomplished by having the patient's chart accompany the patient to the CT department.

PROTOCOL SELECTION

Once an order for an examination has been received by the CT department, a specific examination protocol must be agreed on. The proper selection of protocol is the purview of the radiologist, often with a technologist's input. In some instances, protocol selection is constrained by a specific scanner's capabilities. The overarching goal is to select the protocol that will answer the clinical question(s) posed with the least risk to the patient. Risks to the patient include those attributed to radiation exposure, contrast media reactions, or complications such as bleeding or infection that may arise from procedures such as biopsies or fluid drainage. The protocol selected must consider the patient's ability to tolerate the examination.

BOX 11-2   Key Concept

The selection of protocol should attempt to answer the clinical question(s) posed with the least risk to the patient. Risks to the patient include those attributed to radiation exposure, contrast media reaction, or complications such as bleeding or infection (from more invasive procedures).

In some institutions radiologists review each CT request, consider the patient's medical history, and assign a specific protocol. Technologists will then carry out the selected protocol unless their review of the actual patient (rather than just the paperwork) brings up questions or concerns.

In other facilities radiologists set up specific algorithms for technologists to follow. These might include matching specific clinical indications to specific examination protocols. For example, a clinician's order for a CT Head with the clinical indication of new-onset right facial droop may be mapped to a routine CT examination of the head without the use of intravenous contrast media. These algorithms most often require the technologist to review a number of criteria from the patient's medical history (e.g., laboratory values related to renal function, allergies) before selecting the appropriate protocol. Technologists then only need to seek the radiologists' advice when uncertainties arise.

In either situation it is imperative that technologists understand the criteria used to determine when various protocols are appropriate. They should carefully review the requisition, reading all clinical data provided by the referring clinician. This is an important patient safeguard in that technologists can identify potential errors before an examination is performed. Criteria regarding possible clinical indications for various examinations will be covered in Section IV of this text. Criteria regarding contrast media are discussed in Chapter 12.

ROOM PREPARATION

Before bringing the patient to the examination room, it should be appropriately prepared. Scanner calibrations and tube warm-up procedures should be done while the room is free of both patients and CT staff. The room should be checked for cleanliness, items from previous patients discarded, and supplies stocked and in their designated location. The appropriate equipment, such as head holder or foot extension, should be attached. Positioning devices such as angle sponges should be clean and readily accessible.

Appropriate safety equipment, such as thyroid or breast shields, should be ready for use. On the infrequent occasion that someone other than the patient will remain in the scan room during the examination, appropriate safety equipment (e.g., lead aprons or a lead screen) must be provided.

MEDICAL HISTORY

An appropriate medical history is a vital aspect of any CT examination. It will help to ensure a patient's safety, guide the selection of examination protocol, and offer the radiologist valuable diagnostic information. Figure 11-1 is an example of a patient history form used to collect data for a CT examination.

BOX 11-3   Key Concept

Questions included on the CT history form seek to achieve three goals: patient safety, correct selection of protocol, and providing information useful for interpreting the examination.

At first contact with the patient the technologist must be careful to accurately identify the patient. Many cases have occurred in which technologists confused patients with similar sounding names and performed the wrong examination. When such errors are made, not only is the patient exposed to radiation from an unnecessary examination, there are risks from associating the wrong historical data to the patient (such as administering iodinated contrast to a patient who is known to be allergic to it) and, if the error is not discovered, from having a patient's treatment based on incorrect diagnostic information. At least two methods of verifying a patient's identity is required. For instance the technologist might call the patient by his full name and then ask the patient to recite his birth date and year so that it can be checked against the CT order. Methods such as checking a patient's armband and verifying identity with family members accompanying the patient can be used when the patient is unable to communicate. Hospital patients should not be identified by room number or by the name posted above the patient's bed or on the door of the patient's room.

BOX 11-4   Key Concept

At least two methods of verifying a patient's identity are required.

Patient Safety

The administration of contrast media is contraindicated in some situations. In other situations, contrast media is administered only after a patient is premedicated to reduce the risks of an adverse event. Patients are questioned regarding renal impairment and previous allergies to assess

DEPARTMENT OF RADIOLOGY IN PATIENT QUESTIONNAIRE FOR CT	Birthdate:	Age:
	Name:	
	Reg No:	

Date: _____ Height/Weight _____

Patient history of any of the following:	From Patient Chart			Confirmed by Patient
	Yes	No	Not found	
IV Contrast allergy	☐	☐	☐	☐
Severe food or medication allergy	☐	☐	☐	☐
Pregnant	☐	☐	☐	☐
Breast feeding	☐	☐	☐	☐
Active kidney disease, kidney failure, or dialysis	☐	☐	☐	☐
	Creatinine: value _____ date _____			
	BUN: value _____ date _____			
Thyroid cancer or hyperthyroidism	☐	☐	☐	☐
Myasthenia gravis	☐	☐	☐	☐
Taken Interleukin-2 in the past 2 weeks	☐	☐	☐	☐
	☐	☐	☐	☐
Currently taking Metformin (e.g. Glucophage, Glucovance)				☐
Current order for asthma medication				☐

_____   _____
Signature of person completing questionnaire   Date

_____   _____
Signature of technologist performing the exam   Date

FIGURE 11-1   An example of a patient history form used to collect data for a CT examination.

whether they can safely be given an intravenous contrast agent. Knowing a patient's previous allergies is also necessary should an unexpected reaction occur that necessitates immediate pharmaceutical treatment. Questions regarding hyperthyroidism and other diseases of the thyroid also relate to whether the patient can safely receive an iodinated contrast agent. These issues are discussed more fully in Chapter 12.

BOX 11–5   Key Concept

Questions on the medical history regarding renal function, allergies, and thyroid conditions help to determine whether an iodinated contrast agent will be administered intravenously.

A fetus, exposed to ionizing radiation in utero, is particularly sensitive to its harmful effects (see Chapter 14). Female patients within childbearing age must be questioned as to the possibility that they may be pregnant. If the woman is uncertain, the examination should be delayed while pregnancy status is determined. In the event that the patient is pregnant a careful analysis of the risks and benefits of the examination must be considered. This discussion should include the patient, the referring doctor, and the radiologist.

Protocol Selection

Ideally, enough patient information is provided by the ordering clinician to guide the selection of examination protocol. In addition, some institutions offer electronic health records, or offer readily accessible paper records that can be used to supplement the information provided on the order requisition. Unfortunately, this is not always the case. In many situations, information obtained from the patient once he or she arrives at the imaging center will determine what examination protocol is applied. Questions regarding the symptoms that a patient is experiencing, whether the symptoms are new or chronic, and the onset of those symptoms are frequently used to select the appropriate protocol. Previous examinations should also be noted as these may also influence the protocol selected, or they may be needed as a comparison once the examination is completed.

Diagnostic Information

Many diseases or conditions have similar findings on CT images. A medical history can often aide the radiologist in narrowing down, or pinpointing exactly, the disease or condition from which the patient suffers. For example, because scarring caused by radiation therapy can mimic lung disease, it is helpful to note previous oncology treatments. Questions that include the patient's past surgeries, significant medical issues, and current symptoms augment other clinical data in helping radiologists to accurately interpret CT images.

Laboratory Values

The laboratory values most frequently reviewed before routine CT examinations are blood urea nitrogen (BUN) and serum creatinine. Both of these values provide information about a patient's kidney function, which is important if the patient will receive an intravenous (IV) contrast agent. The normal range of these values can vary slightly from laboratory to laboratory, and also among adult men, adult women, and children. Laboratory reports typically provide guidance as to when a value is outside of the normal limit for a specific patient. However, as a general guide the normal range for BUN is typically between 7 and 25 milligrams per deciliter (mg/dL), and the normal range for serum creatinine is 0.6 to 1.7 mg/dL. Many institutions have a policy for when a radiologist is consulted before intravenous contrast medium is administered to patients in whom the BUN is greater than 30 mg/dL or the creatinine value is greater than 2 mg/dL. The impact of iodinated contrast media on renal function is discussed in detail in Chapter 12.

BOX 11–6   Key Concept

The laboratory values for BUN and serum creatinine provide information about a patient's renal function. This is important if a patient will receive an IV contrast agent.
The laboratory values for PT and PTT provide information about the blood's coagulation ability. This is important for examinations that carry the risk of excessive bleeding, such as biopsies and fluid drainage.

Examinations such as biopsies and fluid drainage carry the risk of excessive bleeding. Before these examinations are performed it is important to check laboratory values that indicate whether there are any problems with the blood's ability to form clots (coagulate). Tests most often used are prothrombin time (PT), partial thromboplastin time (PTT), and platelet count. Again, although the normal range may vary slightly from laboratory to laboratory, a typical range for PT is 11 to 14 seconds, PTT is 25 to 35 seconds, and platelet count is 150,000 to 400,000 cubic millimeters (mm³). Many health conditions (e.g., stroke, heart disease) are treated with medications that inhibit coagulation. Common anticoagulant medications include warfarin (Coumadin), heparin, Plavix, and aspirin. To reduce the risk of excessive bleeding, anticoagulation medications are often temporarily discontinued before an interventional procedure.

Table 11-1 lists laboratory values relevant to CT examinations and their approximate normal ranges.

PATIENT EDUCATION AND INFORMED CONSENT

CT technologists have a professional responsibility to provide patient education. The patient has the right to know about any radiologic procedure they will undergo,

TABLE 11-1   Laboratory Values

Laboratory Test	Approximate Normal Range*	Indicates
Blood urea nitrogen (BUN)	7 to 25 mg/dL	Renal function
Serum creatinine	0.6 to 1.7 mg/dL	Renal function
Prothrombin time (PT)	11 to 14 seconds	Blood coagulation ability
Partial thromboplastin time (PTT)	25 to 35 seconds	Blood coagulation ability
Platelet count	150,000 to 400,000 mm^3	Blood coagulation ability

*The range of normal values varies slightly from laboratory to laboratory and, in many cases, among adult men, adult women, and children. Laboratory reports typically indicate whether a specific value is out of range for that laboratory and that particular patient.

and most often it is the technologist who provides this information. Another aim in providing patient education is to increase patient compliance and facilitate the efficient completion of a high-quality examination.

At a minimum, the technologist should describe

- How the procedure is carried out (e.g., "you will lie on your back on a cushioned table that will move in and out of the CT scanner, which resembles a large donut")
- The approximate length of the procedure
- Whether contrast agents will be administered; if they are planned, then an explanation of how they will be administered (e.g., oral, IV) and any potential side effects is required
- What is expected of the patient (e.g., hold your breath when you hear the command, remain very still, remove metallic objects, change into a patient gown)
- Any follow-up necessary after the examination has been completed

The practice of obtaining consent from a patient before providing a healthcare service stems from the patient's legal and ethical rights to determine what shall be done with his or her own body. When a patient has not provided consent for an examination the technologist who performs the examination may be liable for battery (defined as the nonconsensual touching of another) and the facility may be vulnerable to a malpractice claim. In the medical context, the person committing battery does not have to intend harm.

BOX 11-7   Key Concept

Basic consent is appropriate for most routine, noninvasive healthcare services. Basic consent involves letting the patient know what you plan to do and asking them whether they agree.

Basic (or simple) consent involves letting the patient know what you plan to do and asking them whether they agree. Basic consent is appropriate for most types of radiologic procedures.

The practice of obtaining written consent from the patient for the CT examination, particularly when an intravenous contrast material is to be administered, is common in many facilities. Acquiring a signed consent form documents that the procedure and its associated risks were discussed with the patient. The practice is not universally accepted for routine CT examinations. Opponents believe that the process of reading and signing a consent form can increase patient anxiety and increase the likelihood of an adverse reaction. Further, they believe that the forms offer little protection in cases of litigation.

The goal of informed consent is to provide the patient an opportunity to be an informed participant in his healthcare decisions. It is generally accepted that complete informed consent includes a discussion of the following elements:

- The nature of the procedure
- Reasonable alternatives to the proposed intervention
- The relevant risks, benefits, and uncertainties related to each alternative
- Assessment of the patient's understanding
- The acceptance of the intervention by the patient

In the case of CT examinations of a more invasive nature, such as biopsies, there is universal agreement that a signed consent form is necessary. For the patient's consent to be valid, he must be considered competent to make the decision at hand and his consent must be voluntary. Therefore, when a consent form is required it must be signed by the patient before the administration of any medication used for pain relief or sedation. In the case of pediatric patients, a parent or legal guardian must sign the consent form. Figure 11-2 is an example of a consent form.

IMMOBILIZATION AND PATIENT RESTRAINT DEVICES

A variety of immobilization and restraint devices are used in CT for both patient safety and to improve the quality of the examinations. Oftentimes straps are used to protect patients from falling from the CT table and to remind

<<FACILITY NAME>>
Request and Consent to Medical, Surgical, Radiological or Other Procedures
Page 1 of 2

1. I have spoken with my doctors and I understand my diagnosis and condition.

2. My doctors have recommended the procedures listed on page 2 for diagnosis and/or treatment of my condition. I understand the potential benefits of these procedures. I understand the risks of not having these procedures.

3. I understand there are risks to me if the recommended procedures are done. These risks were explained to me and I understand them. They are listed on page 2.

4. The approximate location of my surgery or other procedures(operative field) has been explained to me and identified on the illustrations(if applicable). Procedures are categorized for identification and marking as follows:

   <u>Operative Field</u> — all procedures involving right/left distinction of the incision, multiple structures such as fingers or toes and self-identifying skin lesions such as single large lesions(e.g.,single café au lait).

   <u>Specific Surgical Site</u> — all procedures requiring specific surgical site verification, such as lymph nodes, non-self-identifying skin lesions, or breast masses; or identification on the day of surgery, such as cochlear implants, donor nephrectomies, or transplants.

   <u>Intraoperative Surgical Site</u> — all procedures requiring intraoperative surgical site verification, such as cochlear implants requiring EEABR (Electrical Evoked Auditory Brainstem Response) testing, spinal level procedures requiring confirmation by x-ray or stereotactic Neurosurgery and other surgical procedures requiring intraoperative site marking such as plastic reconstructive procedures.

   <u>Excluded Sites</u> — The following sites do no require marking: mid-line sternotomy for open heart surgery, C-Sections, laparotomy and laparoscopy that do not involve left/right distinction of the incision, interventional procedures for which the site of insertion is NOT predetermined, such as cardiac catheterization, endoscopic procedures where the scope passes through the oropharynx, nasopharynx, urethra or rectum,transvaginal or transrectal surgery, procedures of the genitalia, penile, scrotal, testicular, or vulvar areas, and breast biopsy with wire localization and dental procedures.

5. I understand that sometimes during a procedure, the doctors may decide that related or additional procedures are also necessary. I request and authorize the <<facility name>> and the providers responsible for my treatment to perform any necessary additional procedures.

6. I understand that there are risks in addition to those listed in any procedure or in the administration of an anesthetic or sedation analgesia. These include severe blood loss, infection, damage to teeth,mouth,throat,or vocal cords,nerve or eye damage, drug reaction, slowing or stopping of breathing, failure of the anesthetic or sedation analgesia, cardiac arrest, risks that cannot be predicted, permanent disability or even death. Knowing these risks, I consent to the recommended and any additional procedures. I also consent to the use of any anesthetic or sedation analgesia that my doctors or the anesthetists believe is necessary.

7. My doctors have explained the possible alternatives to the recommended surgery or other procedure and their risks. I have decided to proceed with the recommended surgery or other procedure.

8. I here by donate and authorize <<facility name>> to won, retain, preserve, manipulate, analyze, or dispose of any excess tissues, specimens or parts of organs that are removed from my body during the procedures described above and are not necessary for my diagnosis or treatment.<<Facility name>> may use or retransfer these items for any lawful purpose, including education and retrospective research on anonymous specimens.

9. I request and authorize <<facility name>> and such doctors, nurses, medical residents and other trainees, technicians, assistants or others as may be assigned to my case to participate in the diagnosis and treatment of my condition. I understand this may also include representatives of companies that sell equipment that may be used in my surgery or procedure. I also understand that <<facility name>> is a teaching facility and that medical and other students can and do participate in procedures as part of their education. By signing this form, I am agreeing to allow medical or other students to participate in my surgery or procedure. This may include performing an examination under anesthesia that is relevant to my operation.

10. I understand that the practice of medicine and surgery is not an exact science. I have been informed of the probability of success but no promises or guarantees have been made or can be made to me about my surgery or procedure.

List any exceptions under the Exceptions section located on page 2.

FIGURE 11-2 An example of a consent form. A signed consent form is necessary before a CT examination of a more invasive nature, such as a biopsy, is performed.

Date: _____ Time: _____ A.M. / P.M.

PLEASE PRINT CLEARLY WHEN COMPLETING THIS SECTION.

1. My diagnoses/conditions are:

**2. My recommended procedures have been explained by
(Physician)** _____ID#: _____
They are:

3. My risks include:

**4. I understand the approximate location of my procedure or
surgical incision (operative field) as identified on the
illustrations.**

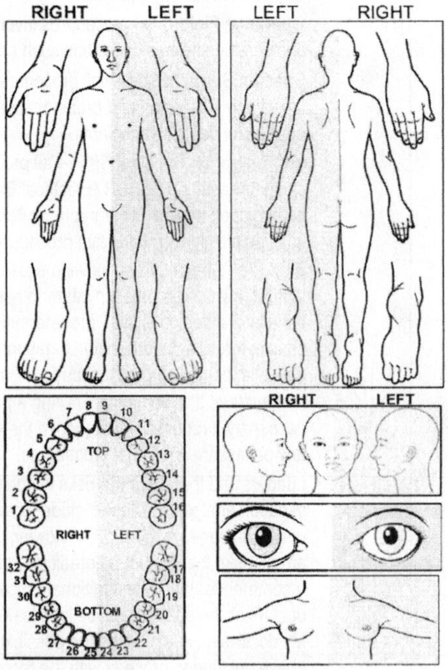

I have read all of the attached information. I have been given the
chance to ask any questions. I understand the answers and have no
other questions. I consent to the following:
PROCEDURE(S)

[ ]   I consent to the procedure(s) listed in #2 above
         (please initial).

Exceptions (to be completed by Provider ONLY): _____
_____
_____
_____
_____

BLOOD TRANSFUSIONS

[X]   Transfusion is not applicable to my operation

_____
Signature of Patient or Legally Authorized Representative (if patient is a minor or unable to sign)

_____
Consent Obtained By:

_____
Date:

BIRTHDATE

NAME

Reg No.

RIGHT   LEFT   LEFT   RIGHT

RIGHT   LEFT

MUST CHECK ONE BOX BELOW:

[ ] **Operative Field:** Check here if the site will be marked
preoperatively on the day of surgery by the Preoperative
Nurse/patient (see page 1).

**Attending performing procedure must initial here to
verify operative field .** ➡ [   ]

**If not initialed, the Attending will be paged to mark the
site preoperatively on the day of the procedure.**

[ ] **Specific Surgical Site:** Check here if the site will be
marked preoperatively on the day of surgery by the
Attending. The Attending will be paged on the day of
surgery (see page 1).

[ ] **Intraoperative Surgical Site:** Check here if the site will
be determined in the operating room on the day of surgery
based on intraoperative testing or intraoperative site
marking (see page 1).

[ ] **Excluded Sites:** Check here if the operative site is
considered an excluded site (see page 1).

FIGURE 11-2   Cont'd.

them to remain still during the procedure. Bean bags can be placed alongside lower limbs to prevent motion that will degrade the CT images. Technologists should be sensitive to the patient's feeling regarding such devices. Before using any immobilization or restraining device the technologist must explain to the patient (or the patient's guardians) the need for the device and show them exactly how it will be used in their care. Whenever possible, basic consent for the use of the device should be given. In some situations consent cannot be obtained, such as for an unaccompanied patient who is unconscious, delirious, or mentally disabled. Technically, a clinician's order is required to use a restraining device for a patient who cannot provide consent. However, the short-term use of restraints to complete an imaging examination is often done without consulting the patient's physician. When restraining devices are used in CT, the following rules should be strictly adhered to:

- The patient must be allowed as much mobility as is safely possible.
- The areas of the body to which immobilizers are applied must be padded to prevent injury to the skin beneath the device.
- Normal anatomic position must be maintained.
- Knots that will become tighter with movement are prohibited.
- The immobilizer must be easy to remove quickly if necessary.
- Neither circulation nor respiration must be impaired by the immobilizer.
- If leg immobilizers are necessary, wrist immobilizers must also be applied to prevent the patient from either unfastening the device or, in an attempt to leave the table or gurney, unintentionally hanging themselves.

ASSESSMENT AND MONITORING VITAL SIGNS

Technologists should begin to assess the patient when they first introduce themselves. It is important to notice the patient's breathing, skin coloration, and overall health before the patient ever lies on the CT table. This will help the technologist notice signs should adverse effects occur during the scan process. Throughout the CT examination the patient should be monitored visually and spoken to frequently using the scanner's intercom system. This reassures the patient and allows the technologist to intervene quickly should problems arise.

Special monitoring devices are not generally required for routine CT examinations performed on stable patients. However, patients from inpatient units may arrive in the CT department already connected to equipment such as monitors or a respirator. Unstable patients and the equipment they arrive with must be watched carefully while in the CT department. Because the CT technologist must

focus on the tasks necessary to perform a high-quality examination, a nurse (or other health professional with appropriate training) should accompany these patients to provide the necessary monitoring and intervene should the need arise.

It is obvious that many of the patients cared for in the CT department are quite ill. In addition to the medical symptoms that necessitated the examination, patients may also have adverse reactions to the intravascular contrast agent used for the examination (more about this in Chapter 12).

Adverse reactions are, for the most part, random and totally unpredictable. Therefore, technologists must be alert for physiologic changes in their patients. The best early indicators of a problem are changes in body temperature, pulse, respirations, and blood pressure. Collectively these are called the vital signs (or cardinal signs). The normal range of vital signs may vary somewhat with age, sex, weight, exercise tolerance, and condition. Other important indicators include pain, pulse oximetry values (indicates blood oxygenation), and pupil size, equality, and reactivity.

BOX 11–8   Key Concept

Vital signs are the best early indicators of a physiologic change in a patient. Vital signs are body temperature, pulse, respirations, and blood pressure.

Body Temperature

Body temperature is most often taken by placing the thermometer in the mouth, the ear (using a tympanic infrared thermometer), the axilla, or the rectum. In the CT department, the thermometer is most often an electronic, battery-operated device with disposable protective sheaths. Other options are tympanic thermometers (also with disposable protective sheaths); disposable, single-use chemical strip thermometers (such as the 3M Tempa-Dot); mercury-free, glass thermometer (a blue tip typically denotes an oral thermometer whereas a red tip denotes a rectal thermometer). Oral, rectal, and tympanic temperature measurements are higher than axillary measurements because the measuring device is in contact with the mucous membrane. Table 11-2 lists the average temperature and the normal range for each temperature site.

Pulse

Each time the heart contracts it forces blood into an already full aorta. The elasticity of the arterial walls allows them to expand to accept the increase in pressure. Pulse is defined as the alternate expansion and recoil of an artery. By counting each expansion of the arterial wall in a given time frame the pulse rate can be determined.

In general, the pulse can be felt wherever a superficial artery can be held against firm tissue, such as a bone.

TABLE 11-2   Average and Normal Range of Body Temperature

Route	Average	Normal Range
Oral	98.7°F (37. 0°C)	96.8° to 100.4°F (36.0° to 38.0°C)
Rectal	99.1°F (37. 7°C)	97.2° to 100.8°F (36.7° to 38.7°C)
Axillary	97.7°F (36.4°C)	95.8° to 99.4°F (35.4° to 37.4°C)
Tympanic*	Calibrated to oral or rectal scales	

*Research is inconclusive as to the accuracy of readings and correlations with other body temperature measurements.[2]

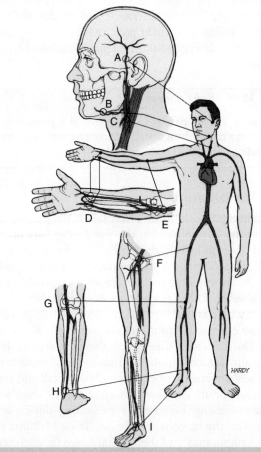

FIGURE 11-3   Locations where pulse can be taken.

Some of the specific locations where the pulse is most easily felt are as follows (Fig. 11-3):

A. Temporal pulse (superficial temporal artery)–just anterior to the ear
B. Facial pulse (facial artery)–the lower margin of the mandible, about one third anterior to the angle
C. Carotid pulse (carotid artery)–along the anterior aspect of the neck, to the right or left of midline

D. Radial pulse (radial artery)–at the thumb side of the wrist
E. Brachial pulse (brachial artery)–on the medial side of the elbow cavity, located between the biceps and triceps muscle, frequently used in place of the carotid pulse in infants
F. Femoral pulse (femoral artery)–in the groin
G. Popliteal pulse (popliteal artery)–behind the knee
H. Pedal pulse (tibialis posterior artery)–posterior ankle, behind medial malleolus
I. Pedal pulse (dorsalis pedis artery)–top of the foot

The patient's blood pressure will impact the ease of palpability of a pulse. If his systolic blood pressure is less than 90 mm Hg, the radial pulse will not be palpable. Less than 80 mm Hg, the brachial pulse will not be palpable. Less than 60 mm Hg, the carotid pulse will not be palpable. Because systolic blood pressure rarely drops that low, the lack of a carotid pulse usually indicates cardiac arrest.

The average adult pulse rate ranges from 60 to 100 beats per minute. However, in athletic adults, a normal pulse rate can range between 45 and 60 beats per minute. The average pulse rate for a child ranges from 95 to 110 beats per minute; infants, from 100 to 160 beats per minute. When a pulse is being counted, the rate, rhythm, and volume should be noted. An irregular pulse is one that has a period of normal rhythm broken by periods of irregularity or skipped beats. The volume (or strength) of the pulse is often described as full and bounding if it seems regular and with good force, or if it is difficult to palpate and irregular it is often described as weak or thready.

Respirations

The respiratory rate is the number of breaths a person takes per minute. It is usually measured when the patient is at rest and simply involves counting the number of breaths for 1 minute by counting how many times the chest rises. Normal respiratory rates vary according to age. Commonly accepted normal ranges are as follows: adults, 14 to 20; adolescent youth, 18 to 22; children, 22 to 28; infants, 30 or greater. The ratio of respiration to pulse is fairly constant at approximately 1 breath to 4 heart beats.

Blood Pressure

Blood pressure may be defined as the pressure exerted by circulating blood on the walls of the vessels. The term blood pressure generally refers to arterial pressure, that is, the pressure measured in the larger arteries. The pressure is determined by the force and amount of blood pumped, and the size and flexibility of the arteries. Blood pressure is continually changing depending on activity, temperature, diet, emotional state, posture, physical state, and medications used. Blood pressure is most commonly measured by a sphygmomanometer (often condensed to sphygmometer), which uses the height of a column of mercury to reflect the circulating pressure. Although many modern blood pressure devices no longer use mercury, values are still universally reported in millimeters of mercury (mm Hg).

The systolic pressure is defined as the peak pressure in the arteries, which occurs near the beginning of the cardiac cycle; the diastolic arterial pressure is the lowest pressure (at the resting phase of the cardiac cycle). Although there are large individual variations, typical values for a resting, healthy adult are approximately 120 mm Hg systolic and 80 mm Hg diastolic. This would be written as 120/80 mm Hg, and spoken as "one twenty over eighty." Hypertension refers to blood pressure that is abnormally high, whereas hypotension refers to blood pressure that is abnormally low. In children the observed normal ranges are lower; in the elderly, they are often higher, largely because of reduced flexibility of the arteries. Sex and race also influence blood pressure values. Debate exists over the optimal blood pressure values that will reduce the risk of cardiovascular disease. However, in the CT department blood pressure is used as an indicator of acute problems; therefore, the technologist need only be concerned about measurements that fall outside of a relatively broad range of values considered "normal." For adults, the normal range of systolic pressure is 90 to 140 mm Hg, diastolic, 60 to 90 mm Hg. For children, the normal range of systolic pressure is 65 to 130 mm Hg, diastolic, 45 to to 85 mm Hg.

BOX 11–9   Key Concept

Systolic pressure is the peak pressure in the arteries; the diastolic pressure is the pressure in the heart's resting phase. Although there is a wide variation, a typical value for a resting, healthy adult is 120 mm Hg systolic and 80 mm Hg diastolic. This is written as 120/80 mm Hg and spoken as "one twenty over eighty."

In radiology, blood pressure is most commonly measured by the auscultatory method that uses a stethoscope and a sphygmomanometer. An inflatable cuff that is attached to a manometer is placed around the upper arm at roughly the same vertical height as the heart. The technologist should take care to use a cuff of the appropriate size (i.e., small cuffs for pediatric patients, larger cuffs for obese patients). The cuff is manually inflated by repeatedly squeezing a rubber bulb until the artery is completely occluded (i.e., gauge reads at least 180 mm Hg). Listening with a stethoscope at the brachial artery at the inside of the elbow, the technologist slowly releases the pressure

in the cuff. When blood begins to flow again in the artery the turbulent flow creates a "whooshing" sound. The pressure at which this sound is first heard is the systolic blood pressure. The cuff pressure continues to be released until no sound can be heard. This point is the diastolic pressure.

SUMMARY

Many critical steps in the CT process occur before the first image is acquired. Safe, clinically useful examinations can only be performed after an appropriate medical history has been taken, the patient has been accurately identified, the examination explained, and the patient consents to the procedure. Safe and effective patient care also necessitates the technologist's understanding of assessment and monitoring techniques.

The steps taken can be summarized as followed:

1. Prepare room
2. Verify order
3. Verify patient identity
4. Obtain medical history
5. Explain examination and obtain consent
6. Continually assess patient

REVIEW QUESTIONS

1. What should be done if there is a discrepancy between the written order and the examination the patient thinks he is scheduled for?
2. Explain how a specific CT protocol is selected.
3. Give one example of information on the patient's medical history that will a) ensure a patient's safety, b) guide the selection of examination protocol, and c) provide the radiologist diagnostic information.
4. What type of information do the following laboratory tests provide: blood urea nitrogen (BUN), serum creatinine, prothrombin time (PT), partial thromboplastin time (PTT), and platelet count?
5. Explain the difference between basic (or simple) consent and informed consent.
6. Name each of the vital signs and give an approximate normal range for an adult patient of each.

REFERENCES

1. Altman GB. Delmar's Fundamental and Advanced Nursing Skill. 2nd Ed. Theomson Learning, 2004.
2. Craig JV, Lancaster GA, Taylor S, Williamson PR, Smyth RL. Infrared ear thermometry compared with rectal thermometry in children: a systematic review. Lancet 2002;360:603–9.

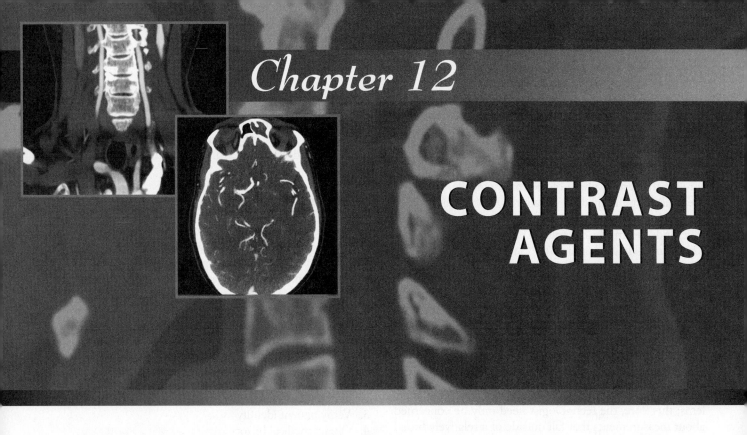

Chapter 12

CONTRAST AGENTS

Key Terms: positive agents • negative agents • osmolality • isotonic • hyperosmolar hypertonic • high-osmolality contrast media (HOCM) • low-osmolality contrast media (LOCM) • isosmolar contrast media (IOCM) • viscosity • ionicity • clearance • half-life • dose • subjective side effects • chemotoxic reactions • idiosyncratic reactions • anaphylactoid • delayed reactions • premedication • contrast media-induced nephropathy (CIN) • acute renal failure (ARF) • homeostasis • glomerular filtration rate (GFR) • serum creatinine (SeCr) • renal failure • renal insufficiency • nephropathy • metformin therapy • hyperthyroidism • thyroid toxicosis • thyroid storm • Graves' disease • blood-brain barrier • interleukin-2 • neutral contrast agents • barium peritonitis

To distinguish adjacent tissues on a CT image, the tissues must have different densities (attenuation). These varying densities will result in distinct attenuation coefficients, which produce an image that clearly displays the different tissues.

In some parts of the body, such as the chest, subject contrast is inherently high. The pulmonary vessels and ribs have significantly different densities from the adjacent aerated lung, which allows easy identification on the image. Unfortunately, not all areas of the body possess this level of inherent tissue contrast. Often, many tissues have quite similar attenuation coefficients. In addition, tumors and other disease processes may have attenuation coefficients that are very similar to their surrounding tissues.

An oral or intravenous administration of a contrast agent is often used to create a temporary, artificial density difference between objects. The goal is to give different tissues, which would ordinarily have similar attenuations, different attenuation coefficients, making them more readily visible on the image. Methods of contrast administration vary widely, but in CT, enhancement falls into the two main categories of intravascular and gastrointestinal. Less commonly, contrast agents can be administered intrathecally (into the subarachnoid space surrounding the spinal cord) or intraarticularly (directly into a joint space). In all categories, contrast agents fill a structure with a material that has a different density than that of the structure. In the case of most agents that contain barium and iodine, the material is of a higher density than the structure. These are typically referred to as positive agents. Low-density contrast agents, or negative agents, such as air or carbon dioxide, can also be used. Certain gastrointestinal agents possess a density similar to that of water and are sometimes referred to as "neutral" contrast agents.

BOX 12–1   Key Concept

Contrast agents fill a structure with a material that has a different density than that of the structure. When the agent is of a higher density than the structure it is referred to as a positive agent. When the agent is of a lower density than the surrounding structure it is referred to as a negative agent.

INTRAVASCULAR CONTRAST AGENTS

Iodinated agents are universally used for a variety of radiology examinations because they are water soluble, easy to administer intravascularly, and have a high safety index. Over the years many different agents other than iodine have been tested for intravascular use, but none have become commercially available for widespread clinical use because of unacceptable toxic side effects.

Properties of Iodinated Agents

Intravascular contrast material has high attenuation compared with human soft tissue, and therefore, wherever it distributes it increases the ability of the enhanced structure to attenuate the x-ray beam. Because of their relatively high atomic number of 53, the iodine atoms in the contrast material are responsible for this increase in attenuation. Adding an iodinated agent to the bloodstream will temporarily increase the beam-attenuating ability of the blood; structures with an adequate blood supply show an increase in attenuation, which is displayed as a change from darker to lighter on the image.

Two tissues must differ by at least 10 Hounsfield units (HU) to be visibly different on a CT scan. Because different tissues often enhance differently, and because intravascular contrast material is handled differently in normal versus abnormal tissue, contrast agents can serve to widen the inherent difference in attenuation. This difference often allows tissues, tumors, and disease processes to be more easily discernible. The proper administration of contrast media can easily provide a 40- to 75-HU increase in the natural difference of attenuation between tissues, thus making them visibly different in the image.

BOX 12-2   Key Concept

Contrast agents can serve to widen the difference in attenuation between adjacent structures because different tissues often enhance differently and because intravascular contrast material is handled differently in normal versus abnormal tissue.

Contrast agent administration varies significantly from other pharmaceuticals that are administered intravascularly. Unlike other medications, iodinated agents are not used for their therapeutic qualities, but rather for their distribution and elimination from the body. The difference is even more dramatic when dose and delivery are considered. Therapeutic agents are given in very small quantities at regularly spaced intervals, whereas relatively large quantities of contrast media are typically given in a bolus lasting only a minute or two, with the intention of having no untoward physical effects. To illustrate the disparity, consider the use of morphine sulfate, given specifically to alleviate pain, at a typical dose of 2 to 10 mg diluted in 5 to 15 mL of sterile water, and

given at regular intervals of 4 hours. Compare this with iodinated contrast agents that are given in a single dose, typically between 100 and 150 mL, and often delivered in less than a minute. Because of these dramatic differences, guidelines for the use of other pharmaceuticals are of little value when applied to the use of intravenous (IV) contrast agents.

Osmolality

Most intravascular drugs are nearly isotonic; that is, they have nearly the same number of particles in solution per unit of liquid as blood. Contrast agents may have up to seven times the number of particles in solution per unit of liquid as blood. The structural property of a liquid regarding the number of particles in solution is known as osmolality. Osmolality is measured in milliosmoles per kilogram (mOsm/kg) of water. The osmolality of blood plasma is approximately 290 mOsm/kg water.

BOX 12-3   Key Concept

Osmolality is a property of intravascular contrast media that refers to the number of particles in solution, per unit liquid, as compared with blood.

High-osmolality contrast media may have as much as seven times the osmolality of blood.

Low-osmolality contrast media has roughly twice the osmolality of blood.

Contrast media that is isosmolar has the same osmolality as blood.

Most brands of iodinated contrast medium have a greater osmolality than blood plasma. Therefore, most contrast agents are said to be hyperosmolar or hypertonic solutions. Older iodinated agents, now less commonly used for intravascular injections, are considered high-osmolality contrast media (HOCM). The osmolality of these agents range from approximately 1,300 to 2,140 mOsm/kg, or about 4 to 7 times that of human blood. In the 1980s contrast agents were introduced with much lower osmolality, from approximately 600 to 850 mOsm/kg, or roughly 2 to 3 times the osmolality of human blood. Hence, these agents have been classified as low-osmolality contrast media (LOCM). Although the exact mechanisms of adverse reactions are still not completely understood, it is certain that the osmolality of the agent does play a role in contrast media safety. Initially, the LOCM were much more expensive than the older HOCM. Because of their high cost, the newer agents were often reserved for use in patients considered to be at a higher risk of adverse reactions. Many different criteria were developed. However, regardless of the criteria used, accurate patient screening and risk stratification was problematic and could not reliably predict which patient might have the rare, life-threatening reaction to iodinated contrast media. As the cost of LOCM decreased, the practice of the universal intravascular use of LOCM has increased.

In 1996, a contrast agent (Visipaque, GE Healthcare, Milwaukee WS) was introduced with an osmolality equal to that of blood. It is referred to as an isosmolar contrast media (IOCM) and is considerably more expensive than LOCM. It has been suggested that isosmolar contrast media may offer some advantages, particularly in patients at risk of renal complications. The effect of all types of contrast medium on renal function will be discussed in detail later in this chapter.

Osmolality is universally recognized as playing a major role in nonallergic reactions to contrast medium. A bolus injection of a hypertonic contrast agent causes a rapid increase in the osmolality of the plasma. The higher the agent's osmolality, the more pronounced the effects of this increase.

Viscosity

Contrast material is much more viscous than most other intravascular agents. Viscosity is a physical property that may be described as the thickness or friction of the fluid as it flows. It is an important property that will influence the injectability of intravascular agents through small-bore needles and intravenous catheters. Molecular structure and concentration affect viscosity; therefore, different brands of iodinated contrast media will possess varying viscosities. The viscosity of the contrast material can be significantly decreased by heating the liquid to body temperature for injection. Warming a contrast agent reduces viscosity in a way similar to warming maple syrup. Finally, the concentration of iodine in the agent affects its viscosity; the higher the concentration of iodine, the more viscous the solution.

BOX 12-4   Key Concept

Viscosity is a physical property of intravascular contrast media. It can be described as the thickness or friction of the fluid as it flows. The brand, temperature, and concentration of the contrast affect its viscosity.

Ionicity

Intravascular contrast agents can be classified as to whether the molecules they contain will separate into charged particles (i.e., ions) when dissolved in an aqueous solution. Ionic contrast agents are composed of molecules that will dissociate into ions when in solution. The molecules contained in nonionic contrast media do not dissociate. Although most nonionic contrast agents also have low osmolality, the two terms are not synonymous. An LOCM may be ionic. Hexabrix (Mallinckrodt, Inc., St. Louis, MO) is an example of a contrast agent that is low osmolality but ionic. Table 12-1 lists many brands of contrast agents, along with their osmolality, viscosity, and whether they are ionic or nonionic.

BOX 12-5   Key Concept

In solution, ionic contrast agents contain molecules that will form ions. The molecules contained in nonionic contrast media do not disassociate.

Although most nonionic contrast agents also have low osmolality, the terms are not synonymous.

Clearance

Once injected, all types of iodinated contrast media undergo very rapid distribution throughout the entire extracellular space. They are not metabolized and are excreted by the body nearly exclusively by the kidney via glomerular filtration. The half-life (i.e., time it takes for half of the dose to be eliminated from the body) in patients with normal renal function is approximately 2 hours.[1]

Dose

To accurately assess the dose of iodinated contrast agent to be delivered, both the iodine concentration and the volume must be considered. The beam attenuation abilities of a given amount of contrast media are directly related to the concentration of iodine. Many concentrations are commercially available. LOCM are measured in milligrams of iodine per milliliter (mgI/mL) of solution, whereas most HOCM are labeled in terms of their percent weight per volume, but the concentration of iodine in mg/mL is easily found in tables or on the vial label. When comparing doses between different contrast concentrations and volumes, it is often useful to look at the total grams of iodine delivered.

Different CT scan protocols require different doses of iodine. These will be listed in the section that deals with imaging protocols. In some instances, the injection rate and the delay from injection to scanning will affect the contrast dose selected for the examination. In addition, the iodine concentration of the contrast will affect the selection of injection flow rate. This is because contrast enhancement in CT depends on the iodine concentration in the vasculature or tissues. In the vessels, this concentration depends on the injection rate of iodine in mg/s. Therefore, a concentration of 400 mg/mL

Clinical Application Box 12-1

Total Iodine Delivered

How many grams of iodine will be delivered when:
125 mL of an agent with a concentration of 240 mgI/mL is injected
   Answer: 125 mL × 240 mgI/mL = 30,000 mgI = 30 gI
100 mL of an agent with a concentration of 300 mgI/mL
   Answer: 100 mL × 300 mgI/mL = 30,000 mgI = 30 gI
150 mL of an agent with a concentration of 370 mgI/mL
   Answer: 150 mL × 370 mgI/mL = 55,500 mgI = 55.5 gI

TABLE 12-1   Contrast Media Characteristics

Product	Chemical Name	Iodine Concentration (mgI/mL)	Osmolality (mOsm/kg H$_2$O)	Viscosity (cP at 37°C)
Intravascular, Nonionic				
Ultravist 240 (Bayer HealthCare)	Iopromide	240	483	2.8
Optiray 240 (Mallinckrodt)	Ioversol	240	502	3.0
Omnipaque 240 (GE Healthcare)	Iohexol	240	520	3.4
Isovue 250 (Bracco)	Iopamidol	250	524	3.0
Visipaque 270 (GE Healthcare)	Iodixanol	270	290	6.3
Oxilan 300 (Guerbet)	Ioxilan	300	585	5.1
Ultravist 300 (Bayer HealthCare)	Iopromide	300	407	4.9
Isovue 300 (Bracco)	Iopamidol	300	616	4.7
Optiray 300 (Malinckrodt)	Ioversol	300	651	5.5
Omnipaque 300 (GE Healthcare)	Iohexol	300	672	6.3
Visipaque 320 (GE Healthcare)	Iodixanol	320	290	11.8
Optiray 320 (Mallinckrodt)	Ioversol	320	702	7.5
Oxilan 350 (Guerbet)	Ioxilan	350	695	8.1
Optiray 350 (Mallinckrodt)	Ioversol	350	792	9.0
Omnipaque 350 (GE Healthcare)	Iohexol	350	844	10.4
Ultravist 370 (Bayer HealthCare)	Iopromide	370	774	10.0
Isovue 370 (Bracco)	Iopamidol	370	796	9.4
Intravascular, Ionic				
Conray (Mallinckrodt)	Meglumine Iothalamate	282	1400	4.0
Reno 60 (Bracco)	Diatrizoate Meglumine	282	1404	4.3
Renografin 60 (Bracco)	Diatrizoate Meglumine and Diatrizoate Sodium	292.5	1450	4.2
Hexabrix (Mallinckrodt)	Ioxaglate Meglumine and Ioxaglate Sodium	300	600	7.5
MD-76 (Mallinckrodt)	Diatrizoate Meglumine and Diatrizoate Sodium	370	1550	10.5
Conray 400 (Mallinckrodt)	Meglumine Iothalamate	400	2300	4.5

injected at 3 mL/s will provide the same enhancement as a concentration of 300 mg/mL injected at 4 mL/s. Specific injection techniques are discussed in Chapter 13.

Undoubtedly, an adequate dose of iodinated contrast is an essential component in producing examinations of consistently high quality. The dose must also be safe for the patient. Although they rarely occur, an overdose of iodinated contrast media is possible. Deaths have occurred as a result of volumes of 250 to 300 mL of undiluted, HOCM, ionic media.[2] The adverse effects of overdosage affect mainly the pulmonary and cardiovascular systems.[3] Because of the risk of overdose, most facilities set guidelines as to the upper limit on the total volume of contrast media given all at once for routine examinations, regardless of the patient's size. Individual factors, such as a patient's level of hydration, can influence what is a safe dose. Therefore, this upper limit is often quite cautious, typically 200 mL of an agent with a concentration of 320 mgI/mL (a total of 64 grams of iodine). It should be noted, however, that specific circumstances may necessitate exceeding this 200-mL guideline. A radiologist is responsible for determining in what instances, and to what extent, a facility's guidelines can be safely exceeded.

Regardless of the type of iodinated contrast agent, the lowest dose necessary to obtain adequate visualization should be used. A lower dose may reduce the possibility of an adverse reaction, particularly those affecting renal function. Seldom does a CT procedure require either the maximum volume or the highest concentration of an iodinated contrast. The combination of volume and concentration to be used should be individualized accounting for factors such as age, body weight, and the size of the vessel into which it will be injected. Other factors include anticipated pathology, degree and extent of opacification required, structure(s) or area to be examined, disease processes affecting the patient, and the specific equipment available.

In most clinical practices, the dose used to perform CT examinations on pediatric patients is calculated by weight. The most common formula used is 2 mL/kg. It is interesting to note that dose formulas are typically abandoned when it comes to scanning adults, and the same dose is

TABLE 12-2 Examples of Dose Variation When a Uniform Contrast Media Dose Is Used on All Adult Patients

Patient Weight in kg (lb)	mL/kg With a Uniform Dose of 100 mL
46 kg (102.5 lb)	2.17 mL/kg
68 kg (149.6 lb)	1.47 mL/kg
91 kg (200.2 lb)	1.09 mL/kg
114 kg (250.8 lb)	0.88 mL/kg
137 kg (301.4 lb)	0.72 mL/kg
160 kg (353 lb)	0.63 mL/kg

given whether the patient is a 100-pound woman or a 350-pound man. Table 12-2 demonstrates the dose variation, in mL/kg, when a uniform dose of contrast agent is given to all adult patients. In this example, a 100-pound woman would receive more than three times the dose per kg as the 350-pound man.

BOX 12-6 Key Concept

The most common formula for calculating the dose of intravascular contrast for pediatric CT studies is 2 mL/kg.

It is unclear how the practice of administering a uniform dose of an IV contrast agent, regardless of the size of the adult patient, became so well established. Did the practice arise from the convenience of using the same dose for each patient? Ultimately, the important question is whether this system is best for the patient. Does a protocol of uniform dosing result in underdosing the heavier patients and overdosing the lighter ones? Studies have been conducted that compared the examination quality from uniform dosing protocols to those that result when a weight-based system is used.[4,5] The results of these studies suggest that the quality of examinations are the same, or better, when a weight-based dosing protocol is used. An example of a weight-based calculation for routine body scanning is 1.5 mL/kg (not to exceed 200 mL). Furthermore, when compared with using a standard dose of 150 mL, a significant cost savings can be realized using a weight-based dose (provided prefilled syringes are not used).

Iodinated Contrast Media During Pregnancy and Lactation

Pregnancy

As a result of concerns about exposing the fetus to ionizing radiation, CT examinations are seldom done during pregnancy. Occasionally, such examinations may be vital for the mother's health. Studies of iodinated contrast agents in pregnancy have been limited, and effects on the human embryo or fetus are unknown. Laboratory and animal tests of HOCM and LOCM, respectively, found no mutagenic or teratogenic effects. Iodinated contrast media

have been shown to cross the human placenta and enter the fetus.

The ACR Committee on Drugs and Contrast Media has reviewed this issue extensively and has prepared a summary of information and recommendations, shown in Table 12-3.

BOX 12-7 Key Concept

There is no proof that contrast agents present a risk to the fetus. However, there is not enough evidence to be certain they pose no risk.

Lactation

Contrast-enhanced CT is sometimes performed on a woman who is breast-feeding. Often the patient expresses concerns regarding the potential adverse effects to the infant from contrast media that is excreted into the breast milk.

Although the literature regarding the excretion of iodinated contrast media is limited, some important facts are known. Less than 1% of the dose of contrast agent given to the mother is excreted into breast milk. Moreover, less than 1% of the contrast medium in breast milk ingested by an infant is absorbed from the gastrointestinal tract. Therefore, the expected dose of contrast medium absorbed by an infant from ingested breast milk is extremely low. For example, if the maternal dose of contrast agent is 150 mL, the breast-fed infant can be expected to ingest just 0.015 mL of the contrast agent.

The ACR committee on Drugs and Contrast Media provides a summary information and recommendations (Table 12-4).

BOX 12-8 Key Concept

A very small percentage of the iodinated contrast medium given to a mother will be excreted into breast milk and absorbed by the infant. Therefore, it is believed to be safe for the mother and infant to continue breast-feeding after receiving a contrast agent.

Adverse Effects of Iodinated Contrast Medium

Iodinated contrast agents are one of the most widely used of all medications. They are also one of the safest.[6] Fatal reactions are extremely rare in both HOCM and LOCM, estimated at 0.9 per 100,000 (<0.001%).[7] Nonetheless, it is well documented that adverse reactions sometimes occur with their use. It is impossible to accurately predict which patients will have an adverse reaction. The drugs and equipment needed to treat acute reactions must be readily available, and staff must be trained to respond quickly.

TABLE 12-3   Administration of Contrast Media to Pregnant or Potentially Pregnant Patients

Iodinated X-ray Contrast Media (Ionic and Nonionic)

Diagnostic iodinated contrast agents have been shown to cross the human placenta and enter the fetus when given in usual clinical doses. No adequate and well-controlled teratogenic studies of the effects of these agents in pregnant women have been performed.

In conjunction with the existing ACR policy for the use of ionizing radiation in pregnant women, we recommend that all imaging facilities should have polices and procedures to reasonably attempt to identify pregnant patients prior to the performance of any diagnostic examination involving ionizing radiation to determine the medical necessity for the administration of iodinated contrast media. If a patient is known to be pregnant, both the potential radiation risk and the potential added risks of contrast media should be considered before proceeding with the study. (Res. 24, 1995, ACR Policy)

Although it is not possible to conclude that contrast agents present a definite risk to the fetus, there is insufficient evidence to conclude that they pose no risk. Consequently, the committee recommends the following:

A. The radiologist should confer with the referring physician and document in the radiology report or the patient's medical record the following:
  1. That the information requested and the necessity for contrast material administration cannot be acquired via other means (e.g., ultrasonography).
  2. That the information needed affects the care of the patient and fetus *during the pregnancy.*
  3. That the referring physician is of the opinion that it is not prudent to wait to obtain this information until after the patient is no longer pregnant.
B. It is recommended that pregnant patients undergoing a diagnostic imaging examination with ionizing radiation and iodinated contrast material provide informed consent to document that they understand the risk-benefits of the procedure to be performed and the alternative diagnostic options available to them (if any), and that they wish to proceed.

Reprinted with permission from The American College of Radiology. Manual on Contrast Media, version 6, 2008:61–3. Available at http://www.acr.org/SecondaryMainMenuCategories/quality_safety/contrast_manual.aspx. Accessed February 9, 2009.

TABLE 12-4   Administration of Contrast Media to Breast-Feeding Mothers

Iodinated X-ray Contrast Media (Ionic and Nonionic)

Background

The plasma half-life of intravenously administered iodinated contrast medium is approximately 2 hours, with nearly 100% of the agent cleared from the bloodstream within 24 hours. Because of its low lipid solubility, less than 1% of the administered maternal dose of iodinated contrast medium is excreted into the breast milk in the first 24 hours. Because less than 1% of the contrast medium ingested by the infant is absorbed from its gastrointestinal tract, the expected dose absorbed by the infant from the breast milk is less than 0.01% of the intravascular dose given to the mother. This amount of contrast medium represents less than 1% of the recommended dose for an infant undergoing an imaging study, which is 2 mL/kg. The potential risks to the infant include direct toxicity and allergic sensitization or reaction, which are theoretical concerns but have not been reported.

Recommendation

Mothers who are breast-feeding should be given the opportunity to make an informed decision as to whether to continue or temporarily abstain from breast-feeding after receiving intravascularly administered iodinated contrast media. Because of the very small percentage of iodinated contrast medium that is excreted into the breast milk and absorbed by the infant's gut, we believe that the available data suggest that it is safe for the mother and infant to continue breast-feeding after receiving such an agent. If the mother remains concerned about any potential ill effects to the infant, she may abstain from breast-feeding for 24 hours with active expression and discarding of breast milk from both breasts during that period. In anticipation of this, she may wish to use a breast pump to obtain milk before the contrast study to feed the infant during the 24-hour period following the examination.

Reprinted with permission from The American College of Radiology. Manual on Contrast Media, version 6, 2008:65–6. Available at http://www.acr.org/SecondaryMainMenuCategories/quality_safety/contrast_manual.aspx. Accessed February 9, 2009.

BOX 12–9   Key Concept

It is impossible to predict which patients will have an adverse reaction to intravenously administered contrast medium. Therefore, CT staff must be trained to respond quickly.

Mechanism of Adverse Reactions

The term "contrast reaction" can be confusing because it is used in a variety of different ways in relation to the effects of iodinated radiologic contrast agents. In some instances, it is used to describe all undesired effects including the many subjective side effects experienced to some degree by most patients to whom contrast is administered. These subjective effects include the feeling of heat, nausea, and mild flushing. In other instances, the term contrast reaction is used to describe the less common, more serious side effects that may require treatment or even be life threatening.

There is variation in the literature between quoted incidences of adverse reactions to contrast media. This is attributable to a number of reasons, but mainly because there is no standard definition of an adverse reaction or standard system to classify their severity. The ACR Manual on Contrast Media provides a severity-based classification that is widely, though not universally, used.

In an effort to simplify the discussion of adverse reactions to injectable contrast media, it is useful to separate reactions into two categories: chemotoxic reactions and idiosyncratic reactions. However, in clinical practice it can be difficult to characterize some reactions into one group or the other.

Chemotoxic reactions result from the physicochemical properties of the contrast media, the dose, and speed of injection. All hemodynamic (i.e., relating to blood circulation) disturbances and injuries to organs or vessels perfused by the contrast medium are included in this category. Contrast-induced nephropathy is an example of a chemotoxic reaction.

Idiosyncratic reactions include all other reactions. These reactions are largely unpredictable, most often occur within 1 hour of contrast medium administration, and are not related to the dose. The mechanisms by which idiosyncratic reactions occur are not precisely understood. The origin of these reactions is rarely, if ever, "an allergy."[8] True allergic reactions result in the production of antibodies. These are not found after reactions to contrast media. In addition, if the reaction were an allergy it would be expected that patients would consistently suffer a similar or more severe adverse event with subsequent contrast injections. But researchers have not found this to be true; instead the incidence of recurrent reactions appears to be relatively low. With intravenous administration, the risk of recurrent reaction in a patient with a prior reaction is 16% to 35% when HOCM[9-12] is used and even lower (approximately 7%) when LOCM is used.[8] Even though the underlying cause is likely different, symptoms of idiosyncratic reactions resemble allergic (or anaphylactic) reactions and are, therefore, often called "allergic-like" or "anaphylactoid" reactions. Even though not completely accurate, the term "contrast allergy" remains in common use.

BOX 12–10   Key Concept
Contrast media reactions can be broadly categorized as either chemotoxic or idiosyncratic in nature.

Children have a lower frequency of contrast reactions than adults.[13] When they do occur, they tend to be idiosyncratic in nature. Infants and young children are unable to verbalize discomfort or symptoms, posing additional challenges for the CT staff. Young patients must be carefully monitored throughout the examination. In addition, pediatric emergency equipment should be available in all locations where intravascular contrast media are administered to children.

Most adverse reactions occur within minutes of injection, but delayed reactions have also been reported. It is not clear whether delayed reactions are idiosyncratic or chemotoxic in nature. It is likely that both factors play a role; that is, some delayed reactions are idiopathic and others chemotoxic. Because delayed reactions are poorly understood and difficult to classify, in this text they are treated separately.

Side effects of intravascular contrast media administration that are common and can be expected to occur in many, if not most, patients are nausea, vomiting, altered taste (often described as metallic), perspiration, warmth, flushing, and anxiety. These side effects are much less common when LOCM are used. In the most common usage of the term, these effects are not considered a contrast reaction; they are generally of no clinical consequence. However, although they do not endanger the patient, some side effects (such as vomiting) may delay the start of scanning and thereby affect the quality of the examination.

Idiosyncratic Reactions

Classifications of Idiosyncratic Reactions Acute idiosyncratic reactions are usually characterized as mild, moderate, or severe. Mild reactions are usually of short duration and self-limiting. Although a mild reaction does not require treatment the patient should be carefully monitored for at least 20 to 30 minutes, as symptoms of a mild reaction may become a more severe reaction. Examples of symptoms of a mild reaction are cough, itching, rash (hives), pallor, nasal stuffiness, minimal swelling in the eyes and face, and facial rash.

Moderately adverse reactions are not immediately life threatening, although they may progress to be so. Symptoms that usually require treatment include respiratory difficulties (bronchospasm, dyspnea, wheezing, mild laryngeal edema), pulse change,* hypertension, and hypotension. Treatment may include diphenhydramine (Benadryl, Johnson & Johnson) for symptomatic hives, leg

---

*Slow pulse, usually accompanied by hypotension, typically represents a vasovagal reaction. Vasovagal reactions are not allergic-like in nature, but because the initial presentation of hypotension must be differentiated from allergic-like hypotension, it is usually included with the allergic-like reactions for convenience.

elevation for hypotension, use of a β-agonist inhaler for bronchospasm, or epinephrine for laryngeal edema.[13]

Severe reactions are potentially or immediately life threatening. Symptoms include substantial respiratory distress, unresponsiveness, convulsions, clinically manifested arrhythmias, and cardiopulmonary arrest. Although life-threatening reactions are rare, it is imperative that all technologists be aware that they can occur and that they require prompt recognition and treatment. Most severe reactions occur soon after administration and can begin with any number of signs and symptoms, ranging from anxiety to diffuse erythema to cardiac arrest.[13] Complete cardiovascular collapse requires prompt cardiopulmonary resuscitation, advanced specialized life-support equipment, and trained personnel. Although idiosyncratic contrast reactions are not truly anaphylactic in origin (because antibodies to contrast agents have not been demonstrated), the clinical presentation is often identical to that of acute anaphylaxis and the treatment is the same; that is to say, the "ABCs" (airway assessment, breathing, and circulation) followed by appropriate advanced cardiac life support (ACLS) treatment.[13]

Incidence and Risk Factors for Idiosyncratic Reactions The majority of idiosyncratic adverse side effects are mild, non–life-threatening events that require only observation, reassurance, and support. The reported rate of all types of reactions for HOCM is from 5% to 12%. Of those, 98% to 99% are classified as mild.[9,14] Reported reaction rates from LOCM are much lower than HOCM, by a factor of approximately four to five times.[8,10] Because death from either HOCM or LOCM is very rare, it is difficult to accurately assess the mortality rate. Some data suggest that there is no significant difference in mortality between the types of contrast agents, but other data suggest a lower mortality with LOCM.[10,11]

Previous Contrast Medium Reaction As previously stated, the mechanism for idiosyncratic reactions to contrast media is not thoroughly understood. Contrast reactions are not true allergic responses, although the symptoms, and therefore, the treatment of these symptoms, are virtually indistinguishable from an allergic response. Why then is it important to make the distinction by referring to idiosyncratic reactions as "allergic-like"? Primarily, the difference is important when considering the risk of subsequent contrast-enhanced examinations in patients who have had a previous reaction to contrast media. In a true drug allergy, the first time a medication is administered the immune system launches an incorrect response against a substance that is harmless in most people. The next time the medication is given the body produces antibodies and histamine. Although first-time exposure may only produce a mild reaction, repeated exposures may lead to more serious reactions. Once a person is sensitized (has had a previous reaction), even a very limited exposure to a very small amount of allergen can trigger a severe reaction. The recommendation is that individuals avoid medications that have caused an allergic reaction, even a mild one, in the past. Idiosyncratic contrast reactions are not true allergies, and repeat administration does not carry the same certainty of a reaction as does repeat exposure to a true allergen. Nonetheless, the reaction rate is higher among individuals who have had a previous reaction to contrast medium compared with those who have no history of a reaction. With HOCM, the risk of a reaction in a patient who reacted previously has been stated to be 16% to 35% [9,12] and to be 11 times greater than the risk in a nonreactor.[14] When a patient who previously reacted to an HOCM is given an LOCM, the risk of a repeat reaction is reduced to approximately 5%.[15] So, although a previous contrast medium reaction is a poor predictor of subsequent reactions, it must still be taken into consideration because it is impossible to know which patients will react. In fact, of the relative risk factors predictive of a contrast reaction, a previous contrast reaction is considered to be the most important.

BOX 12–11   Key Concept

Contrast reactions are not true allergic responses, although the symptoms, and therefore, the treatment of these symptoms, are virtually indistinguishable from an allergic response. This difference is important when considering the risk of subsequent contrast-enhanced exams in patients that have had a previous reaction to contrast media. Only a small percentage of patients will have repeat adverse reactions (although it is impossible to accurately predict which patient will). This is very different from a true allergic reaction which is nearly guaranteed to produce the same, or even more severe, reaction when exposure to the allergen is repeated.

Asthma Asthma is also considered a risk factor. Although there is some variation in the reported incidence, patients with asthma have approximately eight times the risk of reaction to HOCM, and about five times the risk of reaction to LOCM compared with the population of patients without asthma.[10]

Allergies A history of allergy to food, drugs, or other substances is associated with an increased risk of adverse reaction to contrast media. Allergic conditions such as hayfever and eczema are also associated with an increased risk of reaction. In most reports, these are less of a risk than asthma; a twofold risk is commonly cited.[10,12]

Patients with a history of allergy to foods that contain iodine (e.g., seafood) often cause particular concern in the CT department. However, this worry is unfounded. Seafood allergy results from hypersensitivity to a protein within the seafood and has no association with iodine. Many years of data substantiate that allergy to seafood is no more or less significant than allergy to other foods.[9,12,16]

Specific questioning of patients concerning seafood allergies perpetuates the myth and should be avoided. In addition, an allergy to topical iodine skin preparations (e.g., Betadine) does not increase the risk of contrast medium reactions.[12]

BOX 12-12   Key Concept

An allergy to seafood (or other iodine-containing foods) is no more significant than an allergy to other foods. Also, an allergy to topical iodine skin preparation does not indicate an allergy to iodinated contrast media.

Drugs   There is speculation that patients taking β-blockers may be at increased risk for idiosyncratic contrast actions, but this has not been proved. However, it is agreed that the use of β-blockers can impair the response to treatment should a reaction occur.[12]

Prevention of Acute Idiosyncratic Reactions   In patients identified as being at increased risk of adverse reaction to contrast medium, the possibility of performing the CT examination without the benefit of a contrast agent or using an alternative diagnostic method (e.g., ultrasonography, magnetic resonance imaging) should be considered. This decision is outside the technologist's scope of practice. The technologist should bring all relevant information to the attention of a radiologist. If iodinated contrast medium is deemed essential, steps can be taken to reduce the associated risks.

Although the majority of severe reactions occur within the first 20 minutes after contrast medium injection,[12] it is prudent to have high-risk patients remain monitored in the radiology department for 1 hour.

Idiosyncratic reactions are not dose dependent; reactions have resulted from very small volumes of iodinated contrast media. Test injections are of no predictive value and are not recommended.

BOX 12-13   Key Concept

Patients identified as being at increased risk of an adverse reaction to contrast medium should be brought to the attention of the radiologist. If contrast media is deemed essential the patient should be monitored in the radiology department for 1 hour and should receive LOCM.

Use LOCM   The most important method of reducing the risk of idiosyncratic contrast medium reaction is to use LOCM. The risk associated with these agents is four to five times lower than that of HOCM. Patients with a history of contrast reaction to HOCM and subsequently given LOCM had less incidence of adverse reaction than patients without a history of allergy who were given HOCM.[12]

Role of Premedication   There is good evidence that pretreatment with steroids will reduce the rate of idiosyncratic contrast medium reactions when HOCM is given.[12] When LOCM is used there is less certainty that premedication with steroids is helpful in reducing moderate or severe adverse reactions.[6] Available data can be interpreted in different ways: some radiologists believe that steroid pretreatment in conjunction with LOCM is effective only in reducing minor reactions; others conclude that it is likely that moderate and severe reactions are reduced as well.

Pretreatment with steroids does not prevent all contrast reactions; some patients experience contrast reactions despite steroid pretreatment. The goal of pretreating high-risk patients is to reduce their risk. The degree to which that risk is reduced is unknown, although it is generally believed that pretreating high-risk patients reduces their risk.

When the decision to premedicate is made by the radiologist, a variety of regimens can be used. Two common regimens are outlined in Table 12-5. When steroid premedication is used, it is important that the steroids be started at least 6 hours (but preferably 12 hours) before contrast medium administration. Oral administration of steroids seems preferable to intravenous administration, and prednisone and methylprednisolone are equally effective.[13] If the patient is unable to take oral medication, 200 mg of hydrocortisone intravenously may be substituted for oral prednisone. In addition to the steroids, the administration of an H_1 antihistamine (e.g., diphenhydramine), given either orally or intravenously, may reduce the frequency of urticaria, angioedema, and respiratory symptoms.[13]

When there has been a previous reaction to LOCM, the use of a different brand of LOCM has been recommended to lower the risk of a repeat adverse event, although this has not been scientifically substantiated.

TABLE 12-5   Two Frequently Used Premedication Regimens (for Adult Patients)*

Regimen 1: Corticosteroid/antihistamine
13 hours before examination: prednisone 50 mg by mouth
7 hours before examination: prednisone 50 mg by mouth
1 hour before examination: prednisone 50 mg by mouth
1 hour before examination: diphenhydramine (Benadryl) 50 mg by mouth
Use LOCM

Regimen 2: Corticosteroid alone
12 hours before examination: methylprednisolone (Medrol) 32 mg by mouth
2 hours before examination: methylprednisolone (Medrol) 32 mg by mouth
Use LOCM

*Premedication regimens must be initiated by a licensed prescriber and is outside the technologist's scope of practice.

BOX 12-14 Key Concept

Steroid pretreatment is effective in reducing the rate of idiosyncratic adverse effects when HOCM is used. However, data are unclear regarding the effectiveness of steroid pretreatment in conjunction with LOCM. Some radiologists believe it is only effective in preventing minor reactions; others conclude that it also reduces moderate and severe reactions.

Documentation An adverse reaction to contrast medium administration must be appropriately documented. Most facilities have forms designed specifically for such events. Figure 12-1 is an example of such a form. At a minimum, elements that must be captured are 1) amount and type of the contrast injected, 2) signs and symptoms of the reaction, 3) interventions or medications given during the reaction and the patient's response to treatment, and 4) final outcome (e.g., was the patient sent home or admitted to the hospital?).

Before the patient leaves the radiology department, a technologist, radiologist, or radiology nurse should provide instruction to the patient or the patient's family regarding future contrast-enhanced examinations. The patient should be told that they had a reaction to iodine contrast (so that the patient separates it from the gadolinium contrast agent used in magnetic resonance [MR] imaging). Should a future examination requiring iodinated contrast medium be considered, the patient should inform their healthcare provider of the reaction, because this may influence their doctor's decision. Depending on the severity of the reaction and the clinical need for the examination, the clinician may order an alternative examination (e.g. ultrasonography or MR) or she may order pretreatment medication for the patient before the contrast-enhanced CT examination.

Chemotoxic Reactions

Contrast reactions that stem from the contrast agent's pharmacologic properties are broadly referred to as chemotoxic. Like idiosyncratic reactions, the exact mechanisms responsible for all types of chemotoxic reactions are not completely understood. The types of chemotoxic reaction are variable and the underlying etiologies multifactorial. It has been suggested that an agent's chemotoxic effects stem from its molecular capacity to bind protein, resulting in the inhibition of certain enzyme systems that subsequently interfere with normal metabolic pathways by binding cell surface receptor proteins. Pain at the injection site belongs in this category because a combination of hypertonicity and calcium binding can result in vasodilation. A thorough discussion of the pharmacology of contrast agents is beyond the scope of this text. Instead the various types of chemotoxic adverse reactions are discussed, although the underlying mechanisms for the reactions are largely ignored.

Contrast Media-Induced Nephropathy It is well documented that the iodinated contrast agents used in imaging modalities such as angiography and CT affect kidney function.[17-22] It is generally believed that in most cases the effects are confined to a short period of kidney dysfunction that does not produce symptoms and therefore usually goes undetected. However, it is important to note that iodinated agents can result in significant nephrotoxic effects, particularly in patients who are considered to be at high risk for nephropathy. Given the huge number of contrast media-enhanced examinations performed (the worldwide sale of contrast media is approximated at 60 million doses annually[18]), the nephrotoxic effects are a serious concern. Contrast media-induced nephropathy (CIN) has been reported to be the third-leading cause of acute renal failure (ARF) in hospitalized patients.[19] Although often treatable, ARF is a serious complication associated with high mortality.[21,23]

In an effort to better understand the issues surrounding CIN, we 1) review basic renal physiology, particularly those aspects that relate to how the kidneys process iodinated contrast agents; 2) define CIN, including its clinical presentation, incidence, and the factors that place a patient at an elevated risk; and finally, 3) summarize strategies that can prevent cases of CIN.

BOX 12-15 Key Concept

Intravascular contrast agents affect kidney function. In most cases the effects are confined to a short period of kidney dysfunction that does not produce symptoms. However, in some instances iodinated agents can result in significant nephrotoxic effects, particularly in patients who are considered to be at high risk for nephropathy.

Renal Anatomy and Physiology The kidneys play an essential role in maintaining homeostasis. The word homeostasis comes from two Greek words—*homios,* meaning the same, and *stasis,* meaning standing. Therefore, the literal translation of the word is "standing or staying the same." It is important to note, however, that regarding the body, homeostasis is not a static state, but rather the minute-to-minute state of balance of water, electrolytes (such as sodium, potassium, chloride, and bicarbonate), and pH.

All vertebrate animals possess kidneys. In higher animals the kidneys evolved to eliminate toxic nitrogenous wastes (by-products of protein synthesis) and regulate homeostasis. It is remarkable that the kidney must function quite differently in different animals. Fish living in salt water are less "salty" compared with their environment, whereas land animals living in air are in constant threat of drying out because of respiration. In each case, the kidney has adapted to meet the specific need of the organism.

DEPARTMENT OF RADIOLOGY
CONTRAST REACTION REPORT

GENERAL INFORMATION

ID No: _____

Date/Time of Incident: Date _____   Time _____

Inpatient: _____   Outpatient: _____

Previous Incident: Date _____   Type _____

Date/Time Notified Radiology House Officer _____   Attending Radiologist: _____

Attending Physician _____   House Physician _____

DESCRIPTION OF INCIDENT

Contrast Administered _____   Dose _____   Route _____   Length of Time _____

Procedure Done: _____

Patient's Normal Blood Pressure _____   Patient's Normal Pulse _____

Patient's Blood Pressure During Incident _____   Patient's Pulse During Incident _____

Pre-Medication Given: _____

SYMPTOMS AND SIGNS OF REACTION:

CARDIOVASCULAR:

RESPIRATORY:

NERVOUS:

SKIN:

GI TRACT:

OTHERS: _____

MEDICAL REPORT

TREATMENT ADMINISTERED:

None _____ O_2 _____   IV _____   Epinephrine _____

Benadryl _____   Atropine _____   Steroids _____   Aminophylline _____

Cardiopulmonary Resuscitation _____   Other _____

Radiologist Findings: _____
_____

Signature _____   Date _____   Time _____

Q.A.

Was the contrast reaction kit readily available?   _____ Yes   _____ No

Were the contents of the reaction kit adequate for this incident?   _____ Yes   _____ No

Was support equipment, e.g., suction equipment, O_2, etc., readily available?   _____ Yes   _____ No

Did you have enough support in the management of this contrast reaction?   _____ Yes   _____ No

RADIOLOGY DEPARTMENT	CONTRAST REACTION REPORT

FIGURE 12-1   Sample of a contrast reaction report form.

The kidneys are paired organs that lie behind the parietal peritoneum, against the posterior abdominal wall, approximately at the level of the last thoracic and first three lumbar vertebrae. The liver pushes the right kidney down to a level somewhat lower than the left kidney. A heavy cushion of fat normally keeps the kidneys in position. Renal fasciae (connective tissue) anchor the kidneys to surrounding structures to help maintain their normal position.

Medially, each kidney has a concave notch called the *hilum*. Structures enter the kidneys through this notch just as they enter the lung through its hilum. A tough white fibrous capsule encases each kidney.

If a coronal section were made through the kidney, it would reveal an outer layer, or *cortex*, and an inner portion, or *medulla* (Fig. 12-2). The medulla is divided into a dozen or more triangular wedges called *renal pyramids*. The bases of the pyramids face the cortex, and their apices, or renal papillae, face the center of the kidney.

The kidneys represent approximately 0.5% of the total weight of the body, but receive 20% to 25% of the total arterial blood pumped by the heart. The basic functioning unit of the kidney is the nephron, a tube that is closed at one end and open at the other. Each kidney contains from one to two million nephrons. The nephron consists of Bowman's capsule, glomerulus, proximal convoluted tubule, loop of Henle, distal convoluted tubule, and a collecting tubule. Each component provides a specialized function.

The nephron produces urine by filtering out from the blood small molecules and ions and then reclaiming the needed amounts of useful materials. Surplus or waste molecules and ions are discarded as urine.

Renal Function   The overall function of the kidney is often described as clearance, a reference to the ability of the kidney to remove a substance from the blood. Clearance is the volume of plasma that is cleared of a specific substance in a given time. It is difficult to use the clearance rate for a direct measure of kidney function as a result of the lack of a perfect compound to measure.

Estimating Renal Function   One method of estimating kidney function is by calculating the glomerular filtration rate (GFR) and the effective renal plasma flow (ERPF). The administration of a substance called inulin, with subsequent measurement of its clearance from the blood, has been used for the estimation of GFR. Inulin is an ideal filtration marker because it is metabolically inert and cleared only by the kidney. However, analysis of inulin is technically demanding and time-consuming. Similarly, hippuran clearance has been used to measure ERPF. Normal adult GFR is approximately 120 mL/min, and normal ERPF is approximately 500 mL/min.[24] Because these methods are cumbersome to use routinely, other methods are frequently used to monitor kidney function.

Serum Creatinine as an Index of GFR   Creatinine is a by-product of muscle protein metabolism generated by the body at a fairly steady rate and excreted entirely in the urine. Measuring serum creatinine (SeCr or SCr) is a fast and inexpensive way to assess renal function. However, there are significant limitations in using SeCr as an accurate measure of renal function.[24-27]

First, although creatinine is freely filtered by the glomerulus, it is also secreted by the proximal tubule. Hence, the amount of creatinine excreted in the urine is the composite of both the filtered and secreted creatinine. Because of this, creatinine clearance systematically overestimates GFR. This overestimation is approximately 10% to 40% in healthy persons, but is greater and less predictable in patients with chronic kidney failure. Another limitation stems from the fact that creatinine is mainly derived from the metabolism of creatine in muscle; consequently, its generation is proportional to total muscle mass. As a result, mean creatinine generation is higher in men versus women, younger versus older persons, and blacks versus whites. This leads to differences in SeCr according to sex, age, and race, even after adjusting for GFR. Muscle wasting is also associated with reduced creatinine generation; in malnourished patients with chronic kidney disease, muscle wasting produces a lower SeCr than expected for the level of GFR. Creatinine generation is also affected to a certain extent by the consumption of cooked meat, because the cooking process converts a variable portion of creatine to creatinine. Therefore, SeCr is lower than expected for

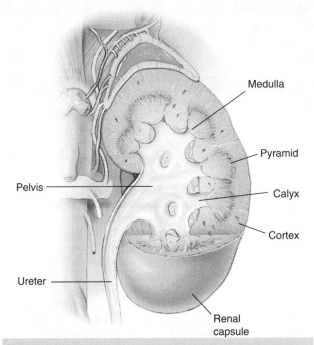

FIGURE 12-2 Coronal section through the right kidney.

the level of GFR in patients following a low-protein diet. Table 12-6 lists factors that affect the accuracy of SeCr in estimating GFR.

Formulas have been developed that incorporate factors such as patient age, weight, and height with the reported SeCr level. Two such formulas, the Cockcroft-Gault and Modification of Diet in Renal Disease (MDRD) study equations, have been proved to provide a reasonably accurate estimate of GFR.[24]

Despite its drawbacks, SeCr is a good reflection of any major drug-induced fluctuation in GFR and remains a useful clinical tool in assessing kidney function.[27]

BOX 12-16   Key Concept

Although it has significant limitations, measuring serum creatinine (SeCr) is a fast and inexpensive way to assess renal function.

Renal Dysfunction   The inability of the kidney to maintain homeostasis can result in the accumulation of nitrogenous wastes (or azotemia) and is referred to as *renal failure*. The exact biochemical or clinical criteria for a diagnosis of renal failure are not clearly defined.[20,25] The term renal failure is distinguished from *renal insufficiency*, in which renal function is abnormal but capable of sustaining essential bodily function. Renal failure is further classified as anuric (absence of urine formation) when urine volume is less than 50 mL for 24 hours; oliguric (diminished urine formation) when the volume is less than 500 mL for 24 hours; and nonoliguric (normal volume of urine formation) when volume is from 500 to 6,000 mL for 24 hours. Urine output greater than 6,000 mL is designated polyuric.

BOX 12-17   Key Concept

Renal failure is the inability of the kidney to filter waste from the blood.

Renal insufficiency is used when renal function is abnormal but capable of sustaining essential bodily function.

Technically, nephropathy denotes any condition or disease affecting the kidney; however, it is sometimes used synonymously with renal impairment.

The term *nephropathy* technically denotes any condition or disease affecting the kidney; however, it is sometimes used synonymously with renal impairment. CIN is an acute impairment of renal function subsequent to the intravascular administration of contrast material (for which alternative causes have been excluded). Although a functional definition varies among different studies, the most common measure is a reported rise in SeCr of more than 25% above baseline or an absolute rise of 0.5 mg/dL within 48 hours of receiving an iodinated contrast agent. Most cases of CIN occur after cardiac catheterization, selective-vessel angiography, or contrast-enhanced CT studies.

BOX 12-18   Key Concept

Contrast-induced nephropathy is an acute impairment of renal function that occurs after the intravascular administration of contrast material (for which alternative causes have been excluded).

Characteristically, the presentation of CIN is an acute, progressive rise in SeCr within 24 hours of contrast administration, although this elevation may take up to

---

TABLE 12-6   Factors Affecting Serum Creatinine Concentration[24]

Factor	Effect on SeCr	Mechanism
Kidney disease	Increase	Decreased GFR (although the increase in SeCr is blunted by increased tubular secretion of creatinine, and reduced creatinine generation)
Reduced muscle mass	Decrease	Reduced creatinine generation: common in children, women, and older and malnourished patients
Ingestion of cooked meat	Increase	Transient increase in creatinine generation, although the increase may be blunted by a transient increase in GFR
Malnutrition	Decrease	Reduced creatinine generation caused by reduced muscle mass and reduced meat intake
Use of cimetidine (Tagament)	Increase	Inhibition of tubular creatinine secretion
Use of flucytosine (an antifungal), some cephalosporins (group of antibiotics)	Increase	Positive interference with iminohydrolase and picric acid assays for creatinine
Ketoacidosis (high level of ketones in the blood, most commonly as a result of hyperglycemia)	Increase	Positive interference with picric acid assay for creatinine

GFR = glomerular filtration rate; SeCr = serum creatinine.

48 hours.[20] The serum creatinine level generally peaks at 4 to 5 days and then begins to return toward baseline within 7 to 10 days. Patients with CIN are usually nonoliguric. In most cases CIN is reversible.[19] However, as in other causes of renal failure, if oliguria does occur, the prognosis is poorer. Urinalysis typically reveals coarse granular casts, renal tubular epithelial cells, and amorphous sediment. Proteinuria may be low grade. Hematuria is not a characteristic of CIN. Urinalysis may show urate or calcium oxalate crystals. To make the diagnosis of CIN, alternative causes must be eliminated. This is an important step because there are many causes (>50) that can trigger the pathophysiologic mechanisms that lead to ARF.[28] Table 12-7 summarizes the clinical presentation of CIN.

CIN Incidence and Risk Factors   In the random population undergoing contrast-enhanced imaging, the incidence of CIN is low, generally thought to be between 1% and 6%.[17,19,22] However, a number of factors, such as renal impairment and diabetes, place patients at a higher risk of CIN. In high-risk patient populations, the incidence of CIN can reach 50%.[17] Unfortunately, it is frequently this higher risk group that is in need of imaging studies. For the past decade clinical investigators have focused on identifying patients at higher risk of developing CIN and developing interventions that may diminish the risk of CIN.

Although most patients who have CIN suffer little morbidity and recover to near-baseline renal function within 7 to 10 days, some patients require temporary dialysis. Even more worrisome, in rare patients CIN precipitates the need for chronic dialysis. Studies have been conducted substantiating the development of CIN leading to longer hospital stays.[29,30] One large retrospective study showed that hospitalized patients who experience CIN had a mortality rate of 34% compared with 7% in control subjects, even after controlling for underlying comorbidities.[23] The development of CIN appears to increase the risk of death from nonrenal causes such as sepsis, bleeding, respiratory failure, and delirium.[20,23]

The cumulative effect of multiple risk factors increasing the risk of CIN has been well-documented.[17,19,20,22–24,31] In one study that evaluated the effect of five factors (contrast volume, albumin, diabetes, serum sodium, and SeCr), CIN occurred in 1.2% of patients with no risk factors, 11.2% of patients with one risk factor, and more than 20% of patients with two or more risk factors.[31] Further, when all risk factors were present, the risk of CIN was 100%. Table 12-8 stratifies patients according to risk factors.

Studies have confirmed that preexisting renal insufficiency is a significant risk factor for CIN.[17–23,28,31] If HOCM is used even patients with mild renal impairment may be at some risk.[32]

Diabetes Mellitus   Diabetes mellitus has long been considered a risk factor for CIN. Although there is some disagreement in the literature, it is generally thought that the diabetic patient with normal renal function is not at a significantly increased risk of CIN. However, a strong association between diabetes mellitus with preexisting renal dysfunction and CIN has been established.[32–37] Analysis of the incidence of CIN in patient groups studied by Rudnick and coworkers[32] yielded the following results: diabetes and normal renal function, 0.6%; renal insufficiency alone, 6%; diabetes and renal insufficiency, 19.7%.

In summary, although patients with diabetes and normal renal function should be evaluated carefully, most appear to be at fairly low risk for having CIN. However, patients with diabetes mellitus and preexisting renal insufficiency represent a group with an extremely high risk of experiencing CIN.

Volume of Contrast Material   Several studies have revealed a direct correlation between the volume of contrast administered and risk of CIN.[22,32–34] Therefore, procedures that require a higher volume of contrast material, such as selective vessel angiography, place a patient at higher risk. In CT it is unusual to administer more than 200 mL of IV contrast in a single day. However, when this

---

TABLE 12-7   Clinical Presentation of CIN

Acute rise in SeCr 24-48 hours following contrast administration

SeCr peaks at 4-5 days and returns to baseline over 7-10 days

Usually nonoliguric

Urinalysis shows coarse granular casts, renal tubular epithelia cells, and amorphous sediment. Low-grade proteinuria may be present. Hematuria is absent. Urate and calcium oxalate crystals may be present.

Alternative causes eliminated.

CIN = contrast media-induced nephropathy; SeCr = serum creatinine.

TABLE 12-8   Identification of Patients at Risk for CIN[19]

High-Risk Patients
Stable creatinine clearance <25 mL/min
Stable creatinine clearance 25–50 mL/min + risk factor(s)
   History of diabetes mellitus
   History of recent administration of iodinated contrast agent
   Anticipated large volume of contrast material
   History of congestive heart failure

Moderate-Risk Patients
Stable creatinine clearance 25–50 mL/min
Stable creatinine clearance 50–75 mL/min + risk factors(s)
   History of diabetes mellitus
   History of recent administration of iodinated contrast agent
   Anticipated large volume of contrast material
   History of congestive hear failure

CIN = contrast media-induced nephropathy.

is being considered, the renal status of the patient will be an important consideration.

Other Risk Factors   It is well accepted that patients who are dehydrated before the imaging examination have an increased risk of CIN. Although multiple myeloma has traditionally been regarded as a risk factor CIN, many researchers now believe that the risk is primarily related to the dehydration of the multiple myeloma patient.[19]

Several other risk factors have been investigated, with no clear consensus at present as to whether they represent independent risk factors for CIN. These factors include patient age, male sex, atherosclerotic disease, and low left ventricular ejection fraction.[19]

Prevention of CIN   Unlike most forms of hospital-acquired ARF, CIN is amenable to preventive measures.[19,38-40] Newer research has provided an increased understanding of the pathogenesis of CIN and the critical roles of renal vasoconstriction and medullary ischemia. This knowledge has resulted in the proposal of several prophylactic approaches. Table 12-9 summarizes the methods recommended for preventing CIN.

Use of LOCM or Isosmolar Contrast Media   The nephrotoxic effects of contrast media are likely caused by chemotoxicity and osmolality. The viscosity of the media may have a role, but this hypothesis is currently unproved. It is well recognized that older HOCM is associated with a higher rate of nephrotoxicity than is LOCM.[19,32,34] At least two studies have indicated that for high-risk patients, isosmolar contrast media offers even more protection from CIN than does LOCM, although other studies state that isosmolar agents confer no protection.[17,18]

Hydration   It has been well documented that hydration decreases the incidence of CIN. On the basis of numerous animal and human studies, it is recommended that all patients receive oral or IV hydration at the time of the contrast-enhanced procedure.[19,30,35,36,41] Patients at risk for CIN should receive IV fluids before and after the imaging procedures.

Volume of Contrast Material   As mentioned earlier, CIN is dependent on the dose of contrast material used.

Therefore, the smallest amount of contrast agent possible should be used for each procedure. In some cases, enhancement profiles may be improved with the use of a saline bolus after the contrast injection, resulting in the reduction of contrast required for a given study. Allowing at least 48 hours to lapse between procedures in which contrast material is used enables the kidneys to recover.[42]

Other Nephrotoxic Medications   Many medications are associated with the development of acute renal failure. When a contrast-enhanced examination is scheduled for a patient at risk for CIN, the patient's physician may wish to temporarily discontinue these medications.[19] Nonsteroidal anti-inflammatory drugs (NSAIDs) and the antiplatelet agent dipyridamole are two examples of nephrotoxic medications.

BOX 12-19   Key Concept

The risk of CIN can be reduced in patients identified as high risk by:

- Using LOCM or IOCM
- Hydrating the patient
- Using the smallest dose of contrast media possible
- Allowing 48 hours to elapse between contrast-enhanced procedures

---

Metformin Therapy   Metformin is an oral medication given to non–insulin-dependent diabetics to lower blood sugar. Metformin is available as a generic drug; it is also sold under a variety of brand names (e.g., Glucophage, Riomet, Fortamet, Glumetza, Diabex, Diaformin). Metformin is also available in combination with other drugs (e.g., Avandamet, ActoplusMet, Metaglip, Glucovance). The most serious adverse effect of metformin therapy is the potential for the development of lactic acidosis in susceptible patients. Although the incidence of metformin-associated lactic acidosis is very low (<1 case per 10,000 patient-years), when it does occur it is fatal in about 50% of patients.[13] Any factors that decrease metformin excretion are risk factors for lactic acidosis. Therefore, renal insufficiency is a risk factor.

Because iodinated contrast agents have been associated with renal dysfunction, the administration of iodinated contrast media to patients taking metformin is a clinical concern. If CIN were to occur, it could indirectly lead to lactic acidosis by causing an accumulation of metformin in the body. Therefore, it is recommended that metformin be temporarily discontinued after any examination involving iodinated contrast. Metformin therapy can be resumed after 2 days, assuming kidney function is normal.[43]

To restate, iodinated contrast media does not cause lactic acidosis. Nor does metformin cause renal impairment. Rather, when renal dysfunction occurs in patients taking metformin the drug can accumulate and result in lactic acidosis.

TABLE 12-9   Methods of Preventing CIN[19,21]

Identify patients at high risk. Patients with diabetes mellitus or other risk factors scheduled for any procedure including IV contrast should have SeCr measured.

Use LOCM or IOCM.

Ensure adequate patient hydration.

Minimize contrast material volume.

Allow at least 48 hours between procedures requiring contrast material.

Discontinue other nephrotoxic medications before the procedure.

CIN = contrast media-induced nephropathy; IOCM = isosmotic contrast media; IV = intravenous; LOCM = low-osmolality contrast media; SeCr = serum creatinine.

Dialysis and Contrast Media   Patients may be started on dialysis after an episode of acute renal failure, with the hope that their kidneys will recover sufficiently so that dialysis can be discontinued. In these situations the conventional wisdom is that iodinated contrast media should not be given. The aim is to avoid any risk of further renal insult, which could diminish residual renal function and result in the renal failure becoming chronic with the need for ongoing hemodialysis.

In patients with end-stage renal failure, concerns are of a different nature. In these situations it is not expected that renal function will return; the need for ongoing dialysis is accepted. Contrast-enhanced CT examinations are often performed with the recognition that the kidneys cannot be damaged further. Patients with end-stage renal failure typically receive hemodialysis three times per week; therefore the contrast media can remain in the blood for prolonged periods. There is concern that such patients are at risk of central nervous system reactions such as convulsions and respiratory depression.

The half-life of iodinated contrast media in patients with normal renal function is approximately 2 hours, but in patients with severe renal dysfunction it can be extended to more than 30 hours depending on the extent of the renal impairment. Contrast media can be efficiently removed from the blood by hemodialysis. Peritoneal dialysis is also effective in removing contrast agents from the body, but takes longer.

It has been suggested that performing dialysis immediately after the administration of contrast media will reduce the rate of complications. However, studies have not proven this to be true. Patients on dialysis who undergo contrast-enhanced CT may continue their routine dialysis schedule.[44]

Other Organ- or System-Specific Adverse Effects

Effects on Thyroid Function   In the absence of thyroid disease the administration of iodinated contrast agents will have no significant impact on thyroid function. In patients with hypothyroidism, particularly those with autoimmune (Hashimoto) thyroiditis, there may be a small, temporary reduction in thyroid function, which does not require additional treatment. However, in patients with a history of hyperthyroidism, iodinated contrast media can intensify thyroid toxicosis (excessive thyroid hormone). In rare cases, iodinated contrast media can precipitate thyroid storm (or thyrotoxic crisis), which is a severe, life-threatening condition resulting when thyroid hormone reaches a dangerously high level.[45]

The two main causes of hyperthyroidism are Graves' disease and a condition known as thyroid autonomy. Iodine deficiency is an important factor in the development of thyroid autonomy. Iodine deficiency is low in the Americas (primarily as a result of iodized salt) but prevalent in other regions, including many European countries.

Contrast media affects patients with hyperthyroidism because of the small amount of free iodide it contains. The majority of iodine contained in contrast media is organically bound and does not impact thyroid function.

Hyperthyroidism is not a common condition in the United States; it is seen much less frequently than hypothyroidism. Nonetheless, patients should be questioned as to their thyroid status before the administration of an iodinated contrast agent. When a patient with a history of hyperthyroidism is identified, this fact should be brought to the attention of the radiologist before proceeding with the examination. If the examination is performed the patient may be instructed to see their endocrinologist for monitoring.

Iodinated contrast material can interfere with the results of a radioactive thyroid uptake study performed in the nuclear medicine department. Therefore, CT studies that use iodinated contrast material should not be scheduled sooner than 2 weeks before a nuclear medicine thyroid study.

Pulmonary Effects   Several potential pulmonary adverse effects have been documented after the IV administration of iodinated contrast agents. These include bronchospasm, pulmonary arterial hypertension, and pulmonary edema. Patients with a history of pulmonary hypertension, bronchial asthma, or heart failure are at increased risk. Pretreatment with steroids has been tried but did not offer any protection. The use of LOCM significantly reduces the risk of pulmonary effects.[46]

Pheochromocytoma   Pheochromocytoma is a neuroendocrine tumor, most often found in the adrenal medulla. These tumors result in the excessive secretion of catecholamines, usually epinephrine and norepinephrine. In patients with pheochromocytoma HOCM has been reported to further increase the level of circulating catecholamines. LOCM does not increase the level of circulating catecholamines and can be used in patients with pheochromocytoma.[47]

Central Nervous System   The blood-brain barrier (BBB) is a semipermeable structure that protects the brain from most substances in the blood, while still allowing essential metabolic function. Iodinated contrast agents will not cross an intact BBB.

The use of iodinated contrast media has been shown to provoke seizures in patients who have diseases that disrupt the BBB. For unknown reasons, the risk of seizures after contrast administration is greater for patients with metastasis to the brain than those with primary brain tumors, although both tumors disrupt the BBB. In these patients, the risk of seizure can be substantially reduced by a one-time oral dose of 5 to 10 mg of diazepam (i.e., Valium), 30 minutes before contrast administration.[48] Seizures that occur can also be controlled with diazepam.

Contrast Extravasation   During routine use of IV contrast material in the CT department, extravasation of contrast medium into the subcutaneous tissue sometimes occurs. The prevention and management of extravasated iodinated contrast media is discussed in Chapter 13.

Delayed Reactions

Delayed reaction to intravascular iodinated contrast media are defined as reactions occurring between 1 hour and 1 week after contrast medium injection. Accurate statistics regarding late reactions are inherently difficult to collect, because as the time interval increases between the contrast medium injection and the onset of symptoms, so does the difficulty of being certain that the symptoms are directly related to the contrast medium. For example, reported symptoms of late reactions after CT examination include headache, skin rash, itching, nausea, dizziness, urticaria, fever, arm pain, and gastrointestinal disturbances. However, when analyzed, all but the skin reactions appeared equally after enhanced and unenhanced CT.[49] In spite of these difficulties, it is certain that delayed reactions do sometimes occur. Skin reactions appear to account for the majority of true late reactions. Most are minor and last only a short time, but severe reactions can occur. The types of skin reactions and their frequencies are similar to those that occur with many other drugs.[49] Types of late skin reactions include maculopapular rash (red spots or bumps), angioedema (weltlike swelling), and urticaria (hives).

Less frequently reported, iodide "mumps" (salivary gland swelling) and a syndrome of acute polyarthropathy (pain in multiple joints) are other possible delayed reactions. These can occur after either HOCM or LOCM and may be more frequent in patients with renal dysfunction.[13]

Patients who are receiving or have received interleukin-2 can have delayed reactions after the administration of contrast media.[13] Interleukin-2 (brand name Proleukin, Chiron Corporation) is an immunotherapy used to treat some cancers (e.g., malignant melanoma, renal cell carcinoma). After the administration of iodinated contrast media, patients may experience symptoms that recall the side effects of the interleukin-2 therapy, such as fever, nausea, vomiting, diarrhea, itching, and rash.

In general, there is no relationship between the volume of contrast administered and the frequency or severity of delayed cutaneous events.[6] Like other types of reactions, delayed reactions occur less frequently with LOCM. The exact nature of delayed reactions is unclear; it is likely that some can be attributed to chemotoxicity whereas others are idiosyncratic in nature. Unlike other contrast-related adverse events, there is some evidence that suggests that delayed cutaneous reaction may be immune-mediated (stemming from a true allergy or an autoimmune response).[8]

GASTROINTESTINAL CONTRAST MEDIUM

In the gastrointestinal tract, contrast medium is essential to distinguish loops of bowel from a cyst, abscess, or neoplasm. For this reason, oral contrast material is used in most CT scans of the abdomen and pelvis. For some indications, the rectal administration of contrast material is useful.

In general, contrast media is classified as positive if it appears bright on the image, and negative if it appears dark on the image. The most common definition classifies gastrointestinal agents as positive or negative depending on the density of the material relative to the walls of the gastrointestinal tract. For example, by this definition water is considered a negative agent, because with an HU of 0, it is less dense than the wall of the gastrointestinal tract. Less commonly, contrast media is classified in accordance to its HU; agents with positive HU values are considered positive agents, those with negative HU values are called negative agents. Using this definition, water is considered a neutral agent.

Options available in oral preparations include barium sulfate solutions, or iodinated water-soluble agents. Options available for rectal preparations include air, carbon dioxide, barium sulfate, or iodinated water-soluble solutions. The ideal agent should provide adequate differentiation of bowel from surrounding structures without creating artifacts. The images in Figure 12-3 demonstrate the use of water, a low HU barium solution, a standard barium sulfate solution, and an ionic, iodinated agent to highlight the gastrointestinal tract.

Barium Sulfate Solutions

Conventional radiography barium suspension cannot be used in CT. Such full-strength solutions would cause unacceptable streak artifacts. These conventional agents cannot simply be diluted for use in CT because of their tendency to settle after ingestion. This tendency leads to irregular opacification of the bowel. Fortunately, products are available specifically for use in CT. The most commonly used are positive agents that contain a 1% to 3% barium sulfate suspension and are specially formulated to resist settling.

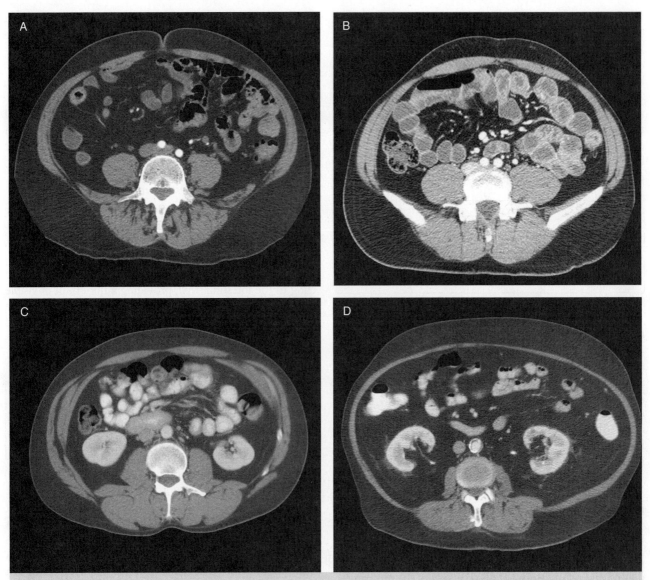

FIGURE 12-3 These images show the various options in oral contrast agents. Water was used for image (A). VoLumen was used for image (B). Barium sulfate suspension was used for image (C). An ionic, iodinated agent was used for image (D). (In all images the patient was also given an IV contrast agent.)

Commercial barium preparations (e.g., Readi-Cat [E Z EM], Baro-Cat [Mallinckrodt]) may include a number of additives to enhance the mucosal coating properties or to improve the taste for oral use.

A higher dose of oral contrast material provides greater bowel opacification. Timing and dose are largely dependent on the area to be opacified. For most examinations a minimum of 500 mL of dilute barium sulfate is given 45 minutes to 2 hours before scanning. An additional 200 mL is given just before scanning to fill the stomach and proximal small bowel.

In patients who cannot take fluids by mouth, a nasogastric tube may be inserted. The contrast medium can be introduced through the tube. If vomiting is a problem, slowing the rate of administration may help.

The typical low-concentration, low-viscosity barium sulfate solutions may not be adequate for an esophageal study. In such cases, high-viscosity, low-concentration, pastes designed for this purpose are recommended.

One disadvantage of positive contrast media is that they make mucosal surfaces more difficult to evaluate after IV administration of contrast material.[50] Another problem is that the density of positive contrast material may create streak artifacts or impede three-dimensional modeling. To overcome these disadvantages a low-HU oral barium sulfate suspension was developed (VoLumen, E Z EM). With just 0.1% barium sulfate, the agent resembles water on CT but provides improved distention (as compared with water), faster transit than positive barium sulfate solutions, and more effective visualization of both the bowel wall and the mucosa. On CT images, VoLumen measures from 15 to 30 HU, a density lower than the wall of the GI tract. Hence, it is most often considered a negative agent as defined by attenuation compared with the bowel wall, but by some definitions it is called a neutral agent.

Barium sulfate should not be given if perforation of the gastrointestinal tract is suspected. Barium leaking into the peritoneal cavity is referred to as barium peritonitis. The mortality rate from this complication is significant. It can be prevented by substituting a water-soluble iodinated oral contrast agent whenever perforation is suspected.

BOX 12–22   Key Concept

Barium sulfate should not be given if perforation of the gastrointestinal tract is suspected. Barium leaking into the peritoneal cavity is referred to as barium peritonitis and is associated with a significant mortality rate.

Barium sulfate is an inert substance that passes through the gastrointestinal tract basically unchanged. Allergic reactions to oral barium sulfate solutions are rare. The product literature reports severe reactions in approximately 1 in 500,000 cases and fatalities in 1 in 2 million cases. It is likely that these reactions can be attributed to the additives in the suspension (e.g., flavorings). Although procedural complications are rare, they include aspiration pneumonitis, barium impaction, and intravasation.[51]

Although definitive answers are not available, fewer complications from aspiration appear to occur with barium sulfate than with high-osmolality iodinated agents.

Iodinated Agents

Both HOCM and LOCM are positive agents that can be diluted and administered orally. Because of the unpleasant taste of HOCM, flavoring is normally added to the solution. A 2% to 5% solution of a water-soluble agent is normally used. Even with these dilute solutions, given orally, iodinated contrast agents usually stimulate intestinal peristalsis. Therefore, patients may experience diarrhea after the ingestion of water-soluble agents. Dosages are similar to those used with barium sulfate. However, water-soluble oral contrast material tends to pass through the gastrointestinal tract slightly faster.

In most situations, HOCM is used for oral administration because is it less expensive than LOCM and provides equivalent gastrointestinal opacification. However, in selective cases LOCM has advantages over HOCM that justify its increased expense. If aspirated, LOCM causes less pulmonary edema than HOCM. Researchers of oral contrast medium in newborns have concluded that LOCM offers a significant reduction in complications compared with barium sulfate or HOCM.[52,53] LOCM should be used in infants and young children under the following conditions: 1) when the possibility of entry of contrast agent into the lung exists; or 2) when the possibility of leaking of contrast agent from the gastrointestinal tract exists.

Studies of older children revealed an additional advantage. Because the LOCM has a neutral taste when diluted, patient cooperation is much greater.

When rectosigmoid abnormality is suspected, rectal administration of contrast material may be necessary. In these cases, 150 to 200 mL of dilute water-soluble agent (1% to 3%) can be given by enema.

Comparison of Positive Oral Contrast Agents

Barium sulfate and water-soluble contrast material cause comparable bowel opacification. Because of the low concentrations used, neither coats the mucosa significantly. Instead, most visible contrast is simply from the agents filling the bowel. Barium sulfate, in small amounts, tends to cling to the intestinal wall, providing a minimum of visible contrast. In comparison, a small quantity of water-soluble oral contrast is usually absorbed by the bowel. Therefore, if a patient is able to drink only a small amount of oral contrast, it is preferable to give them a barium sulfate solution.

BOX 12–23   Key Concept

Barium sulfate and water-soluble contrast material cause comparable bowel opacification. Because of the low concentrations used, neither coats the mucosa significantly.

Water

Water is sometimes used in place of positive contrast agents. As a negative (or neutral) agent, water will not obscure mucosal surfaces, or superimpose abdominal vessels on three-dimensional images. However, water transits quite rapidly and distends the bowel poorly. It will not provide sufficient detail if the bowel is not fully distended.

Air and Carbon Dioxide

Room air or carbon dioxide can be used to produce a very high negative contrast on images of the gastrointestinal tract. Negative contrast agents are particularly useful in CT colonography when adequate colonic distention is critical for effective polyp detection. Poorly distended segments of bowel may be mistaken for carcinoma. Room air or carbon dioxide is administered via a small flexible rectal catheter. Room air is delivered using a standard handheld air bulb insufflator. This air bulb can be controlled either by the patient or the CT technologist. Carbon dioxide is delivered using an automated insufflation system (PROTOCO$_2$L, Bracco Diagnostics, Inc., pictured in Fig. 12-4). Both room air and automated carbon dioxide provide reliable colonic distention. However, carbon dioxide has some advantages over room air in that it is readily absorbed by the body and is eliminated by respiration. It induces less spastic response of the bowel wall and is therefore better

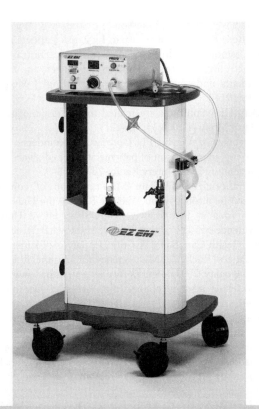

FIGURE 12-4 Automated carbon dioxide insufflation system for CT colonography. Picture courtesy of the Bracco Diagnostics, Inc.

tolerated by most patients.[54] Room air can result in significant postprocedure cramping and discomfort for the patient. In addition, many CT technologists prefer the automated carbon dioxide technique over patient-controlled room air administration. The main reason is that more time is required to coach patients to self-insufflate, whereas automated carbon dioxide requires relatively little patient education to achieve similar results.

The antispasmodic medication, glucagon hydrochloride, is sometimes given by intravenous injection to further improve bowel distention.

INTRATHECAL CONTRAST ADMINISTRATION

Although rarely performed in the CT department, contrast media can be injected into the intrathecal space surrounding the spinal cord. Only certain iodinated contrast media can be safely used intrathecally. Serious adverse reactions have been reported as a result of the inadvertent intrathecal administration of iodinated contrast media that are not indicated for intrathecal use. These serious adverse reactions include death, convulsions, cerebral hemorrhage, coma, paralysis, arachnoiditis, acute renal failure, cardiac arrest, seizures, rhabdomyolysis, hyperthermia, and brain edema. In fact, the U.S. Food and Drug Administration requires the manufacturers of contrast media that

are not intended for this use to mark the packages "not for intrathecal use" or "not for myelography." When a contrast medium is to be administered intrathecally, radiology staff should perform an independent double check to make sure the product they are using is the right one for that purpose. Intrathecal injection is outside the scope of practice of CT technologists.

Patients are frequently sent to the CT department for a postmyelogram CT, while the contrast agent is still in the intrathecal space. Therefore, the contrast agent is injected before the patient arrives for the CT study. To reduce the incidence of headache, keep the patient's head elevated (approximately 30°). The CT examination is typically done from 1 to 3 hours after the intrathecal injection. If the examination is done too soon the contrast material may be too dense and generate streak artifact. Rolling the patient once or twice before scanning is recommended to mix the contrast material that may have settled since the myelogram.

Intraarticular Contrast

Contrast media can be injected directly into a joint space to better visualize the soft tissue structures of the joint. Arthrography can be performed with fluoroscopy in the general radiography department, or more commonly, in MR. However, CT arthrography has the advantage of allowing the simultaneous evaluation of bone and soft tissue. The intraarticular contrast injection is performed by the radiologist, most often under fluoroscopic guidance. Once the contrast has been injected into the joint space the patient is transported to the CT department.

SUMMARY

Contrast agents play an essential role in CT imaging. Without the use of contrast media many structures and disease processes would be indistinguishable. Although there are many diagnostic benefits associated with the administration of contrast media, they also have the potential to cause patients harm. To reduce risks to the patient, technologists must understand important aspects of each of the contrast agents used in the CT department, including their characteristics, dosing guidelines, and possible adverse effects.

REVIEW QUESTIONS

1. Explain how contrast agents are classified as positive, negative, or neutral.
2. Osmolality, ionicity, viscosity and clearance are all properties of iodinated contrast media. Define each property.
3. Why is it important to differentiate contrast reactions from other allergic reactions? In what ways are they similar?
4. What are symptoms of an idiosyncratic reaction to contrast media? What are symptoms of chemotoxic reactions? Into which category do delayed reactions belong?
5. Discuss contrast-induced nephropathy including risk factors and strategies for prevention.

6. Explain why Metformin therapy is a consideration for patients receiving intravenous contrast injections.
7. List the advantages and disadvantages of the various types of oral contrast media.

REFERENCES

1. Morcos SK. Dialysis and contrast media. In: Thomsen HS, ed. Contrast Media: Safety Issues and ESUR Guidelines. 1st Ed. Berlin: Springer, 2005:47.
2. Katzberg RW. The Contrast Media Manual. Baltimore: Lippincott Williams & Wilkins, 1995:68.
3. Daily Med/Current Medication Information resources page. NLM's Medline Plus Web site. Available at: http://dailymed.nlm.nih.gov/dailymed/drugInfo.cfm?id=3515. Accessed December 11, 2007.
4. Yanaga Y, Awai K, Nakayama Y, et al. Pancreas: patient body weight-tailored contrast material injection protocol versus fixed dose protocol at dynamic CT. Radiology 2007;245:475–82.
5. Megibow AJ, Jacob G, Heiken JP, et al. Quantitative and qualitative evaluation of volume of low osmolality contrast medium needed for routine helical abdominal CT. AJR Am J Roentgenol 2001;176:583–9.
6. Bettmann MA. Contrast media: safety, viscosity, and volume. Eur Radiol 2005;15:D62–4.
7. Caro JJ, Trindade E, McGregor M. The risk of death and of severe non-fatal reactions with high- vs low-osmolality contrast media: a meta-analysis. AJR Am J Roentgenol 1991;156:825–32.
8. Bettmann MA, Heeren T, Greenfield A, Goudey C. Adverse events with radiographic contrast agents: results of the SCVIR Contrast Agent Registry. Radiology 1997;203:611–20.
9. Witten DM, Hirsch FD, Hartman GW. Acute reactions to urographic contrast medium: incidence, clinical characteristics and relationship to history of hypersensitivity states. Am J Roentgenol Radium Ther Nucl Med 1973;119:832–40.
10. Katayama H, Yamaguchi K, Kozuka T, Takashima T, Seez P, Matsuura K. Adverse reactions to ionic and nonionic contrast media. A report from the Japanese Committee on the Safety of Contrast Media. Radiology 1990;175:621–8.
11. Lasser EC, Lyon SG, Berry CC. Reports on contrast media reactions: analysis of data from reports to the US Food and Drug Administration. Radiology 1997;203:605–10.
12. Shehadi WH. Adverse reactions to intravascularly administered contrast media. A comprehensive study based on a prospective survey. Am J Roentgenol Radium Ther Nucl Med 1975;124:145–52.
13. ACR Committee on Drugs and Contrast Media. Manual on contrast media, Version 5.0. 5th Ed. Reston, VA: ACR, 2004.
14. Ansell G, Tweedie MC, West CR, Evans P, Couch L. The current status of reactions to intravenous contrast media. Invest Radiol 1980;15(Suppl):S32–9.
15. Siegle RL, Halvorsen RA, Dillon J, Gavant ML, Halpern E. The use of iohexol in patients with previous reactions to ionic contrast material. A multicenter clinical trial. Invest Radiol 1991;24:411–6.
16. Webb JA. Prevention of acute reactions. In: Thomsen HS, ed. Contrast Media: Safety Issues and ESUR Guidelines. 1st Ed. Berlin: Springer, 2005:12.
17. Aspelin P, Aubry P, Fransson SG, Strasser R, Willenbrock R, Berg KJ. Nephrotoxicity in high-risk patients study of iso-osmolar and low-osmolar non-ionic contrast media study investigators. Nephrotoxic effect in high-risk patients undergoing angiography. N Engl J Med 2003; 348:491–9.
18. Berg KJ. Nephrotoxicity related to contrast media. Scand J Urol Nephrol 2000;34:317–22.
19. Waybill MM, Waybill PN. Contrast media-induced nephrotoxicity: identification of patients at risk and algorithms for prevention. J Vasc Interv Radiol 2001;12:3–9.
20. DiFrancesco L, William M. Prevention of contrast-induced nephropathy. In: Wachter RM for the University of California at San Francisco (UCSF)-Stanford University Evidence-based Practice Center, Markowitz AJ, eds. Making Health Care Safer: A Critical Analysis of Patient Safety Practices. Rockville, MD: Agency for Healthcare Research and Quality, 2001:349–357. Available at: http://www.ahcpr.gov/clinic/ptsafety/chap32.htm. Accessed December 12, 2007.
21. Rihal CS, Textor SC, Grill DE, et al. Incidence and prognostic importance of acute renal failure after percutaneous coronary intervention. Circulation 2002;105:2259–64.
22. Maddox TG. Adverse reactions to contrast material: recognition, prevention, and treatment. Am Fam Physician 2002;66:1229–34.
23. Levy EM, Viscoli CM, Horwitz RI. The effect of acute renal failure on mortality. A cohort analysis. JAMA 1996:275:1489–94.
24. Manjunath G, Sarnak MJ, Levey AS. Estimating the glomerular filtration rate. Dos and don'ts for assessing kidney function. Postgrad Med 2001:110:55–62.
25. Grey V, Tange S. Assessment of glomerular filtration rate [The Canadian Society of Clinical Chemists Web site]. Available at: http://www.cscc.ca/articles.php? frm ArticleID=26&staticId=1. Accessed January 23, 2008.
26. Shemesh O, Golbetz H, Kriss JP, Myers BD. Limitations of creatinine as a filtration marker in glomerulopathic patients. Kidney Int 1985;28:830–8.
27. Perrone RD, Madias NE, Levey AS. Serum creatinine as an index of renal function: new insights into old concepts. Clin Chem 1992;38:1933–53.
28. Liano F, Pascual J. Acute renal failure: causes and prognosis. In: Schrier RW, series ed. Atlas of Diseases of the Kidney [text online]. Available at: http://www.kidneyatlas.org/book1/adk1_08.pdf. Accessed January 23, 2008.
29. Solomon R, Werner C, Mann D, D'Elia J, Silva P. Effects of saline, mannitol, and furosemide to prevent acute decreases in renal function induced by radiocontrast agents. N Engl J Med 1994;331:1416–20.
30. Abizaid AS, Clark CE, Mintz GS, et al. Effects of dopamine and aminophylline on contrast-induced acute renal failure after coronary angioplasty in patients with preexisting renal insufficiency. Am J Cardiol 1999;83:260–3.
31. Rich MW, Crecelius CA. Incidence, risk factors, and clinical course of acute renal insufficiency after cardiac catheterization in patients 70 years of age or older. A prospective study. Arch Intern Med 1990;150:1237–42.
32. Rudnick MR, Goldfarb S, Wexler L, et al. Nephrotoxicity of ionic and nonionic contrast media in 1196 patients: a randomized trial. The Iohexol Cooperative Study. Kidney Int 1995;47:254–61.

33. Manske CL, Sprafka JM, Strony JT, Wang Y. Contrast nephropathy in azotemic diabetic patients undergoing coronary angiography. Am J Med 1990;89:615–20.

34. Lautin EM, Freeman NJ, Schoenfeld AH, et al. Radiocontrast-associated renal dysfunction: a comparison of lower-osmolality and conventional high-osmolality contrast media. AJR Am J Roentgenol 1991;157:59–65.

35. Weisberg LS, Kurnik PB, Kurnik BR. Risk of radiocontrast nephropathy in patients with and without diabetes mellitus. Kidney Int 1994;45:259–65.

36. Parfrey PS, Griffiths SM, Barrett BJ, et al. Contrast material-induced renal failure in patient with diabetes mellitus, renal insufficiency, or both. A prospective controlled study. N Engl J Med 1989;320:143–9.

37. Cigarroa RG, Lange RA, Williams RH, Hillis LD. Dosing of contrast material to prevent contrast nephropathy in patients with renal disease. Am J Med 1989;86:649–52.

38. Farrugia E. Drug-induced renal toxicity: diagnosis and prevention. Hosp Med 1998;59:140–4.

39. Solomon R. Radiocontrast-induced nephropathy. Semin Nephrol 1998;18:551–7.

40. Rudnick MR, Berns JS, Cohen RM, Goldfarb S. Contrast media-associated nephrotoxicity. Semin Nephrol 1997;17:15–26.

41. Eisenberg RL, Bank WO, Hedgock MW. Renal failure after major angiography can be avoided with hydration. AJR Am J Roentgenol 1981;136:859–61.

42. Cohan RH, Ellis JH. Iodinated contrast material in uroradiology. Choice of agent and management of complications. Urol Clin North Am 1997;24:471–91.

43. Thomsen HS, Morcos SK. Contrast media and the kidney: European Society of Urogenital Radiology (ESUR) guidelines. Br J Radiol 2003;76:513–8.

44. Deray G. Dialysis and iodinated contrast media. Kidney Int Suppl 2006;69:S25–9.

45. van der Molen AJ. Effects of iodinated contrast media on thyroid function. In: Thomsen HS, ed. Contrast Media: Safety Issues and ESUR Guidelines. 1st Ed. Berlin: Springer, 2005:75–82.

46. Morcos SK. Pulmonary effects of radiographic contrast media. In: Thomsen HS, ed. Contrast Media: Safety Issues and ESUR Guidelines. 1st Ed. Berlin: Springer, 2005:83–92.

47. Mukherjee JJ, Peppercron PD, Reznek RH, et al. Pheochromocytoma: effect of nonionic contrast medium in CT on circulating catecholamine levels. Radiology 1997; 202:227–31.

48. Rosenfeld MR, Dalmau J. Seizures in cancer patients. In: Delanty N, ed. Seizures: Medical Causes and Management. Totowa, NJ: Humana Press, 2002:213.

49. Stacul F. Late adverse reactions to intravascular iodinated contrast media. In: Thomsen HS, ed. Contrast Media: Safety Issues and ESUR Guidelines. 1st Ed. Berlin: Springer, 2005:27–32.

50. Prokop M, van der Molen AJ. Patient preparation and contrast media. In: Prokop M, Galanski M, van der Molen AJ, Schaefer-Prokop CM, Telger TC, trans. Spiral and Multislice Computed Tomography of the Body. New York: Thieme Publishing Group, 2003:91.

51. E-Z-EM [package insert]. Westbury, NY: E-Z-EM, Inc., 2007.

52. Cohen MD. Choosing contrast media for the evaluation of the gastrointestinal tract of neonates and infants. Radiology 1987;162:447–56.

53. Smevik B, Westvik J. Iohexol for contrast enhancement of bowel in pediatric abdominal CT. Acta Radiol 1990; 31:601–4.

54. Shinners TJ, Pickhardt PJ, Taylor AJ, Jones DA, Olsen CH. Patient-controlled room air insufflation versus automated carbon dioxide delivery for CT Colonography. AJR Am J Roentgenol 2006:186:1491–6.

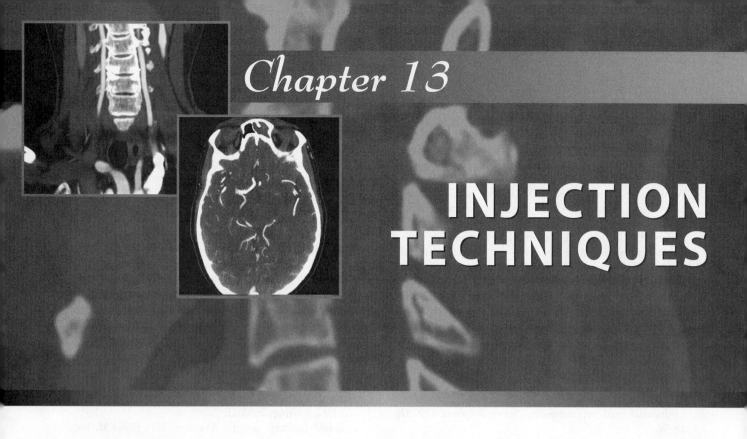

Chapter 13

INJECTION TECHNIQUES

Key Terms: central venous access devices • standard precautions • peripherally inserted central catheters • non-tunneled catheters • tunneled catheters • implantable ports • Huber needles • bolus phase • nonequilibrium phase • equilibrium phase • arteriovenous iodine difference • peak aortic enhancement • peak organ enhancement • nephrographic phase • portal venous phase • drip infusion • bolus injection technique • hand bolus • mechanical injection systems • contrast media extravasation • air embolism • pharmacokinetic factors • time-density curves • bolus shaping • uniphasic injection • biphasic injection • multiphasic injection • automated injection triggering • test bolus • bolus triggering

ACR RECOMMENDATIONS

Once the decision has been made to use intravenous iodinated contrast media for a particular examination, the method of injecting iodinated contrast media will vary depending on available vascular access, the type of examination, and the specific clinical indications for the examination. These factors will determine whether the

injection will be performed by hand or with the use of a mechanical injector. They will also influence the contrast volume used, the flow rate at which the contrast will be injected, the delay between injection and scanning, and whether a saline flush is advantageous.

Subject to the requirements of state law, a radiologist, radiologic technologist, or nurse may administer contrast media. Current American College of Radiology (ACR) recommendations regarding injection of contrast media are included in Box 13-1.[1]

BOX 13–1 Key Concept

The ACR approves of the injection of contrast material and diagnostic levels of radiopharmaceuticals by certified or licensed radiologic technologists and radiologic nurses under the direction of a radiologist or his or her physician designee who is personally and immediately available, if the practice is in compliance with institutional and state regulations. There must be prior written approval by the medical director of the radiology department/service of such individuals. The approval process must have followed established policies and procedures, and the approved radiologic technologists and radiologic nurses need to have documentation of continuing medical education related to the materials being injected and the procedures being performed (ACR Council Policy, 1987; amended 1997).

This chapter examines issues surrounding the intravascular injection of iodinated contrast medium for CT examinations.

VASCULAR ACCESS

Stable intravenous (IV) access is necessary for contrast media administration. In many instances, the IV line must be placed while the patient is in the CT department. In other instances, patients arrive in the CT department with IV access. In addition to standard indwelling peripheral catheters (e.g., BD Angiocath, BD Medical, Franklin Lakes, NJ), patients may arrive with central venous access devices (CVADs). Although CVADs are not optimal for contrast administration, in some cases they are the only option available. Therefore, CT technologists must have a working knowledge of the different types of CVADs, including when and how they can be used to administer iodinated contrast media.

Starting a Peripheral Intravenous Line

Starting an IV line requires a venipuncture technique, in which a needle is inserted into a vein. Before beginning the process the basic consent of the patient is obtained by explaining the procedure and asking whether the patient consents. Aseptic technique must be observed for all intravenous procedures. For the protection of the patient and the healthcare worker, standard precautions* must be strictly adhered to.

> **BOX 13-2   Key Concept**
>
> Aseptic technique must be observed for all intravenous procedures. For the protection of the patient and the healthcare worker, standard precautions must be strictly adhered to.

An indwelling catheter set with a flexible plastic cannula should be used whenever a mechanical injector will be used for contrast media injection. The use of metal needles (i.e., butterfly infusion sets or straight needles) should be avoided in conjunction with mechanical "power" injection as they may contribute to contrast media extravasation and patient injury. Whenever possible, catheters, and other ancillary components in the contrast fluid path to the patient, should be specifically designed for compatibility or have pressure and flow rate compatibility with the parameters that will be programmed for the power

---

*The Centers for Disease Control (CDC) recommends standard precautions for the care of all patients, regardless of their diagnosis or presumed infection status. Standard precautions apply to 1) blood; 2) all body fluids, secretions, and excretions (except sweat), regardless of whether or not they contain visible blood; 3) nonintact skin; and 4) mucous membranes. Standard precautions are designed to reduce the risk of transmission of microorganisms from both recognized and unrecognized sources of infection in hospitals. Standard precautions includes the use of hand washing and appropriate protective equipment such as gloves, gowns, and masks, whenever touching or exposure to patients' body fluids is anticipated. (Adapted from http://www.osha.gov/SLTC/etools/hospital/hazards/univprec/univ.html.)

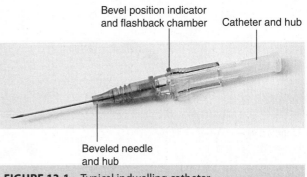

FIGURE 13-1   Typical indwelling catheter.

injection. An indwelling catheter set typically consists of a plastic catheter and hub, a beveled needle and hub, a bevel position indicator, and a flashback visualization chamber (Fig. 13-1). The visualization chamber may contain a reverse spring load to automatically retract the needle when it is removed from the catheter. Regardless of the particular brand of the indwelling catheter, the basic design is the same. A metal needle, ranging in gauge from 25 to 14 (the smaller the number, the larger the bore of the needle), has a tight-fitting plastic catheter placed over it. The catheter is slightly shorter than the needle, so that a short segment of the needle protrudes beyond the catheter.

> **BOX 13-3   Key Concept**
>
> An indwelling catheter set with a flexible plastic cannula should be used whenever a mechanical injector will be used for contrast media injection.

Supplies Needed

Collect the needed supplies before beginning venipuncture, including a tourniquet, tape, sterile gauze, a small cotton ball, saline (in either a syringe or a bag with an IV drip set), disposable gloves, and applicators for preparation of the insertion area. IV start kits are available that usually include all of these items. Choose the gauge of the IV indwelling catheter. The anticipated flow rate of the contrast injection should be appropriate for the gauge of the catheter used. Although 22-guage catheters may be able to tolerate flow rates up to 5 mL/s, a 20-gauge or larger catheter is preferable for flow rates of 3 mL/s or higher. Select two different gauges of catheter, usually a 22-gauge and 20-gauge, to make it easier to adapt to the size of the peripheral vein chosen. After arranging the IV supplies, interview the patient to once again verify their identity and to answer any additional questions they may have.

Choosing the Site

The superficial venous anatomy of the upper extremity allows many choices of a particular vein in which a

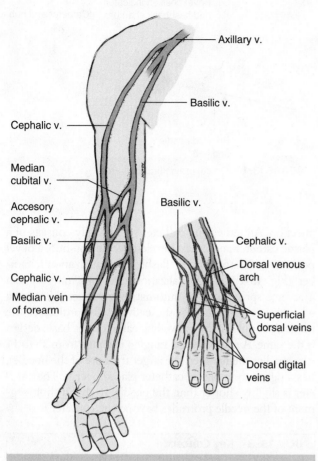

FIGURE 13-2 Major superficial veins of the arm and hand.

peripheral IV line can be placed (Fig. 13-2). An antecubital or large forearm vein is the preferred venous access site when a mechanical injector is used. However, if the patient will be required to lift the arms for scanning, it is important that the patient is able to keep the arm somewhat straight while above the head. Bending at the IV site may kink the IV line and cause it to fail during the injection of contrast media. If a more peripheral site, such as the hand or wrist, is used with a smaller gauge catheter, it may be necessary to limit the flow rate to 2.0 mL/s or less.

Placement

After assembling the supplies, verifying the patient's identity, and selecting the site, venipuncture can be initiated. Apply a tourniquet about 2 inches proximal to the chosen site. If the vein selected for placement does not adequately distend, place a second tourniquet just above the first and hang the arm below the level of the patient's heart. Wearing gloves, prepare the area selected for puncture with the applicator. Use a circular pattern starting in the center and working outward 2 to 3 inches. Allow the area a few moments to dry. Never blow on the site!

Hold the catheter, bevel upward, along the course of the vein from peripheral to central and at a 30° to 45° angle

to the skin with one hand, and gently pull the skin in the direction opposite to that of the needle being placed with the other hand. This will facilitate entry through the skin. Forward resistance is lost once the skin is penetrated. Decrease the angle of the needle and direct it toward the vein. As soon as the needle enters the vein, blood will enter the flashback visualization chamber. Next, advance the needle just a few millimeters into the vessel. Advance the catheter hub slightly away from the needle hub and release the tourniquet set. Continue to advance just the catheter hub three-quarters of the way over the needle, but not completely off of the needle. Place a piece of gauze under the end of the catheter to absorb any small volume of blood that might be lost. Hold direct pressure over the vein just proximal to the insertion site, release the needle from the catheter (setting the needle in plain sight), and attach the saline-filled syringe or connector to the catheter hub. After flushing the IV with the saline to demonstrate the patency of the IV line, cover the site (except the end of the connector) with sterile covering. If there was difficulty in threading the catheter through the vein, try to continue threading the catheter while flushing with saline. This procedure often allows the catheter to pass along the inside lumen without further difficulty.

Secure the connector to the arm by placing a strip of tape beneath the catheter and then bring it forward, crossing over the connector and onto the skin. Secure any extension tubing to the arm with paper tape. When using any sort of extension tubing set, ensure it is rated for use with power injectors or has been rated to tolerate the flow rates and pressures created with power injections. Next, dispose of the sharp needle in the appropriate disposal unit and clean the venipuncture area of any materials, such as packaging and applicators. Gloves are then removed and hands are washed.

Not all attempts to place an IV are successful; many factors can cause a failure. For example, an attempt at puncture can miss the vein. At this point, the needle must be removed and properly disposed of, the bleeding at the site must be stopped, the site must be bandaged, and a new vein proximal to the first attempt must be found. Veins with multiple punctures should be avoided because extravasation may occur through a prior puncture site. Clinical Application Box 13-1 contains a collection of practical venipuncture tips.

Managing Patients With Existing Vascular Access

Patients often arrive in the CT department with vascular access. In some cases the access will be via a standard indwelling peripheral venous catheter, whereas others will arrive with a CVAD. In either situation it is imperative that technologists follow basic rules to ensure the safe administration of a contrast agent.

Using an Established Indwelling Venous Catheter

When a patient arrives in the CT department with an existing indwelling peripheral venous catheter, it must be carefully evaluated before it can be used to administer a contrast agent. An ideal IV access site for administering contrast media 1) is well located (see "choosing the site" above), 2) was established recently (older IV access sites are more likely to extravasate), 3) contains a connecting hub or port that is not accessed (i.e., an intermittent IV line), or if it is accessed, has a saline (0.9% sodium chloride) or a solution of 5% dextrose in water (D5W) running, and 4) does not show evidence of redness, blanching, or swelling in the skin surrounding the puncture site.

Before injecting contrast media ensure the patency of the line by using a small syringe to flush the line with 2 to 5 mL of saline. Because of the potential for chemical incompatibility, contrast media should not be mixed with, or injected in, IV administration lines containing other drugs or total nutritional admixtures. If medications are being given through the port at the time of the examination, an additional bag of saline can be hung (i.e., "piggy-backed") and connected to an open port on the existing IV tubing. Existing medications should be turned off only long enough to complete the contrast injection. The line should be flushed with saline solution before the contrast injection. Once completed, the line should once again be flushed with saline solution before medications are restarted. It is important to restart the patient's medication at the identical preexamination rate.

BOX 13–4   Key Concept

Before injecting contrast media ensure the patency of the line by using a small syringe to flush the line with 2 to 5 mL of saline.

Using a Central Venous Access Device

A CVAD is a venous catheter designed to deliver medications and fluids directly into the superior vena cava (SVC), inferior vena cava (IVC), or right atrium (RA). They provide a painless way of drawing blood or delivering medications to a patient's bloodstream for days, weeks, months, or even years. Compared with a standard indwelling catheter, a CVAD is more durable and does not become as easily blocked or infected. There are several kinds of CVADs. They may contain one, two, or three lumens. Each lumen has an independent catheter port so there is no mixing of injected medications. Catheters may have an open end or closed end. Open-ended peripherally inserted central catheters (PICCs) must be clamped when not in use. Many manufacturers recommend that between uses they be flushed with a heparinized saline flush to maintain the catheter's patency. Closed-end catheters contain a valve that controls fluid flow and prevents reflux of blood into the catheter. Closed-end catheters require only a saline flush to maintain patency.

BOX 13–5   Key Concept

Although CVAD are not optimal for contrast administration, in some cases they are the only option available. Therefore, CT technologists must have a working knowledge of the different types of CVADs, including when and how they can be used to administer iodinated contrast media.

Peripherally Inserted Central Catheters   A PICC is a long catheter that is inserted through the large veins of the upper arm (i.e., cephalic and basilic veins) and advanced so that its tip is located in the lower third of the SVC. PICCs are intended to provide central venous access for several weeks, but can remain in place as long as several months. They can be either single or double lumen. A midline catheter is a similar, but considerably shorter, version that is placed so that it terminates in the upper arm near the axilla. Because midline catheters do not extend into the large central vein, they are considered peripheral, not central catheters. The external appearance of a midline catheter is often difficult to distinguish from a PICC. The type of catheter should be noted in the patient chart.

Many PICC lines cannot tolerate the pressure required to inject contrast media (which is more viscous than most intravenously administered medications) at the high injection rates typical of CT examinations that use mechanical injectors. In these cases it is recommended that a separate IV be inserted for the administration of contrast media. When no other options exist and the PICC must be used for contrast injection, the injection rate must be slowed and the injection should be performed by hand bolus rather than by mechanical injector.

BOX 13–6   Key Concept

Many PICC lines cannot tolerate the pressure required to inject contrast media at the high injection rates typical of CT examinations that use mechanical injectors. When no other options exist and these lines must be used, injection parameters must be adjusted. Some PICC lines have been designed to withstand higher pressure. These are often identifiable by their distinctive colors.

In recent years specific PICC lines have been designed to withstand up to 300 psi–more than enough for power injectors. Many manufacturers produce these special PICC lines in colors that make them readily distinguishable from the traditional PICC lines. Such is the case with the PowerPICC (Bard Access Systems, Salt Lake City, UT), whose deep purple color makes it easy to identify as a PICC line that may be used to instill contrast media at rates up to 5 mL/s by mechanical injector (Fig. 13-3).

The practice for flushing PICCs after contrast administration is variable among facilities. To maintain patency of the PICC and decrease the potential for occlusion, PICCs are typically flushed with normal saline, heparinized saline, or a combination of both.[2] A popular method for PICCs and other CVADs is the SASH method: Saline flush, Administer medication or draw blood, Saline flush, Heparinized saline flush. However, practice will be different if the PICC contains a Luer-activated device. This is a needle-free IV system that is a saline-only device and does not require flushing with heparinized saline after infusion or blood sampling.[2] Technologists should become familiar with their facility's written policy regarding PICC lines.

Non-tunneled and Tunneled Central Venous Catheters   Non-tunneled central catheters are a larger caliber than PICCs because they are designed to be inserted into a relatively large, more central vein such as the subclavian, jugular, or (less commonly) a femoral vein. Non-tunneled catheters usually have three ports, are open ended, and typically remain in place for a few days to 2 weeks.

Tunneled central venous catheters (CVCs) are inserted into the target vein (often the subclavian) by "tunneling" under the skin. This reduces the risk of infection, because bacteria from the skin surface are not able to

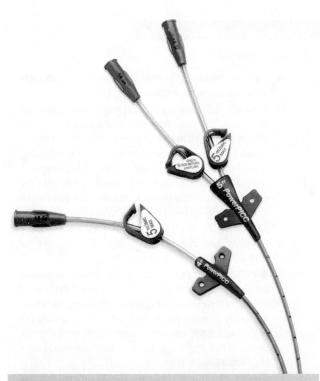

FIGURE 13-3 The easily identifiable PowerPICC (Bard Access Systems, Salt Lake City, UT) is designed to withstand higher pressure, so that it can be used to administer iodinated contrast media using mechanical injectors at flow rate up to 5 mL/s.

travel directly into the vein. The tunneled catheter has a cuff that stimulates tissue growth that will help hold it in place in the body. Examples of tunneled catheters include Hickman, Broviac, and Groshong catheters. The tunneled catheter is the best choice when access to the vein is needed for long periods of time and when the line will be used many times each day. It is secure and easy to access.

Implantable ports consist of a single- or double-lumen reservoir attached to a catheter. The reservoir hub is implanted in the arm or chest subcutaneous tissue, and the catheter is tunneled to the accessed vein. No external device is visible. The outline of the device may be seen and felt as a small round elevation on the skin. Implanted ports are typically used for long-term intermittent access such as that required for chemotherapy. Among central venous catheters, ports have the lowest incidence of infection because they are completely buried under the skin and there is no site for microorganisms to enter.[3] The port is accessed by use of a special noncoring hooked needle (also called Huber needles). If the access needle is not well placed in the reservoir, fluid injected into it could extravasate into the adjacent subcutaneous tissues. Accessing and de-accessing an implanted port requires special training and is beyond the scope of a CT technologist. However, once a port is properly accessed it can be used for infusion.

No established guidelines exist for using CVCs for the mechanical infusion of contrast media. Therefore, whenever possible, a standard peripheral IV access is preferred for contrast media injection. However, using central lines for injecting contrast medium may be the only option in some cases. In general, most CVCs may be infused at rates of 1.5 to 2 mL/s.[4] More rapid injection could potentially result in catheter perforation. When using power injectors with real-time pressure monitoring capabilities, the operator should watch for any deviation from the pressure norms, which could indicate possible occlusion or other adverse events related to catheters. When a CVC is used the technologist should carefully examine the insertion site and report any drainage, oozing, redness, or swelling to the radiologist before injecting into the line. Just as with any form of IV access, cleansing solution should be used to clean all junctions and connections. All cleansing solutions should be allowed to completely dry to provide maximum disinfection. The injection cap cannot be touched once it has been cleaned. Only sterile devices or needles are used to access CVADs. Before administering any substance, the patency of a central line must be verified. This can be done by demonstrating blood aspiration. The inability to aspirate blood can indicate catheter malposition or occlusion. To aspirate a central line, clean the injection cap and attach an empty 10-mL syringe. Gently pull back on the plunger; just enough to see blood, then flush with normal saline solution. If there is any doubt concerning the patency of a CVC, do not inject into the catheter. If there is resistance to flushing a CVC, no further injection attempt should be made as doing so may cause the catheter to rupture. After injection the catheter should be flushed with 10 mL of normal saline. Close the slide clamp while injecting the last 0.5 mL of solution to ensure that the catheter will be full of flush solution and minimize the likelihood of blood backing up into the catheter.[5]

As with PICCs, institutions vary in their policies regarding the use of CVCs for contrast medium infusion. For example, some facilities prohibit the use of ports for contrast infusion, whereas it is common practice in others. The infusion of contrast media for CT using mechanical injectors through CVCs is feasible and safe when established institution guidelines and injection protocols are followed. This provides an acceptable alternative in patients without adequate peripheral IV access when the rapid injection of contrast media is needed.

There are also several types of large-bore tunneled catheters used for dialysis. These should never be used for contrast media injection.

Manufacturers label the external portion of catheters by printing its size and type on the catheter hub or external

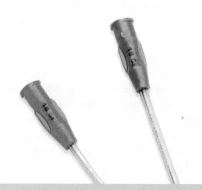

FIGURE 13-4 The size and type of the central venous catheter is printed on the catheter hub or external tubing. Image courtesy of Navilyst Medical, Inc.

tubing (Fig. 13-4). If the catheter type is in doubt, do not use it to inject contrast media.

BASIC PRINCIPLES OF INTRAVENOUS CONTRAST ADMINISTRATION

The proper injection parameters are critical in many CT protocols. Injection parameters that must be considered include the volume and concentration of contrast, the flow rate(s) at which the contrast will be delivered, programmed pressure limiting, and the timing between the start of the injection and the start of scanning. Documentation of intravenous contrast administration is a legal necessity and should include the name of the agent, the dose (volume and concentration), the flow rate(s), and the injection site. Any adverse effects and their treatments must also be documented (Chapter 12). When documenting information, technologists should use only approved abbreviations and forms, sign all documentation, and only record facts they observed.

Although the usefulness of IV contrast agents is universally accepted, much controversy exists over the optimal method of administering contrast material. The overarching goal is to select parameters that will consistently improve images and will facilitate reproducible studies. The latter is important because CT is often used for follow-up care and in cancer staging. It is difficult to determine whether a lesion has actually changed in size (even if it appears so on the image) if the technical factors used during scanning vary widely from study to study. Improved image quality and the ability to reproduce a study will ultimately lead to increases in disease detection and improved diagnosis. Technologists should understand, at least in broad terms, the issues that surround the choice of injection parameters. To that end the discussion starts with a broad view of how contrast media enhances tissues then moves to the more specific as we consider the route and pace of a bolus injection of contrast medium as it travels through the body.

General Phases of Tissue Enhancement

Three general phases of tissue enhancement are commonly discussed in CT: the bolus phase, the nonequilibrium phase, and the equilibrium phase. The difference among these phases is predominantly determined by the rate at which the contrast material is delivered and the time that elapses from the start of the injection and when scanning is initiated. The phases are frequently compared by the arteriovenous iodine difference (AVID). In practice this is done by comparing a Hounsfield unit (HU) measurement taken within the aorta to that of a measurement taken in the inferior vena cava (Fig. 13-5). The radiographic attenuation in HU serves as a surrogate measure of iodine (i.e., contrast) concentration.

BOX 13–10   Key Concept
Three general phases of tissue enhancement are commonly discussed in CT: the bolus phase, the nonequilibrium phase, and the equilibrium phase. The difference among these phases is predominantly determined by the rate at which the contrast material is delivered and the time that elapses from the start of the injection and when scanning is initiated.

The bolus phase is that which immediately follows an IV bolus injection. It is characterized by an attenuation difference of 30 or more Hounsfield units between the aorta and the inferior vena cava (Fig. 13-6). In the bolus phase of contrast enhancement, the arterial structures are filled with contrast medium and brightly displayed on the image. Hence, this phase is also commonly called the arterial phase. Contrast media has not yet filled the venous structures. CT angiography images are taken while contrast is in the bolus phase.

The second phase is the nonequilibrium phase. It follows the bolus phase and is characterized by a difference of 10 to 30 HU AVID (Fig. 13-7). The contrast agent is still much brighter in the arteries than in the parenchyma of organs, but now the venous structures are also opacified. Hence, it is also called the venous phase. This phase begins approximately 1 minute after the start of the bolus injection and lasts only a short time, approximately 1 minute. This window can be manipulated to some degree by varying conditions such as the volume and flow rate of the injected contrast medium. Most routine (nonangiographic) body images are acquired while contrast is in the nonequilibrium phase.

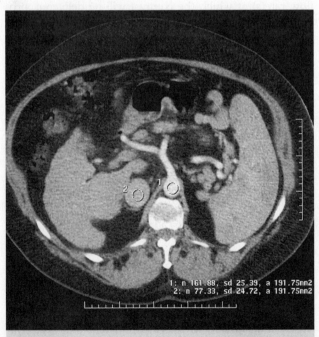

1: m 161.88, sd 25.39, a 191.75mm2
2: m 77.33, sd 24.72, a 191.75mm2

FIGURE 13-5 The AVID is often used to compare phases of contrast media enhancement. This is done by comparing a Hounsfield unit (HU) measurement taken within the aorta to that of a measurement taken in the inferior vena cava.

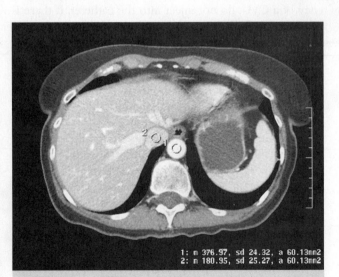

1: m 376.97, sd 24.32, a 60.13mm2
2: m 180.95, sd 25.27, a 60.13mm2

FIGURE 13-6 The bolus phase of contrast enhancement immediately follows an intravenous bolus injection. Arterial structures are filled with contrast medium and brightly displayed on the image. Contrast media has not yet filled the venous structures. Image courtesy of the University of Michigan Health Systems.

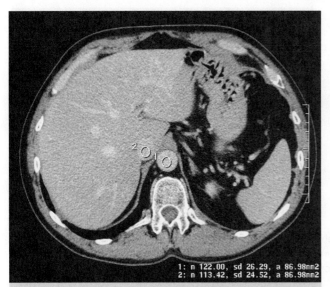

FIGURE 13-7 The nonequilibrium phase follows the bolus phase. While contrast media is still seen brightly in the arteries, vascular structures are also enhanced. Image courtesy of the University of Michigan Health Systems.

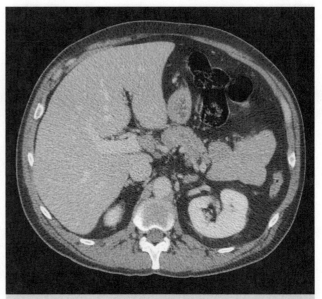

FIGURE 13-8 This image taken in the equilibrium stage of contrast enhancement was acquired approximately 5 minutes after the contrast injection. In this phase the contrast media is largely emptied from the arteries, is diluted in the veins, and has soaked the organ parenchyma. Image courtesy of the University of Michigan Health Systems.

The last phase of tissue enhancement after the IV injection of contrast media is known as the equilibrium (or delayed) phase. It can begin as early as 2 minutes after the bolus phase or after a drip infusion. In this phase contrast media is largely emptied from the arteries, is greatly diluted in the veins, and has soaked the organ parenchyma. In this phase, intravascular structures and interstitial concentrations of contrast material equilibrate and decline at an equal rate. It is characterized by an attenuation difference between the aorta and the inferior vena cava of less than 10 HU (Fig. 13-8). The equilibrium phase is the worst phase for acquiring scans of the body, particularly the liver. Compared with noncontrast examinations, visualization of tumors in the liver is improved in both the bolus and nonequilibrium phases, but not in the equilibrium phase. In some instances scanning in the equilibrium phase is worse than simply scanning without IV contrast enhancement. Because in this phase contrast material disperses more equally in the hepatic parenchyma and the tumor's interstitial space, the tumor can become isodense (i.e., the same density as the surrounding tissue) and be indistinguishable. Therefore, scanning in the equilibrium phase does not improve visualization of hepatic tumor compared with a precontrast examination and carries a considerable risk of tumor enhancement.[7] Figure 13-9 illustrates how hepatic abnormalities can become less conspicuous when scans are acquired in the equilibrium phase.

Historically, CT scan acquisition was much slower, making it impossible to obtain all scans through the liver before contrast media reached equilibrium. In these situations liver lesions were often difficult, or impossible, to detect with only the contrast-enhanced study. For this reason patients were often first scanned without contrast enhancement through the liver, then the entire abdomen was scanned after the injection of contrast media. New scanners are much faster and all scans can easily be obtained before the equilibrium phase. As a result, precontrast scans are now seldom needed for routine abdomen studies.

The exact timing of the start and end of each of the three phases are affected by many factors, including injection parameters and the condition of the patient, particularly the patient's cardiac output. In addition, the bolus and the nonequilibrium phases are often further divided. The terms early arterial phase, late arterial phase, hepatic arterial phase, late hepatic arterial, portal venous phase, hepatic venous phase, early delayed hepatic phase, late delayed hepatic phase, corticomedullary phase, nephrographic phase, and excretory phase can be found in the literature. Frequently the various terms are used inconsistently. Table 13-1 lists some commonly used terms describing different contrast phases.

Contrast material remains concentrated in organs and vessels for a very short time. Injection protocols are designed by first determining the time window from when contrast material is likely to first arrive in the organ or vessel of interest to when most of the contrast has vacated. Once this is estimated, equipment can be programmed so that scans are acquired within the window.

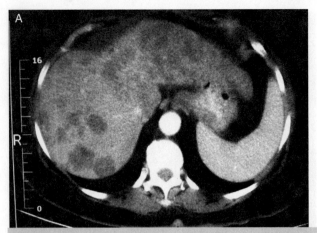

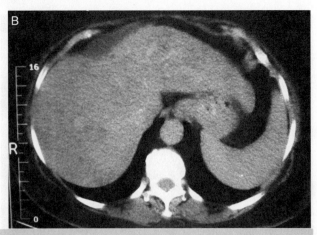

FIGURE 13-9   Image (A) was taken within the nonequilibrium phase of contrast enhancement, and conspicuous hepatic abnormalities are seen. Image (B), at the same location but taken just 2 minutes later, in the equilibrium phase of contrast enhancement, shows that tumors can become isodense and considerably less conspicuous.

TABLE 13-1   Terms Used to Describe Contrast Phases and Approximate Times*

Early arterial phase	15–25 s
Late arterial phase	35–45 s
Hepatic arterial phase	17–25 s
Late hepatic arterial phase	40–55 s
Portal venous phase	65–80 s
Hepatic venous phase	75–85 s
Early delayed hepatic phase (i.e., vascular equilibrium)	3–5 min
Late delayed hepatic phase (i.e., parenchymal equilibrium)	10–15 min
Parenchymal pancreatic phase	40–60 s
Enteric phase	40–50 s
Corticomedullary phase	30–70 s
Nephrographic phase	80–130 s
Excretory phase	3–15 min
Systemic venous phase (inferior vena cava)	3 min

*Frequently the various terms are used inconsistently; there is no consensus regarding the exact times after a bolus contrast injection these phases are reached. In addition, both injection parameters and patient factors will have a significant impact on when each of the phases occur.

Because patient factors can significantly influence the estimated window, tools such as bolus triggering and timing a test bolus are often incorporated into specific examination protocols. These tools will be covered later in this chapter.

The route that intravenously administered contrast medium takes from the site of injection to the various target organs is quite long. Along the way is a relatively predictable sequence of vascular and organ enhancement with various mixing processes. To mention just a few points along the way, the contrast material flows from the injection site vein into the vena cava, enters the right atrium, passes the pulmonary circulation and finally arrives in the aorta. Along the way to the right atrium the contrast mixes with nonopacified blood. Once the agent reaches the right ventricle, the mixing of opacified and nonopacified blood is complete. The contrast material enters the aorta during the arterial phase, then passes through draining veins that either join the vena cava or enter the portal venous system. Contrast material in the portal system enhances the liver parenchyma (the organ's tissue; as opposed to the vascular structures) and drains into the liver veins before it reaches the right atrium again. As the contrast material flows back to the right heart from various organs, recirculation effects occur. Typical contrast arrival times for various organ systems are shown in Table 13-2 and Figure 13-10. It is important to note that arrival time indicates when contrast material is likely to first be present in the organ or vessel. Therefore, arrival time represents the earliest possible time to acquire scans; images acquired before the contrast arrival times will appear unenhanced.

Contrast enhancement typically reaches a near-peak in the aorta from 15 to 22 seconds after the start of the injection. The time it takes to reach peak attenuation is affected by the cardiac output of the patient. As more contrast medium reaches the aorta, the aortic enhancement rises only slightly more, creating a type of plateau. The peak aortic enhancement is reached at the end of this phase when all of the contrast has been delivered, then drops off dramatically. The plateau can be extended by adding a saline flush, which will push forward the contrast material left in the tubing and in the veins leading to the aorta. Scanning within this enhancement plateau is ideal for imaging the arteries. Because the true peak enhancement point is short-lived (often <2 seconds), variable, and difficult to predict, scanning protocols are most often designed so that

TABLE 13-2   Contrast Arrival Times After Injection Into the Right Cubital Vein

Right atrium	6–12 s
Main pulmonary artery	9–15 s
Left atrium	13–20 s
Aorta	15–22 s
Carotids	16–24 s
Renal arteries	18–27 s
Femoral arteries	22–33 s
Jugular vein	22–30 s
Renal veins	22–30 s
Suprarenal IVC	24–32 s
Infrarenal IVC	120–250 s
Splenic vein	30–45 s
Mesenteric veins	35–50 s
Liver veins	50–80 s
Femoral veins	120–250 s

From Prokop[6] with permission.
IVC = inferior vena cava.

BOX 13–11   Key Concept

Routine brain scanning (for metastases or primary central nervous system tumors) provides a notable exception to the general rules of contrast media injection. The enhancement of most brain lesions is caused by blood-brain barrier disruption, not the intrinsic vascularity of the tissue. Therefore, the injection rate is not important, and scan delay is primarily important in that scans are not performed too soon after injection.

Methods of Contrast Media Delivery

The two methods of administering contrast material are the drip infusion and bolus techniques.

Drip Infusion

In the drip infusion technique, an IV line is initiated and contrast medium is allowed to drip in during a period of several minutes. Scanning begins after most, or all, of the contrast agent is administered (roughly 2 to 3 minutes). Because this method relies on gravity the actual flow rate delivered is quite variable and affected by many factors (e.g., bottle height, contrast volume, tubing length, IV catheter size, contrast media viscosity). This variability prevents the injection from being uniformly reproduced in subsequent follow-up studies. This method is not recommended for scans of the neck, chest, abdomen, or pelvis because all of the scans acquired with this technique are taken in the equilibrium phase. The drip infusion method is the least effective injection method for abdominal imaging, and in some respects, is even inferior to scanning without contrast enhancement. The drip infusion method cannot produce peak enhancement of sufficient magnitude for CT angiography. However, it can be used for routine brain scanning (for metastases or primary central nervous system tumors) because there is no need for a high injection rate and a scan delay of at least 4 minutes is typical.

Bolus Techniques

The bolus technique of contrast enhancement uses scanning after a rapid injection of contrast material. A volume of contrast of 50 to 200 mL is injected at a rate (or combination of rates) between 1 and 6 mL/s; scanning begins after a short delay. The interval between the initiation of the injection and the start of scanning (the scan delay) is critical. The contrast bolus can be delivered by hand (using syringes) or by a mechanical injection system.

Hand Bolus Technique   When contrast media is injected by hand the flow rate is subject to many factors, including syringe size, contrast viscosity, IV catheter size, and operator strength. Smaller size syringes require less operator strength to inject but must be serially disconnected when empty and reattached with replacement syringes. This delay will cause a drop in the peak enhancement. Higher viscosity agents and smaller indwelling catheters

images are acquired within the plateau (which typically lasts 10 to 15 seconds) and not at the peak.

Most organs have an exclusively arterial blood supply. The peak organ enhancement for such organs (e.g., pancreas, bowel, bladder) occurs about 5 to 15 seconds after peak aortic enhancement.[6] The kidneys are an exception because their excretion of contrast medium must also be considered. Kidney scans are often acquired in the nephrographic phase, which is 80 to 120 seconds after injection. This can be accomplished by incorporating a slight scan delay between scans of the liver and that of the kidney.

The liver has a dual blood supply. It is supplied primarily by the portal vein, contributing approximately 75%; the remainder is supplied by the hepatic artery. Although liver scanning is sometimes repeated to capture more than one phase of contrast enhancement, at a minimum it should be scanned in the portal venous phase. This phase occurs approximately 60 seconds after a bolus IV injection and, by definition, includes both arterial and venous enhancement.

Routine brain scanning (for metastases or primary central nervous system tumors) provides a notable exception to the general rules of contrast media injection. The enhancement of most brain lesions is caused by blood-brain barrier disruption, not the intrinsic vascularity of the tissue. Therefore, the injection rate is not important, and scan delay is primarily important in that scans are not performed too soon after injection. A scan delay of 4 minutes or greater is typical to allow sufficient time for contrast to leak across a disrupted blood-brain barrier into the abnormal tissue. However, nonroutine brain scanning such as CT angiography or CT brain perfusion studies require careful adherence to contrast injection protocols.

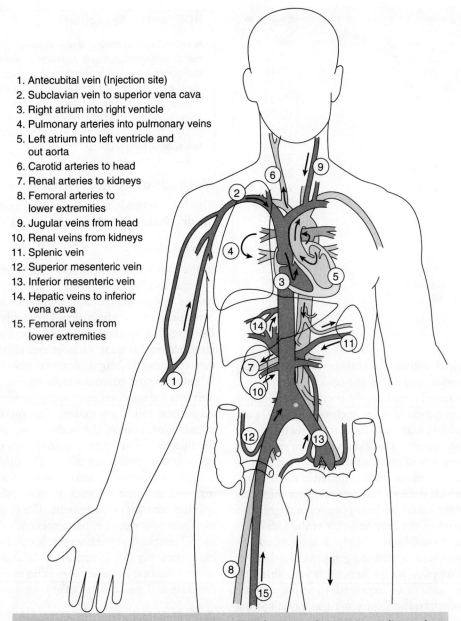

1. Antecubital vein (Injection site)
2. Subclavian vein to superior vena cava
3. Right atrium into right venticle
4. Pulmonary arteries into pulmonary veins
5. Left atrium into left ventricle and out aorta
6. Carotid arteries to head
7. Renal arteries to kidneys
8. Femoral arteries to lower extremities
9. Jugular veins from head
10. Renal veins from kidneys
11. Splenic vein
12. Superior mesenteric vein
13. Inferior mesenteric vein
14. Hepatic veins to inferior vena cava
15. Femoral veins from lower extremities

FIGURE 13-10 The route that intravenously administered contrast medium takes from the site of injection to the various target organs is quite long and relatively predictable.

will require more operator strength for injection. The advantages of the hand bolus method are that it is relatively inexpensive and does not require any special equipment to implement. In addition, it allows the injection site to be closely observed so that the injection can be immediately stopped should there be signs of extravasation of contrast into the soft tissue. As mentioned earlier, this is often the recommended method for injecting into standard PICC lines. However, there are many disadvantages to the hand bolus method: the operator will be exposed to scatter radiation from standing in the room during the scanning process, and because someone must stay in the scan room this method requires two operators.

Probably the primary disadvantages are that the flow rate is variable because of the factors mentioned earlier and the scan delay cannot be precisely controlled; these two factors result in inconsistent images that are not readily reproducible in subsequent studies. So although the hand bolus method is an improvement over the drip infusion method, significant disadvantages limit its use to special circumstances.

Mechanical Injection Systems Mechanical injection systems are standard in CT suites because they deliver the precise flow rates and volumes specified by the operator, regardless of the viscosity of the solution and the gauge of the indwelling catheter. Injections are consistent and can be reproduced in subsequent examinations (providing parameters from studies are properly recorded and repeated). In addition, mechanical injectors are programmable, providing broad clinical utility for a wide range of indications.

BOX 13–12 Key Concept

Mechanical injection systems are standard in CT suites because

- They deliver precise flow rates and volumes
- Injections are consistent and can be reproduced in subsequent examinations
- They are programmable, providing broad clinical utility for a wide range of indications

---

Mechanical injectors, or power injectors as they are frequently called, are made by a variety of manufacturers, come in different models, and offer various features. CT injectors may have a single head for affixing the syringe (Fig. 13-11A) or they may accommodate two syringes (Fig. 13-11B). Dual-head injectors are designed so that saline can be given immediately before or after the contrast media injection. Most models of mechanical injec-

tor include a programmable pressure limit. This allows the operator to set an upper pressure limit, along with an injection rate. Contrast medium is then administered at the selected rate, unless the pressure reaches the maximum psi (pounds per square inch) set. If the pressure reaches the selected limit, the injector reduces the flow rate to prevent exceeding the pressure limit and an alarm sounds to notify the operator. Pressure limiting is designed to protect the integrity of the disposable components (e.g., IV tubing) used in the injection fluid path. Pressure is a result of the force required to overcome the resistance of pushing the contrast from the relatively large syringe barrel, through the patient connector tubing, any ancillary devices, and ultimately the catheter, at the required flow rate. Pressure is greatest at the point where the largest diameter merges to a far smaller diameter, in this case, the syringe tip. From that point to a point halfway down the length of the connecting tubing the pressure will drop by half, whereas at the tip of the catheter, pressure drops to near zero. A common reason for reaching the pressure limit is when the IV tubing becomes kinked, restricting the flow of contrast media. Another common culprit for reaching the pressure limit is the use of components in the fluid path that are not compatible with power injectors and the flow rates and pressures they generate. Another key factor in pressure limiting is contrast viscosity. As mentioned previously, higher iodine concentrations possess a higher viscosity,

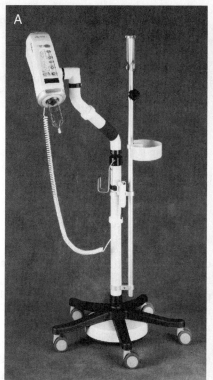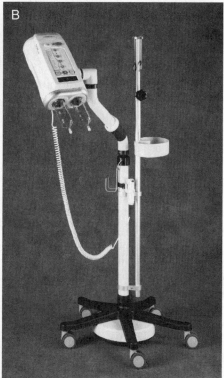

FIGURE 13-11 CT injectors may have a single head for affixing the syringe (A) or they may accommodate two syringes (B). Dual-head injectors are designed so that saline can be given before or after the contrast injection. Photos courtesy of Medrad, Inc.

particularly at room temperature. Contrast viscosity can be dramatically reduced, in some cases by nearly half, by simply warming contrast to body temperature (37°C).

BOX 13–13   Key Concept

When using mechanical injector for IV contrast administration, precaution must be taken to reduce the risk of serious extravasation of the contrast medium into the soft tissue.

Another feature available on some models is a device designed to aid in the detection of contrast medium extravasation. Extravasation is the leakage of fluid from a vein into the surrounding tissue during IV administration. There is particular concern that mechanical injectors may increase the severity of extravasation when extravasations occur. Because mechanical injectors typically deliver contrast at fast flow rates and the operator may not remain in the examination room throughout the injection to quickly intercede should signs of extravasation appear, there is worry that a large volume of contrast extravasation could more readily occur when a mechanical injector is used. However, when appropriate precautions are taken, the risk of serious extravasation can be substantially reduced. The extravasation detection feature available on some injector models is designed to augment, rather than supplant, such precautions. Guidelines are provided in Clinical Application Box 13-2.

Another potential safety feature available with some power injectors is the ability to perform a saline test injection before the delivery of contrast bolus injections. The saline may be programmed at the same flow rate as the contrast bolus, thereby more closely replicating an actual injection, and allowing the technologist additional time to monitor the viability of an IV site.

Although it rarely occurs, when a mechanical injector is used, large air embolism can result from the incorrect preparation and inadequate connection of the injector syringe and tubing. Air embolism can occur during any IV injection. Small quantities of air can be absorbed by the body, so small air emboli may never be detected if patients are asymptomatic. However, large air emboli can cause seizures, permanent neurologic damage, or occasionally death. These large air emboli occur only as a result of human error. Safeguards have been built into injection systems that are successful in preventing most errors of this type. When mistakes occur, they usually are a result of a disruption in the routine of preparing the injector. For example, in preparing for the next patient, the technologist must dispose of the empty syringe from the previous patient and replace it with a new syringe that is prefilled with contrast medium. In these injection systems, the plunger must be retracted before the empty syringe can be removed. The technologist does this, but before he can replace the empty syringe with a full one, the phone rings and he is called away. His

---

Clinical Application Box 13-2

Guidelines for Preventing Contrast Medium Extravasation (and reducing the risk of serious sequelae, should they occur)

In the CT department, extravasation of contrast medium into the subcutaneous tissue sometimes occurs. Mechanical injectors produce the best results and are therefore the most common delivery method. However, if appropriate precautions are not taken, extravasation is likely to be more common and more severe with the routine use of a mechanical injector. Every effort should be made to avoid contrast medium extravasation because the results may be serious, particularly when HOCM is used.

Most extravasations involve small volumes and are not clinically significant. Slight swelling and erythema may develop and usually subside without complication. However, severe tissue necrosis and ulceration may occur. Infants, young children, and unconscious and debilitated patients are at higher risk of contrast media extravasation.[7] LOCM is less injurious to cutaneous and subcutaneous tissue than HOCM.[8]

There is no universally accepted treatment for contrast extravasation. Treatment may include local application of heat for the first 6 hours, then application of cold; local injection of isoproterenol or propranolol; local injection of steroids; and surgical drainage. The result of the various courses of treatement is mixed, and the best method of reducing injury is prevention. Strict adherence to the following guidelines will substantially reduce the risk of contrast extravasation:

1. Use an indwelling catheter set with a flexible plastic cannula; 18 to 20 gauge is preferred. The use of metal needles (i.e., butterfly infusion sets or straight needles) should be avoided.
2. Monitor the injection site, preferably a medially directed antecubital vein, during the initial moments of injection. Swelling at the site of injection indicates extravasation, and the injection should be stopped immediately.
3. Warm the contrast medium to body temperature. Prewarming of the contrast material can help to reduce the viscosity so that it can flow more easily through indwelling IV catheters
4. Use LOCM.

---

coworker steps in to finish the process and, thinking that the syringe has already been replaced, connects it to the patient's IV line. Instead of injecting 120 mL of contrast media, the technologist injects a full syringe of air into the patient.

At least one injector manufacturer has incorporated automation to further reduce the possibility of air emboli. Injectors with this feature will automatically retract the injector position when the syringe is removed, returning it to the home position, before a new syringe is attached.

When a new, unused syringe is attached to the injector, it will automatically drive the piston forward to the load position, thus always avoiding an empty syringe being in place on the injector with the ability to inject air into the patient.

In addition, some syringes contain visual indicators that provide clear and immediate indications as to whether a syringe contains fluid or air.

The exact process of preparing the injector varies depending on the type of injection system, whether the facility uses prefilled syringes, and the specific injection protocol. Therefore, each facility should develop a clear protocol for preparing the mechanical injector(s) used in that department. The protocol should clearly specify the steps taken to prepare the injector for use. Clinical Application Box 13-3 provides an example of a protocol developed for a department that uses a single-head injection system and prefilled syringes.

In summary, the use of mechanical injectors produces the best results. However, precautions must be taken to prevent contrast media extravasation and care must be taken in the preparation and connection of the injector and cannula to avoid the risk of large air emboli. Table 13-3 lists the advantages and disadvantage of the various methods of intravascular contrast administration.

Factors Affecting Contrast Enhancement

Many factors affect the degree of contrast enhancement in human tissue. These factors can be broadly categorized as pharmacokinetic factors, which are largely controllable, and patient or equipment factors, over which technologists have little, or no, control.

Pharmacokinetic Factors

Pharmacokinetic factors include contrast medium characteristics (e.g., iodine concentration, osmolality, viscosity), contrast media volume, flow rate, flow duration, scan delay time, and total scan time.

Contrast Medium Characteristics   Contrast medium characteristics were discussed in detail in Chapter 12. However, one characteristic, that of contrast concentration, bears further elaboration in the context of how it affects injection protocols. Although many concentrations are commercially available, most facilities use one concentration for the majority of their CT examinations. Higher concentration agents may be reserved for specialized studies, such as CT angiography.

Contrast enhancement depends on the iodine concentration in the vasculature or tissues. In the vessels, this concentration depends on the injection rate of iodine in mg/s. Therefore, a concentration of 400 mg/mL injected at 3 mL/s will provide the same total iodine as a concentration of 300 mg/mL injected at 4 mL/s. In spite of the relatively equal enhancement they produce, there are

---

Clinical Application Box 13-3

Example of a Department's Mechanical Injector Protocol

Introduction

Following established procedure can dramatically reduce the number of adverse incidents related to IV injection. This is primarily true because as personnel become accustomed to a given routine, any deviation from the routine will serve as a red flag and cause the technologist to reexamine and double-check the system in question. Nowhere is this more true than in procedures involving the use of mechanical injectors. The potential of introducing an air embolus into the patient is quite real. Although rare, the consequences of such a mistake can be catastrophic. This risk can be greatly reduced when ALL personnel follow the same strict guidelines.

Before Injection

After establishing that the use of an iodinated contrast agent is appropriate (i.e., checking the doctor's order, the patient's identity, allergies, and blood work if available):

- The injector should be loaded using a prefilled syringe from the contrast warmer.
- The syringe is locked into place.
- The connector tubing is attached to the syringe. A locking cannula (e.g., BD Interlink plastic cannula [Baxter]) is connected to the tubing.
- The contrast is bled through the connector tubing and the cannula. Unless the cannula is to be immediately hooked to the patient's IV, the cannula cap must be replaced to prevent contamination of the sterile set.
- Once the injector is loaded and the air bled from the line, the syringe should be **pointed toward the ground**. This is a visual indicator for other personnel that the injector has been loaded.

Injection

- The injection site should be visually monitored for the first few seconds of the injection.
- Anytime the alarm on the injector sounds, the injector and injection site should be visually inspected before proceeding.

After Injection

The possibility of accidental air embolus can be significantly reduced by strict adherence to at least one of the following procedures:

- When the injector tubing is disconnected from the patient's IV, the injector head is **turned so that the syringe points toward the ceiling**—providing a visual clue that the syringe has been used.
- Cut the connector tubing—this will allow other team members to immediately know that the syringe has been used and needs to be replaced. It will also make it impossible to accidentally reconnect a used syringe.
- Do not withdraw the plunger from the syringe unless the syringe will be removed from the mechanical injector at that time.

TABLE 13-3   The Advantages and Disadvantage of Various Methods of Contrast Media Injection

Method	Pros °	Cons
Drip infusion	Inexpensive	Minimal flow rate Inconsistent images Nonreproducible May mask abnormalities Never reach peak enhancement
Hand bolus	Inexpensive Increased flow rate (compared with drip infusion) Can be used with all PICCs and CVADs	Scatter radiation to technologist Variability of flow rates Inconsistent images Nonreproducible Requires two operators

Mechanical injection system	Consistent images
	Reproducible
	Precise flow rates and volumes
	
	Programmable for uniphasic, biphasic, or
	   multiphasic injection protocols
		Capital investment required for
		   equipment purchase
		If proper injection guidelines are
		   not followed more serious
		   extravasation may result
		Incorrect preparation could result
		   in large air embolism

CVAD = central venous access device; PICC = peripherally inserted central catheter.

advantages and disadvantages associated with different concentration agents.

To maintain the same vascular and organ enhancement, lower concentrations of contrast medium require an increase in the injection rate and an increase in the volume (to maintain the same iodine dose). When IV access is not ideal (e.g., small-gauge catheter in the back of the hand), extravasation of contrast material is more likely when a higher injection rate is used. In addition, although uncommon, the increased contrast volume may impose an excessive volume load on some patients. This may be of concern in the rare instance when users make their own dilutions by adding saline solution or injectable distilled water to contrast media. Excessive dilution of contrast media with distilled water may produce hypotonic solutions, with an associated risk to the patient of edema.[6]

Lower concentrations of contrast medium have the advantage of possessing slightly lower osmolality, which is associated with fewer adverse effects. Theoretically, lower concentration solutions will produce fewer high-contrast (streak) artifacts in the injected vein. This is particularly important in the chest where streak artifacts are often created by dense contrast in the central veins (Fig. 13-12). Some power injectors offer the ability to inject contrast and saline simultaneously as a means of decreasing streak artifacts and optimizing image quality, while still delivering high-density contrast to the area of diagnostic interest.

In comparison, injecting a higher concentration agent (≥350 mg iodine/mL) will deliver the same amount of iodine at a lower flow rate. The same or higher flow rate provides a concentrated bolus that is well suited for examinations with a short scan duration (e.g., CT angiography), particularly when multislice scanners are used.

The viscosity of a contrast agent increases with its iodine concentration. Prewarming of the contrast material to body temperature can help to reduce the viscosity so that it can flow more easily through indwelling IV catheters. The value of a saline flush is increased when higher concentration agents are used because the more viscous contrast material will remain longer in the venous injection path.

Contrast Media Volume, Flow Duration, Flow Rate As scanner technology evolved from axial scanning to SDCT to MDCT, scan duration has dramatically decreased. This increased speed has had an impact on the volume of contrast media used for typical CT studies. When scanners were slower, a larger volume of injected contrast served to extend the flow duration and expand the window of opportunity for acquiring scans while tissues were optimally enhanced. Shorter acquisition times often allow the contrast volume to be reduced. The degree to which contrast volume can be decreased depends on the study, however. Whether, and how much, contrast volume can be cut during liver imaging is controversial. A certain amount of iodine is needed to achieve adequate parenchymal enhancement; dropping below that volume will reduce lesion conspicuity.

The rate that contrast media is injected largely determines the time needed for it to reach peak enhancement and will influence how dramatically enhancement falls off once this peak is reached. The effects of varying these factors are more pronounced for aortic enhancement

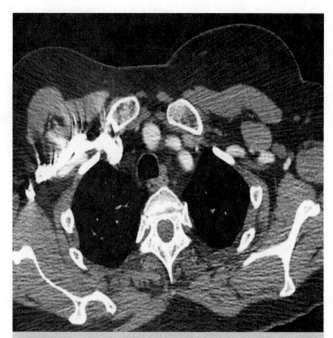

FIGURE 13-12 High-concentration contrast media has the disadvantage of producing more high-contrast (streak) artifacts in the injected vein. This is particularly important in the chest where streak artifacts are often created by dense contrast in the central veins. Image courtesy of the University of Michigan Health Systems.

than for hepatic enhancement. The consequences of varying contrast dose (determined by contrast volume and concentration) and flow rate can be graphically depicted using a time-density curve. The x axis of the graph depicts the time elapsed (in seconds) after the start of injection, whereas the y axis charts the relative enhancement levels achieved, in Hounsfield units (Figs. 13-14 through 13-17). Computer simulations and porcine models help to isolate the consequences of varying specific injection parameters.[9,10] The time-density curves included in this section are intended to illustrate the relationship between contrast media dose, injection flow rate, scan delay, and scan duration.

BOX 13-14   Key Concept

The rate at which contrast media is injected and the volume of contrast used significantly affect the time needed for the contrast to reach peak enhancement. These effects are more pronounced for aortic enhancement than for hepatic enhancement. Therefore, precise injection parameters, particularly scan delay, are more important for CT angiography than for routine body imaging.

The time-density curves in Figure 13-13 demonstrate the effects of varying contrast dose (maintaining concen-

tration but increasing volume) on aortic enhancement (Fig. 13-13A) and hepatic enhancement (Fig. 13-13B). In this simulation both the flow rate and iodine concentration were held constant. The graphs compare the enhancement achieved after three injection volumes, 75 mL, 125 mL, and 175 mL. We see that for a constant injection rate, as the contrast dose is increased (by increasing contrast volume), the magnitude of the peak enhancement increases and the time required to reach that peak also increases.[11] Furthermore, for any given level of desired enhancement, that level is maintained longer as contrast volume increases.

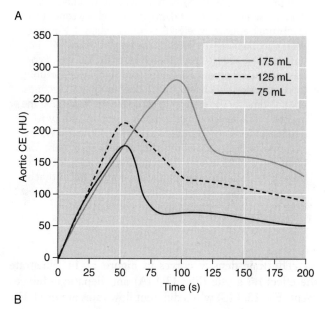

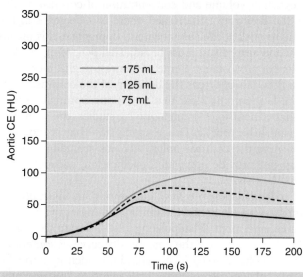

FIGURE 13-13 Time-density curves demonstrate the effect of varying contrast dose on aortic (A) and hepatic (B) contrast enhancement (CE).

Contrast Volume, Scan Duration

Using the graph from Figure 13-13A, consider the following hypothetical scenario:

Radiologists at your facility determine that aortic enhancement level for scan acquisition for a specific CT angiography study be at least 200 HU. The scanner at your facility can complete the programmed images in 14 to 20 seconds. Assuming that the graph in Figure 13-13A reflects the injection protocol flow rate used at your facility, what volume of contrast (of the three depicted in the graph) should be used for these studies?

Answer: 125 mL. Using the graph we can predict that the target rate of 200 HU for aortic enhancement will be reached at approximately 50 seconds after injection. Injecting 125 mL of contrast medium, the enhancement level will continue to climb until approximately 75 seconds, when it will peak. After approximately 85 seconds the enhancement will drop to below the 200 HU level. Therefore, using 125 mL of contrast media will produce a window of scanning opportunity (aortic contrast enhancement ≥ 200) of roughly 35 seconds, enough time for the scanner to complete the images. At the injection rate depicted by the graph, 75 mL will not provide a sufficient level of contrast enhancement. Although 175 mL of contrast will result in a both a higher peak aortic enhancement and a wider window for acquiring the scan, neither of these is necessary for the specific application. Recall that an overarching goal of IV contrast injection is to use the lowest dose necessary to obtain adequate visualization.

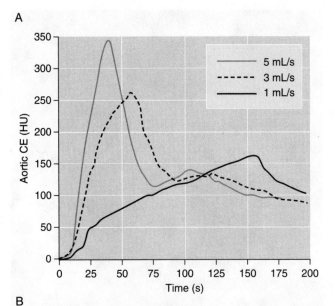

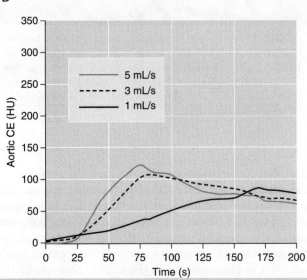

FIGURE 13-14 The time-density curves demonstrate the effect of varying flow rate on aortic (A) and hepatic (B) contrast enhancement (CE) when different flow rates are used. For a constant volume and concentration of contrast media, as the flow rate is increased, there is a decrease in the time to peak aortic enhancement.

The time-density curves in Figure 13-14 illustrate the effect on aortic (Fig. 13-14A) and hepatic enhancement (Fig. 13-14B) when different flow rates are used. For a constant volume and concentration of contrast media, as the flow rate is increased, there is a decrease in the time to peak aortic enhancement. In practice, this means that the scan delay must be adjusted according to flow rate. For a constant volume of contrast media, increasing the flow rate shortens the duration of the contrast injection. It should be clear that to capture optimal vascular enhancement for CT angiography studies, the scan timing must be precise. Image acquisition that is too soon will miss the contrast bolus, whereas scanning too late may not provide adequate opacification, particularly of small vessels.

Manipulating the flow rate during an injection can improve the likelihood of scanning during optimal vascular enhancement. Manipulating the flow rate to change the characteristics of the time-density curves is sometimes called "bolus shaping." The typical time-density curve for aortic enhancement using a single injection flow rate (uniphasic), such as that depicted by the black line in the graph in Figure 13-15, is not ideal for CT angiography. A uniphasic injection results in a single peak of aortic enhancement that is generally much greater than necessary, but of a very short duration. Ideally, injection techniques would achieve an adequate level of aortic enhancement and then maintain that level for a longer period of time, depicted by the blue line in the graph in Figure 13-15. This would increase the window of opportunity for scanning, allowing the scan timing to be less precise. This is particularly useful when using a slower scanner, when using very narrow collimation, or when scanning a longer area. In addition, more uniform vascular enhancement is beneficial for postprocessing. In practice, bolus shaping is accomplished by beginning the injection with a relatively high flow rate and then decreasing the flow rate throughout the remain-

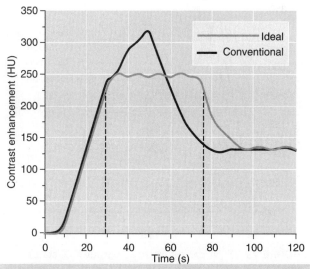

FIGURE 13-15 Typical time-density curves for aortic enhancement using a single injection rate result in a single peak of aortic enhancement that is greater than necessary, but of a very short duration (black line). Ideally, injection techniques would achieve an adequate level of aortic enhancement and then maintain at that level for a longer time (gray line). This would allow the scan timing to be less precise.

Clinical Application Box 13-5

Contrast Flow Rate, Scan Delay

Using the graph from Figure 13-14A, consider the following hypothetical scenario:

The injection protocol for a specific CT angiography study calls for a 5 mL/s injection rate and a scan delay of 20 seconds. According to the graph how should the scan delay be adjusted if the patient's IV access limits the injection rate to 3 mL/s?

Answer: The scan delay should be increased to 40 seconds. Using the graph we see that 20 seconds after beginning the contrast injection at a flow rate 5 mL/s, aortic enhancement is expected to reach approximately 225 HU. If the flow rate is slowed to 3 mL/s, the graph indicates that it will take approximately 40 seconds for aortic enhancement to reach this point.

Note: This exercise is intended to illustrate the relationship between contrast flow rate and scan delay. In practice, bolus triggering or the use of a timing bolus is often used to better tailor the scan initiation to specific patient circumstances.

der of the injection period. When two flow rates are used the technique is often referred to as biphasic; when more than two flow rates are used the technique is referred to as multiphasic. Often the final flow rate is to deliver a saline flush. This allows the entire volume of contrast media to be used as the saline pushes forward any contrast that remains in the injection veins. In some instances bolus shaping can allow a reduction in contrast volume. This is possible when it is used with a fast scanner or when the scan area is relatively limited. However, for most clinical applications a uniphasic contrast injection with a constant flow rate is sufficient.[6]

BOX 13-15   Key Concept

For most clinical applications a uniphasic contrast injection with a constant flow rate is sufficient.

Although considerably less pronounced, many of the same principles apply to hepatic enhancement (Figs. 13-13B and 13-14B). That is, increasing the dose will increase the magnitude of the hepatic enhancement and increasing the flow rate will shorten the time to peak enhancement. However, compared with aortic enhancement the slope of the contrast-timing curves for hepatic enhancement is less steep with a longer horizontal portion during which contrast enhancement remains relatively constant. In practice this allows a wider window of opportunity for scanning; therefore, the timing of scans for routine abdominal imaging does not need to

be as precise as those designed to capture peak aortic enhancement.

Patient Factors Affecting Contrast Enhancement

Many patient factors have important effects on contrast enhancement. These include the patient's age, sex, weight, height, cardiovascular status, renal function, and the presence of other disease.[9] Although patient factors are largely uncontrollable, it is important to recognize their potential effects on contrast enhancement. In some cases injection parameters can be adjusted to help mitigate patient factors.

The patient's weight has a pronounced effect on the degree of aortic and parenchymal enhancement. Figure 13-16 displays a time-density curve for each of a number of simulations of patients with different body weight, when all other factors are held constant.[11] Notice that although peak enhancement is reached at nearly identical times, as patient weight increases the magnitude of contrast enhancement diminishes. In large patients arterial enhancement can be increased by increasing the injection rate (by either increasing the flow rate or increasing the iodine concentration). Because hepatic parenchymal enhancement is determined primarily by the total iodine dose, increasing the dose can also improve hepatic enhancement in large patients. For this reason, some institutions used a weight-based system for determining the contrast media dose for routine body scans.

A patient's cardiac output status can have a significant effect on the time it takes injected contrast media to reach peak aortic enhancement. As cardiac output is reduced, there is a progressively longer delay in the time required

A

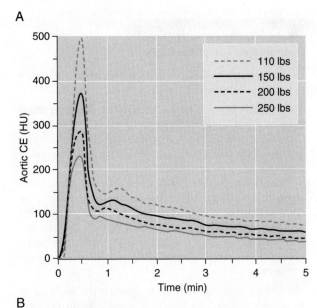

B

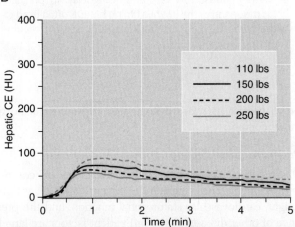

FIGURE 13-16 The time-density curves demonstrate the effect of body weight on aortic (A) and hepatic enhancement (B). Although peak enhancement is reached at nearly identical times, as patient weight increases the magnitude of contrast enhancement (CE) diminishes.

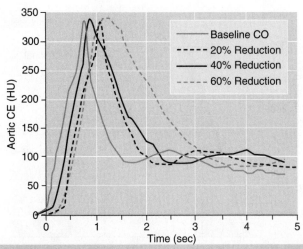

FIGURE 13-17 A patient's cardiac output (CO) status will affect the time it takes injected contrast media to reach peak aortic contrast enhancement (CE). As cardiac output is reduced, there is a progressively longer delay in the time required for the contrast bolus to reach the aorta.

for the contrast bolus to reach the aorta, thus delaying peak aortic enhancement (Fig. 13-17). This requires the scan delay to be extended in proportion to the degree of cardiac impairment; practically, this can only be done by using a method (i.e., test bolus, or bolus-tracking) that individualizes the scan delay to the patient.

Equipment Factors Affecting Contrast Enhancement

Contrast administration and scan timing must also be modified according to the type and capabilities of the CT scanner used. For instance, the scan duration is considerably less for a 64-detector row scanner than for a single-detector row scanner. As a general rule, the scan delay is increased as scan duration decreases. Adding 5 to 20 seconds to the scan delay helps to ensure imaging occurs during peak arterial enhancement. In this way, it

is possible to keep all other contrast injection parameters constant, thereby achieving the same aortic enhancement curves, by simply adjusting the scan delay according to scanner speed. For some applications, a faster scanner may allow the use of a smaller volume of contrast material. As stated previously, when the volume is decreased, the peak enhancement level decreases (Fig. 13-13). Therefore, injection rate or iodine concentration is typically increased to compensate.

Automated Injection Triggering   Two methods exist for individualizing the scan delay; the injection of a test bolus and bolus triggering. Both techniques require the CT scanner to have specialized software. These methods are particularly useful for vascular imaging, in which it is critical that the timing of scan acquisition coincide with peak contrast enhancement. These methods effectively accommodate individual differences in circulation time caused by heart rate, age, and illnesses.

BOX 13-16   Key Concept

Two methods exist for individualizing the scan delay to adjust for patient factors, the injection of a test bolus and bolus triggering. Both techniques require the CT scanner to have specialized software.

Test Bolus   This method consists of administering 10 to 20 mL of contrast medium by IV bolus injection and performing several trial scans to determine the length of time from injection to peak contrast enhancement in a target region, such as the aorta. Using a mechanical injector, the test injection is delivered at the same rate as the diagnostic scans. Trial scans are taken using the lowest

A

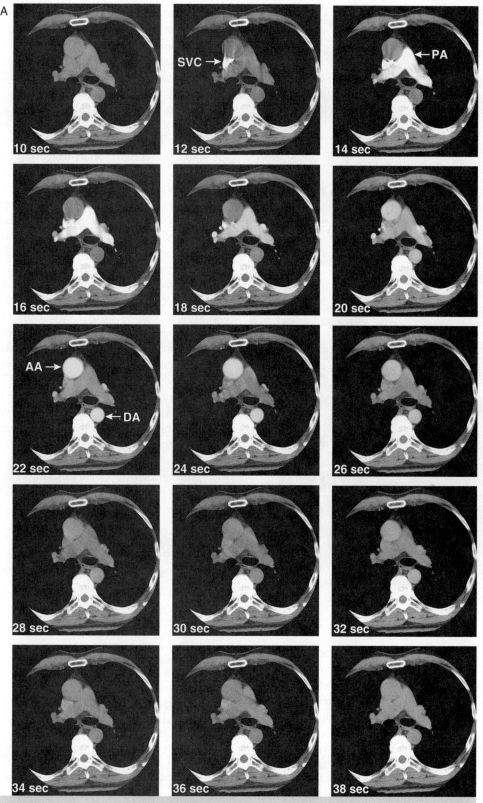

FIGURE 13-18 The timing bolus technique uses a small bolus of contrast to determine the contrast transit time. Images just below the carina are acquired every 2 seconds starting 10 seconds after injection of 20 mL of iodinated contrast material. Arrows show passage of contrast material through superior vena cava (SVC) at 12 seconds, pulmonary artery (PA) at 14 seconds, and ascending aorta (AA) and descending aorta (DA) at 22 seconds. A region of interest is placed within the descending aorta; the graph confirms the visual observation that the highest enhancement level occurred on image 7, which corresponds to 22 seconds after the contrast injection.

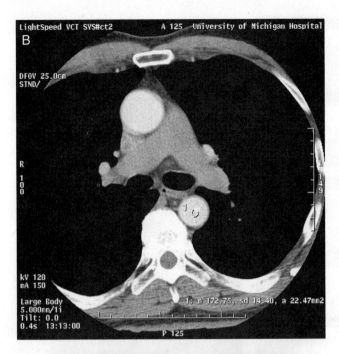

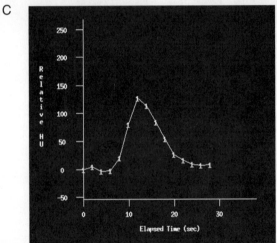

FIGURE 13-18 Cont'd

are obtained every 2 seconds, scan time can be calculated from the test injection using the following: trial scan delay + (2 × the image showing maximum enhancement) + 3 seconds. Special test bolus software helps to simplify the process by graphing the time of the trial injection against the level of contrast enhancement (Fig. 13-18). Clinical Application Box 13-6 provides an example of a test bolus using software on a General Electric CT scanner.

Bolus Triggering This method of individualizing the scan delay is called bolus-triggering, bolus-tracking, or automated triggering. It is a more efficient method than the test bolus because it uses the contrast bolus itself to initiate the scan. This technique uses a series of low-radiation scans to monitor the progress of the contrast bolus. To accomplish this, a single cross-sectional slice is taken and an area of interest is defined. The injection is initiated, and low-radiation scans begin from 8 to 10 seconds later. These scans are sometimes referred to as "monitor scans." Once an adequate level of enhancement is achieved (determined visually or by a cursor placed on the area of interest), the table moves to the starting level and scanning begins. Scanning can be triggered automatically by setting a predetermined threshold CT number or it can be initiated manually by the technologist (Fig. 13-19).

Because the table must move to the correct position and the mAs be set to the appropriate level for diagnostic scanning, there is a 3- to 9-second delay between the last monitor scan and the start of scanning. This lag time is seen by many as a significant drawback to the technique. Recognizing the delay, many facilities use a relatively low

possible mAs settings, typically at 2-second intervals, at the same slice location, for 20 to 30 seconds (i.e., 10 to 15 scans). Trial scans begin from 8 to 15 seconds after the start of the injection, depending on the patient's presumed circulatory status. Hence, trial scans of younger patients with no history of heart disease would begin 8 seconds after the start of the injection, whereas the trial scan of an older patient with known congestive heart failure requires a longer delay. The test bolus is evaluated by identifying the image that shows the maximum enhancement in the target region. The optimal scan delay time for the actual study is presumed to be equal to the time that elapsed from the start of the test injection to that of the image showing maximum enhancement. Experience shows that the best results are achieved by adding 3 seconds to this calculated delay. Therefore, when the test injection images

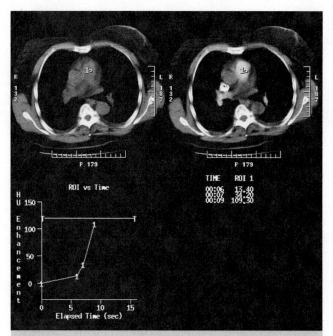

FIGURE 13-19 The bolus triggering technique uses a series of dynamic, low-dose axial scans to track the bolus of contrast material. A single slice is obtained to include the vessel in which the contrast will be tracked, in this case, the main pulmonary artery. The imaging sequence is initiated when the contrast enhancement reaches a predefined value, usually 100 HU. In this instance the automatic trigger was set for 125 HU as a fail-safe; the scan was manually initiated when the 100-HU threshold was reached.

trigger threshold (approximately 50 HU) or manually start the scan as soon as the contrast material is seen in the target region.

An important drawback to bolus triggering is that a technologist cannot stay with the patient for even a short time after the contrast injection begins or they will be exposed to radiation from the monitor scans. The policy at many facilities is for the technologist to remain with the patient for the first few seconds of the injection to watch for extravasation by manually palpating the injection. Although a test injection with saline before the scan can help to verify the patency of the IV line, sometimes extravasation will still occur during the contrast injection. For this reason, bolus tracking is typically reserved for vascular imaging but not for routine examinations of the chest or abdomen, for which timing is not as critical. For routine studies, most facilities rely on preset scan delays. An example of bolus triggering using software on a General Electric CT scanner is included in Clinical Application Box 13-7.

With some newer, more advanced injector systems, many of the above strategies and calculations for designing patient-specific protocols are being calculated by the injector. At least one injector manufacturer now has built-in software that accounts for patient varia-

Clinical Application Box 13-7

Using Bolus Triggering Software

The steps to perform a test bolus may vary somewhat depending on the specific software manufacturer. This example is from a General Electric scanner.

1. Obtain scout views.
2. Obtain a single slice at the area of interest. To reduce the time needed for the table to move to the examination starting location, select a slice within the area of interest that is nearest to the start location as possible.
3. Plan the diagnostic study.
4. Set the trigger threshold, or prepare to manually start the scan sequence.
5. Start the contrast injection. When the area identified on the monitor scans reaches the threshold start the scan.
6. While the table is moving to the start location, instruct the patient to hold his breath (for body studies).

tion in weight, time to peak, scan duration, and contrast iodine concentration and can prescribe an individualized injection protocol designed to optimize enhancement. Further developments will, no doubt, be forthcoming in this area.

SUMMARY

As CT scanners have evolved, the use of intravascular contrast media has become more complex. Contrast media administration requires more tailoring than in the past. Injection techniques must be carefully evaluated so that injection protocols can be developed that suit the specific needs of the facility. Technologists must recognize the many variables surrounding contrast administration so that they can assist radiologists in developing injection protocols and to ensure that the protocols are appropriately followed.

REVIEW QUESTIONS

1. List the qualities of an IV access site that would make it ideal for administering contrast media.
2. In what circumstances can a peripherally inserted central catheter safely be used for contrast media injection?
3. Describe the three general phases of tissue enhancement.
4. What does "contrast arrival time" mean? What will result if scanning takes place prior to that time?
5. Describe the different methods of intravenous contrast media delivery. List the advantages and disadvantages of each method.
6. What safety measures should be followed when using a mechanical injection system to administer contrast media?
7. Explain how variations in contrast dose and flow rate affect aortic enhancement. Is hepatic enhancement affected in the same way?

8. Describe the two methods available for individualizing the scan delay. List the advantages and disadvantages of each method.

REFERENCES

1. ACR Committee on Drugs and Contrast Media. Manual on Contrast Media, Version 5.0. 5th Ed. Reston, VA: ACR, 2004.
2. Bower L, Speroni KG, Jones L, Atherton M. Comparison of occlusion rates by flushing solutions for peripherally inserted central catheters with positive pressure Luer-activated devices. J Infus Nurs 2008;31:22–7.
3. Funaki B. Central venous access: a primer for the diagnostic radiologist. AJR Am J Roentgenol 2002;179:309–18.
4. Rivitz SM, Drucker EA. Power injection of peripherally inserted central catheters. J Vasc Interv Radiol 1997;8: 857–63.
5. Miller PA. Central venous access devices. J Radiol Technol 2006;77:297–305.
6. Prokop M, van der Molen AJ. Patient preparation and contrast media application. In: Prokop M, Galanski M, van der Molen AJ, Schaefer-Prokop C, eds. Spiral and Multislice Computed Tomography of the Body. Stuttgart, Germany: Thieme, 2002:97–100.
7. Bellin MF, Jakobsen JA, Tomassin I, Thomsen HS, Morcos SK. Contrast medium extravasation injury: guidelines for prevention and management. Eur Radiol 2002;12:2807–12.
8. Leder RA, Dunnick NR. Contrast media use in computed tomography. In: Katzberg RW, ed. The Contrast Media Manual. Baltimore: Williams & Wilkins, 1992:68.
9. Bae KT, Heiken JP, Brink JA. Aortic and hepatic contrast medium enhancement at CT. Part I. Prediction with a computer model. Radiology 1998;207:647–55.
10. Bae KT, Heiken JP, Brink JA. Aortic and hepatic contrast medium enhancement at CT. Part II. Effect of reduced cardiac output in a porcine model. Radiology 1998;207:657–62.
11. Heiken JP. CTA of the abdominal aorta guides stent-grafting. Appl Radiol 2004;33:37–44.

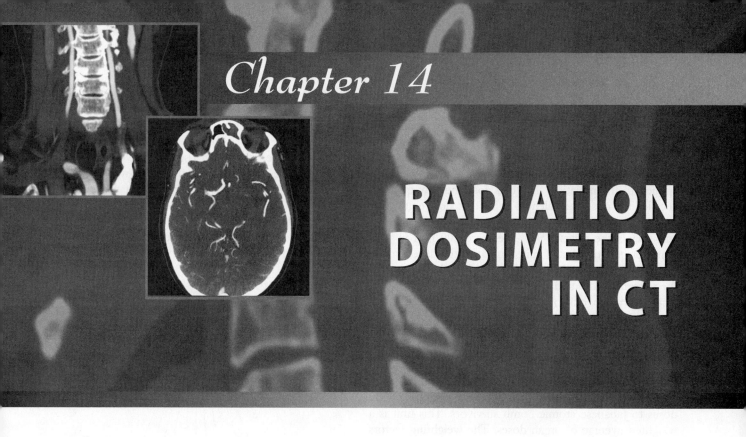

Chapter 14

RADIATION DOSIMETRY IN CT

Key Terms: roentgen (R) • radiation absorbed dose (rad) • International System of Units (SI) • gray (Gy) • centigray (cGy) • quality factor (Q) • roentgen equivalents man (rem) • sievert (Sv) • effective dose • effective dose equivalent • z axis dose distribution • radiation profile • tails • multiple scan average dose (MSAD) • computed tomography dose index (CTDI) • $CTDI_{100}$ • $CTDI_w$ • $CTDI_{vol}$ dose-length product (DLP) • overbeaming • organ dose • automatic tube current modulation

BASIC DOSE CONCEPTS

It is the responsibility of each imaging professional to understand the benefit versus the risks of any procedure and attempt to maximize the positive and minimize the negative.

The rational use of CT relative to patient care involves two components: appropriate patient selection and minimization of the radiation dose without compromising diagnostic image quality. In an effort to address the need for appropriate patient selection, the American College of Radiology (ACR) has created guidelines that are widely available. Although appropriate patient selection is essential, it falls primarily to the radiologist to enforce ACR guidelines. Therefore, this chapter will focus mainly on the second component of the rational use of CT, that is, strategies to minimize dose while maintaining image quality.

To understand the many interrelated factors involved, we begin by reviewing basic radiation dose concepts as they relate to CT. We start with definitions of commonly used terms, then progress to a discussion of how dose is calculated in traditional axial studies. Using this knowledge as a background, we then discuss the effects of various technical CT factors on radiation dose.

Measurement Terminology

The ionizing radiation used in CT is an x-ray with maximum energy from 120 to 140 keV and an average energy near 70 keV.* The unit of x-ray exposure in air is the roentgen (R). When the x-rays from a CT scanner strike a patient and interact with tissue, most of the energy is absorbed, and some of it passes through to the detector.

The unit of absorbed dose is called the radiation absorbed dose, or rad. This unit describes the amount of energy absorbed per unit mass. The International System of Units (abbreviated SI from the French Le Système International d'Unités) is a newer system that is used internationally, both in everyday commerce and in science. The SI unit of absorbed dose is the gray (Gy). There are 100 rad in 1 Gy. A centigray (cGy) equals 1 rad.

---

*Physicists measure the energies of fast-moving particles like those in x-rays, cosmic rays, and particle accelerators in units called electron volts (eV). An eV is the amount of energy that one electron gains when it is accelerated by an electrical potential of 1 volt. (A flashlight battery has about 1.5 volts.) 1 keV = 1,000 eV.

In recognition of the health effects of x-rays, another conversion factor, called the quality factor (Q), is applied to the absorbed dose. This factor accounts for the different biologic effects produced from different types of ionizing radiation. The quality factor is 1 for the diagnostic x-rays that are used in CT. When the quality factor has been applied to the radiation absorbed dose the new quantity is called the dose equivalent. The unit for dose equivalent is the rem, or roentgen equivalent man. The SI equivalent unit is the sievert (Sv). There are 100 rem in 1 Sv. A newer quantity that is quite similar to the dose equivalent is called the equivalent dose (H). It is the product of the absorbed dose and a radiation weighting factor (w_R). The w_R is analogous to the Q. The unit for the equivalent dose is also the rem or the Sv.

Another measurement, referred to as effective dose, or effective dose equivalent, attempts to account for the effects particular to the patient's tissue that has absorbed the radiation dose. It extrapolates the risk of partial body exposure to patients from data obtained from whole body doses to Japanese atomic bomb survivors. This unit is a weighted average of organ doses. The weighting factors are set for each radiosensitive organ in Publication 60 of the International Commission on Radiological Protection.[1] Effective dose is reported in Sv or rem. Although methods to calculate the effective dose have been established, they depend on the ability to estimate the dose to radiosensitive organs from the CT procedure. Unfortunately, determining the radiation dose to these organs is problematic and is a barrier to accurate calculation of the effective dose.[2]

BOX 14-1   Key Concept

Unit of Radiation Dose
Roentgen (R): exposure in air
Radiation absorbed dose (rad): unit of absorbed dose
Gy: Le Système International d'Unités (SI) 1 cGy = 1 rad
Quality factor (Q), and radiation weighting factor (w_R): accounts for different types of radiation
Roentgen equivalent man (rem): unit that represents quality factor being applied to rad
Sievert (Sv): SI unit for the rem

Dose Geometry

In conventional film-screen radiography, the skin of the entrance plane receives 100% of the radiation, and the percentage falls rapidly as the x-ray beam is attenuated by the patient's tissue. By the time the beam exits the patient, most of the radiation has been absorbed or scattered (Fig. 14-1). In conventional radiography, it is common for the exit dose to be only 1% (or 1/100) that of the entrance dose.

In CT, the difference between the dose at the center and the dose at the periphery is not nearly as great as that of conventional radiography. In fact, in CT studies of the head, the dose to the skin is close to that in the center of the slice. The dose is more uniform in CT than in general radiography for two reasons. First, in CT, the beam is heavily filtered as it exits the x-ray tube. This means that fewer low-energy (or "soft") photons remain. Because the beam is "harder" than that used in conventional radiography, a lower percentage of the beam will be absorbed or scattered as it passes through patient tissue. In addition, the CT exposure comes from all directions, creating a more uniform exposure (Fig. 14-2).

The uniformity of the dose decreases as the scan field of view and patient thickness increase. Therefore, body

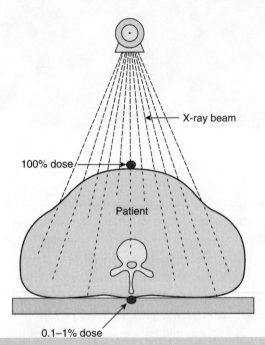

FIGURE 14-1 In conventional radiography, the exit dose may be only 1% of the entrance dose.

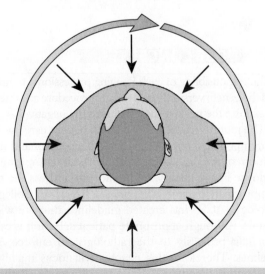

FIGURE 14-2 Rotational nature of CT beam.

scans are less uniform than head scans. The central dose for a body scan is approximately one-third to one-half that of the peripheral dose (Fig. 14-3). To a great degree, this phenomenon accounts for the fact that, for a given set of machine parameters (mAs, slice thickness, and pitch), organ doses are clearly higher for children compared with (larger) adults. To elaborate, consider an organ located on the proximal side of the body relative to the x-ray source. This organ will get roughly the same dose in both adult and child. As the x-ray source rotates, that same organ will be on the distal side of the body relative to the x-ray source; now that organ is partly shielded by the body tissue proximal to it, reducing the organ dose. But this dose-reducing, partial shielding will be much less for a thin individual, such as a child, compared with a thicker adult. Thus, organ doses for children are larger than those for adults.[3]

Z Axis Variations

In addition to the variations within the scan plane, variations along the length, or z axis, of the patient, are described by the z axis dose distribution (or radiation profile). To understand this concept, let us first look at a traditional axial scan sequence (a full gantry rotation at one table position) with contiguous slices (slice thickness

is equal to the table increment; therefore, no overlapping slices, no gapped slices). If there were no scatter radiation, the exposure would be equal throughout the study. For the sake of illustration, let's assume that there is no scatter inherent in CT. In this case, if a single CT slice delivered a dose of 1 cGy, then the total exposure from a 30-slice CT examination that was performed with contiguous slices would also deliver 1 cGy. This would be true because no area of the patient is exposed more than once.

In reality, there is some scatter inherent in CT. However, it is important to recognize that, although there is some radiation that is scattered, the overall amount is low, and the distance it travels is quite short, particularly when compared with conventional radiography. In this discussion of scatter, we are considering scatter that affects adjacent slices. Therefore, we are referring to a distance of only 1 to 10 mm. In CT, the amount of scatter that travels

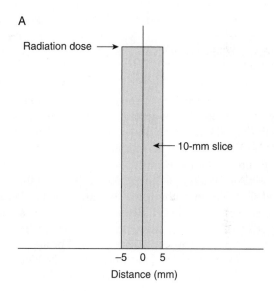

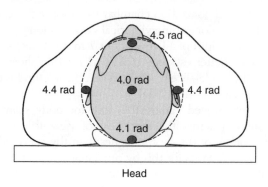

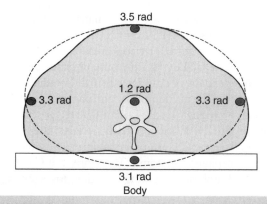

FIGURE 14-3 The center of the patient can receive nearly as much radiation as the periphery for head scans. However, this is not as true for body scans because the dose uniformity decreases as the scan field of view and patient thickness increase.

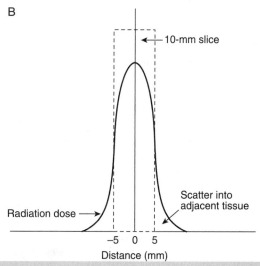

FIGURE 14-4 A. Ideal radiation profile, if no scatter radiation existed. **B.** Actual profile because radiation spreads to tissue outside the designated slice as a result of scatter.

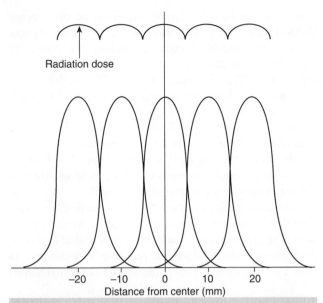

FIGURE 14-5 The radiation dose from multiple scans accounts for scatter overlap from each neighboring slice to the radiation dose of the central slice.

greater distances, such as to the door of the scan room, is very small. However, to accurately assess the z axis dose distribution, the radiation that scatters into adjacent slices must be added to the dose to a single slice.

Figure 14-4A represents an ideal slice with no scatter. In this ideal situation, all the radiation falls within the designated slice. However, this is not the case in reality, because there is some scatter in CT. Because of this scatter, some of the radiation spreads to tissue outside the designated slice. Figure 14-4B represents a true slice profile. The areas of scatter into adjacent tissue are sometimes called tails. Figure 14-5 represents a slice profile that results from multiple scans.

As illustrated, the total dose will be higher when multiple scans are performed. How much the scatter will contribute to the dose depends on factors such as patient size and physical makeup and the kVp used. In general, the tails will contribute approximately 25% to 40% additional dose to the entire study. Therefore, if a single slice of the chest delivered a dose of 4 cGy, the entire dose from 30 contiguous slices would range from approximately 5 cGy (i.e., 4 cGy + 1 cGy) to 5.6 (i.e., 4 cGy + 1.6 cGy). As compared with the dose from a single slice, the overall radiation dose will be higher when multiple scans are performed.

Because most CT applications involve multiple adjacent slices, dose is usually calculated from multiple scans. Measurements are made at the center of the slice and several points around the periphery with plastic phantoms. This procedure accounts for the effect of scatter from the tails of each slice into the neighboring slices. Again, total dose is the central slice radiation dose, plus the scatter overlap (or tails). This is called the multiple scan average dose (MSAD). The MSAD will increase if slices overlap and decrease if there are gaps between slices.

Another type of radiation dose measurement in CT is the computed tomography dose index (CTDI). This allows an estimate of the MSAD to be accomplished with a single scan.[4] The CTDI is what manufacturers report to the U.S. Food and Drug Administration (FDA) and prospective customers regarding the doses typically delivered for their machines. The CTDI can only be calculated if slices are contiguous, that is, there are no overlapping or gapped slices. If there is slice overlap or gaps, the CTDI is multiplied by the ratio of slice thickness to slice increment. This would technically be the MSAD, because the CTDI conditions would no longer exist. Equipment manufacturers report CTDI doses for typical head and body imaging techniques. These are equivalent to the dose a patient receives if multiple adjacent slices are acquired.

Medical physicists usually use a special dosimeter called a pencil ionization chamber to measure the CTDI. This 100-mm-long thin cylindrical device is long enough to span the width of 14 contiguous 7-mm CT slices. This provides a better estimate of MSAD for thin slices than that of the single-slice method. When this method is used it is referred to as the $CTDI_{100}$.

As mentioned earlier, the dose for body scans are not uniform across the scan field of view–the dose at the periphery of the slice is higher than the central dose. The $CTDI_w$ adjusts for this by providing a weighted average of measurements at center and the peripheral slice locations (i.e., the x and y dimensions of the slice). The $CTDI_{vol}$ radiation dose parameter takes the process a step further by taking account the exposure variation in the z direction. For helical sequences the $CTDI_{vol} = CTDI_w$/pitch. The $CTDI_{vol}$ is now the preferred expression of radiation dose in CT dosimetry. The $CTDI_{vol}$ is a measure of exposure per slice and is independent of scan length. If the irradiated length of the scan is to be accounted for, the parameter used is the dose-length product (DLP): DLP = $CTDI_{vol}$ × scan length. Although the DLP more closely reflects the radiation dose for a specific CT examination, its value is affected by variances in patient anatomy. Therefore, the $CTDI_{vol}$ is a more useful tool for comparing radiation doses among different protocols.

Comparison of Dose From CT With Dose From Conventional Radiographic Studies

Because the modalities are significantly different, a simple comparison between doses delivered from CT and those delivered from film-screen radiography cannot be conducted. These two imaging modalities are significantly different in principle and purpose and also have different imaging requirements. However, it is important for technologists to have a general idea of the dose being delivered to the patient and how it relates to other modalities.

CT is an excellent low-contrast discriminator because of the highly collimated x-ray beams and low amount of scatter that reaches the detector. Film-screen systems are inferior in their low-contrast sensitivity. Film is unable to discriminate objects that have less than 10% contrast with their background material. Conversely, CT can typically resolve and display visual differences between small objects that have only a minimal difference in density, as little as 0.1% to 0.5%. This capability allows visualization of soft tissue masses that are not seen with film-screen systems. However, there is a price to be paid to produce good low-contrast images. An adequate radiation dose, or photons per pixel, must be provided to suppress image noise. As a result, the radiation dose for CT examinations is substantially higher when compared with film-screen radiography (Table 14-1).

BOX 14–4   Key Concept

The price that is paid for the excellent low-contrast resolution seen on CT images is a relatively high radiation dose.

In the example given in Table 14-1, the skin (surface) dose is approximately 10 times higher in CT, and the average absorbed dose is approximately 100 times higher. Special procedures such as angiography and interventional radiography may produce radiation doses near or exceeding those from CT. Actual doses are highly variable and are affected by many factors, including type and manufacturer of scanner.

Further perspective can be gained from the seventh in a series of publications from the National Academies concerning radiation health effects called the Biologic Effects of Ionizing Radiation (BEIR VII). People in the United States are exposed to average annual background radiation levels of about 3 mSv: exposure from a chest x-ray is about 0.1 mSv, and exposure from a whole body CT scan is about 10 mSv.[5]

Factors Affecting Dose

Radiation Beam Geometry

Theoretically, a rotation arc of only 180° is all that is required to satisfy most construction algorithms. Most scanners use a 360° tube arc to compensate for radiation beam divergence and patient motion. The extra scanning information improves image quality but increases radiation dose. Additionally, overscanning, which is the process of using more than a 360° tube arc, is sometimes used–particularly in fourth-generation CT systems. Overscanning is also necessary for interpolation of projections in MDCT. Overscans will increase the radiation dose.

Filtration

Filtration affects the radiation dose by removing some of the soft (i.e., low-energy) x-rays. These low-energy x-rays are quickly absorbed by the patient. Photons are needed to penetrate the patient and strike the detectors, but some of them must be absorbed to produce radiographic contrast. Adding metal filters to the beam permits selective removal of x-rays with low energy and reduces the radiation dose while maintaining contrast at an acceptable level.

Detector Efficiency

Detector absorption efficiency affects radiation dose to the patient. Less-efficient detectors will require a higher radiation exposure to produce an adequate image. Solid-state detectors are from 90% to 100% efficient, whereas the xenon gas detectors used in older model scanners are significantly less efficient at absorbing x-rays.

Slice Width and Spacing

In considering a single cross-sectional slice, as slice thickness increases, the volume of tissue irradiated increases, and the dose may increase slightly to the adjacent slices. However, for multiple slice examinations, decreasing slice thickness and using contiguous slices will increase the MSAD because of the increased amount of scatter radiation to adjacent slices. Also, to maintain image quality at the same level, additional radiation is needed for thinner slices. Multiple slice examinations using overlapping slices will produce a higher overall dose, whereas gapped slices will produce a lower overall dose.

Although the effects of beam collimation are small for single-detector row scanners, that is not the case with MDCT. Reports from studies of early versions of MDCT systems revealed a significant dependence on x-ray beam collimation.[6] These effects are from penumbra. To have the same x-ray intensity reach all of the detectors in an MDCT system, the collimators must be opened slightly

---

TABLE 14-1   Approximate Dose Comparison Between General Radiography and CT

General Radiography	Computed Tomography
AP abdomen	Abdominal study
Surface dose = 0.3–0.6 cGy	Surface dose = 2–4 cGy
Central dose = 0.03–0.01 cGy	Central dose = 1–2 cGy

more, allowing the x-ray penumbra to fall outside the active detectors (Fig. 14-6). This is referred to as overbeaming. This contributes to the patient dose but is not used to create an image. The effect is more pronounced for smaller collimator openings.

Pitch

The spacing of CT slices obtained with a spiral (or helical) scan process is called pitch. The pitch is defined as the table distance traveled in one 360° rotation divided by the collimated width of the x-ray beam. For a single-slice helical CT, a pitch of 1 means that the slices are adjacent and not overlapped. Helical scans performed with a pitch of 1 deliver approximately the same dose as that of conventional axial CT studies–provided the kVp and mAs values are the same for each mode. Selecting a pitch greater than 1 will spread the radiation more thinly over the slices. That is, although there are no areas along the z axis that are skipped completely, the gantry will not make a full rotation in a given slice location. The pitch has a direct influence on patient radiation dose because as pitch increases, the time that any one point in space spends in the x-ray beam is decreased. Table 14-2 shows the relationship between radiation dose and various pitch selections. The values presented in Table 14-2 represent variations in pitch with all other technical parameters held constant on a single-detector row CT scanner.

For MDCT scanners, the pitch values must be interpreted differently.[6] For example, the table may be incremented 30.0 mm per rotation to image several simultaneous 10.0-mm slices; however, if the CT system collimates the x-ray beam for four 10.0-mm slices simultaneously (effective pitch, 30 mm/4 × 10 mm = 0.75), there is an overlap of irradiated tissue. However, MDCT scanners typically have several modes that allow the technologist to

TABLE 14-2   Changes in CTDI$_{vol}$ in Head and Body Phantoms as a Function of Pitch*

Pitch	CTDI$_{vol}$ in Head Phantom (mGy)	CTDI$_{vol}$ in Body Phantom (mGy)
0.5	80	36
0.75	53	24
1.0	40	18
1.5	27	12
2.0	20	9

Reprinted with permission from McNitt-Gray.[2]
*All other factors were held constant at 120 kVp, 300 mA, 1 s, and 10 mm. Results are from a single-detector row CT scanner.

TABLE 14-3   Changes in CTDI$_{vol}$ in Head and Body Phantoms as a Function of Collimation for an MDCT Scanner*

Collimation (mm)	Total Beam Width (mm)	CTDI$_{vol}$ in Head Phantom (mGy)	CTDI$_{vol}$ in Body Phantom (mGy)
4 × 1.25	5	62	33
2 × 2.5	5	62	33
1 × 5	5	62	33
4 × 2.5	10	46	24
2 × 5	10	46	24
4 × 5	20	40	20

Reprinted with permission from McNitt-Gray.[2]
*All other factors were held constant at 120 kVp, 300 mA, 1 s, and 10 mm. Results are from a multidetector row CT scanner.

select whether to overlap slices or extend the pitch. Generally, the radiation doses to patients are approximately 30% to 50% greater with earlier models of MDCT, primarily as a result of overbeaming, positioning of the x-ray tube closer to the patient, and possible increased scattered radiation with wider x-ray beams.[7] Table 14-3 shows the results when the collimation is changed while all other parameters are held constant.

Scan Field Diameter

As mentioned earlier, the scan field diameter affects the dose. Phantoms are frequently used to measure radiation dose. Phantoms of two diameters–16 and 32 cm–are used to simulate head and body scans, respectively. Each of the phantoms is created from the same material that is designed to simulate soft tissue. Holding all technical factors constant, a scan of the head phantom will result in a higher radiation dose than that of the body phantom. This is demonstrated by the data in Tables 14-2 and 14-3, in which the same technical factors were used for each phantom. Therefore, the primary difference in results between the head and body phantoms is size. Each of the

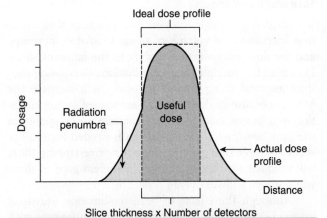

FIGURE 14-6 To have the same x-ray intensity at each of the detectors in an MDCT scanner, the collimators must be opened slightly more so that the x-ray penumbra falls outside the detectors. This contributes to the radiation dose to the patient but dose not contribute to the image created.

tables shows that the smaller object always absorbs the higher dose and that the difference is at least a factor of two. Thus, smaller patients would be expected to absorb much higher amounts of radiation than larger patients.

This effect is primarily attributed to the fact that total exposure is made up of both entrance radiation and exit radiation. For smaller patients, the patient has less tissue to attenuate the beam, which results in a much more uniform dose distribution. Conversely, for a larger patient, the exit radiation is much less intense as a result of its attenuation through more tissue.

Radiographic Technique

As in general radiography, the technique used to create the CT image affects radiation exposure to the patient. The higher the mAs and kVp settings used to create the image, the higher the dose to the patient.

The relationship between mAs and dose is linear. That is, if the mAs settings were doubled, the doses and risks would be doubled. Likewise, if the mAs settings were halved, the doses—and therefore the risks—would be halved. However, a reduction in dose is associated with a subsequent increase in image noise. For example, first assume that the minimum dose to obtain acceptable image quality has been determined. If this dose is halved by halving the mAs, a noise increase of 41% can be expected.[6]

X-ray tube potential (or kVp) also affects the radiation dose, although the effect is not linear. With the mAs kept constant, changing from 120 kVp to 140 kVp increases the radiation dose approximately 30% to 45%.

Patient Size and Body Part Thickness

Large patients or thick body parts require radiographic techniques that increase the radiation dose to avoid an unacceptable level of image noise. In addition, the patient size and body composition may affect the degree of scatter radiation.

Repeat Scans

Areas of the patient that are rescanned to visualize various stages of intravenous contrast enhancement or for other technical or clinical reasons receive additional radiation. The effect is cumulative.

Collimation

Lead collimators are used near the x-ray tube to control the size of the beam striking the patient. If the beam were not controlled to match the detector size, there would be additional scatter radiation to degrade the image; this scenario would result in a higher radiation dose to the patient. Collimators may also be used near the detectors for scatter rejection and aperture use.

Localization Scans

The localization scan performed before scanning, which is often referred to as the scout image, delivers a very low dose. The radiation dose for the scout image is much lower than that used to produce cross-sectional slices.

WHY THE GROWING CONCERN?

The management of radiation dose and image quality in CT has been a matter of concern since the introduction of the first scanners into clinical practice in the early 1970s. However, they are especially important now in view of the increased number of clinical applications, implementation of modern MDCT technology, proliferation of CT-guided procedures, early clinical trends toward screening studies, and the recent controversy concerning the connection between pediatric CT studies and an increased incidence of cancer.[3]

Commonly Used and Relatively High Radiation Doses

CT scanning is a relatively high-dose procedure that contributes disproportionately to the overall radiation dose from all radiologic sources. According to the estimates of Mettler and coworkers,[8] CT examinations represented approximately 11% of all diagnostic radiologic procedures but accounted for 67% of the effective dose from diagnostic radiologic procedures. This unbalanced distribution of dose is simply because the dose associated with CT is higher than that from other radiologic examinations.[8,9] To offer the reader a point of comparison, the radiation dose from one abdominal CT scan has been commonly reported to be equivalent to that of 100 to 250 chest radiographs.[8,10,11]

BOX 14–5 Key Concept

CT scanning is a relatively high-dose procedure that contributes disproportionately to the overall radiation dose from all radiologic sources.

Recent high-speed MDCT technology creates more-defined images in shorter times and has allowed for new clinical indications such as CT angiography. In addition, the faster scan speed has reduced the need for sedation in pediatric patients, thus spurring this modality's use in that population. However, such advantages come with a price. Comparing MDCT with older, single-detector row helical scanners, effective radiation dose is estimated to be 27% to 35% higher with MDCT, whereas organ dose (i.e., kidneys, uterus, ovaries, and pelvic bone marrow) is estimated to be 92% to 180% higher.[12,13] Hence, new CT technology results in two concerns: 1) expanded technology resulting in more CT studies being performed, and 2) higher radiation doses associated with the newer scanners.

New Information Concerning the Effects of Low-Dose Radiation

In the year 2000, new information concerning the effects of low-dose radiation on atomic bomb survivors who were irradiated as children prompted a change of thinking among both physicists and healthcare professionals. Research findings have shown that the effective doses with diagnostic CT have been shown to be similar to those received by Japanese survivors of the atomic bomb; these survivors had a small but statistically significant increased risk of developing cancer as a result of the radiation.[14] On the basis of predictions from the aforementioned data, radiation doses from typical pediatric CT studies may cause the eventual cancer-related death of 1 in 1,000 children examined.[15,16]

A Need for Education

A number of papers have called attention to the need for additional education on the part of just about everyone involved in health care, particularly when it comes to the care of children. Parents, pediatricians, technologists, and even radiologists often lack basic information regarding the dose delivered during CT examinations.

Inappropriate Scanning Parameters

One aspect of the problem was brought to light by a 2001 study in which Paterson and coworkers[17] evaluated the technical parameters used in outside CT examinations that were submitted to Duke University for a second opinion. Technical parameters that can be adjusted to lower doses in children—such as tube current (mA) and pitch—were reviewed. The authors found that most children were routinely being imaged with parameters suited for adults and that adjustments were not being made to compensate for the smaller size of children. In their study population no adjustments were made on the basis of patient age or size; mA settings were no less for the youngest infants and children than those used for teenaged patients. In fact, Paterson and coworkers[17] found that many infants were being imaged at a tube current greater than that used for adolescent patients for both chest and abdominal CT examinations. The mean tube current of the CT examinations in the study was 213 milliamperes (mA) with no adjustment for patient age.[17] The results suggested that pediatric patients were being exposed to unnecessarily high radiation doses from CT.

A lack of attention to the technical parameters used in CT examinations can be profound. When the radiation doses used in adult protocols are used in neonates or young children, the effective dose is up to 50% greater.[18] A more recent study in 2003 by Hollingsworth and coworkers[19] showed that progress is being made. In this study it was found that most pediatric radiologists practicing in children's or university hospitals do practice age-adjusted helical CT. Another encouraging finding by Hollingsworth et al.[19] was a trend of using increased tube current with increased age as well as an overall tendency to use a lower tube current for chest CT compared with abdominal CT in each age group. These practices are recommended for pediatric patients and were notably absent from the prior survey of techniques by Paterson and coworkers.[17] However, 11% to 26% of CT examinations performed on children younger than 9 years use more than 150 mA. Additionally, it was found that 20% to 25% of radiologist respondents did not know the specific parameters used for their examinations. Hollingsworth and coworkers[19] conclude that "Although the need for age-specific scanning is receiving more attention than it did previously, a substantial number of CT examinations in children are performed with relatively few adjustments. These data indicate the need for continued size-based scanning and education about the issues of radiation dose and pediatric CT techniques." There is also an abundance of evidence in the radiology literature that concludes that, in many circumstances, CT exposure doses could also be significantly reduced in adults.[20-22]

BOX 14–6   Key Concept

When the radiation doses used in adult protocols are used in neonates or young children, the effective dose is up to 50% greater. It is critical that technologists adjust scan parameters to suit the patient's size!

Extra Images

Another matter of concern is that of "extra" images contributing to the overall radiation dose of a CT examination. Extra images are defined as those images obtained beyond the desired area of interest. A retrospective study was conducted to determine the number and usefulness of images acquired beyond the intended anatomic area of interest with abdominal or pelvic CT.[23] Assuming other scanning parameters are held constant, the effective radiation dose is directly proportional to the scan volume. Therefore, restriction of the scan volume to the area of interest can help avoid unnecessary radiation. Researchers conducting this study found that a substantial number of extra images are acquired beyond the borders of the area of interest with abdominal or pelvic CT examinations. These extra images added approximately 10% to the patient's radiation dose from the examination. Study results showed that extra images are routinely obtained, both above the diaphragm and below the pubic symphysis, regardless of the clinical indications, patient age, or patient sex. It is noteworthy that the researchers who conducted this study also found that most extra images acquired contributed no additional information. Findings from extra images affected diagnosis in only 1 of 106 (<1%) cases.[23] However, the researchers did acknowledge factors that may, in some cases, justify the inclusion of images beyond the strict area of interest:

"At the supradiaphragmatic level, the acquisition of extra images may be justified to ensure that the entire liver and spleen are included in one phase of contrast enhancement. However, in a small number of cases in our study, as many as 36 extra images were acquired, a fact that may suggest a lack of attention in the selection of scan volume. Infrapubic extension of routine abdominal and/or pelvic CT examinations without appropriate clinical request or reason, especially given the risks of radiation to the gonads, cannot be as easily justified. Likewise, although the acquisition of extra images might be acceptable in uncooperative or breathless patients, we found that it adds no diagnostic information to that provided by images in the area of interest for routine abdominal and/or pelvic CT and should be restricted when not indicated or requested for specific clinical reasons. Indeed, it is important for radiologists and technologists to understand that the extension of image acquisition beyond the region of interest is associated with an additional radiation dose and that they share the responsibility of ensuring that scanning is restricted to the region of interest."[23]

BOX 14-7   Key Concept

Extra images are defined as those images obtained beyond the desired area of interest. They contribute to patient dose without adding useful diagnostic information.

Lack of Awareness

Another study by Lee and coworkers[24] was designed to determine the awareness level concerning radiation dose and possible risks associated with CT scans among patients, emergency department (ED) physicians, and radiologists. In this study each of the three groups (patients, ED physicians, radiologists) were surveyed and asked to estimate the radiation dose for one CT examination versus the dose for one chest radiograph (CR). Respondents could choose

from the following categories: one CT examination is less than or equal to one CR examination; one CT examination is greater than one CR examination, but less than 10 CR examinations; one CT examination is greater than 10 CR examinations but less than 100 CR examinations; one CT examination is equal to from 100 to 250 CR examinations; one CT examination is equal to or greater than 500 CR examinations (Table 14-4). Researchers in this study referred to the category of 100 to 250 as the accurate range. Other questions were also asked that were specific to each group. For instance, patients were asked whether the risks and benefits of the CT scan had been explained to them, and ED physicians were asked whether they had outlined the risks and benefits of the CT scan to their patients. The results from this survey are surprising. Only 7% of patients reported being informed of the risks and benefits before their CT examinations. None of the estimates given by the patients were in the accurate range; all patients significantly underestimated the radiation dose delivered by a CT examination. Twenty-two percent of ED physicians surveyed reported dose estimates in the accurate range. Four percent thought the dose to be higher than it actually was, whereas 73% underestimated the dose. Perhaps most surprising, of radiologists surveyed, only 13% reported dose estimates in the accurate range; 10% overestimated CT dose, whereas 76% underestimated dose. For both ED physicians and radiologists, there was no statistically significant relationship between years in practice and dose estimates. Lee and coworkers[24] concluded that "patients are not given information about the risks, benefits, and radiation dose for a CT scan. Patients, ED physicians, and radiologists alike are unable to provide accurate estimates of CT doses regardless of their experience level."

To summarize, the growing concern about the risks associated with diagnostic CT examinations can be linked to five main factors: 1) higher use; 2) new scanners that often deliver higher radiation doses; 3) new information correlating the effects of low-dose radiation to a higher

TABLE 14-4   Dose Estimates for One CT Scan vs One Chest Radiograph*

Respondent Group	CT ≤ CR	CT >CR < 10 × CR	CT ≥ 10 × CR < 100 × CR	CT = 100–250 × CR†	CT ≥ 500 × CR
Patients (N = 67)	19 (28)	43 (64)	5 (7)	0 (0)	0 (0)
ED Physicians (N = 39)	3 (7)	20 (44)	10 (22)	10 (22)	2 (4)
Radiologists (N = 39)	2 (5)	22 (56)	6 (15)	5 (13)	4 (10)

Reprinted with permission from Lee et al.[24]
*Numbers not in parentheses are the number of respondents. Numbers in parentheses are percentages.
†Accurate range.
CR = chest radiograph; CT = computed tomograph; ED = emergency department.

lifetime cancer risk; 4) lack of knowledge concerning the radiation dose among radiologists, technologists, attending physicians, and patients; and 5) studies showing that some facilities are not adjusting scanning parameters for pediatric patients, therefore exposing infants and children to a higher-than-necessary radiation doses.

PERCEPTION OF RISK

As mentioned earlier, there is a small but statistically significant increase in cancer deaths over the lifetime of individuals who undergo CT examinations in childhood. The estimated lifetime cancer mortality risk attributable to a pediatric radiation exposure (one person in one thousand people scanned during childhood) is greater than that found in a similar study of adult exposure.[14] These data only examine cancer deaths, not cancer occurrence. Many people who develop cancer are successfully treated and do not die of their cancer. Therefore, the incidence of cancer will most likely be shown to be greater (perhaps more than double) than the mortality figures.[14,25]

It is important to put the increased risk that pediatric radiation exposure poses into perspective so that we are better able to effectively communicate with patients and their families. Inherent in the discussion of risk is an understanding that the public may have a different perception of risk than that of scientists or researchers. In general, scientists define risks according to the language and procedures of science itself. They consider the nature of the harm that may occur, the probability that it will occur, and the number of people who may be affected. In contrast, the general public is less aware of probabilities and the size of a risk and much more concerned with broader, qualitative attributes, such as whether the risk is voluntarily assumed, whether the risks and benefits are evenly distributed, whether the risk is controllable by the individual, whether a risk is necessary and unavoidable, and whether there are safer alternatives.[26] Some of the factors identified by experts as influencing the public's perception of risk are as follows:

- Catastrophic potential–People are more concerned about incidents that kill many people at the same time (e.g., airplane crashes) than about fatalities and injuries that are scattered or random in time and space (e.g., automobile accidents).
- Familiarity–People are more concerned about unfamiliar risks (e.g., ozone depletion) than familiar risks (e.g., household accidents).
- Understanding–People are more concerned about poorly understood activities (e.g., exposure to radiation) than those that may be understood (e.g., slipping on ice).
- Scientific uncertainty–People are more concerned about risks that are scientifically unknown or uncertain (e.g., genetically modified crops) than risks that are well known to science (e.g., car crashes).
- Controllability–People are more concerned about risks that are not under personal control (e.g., pesticides on food) than those that are under personal control (e.g., driving a car).
- Voluntariness of exposure–People are more concerned about risks that are imposed (e.g., residues in food) rather than voluntarily accepted (e.g., smoking cigarettes).
- Impact on children–People are more concerned about risks that are perceived to disproportionally affect children.

Recognizing these factors can help us understand that our judgment of risk is often not particularly rational. For example, many individuals are afraid of flying for which the risk of death is one in a million on a commercial airline flight; yet these people will readily accept a hundred times greater risk by driving a car every day.

Taking into account that the perception of risk is greatly affected by many circumstances, some generalizations can still be made. A yearly risk of death of one in a million is generally ignored (e.g., being struck by lightening), whereas a risk of death of one in a hundred is totally unacceptable (e.g., accident and disease in coal miners at the turn of the century). The risk level associated with pediatric CT falls into the more ambiguous intermediate level. This level of risk can be considered acceptable if 1) the individual is aware of the risk; 2) the individual receives some commensurate benefit; and 3) everything reasonable has been done to reduce the risk.[14]

BOX 14-8   Key Concept

This level of risk associated with a CT examination can be considered acceptable if
1. the individual is aware of the risk
2. the individual receives some commensurate benefit
3. everything reasonable has been done to reduce the risk

These general principles of risk are applied to the specific case of pediatric CT through the following recommendations:[14]

1. The patient–or the parent in the case of a patient who is a child–should be told of the small risk involved.
2. The procedure should be restricted to cases in which it is specifically indicated and conveys a commensurate diagnostic benefit that is difficult to obtain by any other means. Pediatric CT involves too large a dose to be used indiscriminately as a screening procedure.
3. Every effort should be made to decrease the radiation dose by adjusting the kVp and mAs to a suitable level according to the size of the child being scanned. "One size fits all" is no longer appropriate now that the risks have been identified.

SPECIAL CONSIDERATIONS FOR THE PEDIATRIC POPULATION

There are three primary factors of special relevance to the use of CT in pediatric radiology: increased sensitivity, higher effective dose, and increasing use.

Increased Sensitivity

Children are much more radiosensitive than adults.[3,14,15,25,27-29] For example, a 1-year-old infant is approximately six times more likely than a 50-year-old adult to develop a malignancy from the same dose of radiation.[5] There are two reasons for this increased sensitivity. One is that because of their younger age, children have more time to develop cancer than do adults. Remembering that the latency time for cancer induction in the dose ranges used in CT is estimated to be between 10 and 30 years,[7] it is clear why radiation exposure to a child is of greater concern than that to an adult. It is also worth recalling that exposure is cumulative; data have revealed that 30% of patients who undergo CT have at least three scans, 7% have at least five scans, and 4% have at least nine scans.[23] Each CT examination (including multiple series per examination) contributes to the patient's lifetime (a newborn baby has an expected life span of more than 75 years) exposure. Radiation for older adults and the elderly does not carry the same cancer risk because many radiation-induced cancers, particularly solid malignancies, will not be evident for decades and thus would develop beyond the life span of many of these older persons. Also, children seem to be inherently more sensitive to radiation simply because they have more dividing cells and thus suffer more adverse radiation effects on dividing cells.[3] Recent research shows that children are four to six times more sensitive to the effects of radiation than middle-aged adults.

BOX 14–9   Key Concept

Children are more radiosensitive than adults. Girls are more radiosensitive than boys.

Higher Effective Dose

Even when machine parameters—most notably milliampere-seconds (mAs) and kVp—are individualized, organ doses are larger in a child compared with an adult (assuming the adult is larger).[3] This is attributable to the absence of partial shielding by intervening tissues, as described earlier in the chapter.

Increasing Use

The use of helical CT is increasing even faster in children than in adults.[8] This trend is probably because of improved scanner capabilities, a general increased reliance on imaging, and the malpractice environment. However, these factors can lead to the temptation to use CT as a screening procedure.

Radiation Dose to the Fetus

A fetus, exposed to ionizing radiation in utero, is also particularly sensitive to its harmful effects. The reasons are the same as those outlined earlier in our discussion of radiation exposure to the pediatric population. The radiosensitivity of a developing fetus is greatest from conception to 3 months' gestation because this is the time of organ and neural crest development.[30] The ACR recommends that when imaging is required in the evaluation of the pregnant woman, nonionizing techniques, such as sonography and MRI, be used as the first choice.[31] However, because sonography is often limited in pregnant women and because CT is widely available, CT is often used for such indications as suspected pulmonary embolus (PE), appendicitis, renal colic, or trauma.[32]

BOX 14–10   Key Concept

The radiosensitivity of a developing fetus is greatest from conception to 3 months' gestation because this is the time of organ and neural crest development.

Fetal radiation doses from maternal body CT have been measured for conventional axial CT scanners, single-detector helical CT scanners, and 16-slice MDCT scanners. Radiation doses to the fetus from 64-MDCT scanners have not yet been reported.

The major concerns regarding risks to the fetus with the low levels of exposure associated with body CT are neurologic and carcinogenic in nature. Recent reports state that standard body protocols using 16-slice MDCT scanners should not result in significant neurologic impairment.[32] However, the correlation between prenatal radiation exposure and carcinogenesis is less clear. The doses delivered in some body protocols could theoretically double the chance of developing childhood cancer. It is estimated that the overall risk of childhood cancer for a fetus from a CT scan of the mother's appendix using MDCT is approximately 2 in 600, as opposed to approximately 1 in 600 for the general pediatric population.[32] Although the risk remains low, it is twice that of background radiation.

For CT protocols that do not result in direct fetal exposure (such as thoracic imaging protocols used for the diagnosis of PE), the dose is lower. Older reports compared the fetal dose from single-detector CT scanners with that of ventilation-perfusion scanning (an alternative method of diagnosis PE) and found the radiation dose from CT to be lower. Newer research using MDCT reports that this is no longer true; these scanners result in a fetal dose that is greater than or equivalent to that of ventilation-perfusion scanning.[32]

The risk-benefit ratio of performing a CT study of the body on a pregnant woman in the first trimester must be carefully weighed. Knowledge of fetal dose and associated risk estimates is critical to an accurate assessment.

STRATEGIES FOR REDUCING DOSE

General Strategies

Because a combination of factors is responsible for the total radiation dose delivered to the patient during a CT examination, a variety of methods for reducing dose are available. The following options can be used in any combination according to the specific clinical situation. Ideally, appropriate strategies are chosen and used in conjunction to reduce the dose as much as possible without sacrificing the image quality necessary to answer the clinical questions posed.

Adjusting mAs

At this point in the discussion of radiation dose, the need to adjust mAs to suit individual patient size should be apparent. Small bodies require a lesser dose, and large bodies require a greater dose. Numerous authors have documented the ability to adjust mAs, and therefore dose, without compromising image quality.[33–35] Although some researchers have used the patient's weight to adjust mAs,[33–35] others prefer using the diameter of the patient to determine optimal mAs setting.[33] Both approaches have proved successful.

Automatic Tube Current Modulation More recently manufacturers have provided users with another method to reduce patient dose. Some systems have an option that will make changes in tube current (mA) based on the estimated attenuation of the patient at a specific location. The estimations are derived from scout views done in both the anteroposterior and lateral projections or from the previous slices. From these views, the mA will be programmed to vary by location along the length of the patient. The exact details of the option vary by manufacturer.

Avoid Increasing kVp

Increasing the x-ray tube potential increases both the radiation dose and penetration of the x-rays through the body. In general, increases beyond 120 kVp should be avoided, except when imaging obese patients.[7] However, an increase in kVp could be accompanied by a reduction in tube current to offset the increased dose.

Increased Pitch

Another useful method for reducing radiation dose with helical scanning is to increase the pitch of the examination. Vade and co-workers[37] showed that increasing the pitch from 1.0 to 1.5 decreased the dose by 33% without any apparent loss of diagnostic information.

Limit the Use of Thin Slices

Using a large number of thin adjacent CT slices results in 30% to 50% more radiation dose to the patient than using fewer thicker slices to scan the same anatomy.[7,38] Although it is not always possible to avoid using thin slices, technologists and radiologists should be aware of the consequences.

Limit Repeat Scans

Because the effects of repeat scans of the same area are cumulative, redundant or multiphase studies should be performed only when clinically indicated. Numerous authors have shown that detection of liver lesions can be improved by multiple scans taken during different phases of contrast injection. Although multiphasic studies are clearly indicated to evaluate for liver abnormalities, they should not be done in all circumstances.[36] Additionally, it has been recommended that triple-phase studies for the evaluation of kidney lesions be reserved for patients in whom a question arises on a routine study or other examination rather than as a standard protocol.[36]

Newer Reconstruction Methods

A newer method of image reconstruction known as iterative reconstruction has been recently introduced for the use in CT image reconstruction and, compared with standard filtered back-projection methods, can reduce the dose by as much as 50% (Chapter 3).

Strategies for Dose Reduction in Pediatric Patients

Like that of adults, strategies for reducing the dose in children involve two components: appropriate patient selection and appropriate technical parameters that will minimize the dose without compromising diagnostic quality. These strategies are summarized in Table 14-5. Although technologists play an essential role in dose-reduction strategies for CT scanning of infants and children, it is ultimately the responsibility of the radiologist to see that such strategies are implemented.

TABLE 14-5 Strategies for Reducing CT Radiation Dose

Appropriate Patient Selection
    Confirm CT is necessary
    Consider alternative modalities

Appropriate Technical Parameters
    Limit the region covered
    Minimize the use of multiphase examinations
    Adjust mAs based on size
    Adjust mAs based on region
    Adjust mAs based on clinical indication
    Consider an increase in pitch
    Limit the use of thin slices
    Use new equipment options that automatically adjust dose during scanning
    Consider patient shielding

Use CT Only When Clinically Indicated

The first step in minimizing radiation exposure in children is to decide that CT is in fact the best method of answering the specific clinical question. Perhaps 40% of all pediatric CT examinations are not clearly indicated.[25] Communication between pediatric healthcare providers and radiologists is critical in deciding whether a CT examination is appropriate. Technologists play a critical role in this communication process by bringing to the radiologist's attention any order that seems inappropriate or unnecessary. Armed with sufficient clinical information, radiologists may offer an alternative such as ultrasonography or magnetic resonance imaging (MR) that does not use ionizing radiation. In some institutions a lack of accessibility poses a barrier to the use of other imaging methods. If modalities such as MR are to be viable alternatives they must be as easy to schedule as CT examinations. If it is decided that CT is indeed the best modality, the clinical information provided can help in customizing the CT scan.

Customize the CT Examination

One way of tailoring the examination to the specific diagnostic need is for the radiologist to limit the examination to the region in question. For example, routine scanning of the pelvis as part of an abdominal CT is not always necessary; in this way, exposure to the gonads will be reduced or eliminated.[39] There are many potential situations wherein limited CT could be used. For example, in follow-up examinations, the region scanned could be limited to just the area of interest (e.g., pseudocyst, lung, or abdominal abscess).

Limiting the use of multiphase examinations is another important consideration. Essentially, every additional phase increases the radiation dose by the multiple of the total number of phases. In body scanning, it has been reported that multiphase scanning is used in approximately 30% of children, many times with three phases.[17] Justification for the routine use of multiphase examinations in infants and children has been questioned.[29,39] Frush[29] reported that "the indications for scanning through a region more than once are few," and "if the use of multiphase examinations were limited, the overall radiation would be at least 15% lower." In the rare instance (<3% of body scans)[39] for which multiple phases are necessary, scan parameters–including length of scan, slice thickness, and tube current–should be adjusted to minimize the additional radiation received.

Technical Parameters

All of the strategies outlined earlier can also be used to reduce the dose to pediatric patients. Because of a child's increased sensitivity to radiation, additional strategies are suggested for consideration. Again, it is expected that appropriate strategies are chosen and used together to reduce the dose as much as possible without sacrificing the image quality necessary to answer the clinical questions posed. It is in the mastery of the issues associated with the adjustment of each technical factor that technologists can play a unique and vital role in limiting the radiation dose to pediatric patients.

Adjust mAs   Appropriate selection of mAs is important for all patients, but it is imperative in children. Patient size is the primary criteria in the selection of mAs, but the region scanned and the clinical indication that prompted the scan are also considerations.

The mAs setting selected should also be based on the region scanned. Lower tube currents are adequate in evaluating lung parenchyma.[29,39,40] Because bone intrinsically has high contrast, the tube current should be lowered when a bone is of primary interest.[29]

The cost of reducing mAs below a threshold point is that the signal-to-noise ratio decreases because the number of image-forming photons decreases. The resulting noisier images have decreased low-contrast resolution. In many cases, this decrease in image quality will affect diagnosis, but in some cases the reduction may be acceptable. For example, in a child for whom a large abnormality is being evaluated, such as a retroperitoneal hematoma or an abscess, the noisier image will probably be sufficient. Therefore, tube current should be adjusted for patient size, region scanned, and scan indication.

Patient Shielding

Although lead shielding is standard in general radiography, it is less beneficial in CT. Because of narrow collimation, radiation to areas outside that of the selected scan area is minimal and usually attributable to the internal scattering of photons that are unaffected by surface shielding. However, a recent investigation suggested that shielding of the breast tissue and thyroid gland can be a valuable dose-reduction strategy.[41] The scout image displayed in Figure 14-7 shows

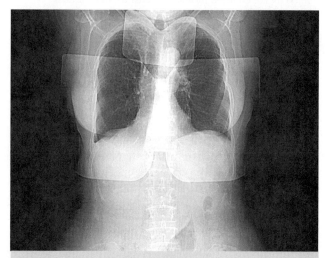

FIGURE 14-7 This scout image shows evidence of both thyroid and breast shields. These shields are a valuable dose-reduction strategy.

evidence of both types of shields. Perhaps equally important, patient shielding may play a role in the perception of risk; that is, it would assure the patient (or child's family) that every effort was being taken to reduce the radiation dose.

SUMMARY

CT is a valuable imaging modality. Because CT is associated with a relatively high radiation dose, it therefore involves some risk. In cases in which CT is positively indicated, the risk is far outweighed by the potential benefit. However, healthcare providers must do everything in their power to avoid delivering excessive radiation. This is particularly true when scanning children, given the increasing use of CT in the pediatric population, children's greater sensitivity, and the accumulating data about the risks of cancer development after low-level radiation. Strategies include appropriate patient selection; adjusting the scan protocol to meet the clinical need; and adjusting the technical factors based on the size of the patient, the region being scanned, and the indication.

REVIEW QUESTIONS

1. Name the two main components in the rational use of CT relative to patient care.
2. How is exposure uniformity related to the fact that, for a given set of technical parameters, organ doses are higher for children compared with adults?
3. Explain how the dose from an examination consisting of multiple adjacent scans is calculated. How do the "tails" affect the total dose?
4. List the factors that affect the radiation dose.
5. What factors contribute to the concern regarding the radiation dose delivered from a CT examination?
6. Regarding the risks associated with pediatric CT, list the three recommendations that should be followed by healthcare professionals.
7. Why are children more radiosensitive than adults?
8. What are the major risks to the fetus with the low levels of exposure associated with body CT?
9. List all of the possible methods for reducing the dose from CT.
10. Is patient shielding effective in reducing the dose from CT?

REFERENCES

1. International Commission on Radiation Protection. 1990 recommendations of the International Commission on Radiological Protection. Publication 60. Ann ICRP 1991;21. Oxford, England: Pergamon.
2. McNitt-Gray MF. AAPM/RSNA physics tutorial for residents: topics in CT. Radiation dose in CT. Radiographics 2002;22:1541-53.
3. Brenner DJ. Estimating cancer risks from pediatric CT: going from the qualitative to the quantitative. Pediatr Radiol 2002;32:228-31.
4. Bushberg JT, Seibert JA, Leidholdt EM, Boone JM. The Essential Physics of Medical Imaging. Lippincott Williams & Wilkins, 2002.
5. Committee to Assess Health Risks from Exposure to Low Levels of Ionizing Radiation, National Research Council, Board on Radiation Effects Research. Health Risks from Exposure to Low Levels of Ionizing Radiation: BEIR VII Phase 2; 2006. National Research Council of the National Academies. National Academies Press. Washington, DC. Available at: http://www.nap.edu/catalog.php?record_id=11340#toc. Accessed September 4, 2008.
6. McCollough CH, Zink FE. Performance evaluation of a multi-slice CT system. Med Phys 1999;26:2223-30.
7. Nickoloff EL, Alderson PO. Radiation exposures to patients from CT: reality, public perception, and policy. AJR Am J Roentgenol 2001;177:285-7.
8. Mettler FA Jr, Wiest PW, Locken JA, Kelsey CA. CT scanning: patterns of use and dose. J Radiol Prot 2000;20:353-9.
9. Shrimpton PC, Edyvean S. CT scanner dosimetry. Br J Radiol 1998;71:1-3.
10. Dixon AK, Goldstone KE. Abdominal CT and the Euratom Directive. Eur Radiol 2002;12:1567-70.
11. Dixon AK, Dendy P. Spiral CT: how much does radiation dose matter? Lancet 1998;352:1082-3.
12. Thomton FJ, Paulson EK, Yoshizumi TT, Frush DP, Nelson RC. Single versus multi-detector row CT: comparison of radiation doses and dose profiles. Acad Radiol 2003;10:379-85.
13. Yates SJ, Pike LC, Goldstone KE. Effect of multislice scanners on patient dose from routine CT examination in East Anglia. Br J Radiol 2004;77:472-8.
14. Hall EJ. Lessons we have learned from our children: cancer risks from diagnostic radiology. Pediatr Radiol 2002;32:700-6.
15. Brenner DJ, Elliston CD, Hall EJ, Berdon WE. Estimated risks of radiation-induced fatal cancer from pediatric CT. AJR Am J Roentgenol 2001;176:289-96.
16. Benz MG, Benz MW. Reduction of cancer risk associated with pediatric computed tomography by the development of new technologies. Pediatrics 2004;114:205-9.
17. Paterson A, Frush DP, Donnelly LF. Helical CT of the body: are settings adjusted for pediatric patients? AJR Am J Roentgenol 2001:176;297-301.
18. Ware DE, Huda W, Mergo PJ, Litwiller AL. Radiation effective doses to patients undergoing abdominal CT examinations. Radiology 1999;210:645-50.
19. Hollingsworth C, Frush DP, Cros M, Lucaya J. Helical CT of the body: a survey of techniques used for pediatric patients. AJR Am J Roentgenol 2003;180:401-6.
20. Itoh S, Ikeda M, Arahata S, et al. Lung cancer screening: minimum tube current required for helical CT. Radiology 2000;215:175-83.
21. Tack D, Sourtzis S, Delpierre I, de Maertelaer V, Gevenois PA. Low-dose unenhanced multidetector CT of patients with suspected renal colic. AJR Am J Roentgenol 2003;180:305-11.
22. Rogers LF. Low-dose CT: how are we doing? AJR Am J Roentgenol 2003;180:303.
23. Kalra MK, Maher MM, Toth TL, Kamath RS, Halpern EF, Saini S. Radiation from "extra" images acquired with abdominal and/or pelvic CT: effect of automatic tube current modulation. Radiology 2004;232:409-14.
24. Lee CI, Haims AH, Monico EP, Brink JA, Forman HP. Diagnostic CT scans: assessment of patient, physician, and

radiologist awareness of radiation dose and possible risks. Radiology 2004;231:393–8.

25. Slovis TL, ed. Multidisciplinary conference organized by the Society of Pediatric Radiology. The ALARA concept in pediatric CT–intelligent dose reduction. Pediatr Radiol 2002;32:217–313.

26. Powell D. An introduction to risk communication and the perception of risk. 1998. Available online at http://www.foodsafetynetwork.ca/en/article-details.php?a=3&c=17&sc=130&id=491. Accessed September 4, 2008.

27. Slovis TL. CT and computed radiography: the pictures are great, but is the radiation dose greater than required? AJR Am J Roentgenol 2002;179:39–41.

28. Trott KR. Radiation risks from imaging of intestinal and abdominal inflammation. Scand J Gastroenterol Suppl 1994; 203:43–7.

29. Frush DP. Pediatric CT: practical approach to diminish the radiation dose. Pediatr Radiol 2002;32:714–7.

30. Wagner LK, Lester RG, Saldana LR. Exposure of the Pregnant Patient to Diagnostic Radiation: A Guide to Medical Management. 2nd Ed. Madison, WI: Medical Physics Publishing, 1997:93.

31. ACR appropriate criteria. Reston, VA: American College of Radiology, 1999:1–8.

32. Hurwitz LM, Yoshizumi T, Reiman RE, et al. Radiation dose to the fetus from body MDCT during early gestation. AJR Am J Roentgenol 2006;186:871–6.

33. Ravenel JG, Scalzetti EM, Huda W, Garrisi W. Radiation exposure and image quality in chest CT examinations. AJR Am J Roentgenol 2001;177:279–84.

34. Ware DE, Huda W, Mergo PJ, Litwiller AL. Radiation effective doses to patients undergoing abdominal CT examinations. Radiology 1999;210:645–50.

35. Rusinek H, Naidich DP, McGuinness G, et al. Pulmonary nodule detection: low-dose versus conventional CT. Radiology 1998;209:243–9.

36. Rogers LF. Radiation exposure in CT: why so high? AJR Am J Roentgenol 2001;177:277.

37. Vade A, Demos TC, Olson MC, et al. Evaluation of image quality using 1:1 pitch and 1.5:1 pitch helical CT in children: a comparative study. Pediatr Radiol 1996;26:891–3.

38. Nickoloff E. Current adult and pediatric CT doses. Pediatr Radiol 2002;32:250–60.

39. Frush DP, Donnelly LF, Rosen NS. Computed tomography and radiation risks: what pediatric health care providers should know. Pediatrics 2003;112:951–7.

40. Lucaya J, Piqueras J, Garcia-Pena P, Enriquez G, Garcia-Macias M, Sotil J. Low-dose high-resolution CT of the chest in children and young adults: dose, cooperation, artifact incidence, and image quality. AJR Am J Roentgenol 2000; 175:985–92.

41. Fricke BL, Donnelly LF, Frush DP, et al. In-plane bismuth breast shields for pediatric CT: effects on radiation dose and image quality using experimental and clinical data. AJR Am J Roentgenol 2003;180:407–11.

Section III

CROSS-SECTIONAL ANATOMY

CHAPTER 15 • **Neuroanatomy**

CHAPTER 16 • **Thoracic Anatomy**

CHAPTER 17 • **Abdominopelvic Anatomy**

CHAPTER 18 • **Musculoskeletal Anatomy**

INTRODUCTION

A radiologic technologist practicing in any field of radiology must understand basic human anatomy and physiology in order to perform his or her duties. Those working in CT or MRI must also be able to identify normal anatomic structures on cross-sectional images. This requires an adaptation in thinking; special attention must be paid to the relationships among structures. There are many excellent resources available that provide comprehensive images from the entire head and body, allowing readers to learn, identify, and recall anatomic structures in cross section. Some of these resources are listed here.

The aim of this section is to provide an introduction to cross-sectional anatomy by presenting just a few representative slices from some of the most common examinations performed in the CT department. Each cross-sectional image is accompanied by a drawing, in shades of gray, to help identify structures. All the drawings have been done according to the same gray scale. Regardless of where they are found in the body, air is depicted as black; bone is white. Within these extremes, shading varies for tissues, organs, and abnormalities. Each cross-sectional image is also accompanied by a reference image to help the reader imagine its location in the body.

Because only representative slices are included, the slices displayed are not adjacent. Compared with an actual CT examination that includes contiguous slices, the reader is at a considerable disadvantage in accurately identifying specific structures from a single image. (Note: questions contained in the certification examination for CT asking the examinee to identify anatomic structures most often provide only a single cross-sectional image. Therefore, this format, although not reflecting actual practice, does mirror that commonly used for the CT examination.)

In actual practice, whenever there is doubt the viewer should analyze adjacent superior and inferior images and compare the structures in question.

Resources:

Madden ME. Introduction to Sectional Anatomy. Philadelphia: Lippincott Williams & Wilkins, 2001.

Kelley LL, Peterson C. Sectional Imaging for Imaging Professionals. St. Louis: Mosby/Elsevier, 2006.

Dean D, Herbener TE. Cross-Sectional Human Anatomy. Philadelphia: Lippincott Williams & Wilkins, 2000.

HEAD

Brain

Routine scans of the brain usually begin at the base of the skull and continue superiorly. Depending on the clinical indication, the scans may be done without IV contrast enhancement, with IV contrast enhancement, or without and with IV contrast enhancement. The images included below include IV contrast enhancement.

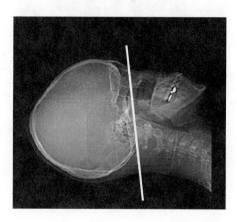

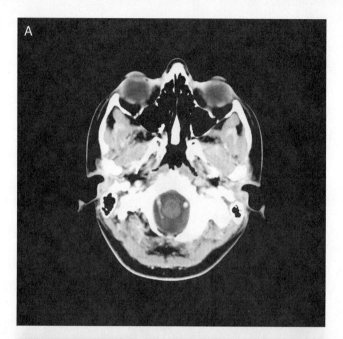

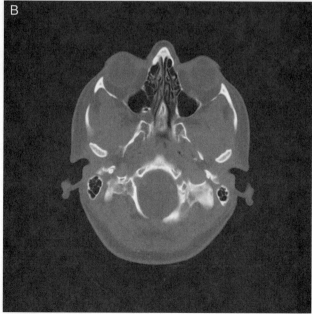

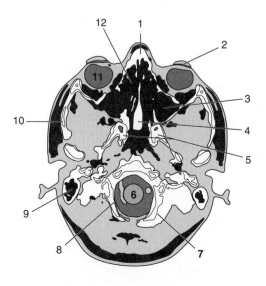

1. Nasal bones	7. Occipital bone
2. Eye, lens	8. Vertebral artery
3. Maxillary sinus	9. Mastoid air cells
4. Vomer	10. Zygoma
5. Sphenoid bone	11. Eye, globe
6. Medulla oblongata	12. Ethmoid sinus

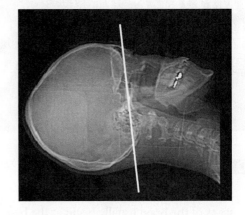

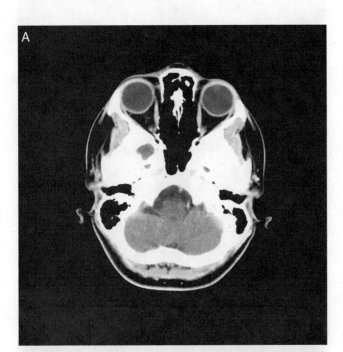

A

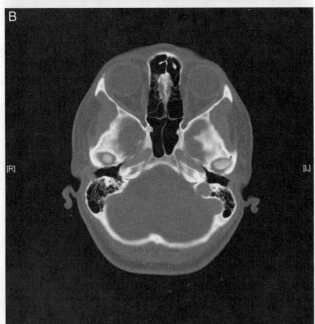

B

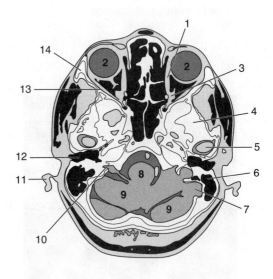

1. Medial rectus m.
2. Globe of eye
3. Optic n.
4. Sphenoid bone, greater wing of
5. Mandibular condyle
6. Mastoid air cells in left temporal bone
7. Sigmoid sinus
8. Pons
9. Cerebellum
10. Internal auditory canal
11. Auricle
12. External auditory meatus
13. Lateral rectus m.
14. Zygoma

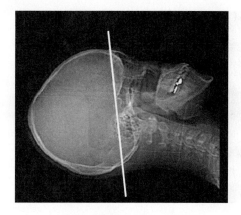

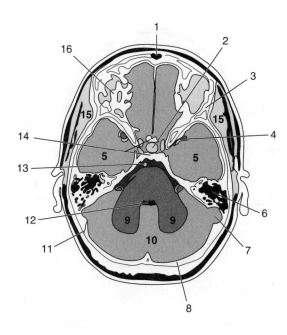

1. Frontal sinus
2. Pituitary
3. Sphenoid bone
4. Middle cerebral a.
5. Temporal lobe
6. Mastoid air cells
    in left temporal bone
7. Sigmoid sinus
8. Occipital bone
9. Cerebellar peduncles
10. Cerebellum
11. Right lamboid suture
12. Fourth ventricle
13. Basilar a.
14. Sella tursica
15. Temporalis m.
16. Frontal bone, orbital roof

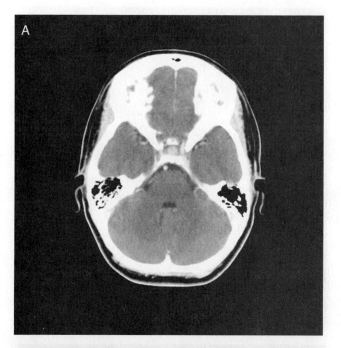

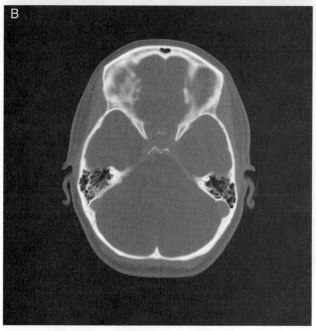

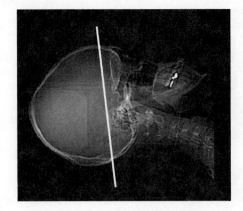

A

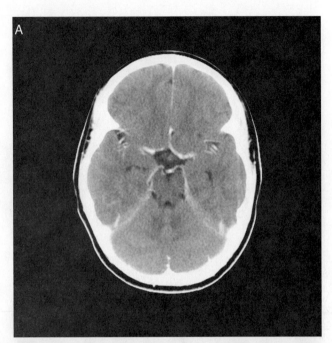

B

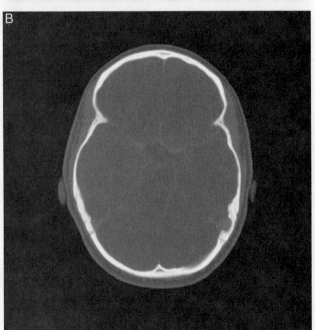

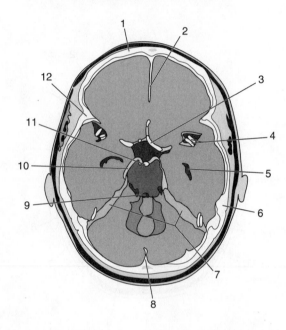

1. Frontal bone
2. Falx cerebri
3. Anterior cerebral a.
4. Middle cerebral a.
5. Lateral ventricle, temporal horn
6. Parietal bone
7. Cerebellum, tentorium
8. Internal occipital protuberance
9. Fourth ventricle
10. Posterior cerebral a.
11. Basilar a.
12. Temporal bone

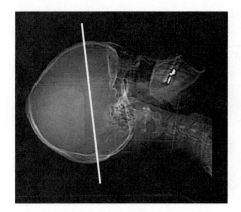

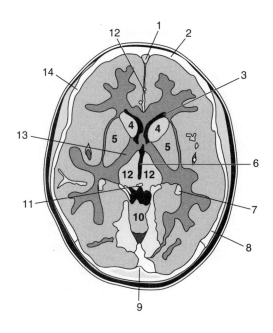

1. Superior sagittal sinus
2. Frontal bone
3. Lateral ventricle, anterior horn
4. Caudate nucleus, head
5. Putamen/Globus pallidus
6. Third ventricle
7. Choroid plexus
8. Parietal bone
9. Internal occipital protuberence
10. Cerebellar vermis
11. Pineal body
12. Thalamus
13. Internal capsule
14. Temporal bone

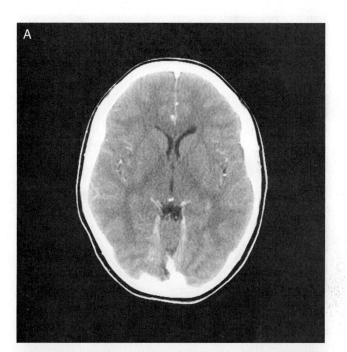

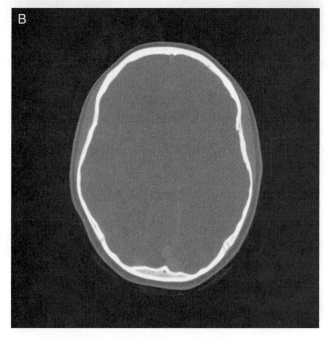

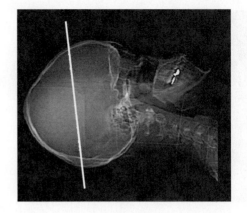

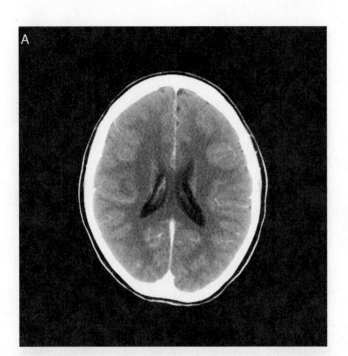

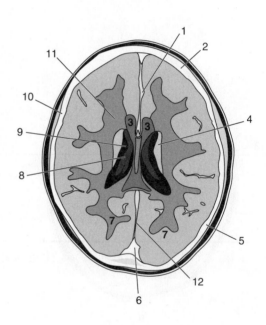

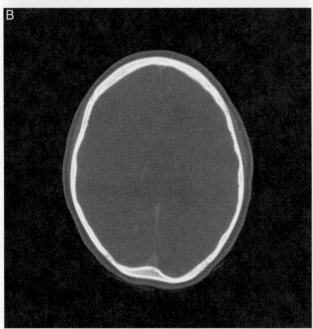

1. Falx cerebri
2. Frontal bone
3. Corpous callosum
4. Caudate nucleus, body
5. Parietal bone
6. Confluence of sinuses (torcula)
7. Occipital lobe
8. Choroid plexus
9. Lateral ventricle, body
10. Temporal bone
11. Corona radiata
12. Straight sinus

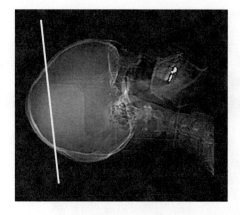

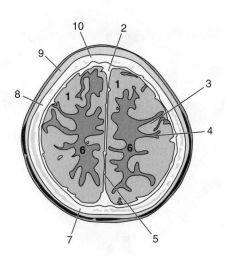

1. Frontal lobe
2. Superior sagittal sinus
3. Precentral gyrus
4. Central suicus
5. Falx cerebri
6. Parietal lobe
7. Parietal bone
8. Temporal bone
9. Scalp
10. Frontal bone

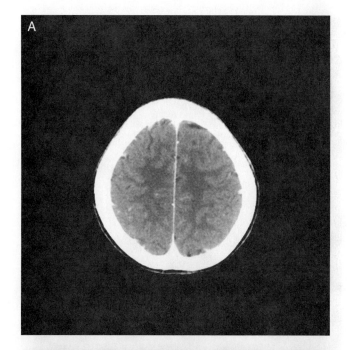

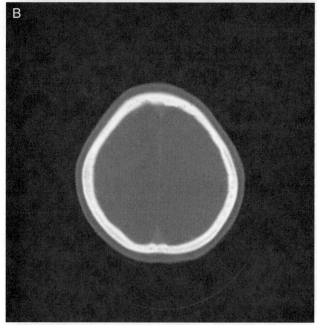

Sinuses

Sinus screening is intended as an inexpensive, accurate, and low radiation dose method for confirming the presence of inflammatory sinonasal disease. If confirmed and the patient will then have endoscopic sinus surgery, the coronal images provide a "roadmap" for the surgeon. When the clinical indication is recurrent or chronic sinusitis, the study is done without IV contrast enhancement and scanning is done in the coronal plane. Other clinical indications may require the administration of IV contrast or additional scans in the axial plane.

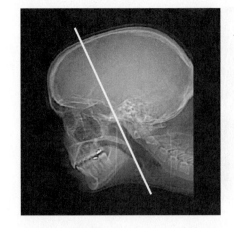

Sinuses (Coronal)

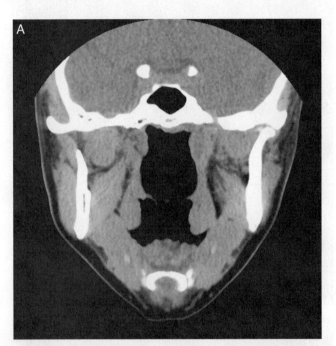

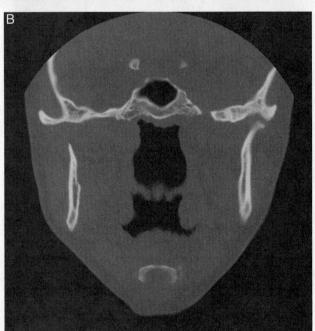

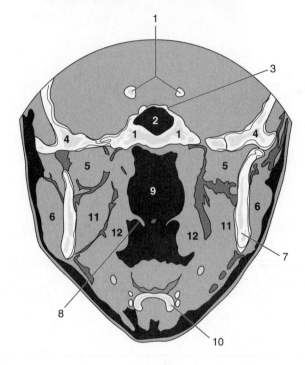

1. Sphenoid bone	7. Mandible
2. Sphenoid sinus	8. Aryepiglottic fold
3. Sella tursica, floor	9. Pharynx
4. Zygoma	10. Hyoid bone
5. Medial pterygoid m.	11. Lateral pterygoid m.
6. Masseter m.	12. Pharyngeal constrictor

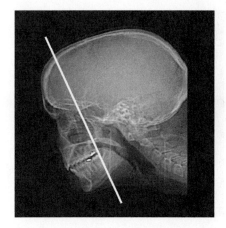

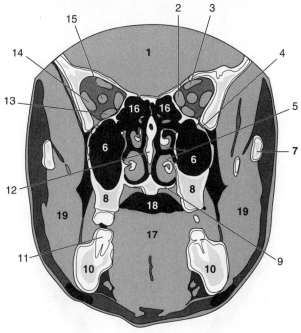

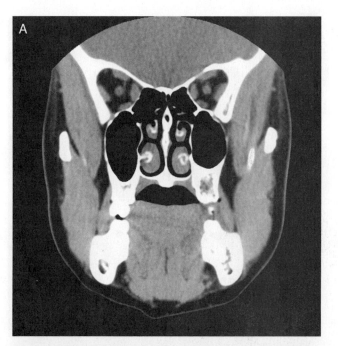

A

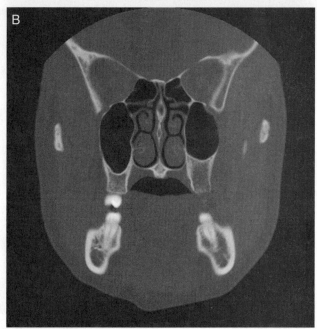

B

1. Frontal lobe
2. Medial rectus m.
3. Superior rectus m.
4. Infraorbital fissure
5. Nasal conchae
6. Maxillary sinus
7. Zygoma
8. Maxillary bone
9. Hard palate
10. Mandible
11. Tooth
12. Nasal bone (nasal septum)
13. Inferior rectus m.
14. Lateral rectus m.
15. Optic nerve/ canal
16. Sphenoid sinus
17. Tongue
18. Oral vestibule
19. Masseter m.

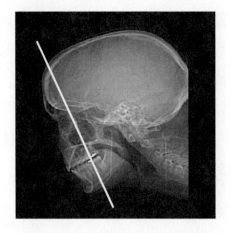

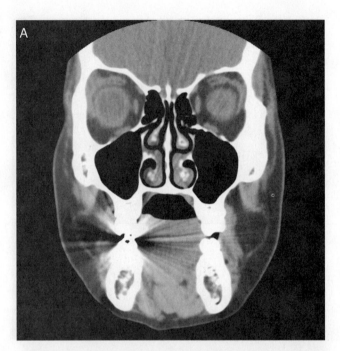

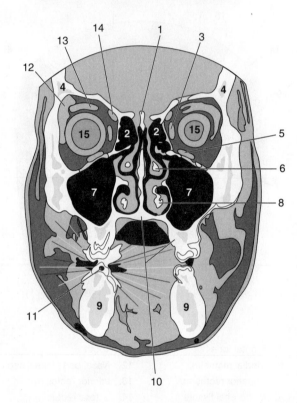

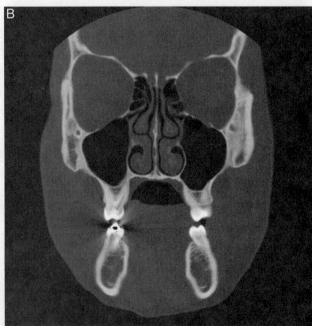

1. Crista galli
2. Ethmoid sinus
3. Medial rectus m.
4. Frontal bone
5. Inferior rectus m.
6. Middle nasal turbinate
7. Maxillary sinus
8. Inferior nasal turbinate
9. Mandible
10. Maxillary bone, hard palate
11. Dental filling (spray artifact)
12. Lacrimal gland
13. Superior rectus m.
14. Superior oblique m.
15. Eye, globe

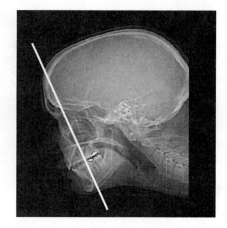

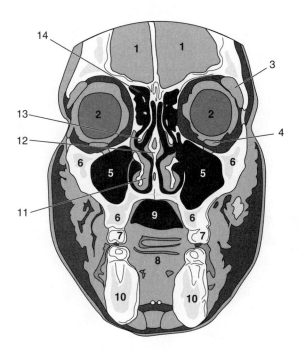

1. Frontal lobe
2. Eye, globe
3. Lacrimal gland
4. Inferior rectus m.
5. Maxillary sinus
6. Maxillary bone
7. Tooth
8. Tongue
9. Oral vestibule
10. Mandible
11. Inferior nasal chonchae
12. Nasal bone (nasal septum)
13. Middle nasal chonchae
14. Ethmoid sinus

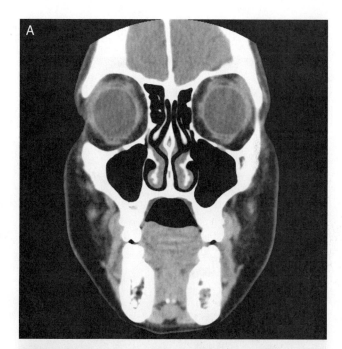

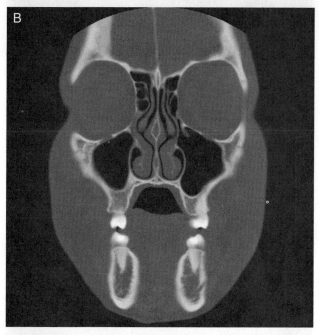

Temporal Bones

The organs of hearing and balance are located in the petrous ridge of the temporal bone. Because these organs are tiny, thin slices are used. Once the scan data are acquired, the two petrosal bones are reconstructed separately so that the display field of view can be reduced to ensure optimal resolution. Most protocols include scans in both the coronal and axial planes; the use of IV contrast varies according to the clinical indication.

Temporal Bones (Coronal)

1. Epitympanum
2. Malleus
3. Facial canal
4. Cochlea
5. Internal auditory canal
6. Tympanic cavity
7. Mastoid air cells
8. Temporal bone
9. Semicircular canals
10. Hypoglossal canal
11. Occipital condyle
12. Jugular fossa

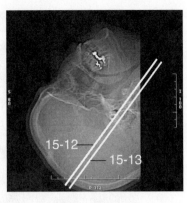

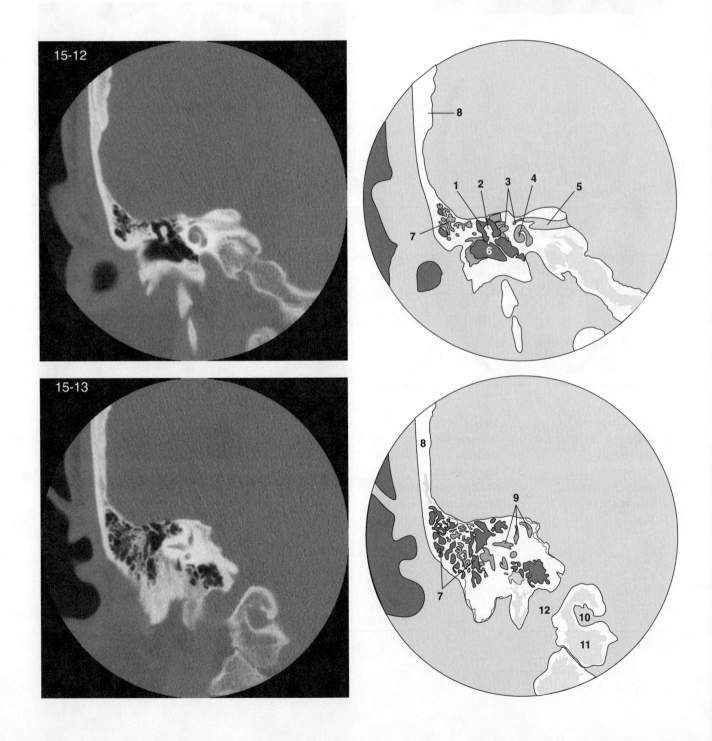

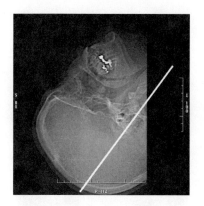

1. Internal auditory canal
2. Superior semicircular canal
3. Lateral semicircular canal
4. Epitympanum
5. Incus
6. External auditory canal
7. Styloid process
8. Tympanic cavity
9. Oval window

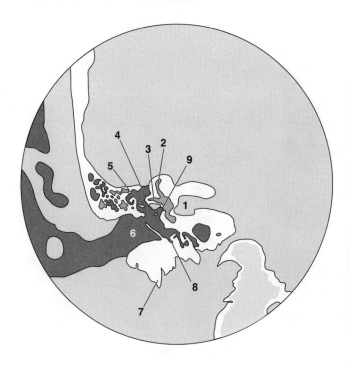

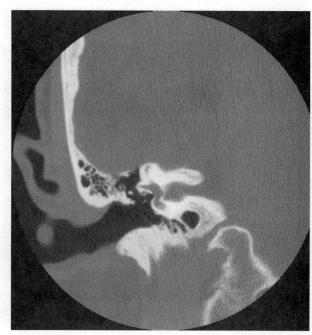

Temporal Bones (Axial)

1. Mandible, condyle
2. Sphenoid sinus
3. Clivus
4. Carotid canal
5. Sigmoid sinus
6. Mastoid air cells
7. External auditory canal
8. Jugular foramen
9. Auditory ossicle: malleus
10. Auditory ossicle: incus
11. Carotid canal
12. Internal auditory canal
13. Vestibule
14. Semicircular canal
15. Cochlea

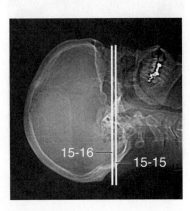

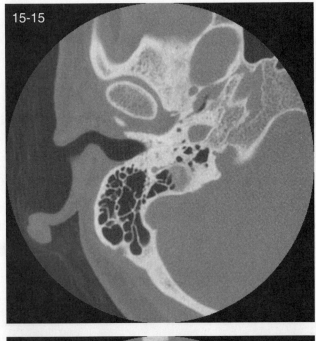

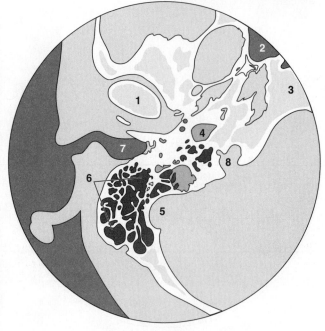

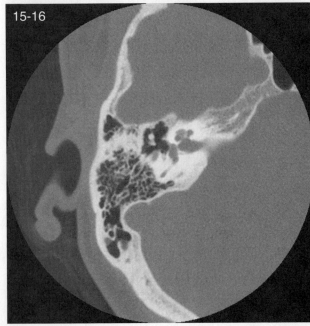

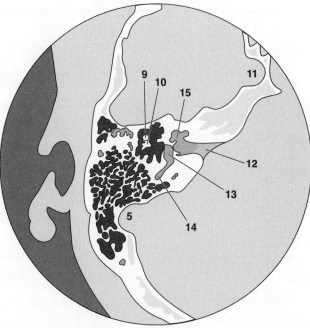

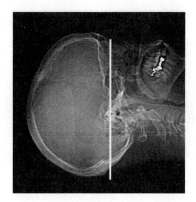

1. Temporal lobe
2. Superior semicircular canal
3. Mastoid antrum
4. Posterior semicircular canal
5. Sigmoid sinus
6. Temporal bone
7. Occipital bone

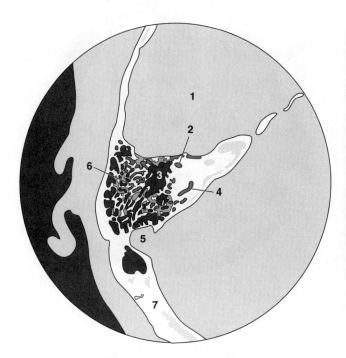

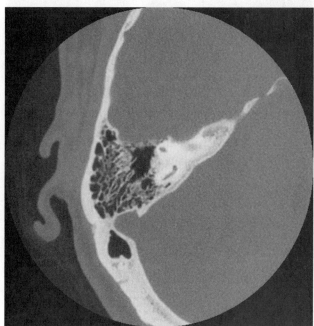

NECK

Unless contraindicated, CT examinations of the neck are done with the IV administration of contrast media. Artifacts caused by dental work often obscure surrounding structures at some levels. Some facilities split the data acquisition into two groups so that the gantry can be angled to reduce artifact. However, many MDCT systems do not allow the gantry to be angled in the helical mode, so this is not always possible.

1. Maxillary bone
2. Oral vestibule
3. Masseter m.
4. Mandible, ramus
5. Atlas, anterior arch
6. Dens
7. Spinal cord
8. Internal jugular v.
9. Mastoid tip
10. Parotid gland
11. Retromandibular v.
12. Internal carotid a.
13. Pharynx
14. Genioglossus m.
15. Vertebral a.
16. Vertebra, spinous process
17. Longus colli muscles
18. Rectus/oblique capitus m.
19. Splenius capitus m.
20. Pterygoid m.

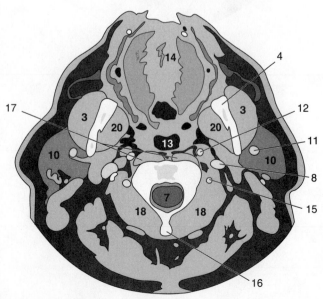

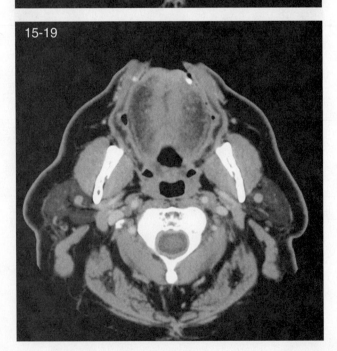

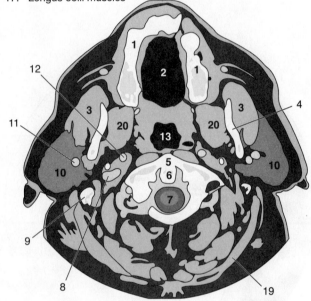

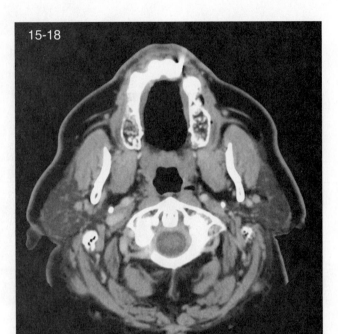

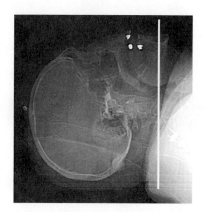

1. Genioglossus m.
2. Tongue
3. Mandible
4. Pharynx
5. Left external carotid a.
6. Internal jugular vv.

7. Left internal carotid a.
8. Vertebral body
9. Right vertebral a.
10. Sternocleidomastoid m.
11. Submandibular gland

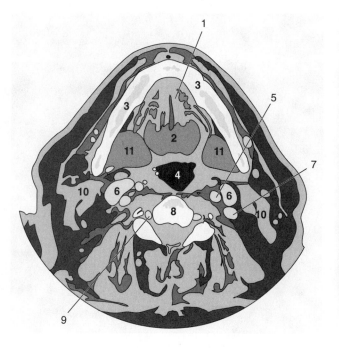

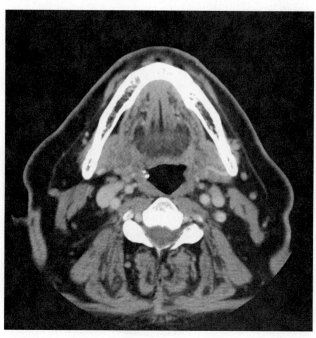

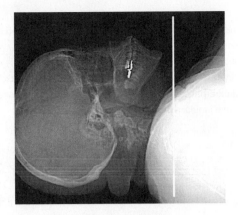

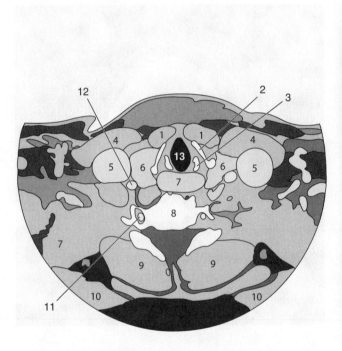

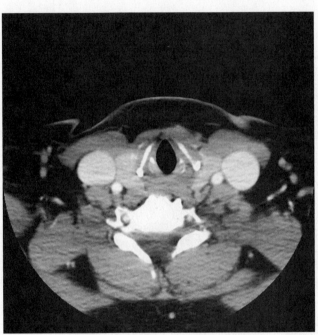

1. Sternohyoid/Sternothyroid mm.
2. Thyroid cartilage
3. Cricoid cartilage
4. Sternocleidomastoid m.
5. Jugular vv.
6. Thyroid gland
7. Esophagus
8. Vertebral body
9. Erector spinae m.
10. Trapezius m.
11. Right vertebral a.
12. Right common carotid a.
13. Pharynx

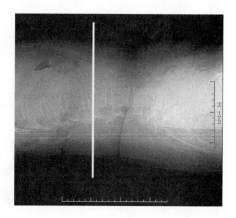

SPINE

CT of the spine is most often performed without IV contrast media administration. However, scans of the spine are often obtained after intrathecal contrast material is given for a myelography study.

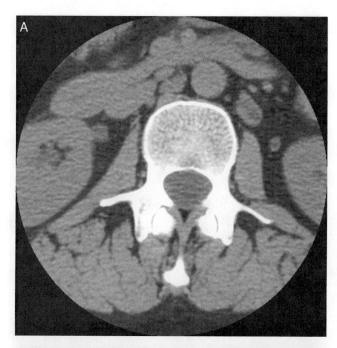

A

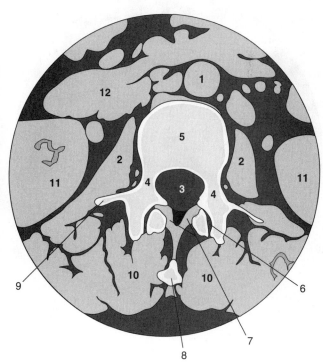

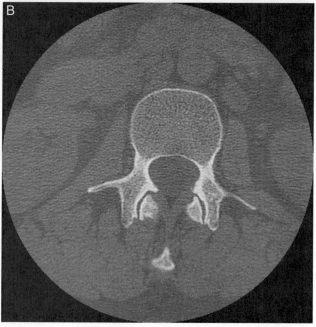

B

1.	Aorta	7.	Ligamenta flava
2.	Psoas m.	8.	L1, spinous process
3.	Dural sac	9.	L2, transverse process
4.	Pedicle	10.	Erector spinae m.
5.	Lumbar vertebra 2	11.	Kidneys
6.	Articular facet	12.	Jejunum/ileum

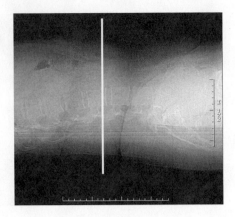

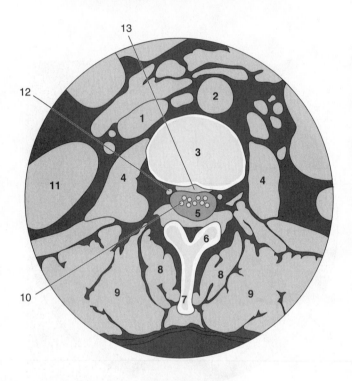

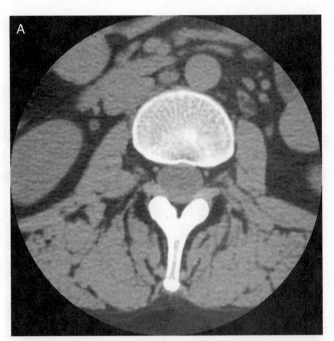

1. Inferior vena cava
2. Aorta
3. L2, vertebral body
4. Psoas m.
5. Dural sac
6. L2, lamina
7. L2, spinous process
8. Multifidus m.
9. Erector spinae m.
10. Cauda equina (in dural sac)
11. Right kidney
12. Nerve root (exiting)
13. Posterior longitudinal lig.

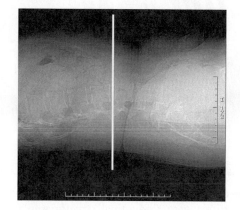

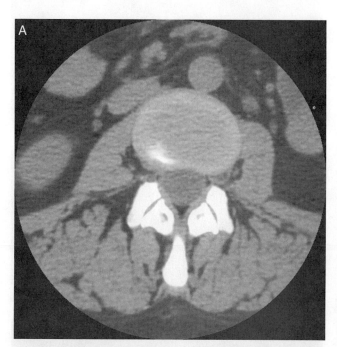

A

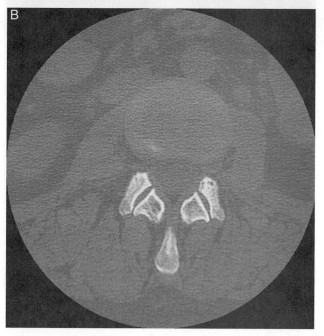

B

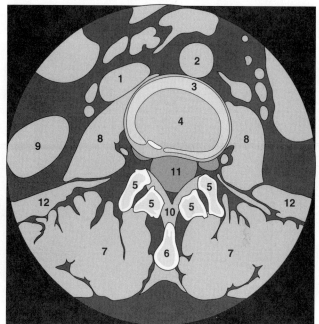

1. Inferior vena cava
2. Aorta
3. Anulus fibrosus
4. Intervertebral disk L2/L3
5. Articular processes
6. L2, spinous process
7. Erector spinae m.
8. Psoas m.
9. Right kidney
10. Ligamenta flava
11. Dural sac
12. Quadratus lumbrum m.

CHEST

A routine chest protocol includes both soft tissue and lung windows to evaluate mediastinal structures in conjunction with lung tissue. Scans extend from the lung apices to under the diaphragm (including the adrenals when there is history of certain carcinomas). The administration of IV contrast media is dependent on the clinical indication and the preference of the radiologist. Demarcation of the esophagus can be improved by giving an oral barium suspension shortly before starting the scan.

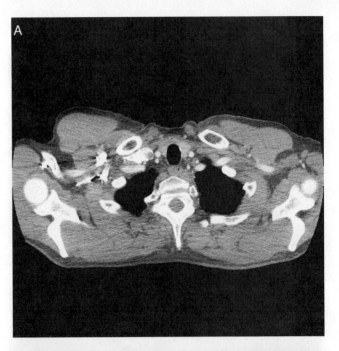

A

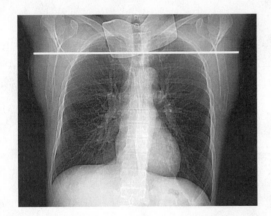

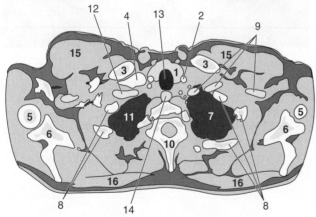

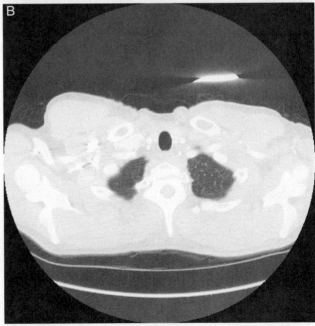

B

1. Thyroid
2. Left common carotid a.
3. Clavicle
4. Right subclavian v.
5. Humeral head
6. Scapula
7. Left lung, upper lobe
8. Rib
9. Left subclavian a.
10. Vertebra
11. Right lung, upper lobe
12. Right subclavian a.
13. Trachea
14. Esophagus
15. Pectoralis major m.
16. Trapezius m.

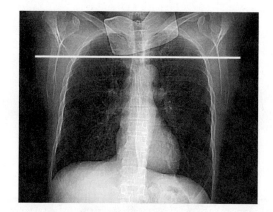

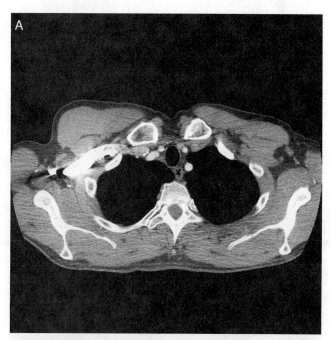

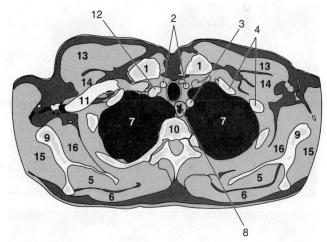

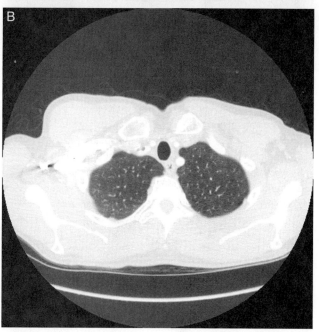

1. Clavicle, head
2. Common carotid aa.
3. Left subclavian a.
4. Ribs
5. Supraspinatus m.
6. Trapezius m.
7. Lung
8. Esophagus
9. Scapula
10. Vertebra
11. Right subclavian v.
12. Right subclavian a.
13. Pectoralis major m.
14. Pectoralis minor m.
15. Infraspinatus m.
16. Subscapularis m.

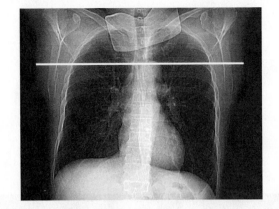

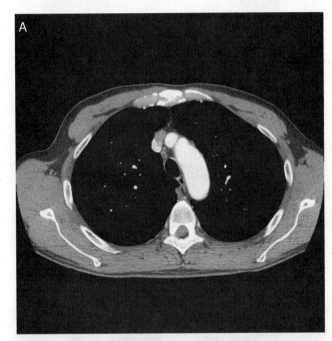

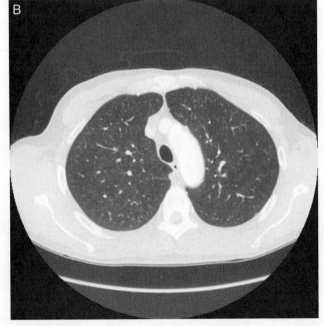

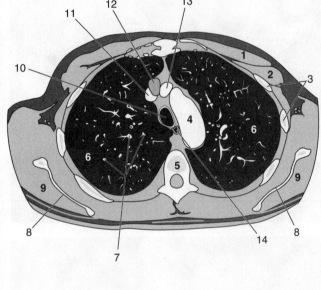

1. Pectoralis major m.
2. Pectoralis minor m.
3. Ribs
4. Aortic arch
5. Vertebra
6. Lung
7. Pulmonary vessels
8. Scapula
9. Infraspinatus m.
10. Trachea
11. Right brachiocephalic v.
12. Left brachiocephalic v.
13. Brachiocephalic a.
14. Esophagus

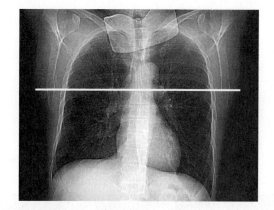

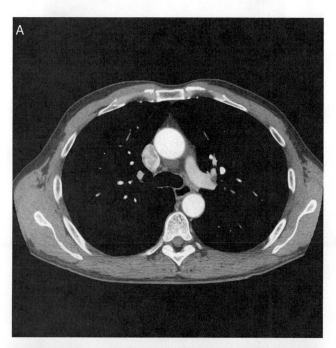

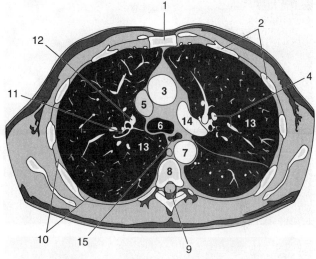

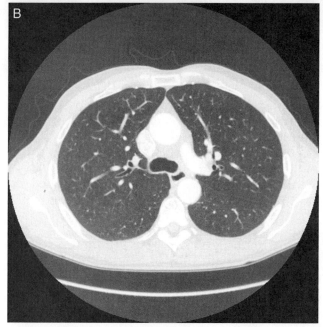

1. Sternum
2. Rib
3. Ascending aorta
4. Pulmonary vessels
5. Superior vena cava
6. Trachea bifurcation (carina)
7. Descending aorta
8. Vertebra
9. Thecal sac with spinal cord
10. Intercostal m.
11. Right upper lobe segmental bronchus
12. Right superior pulmonary v.
13. Lung
14. Left pulmonary a.
15. Esophagus

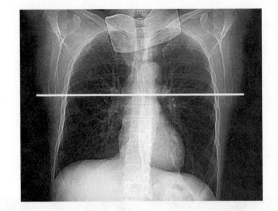

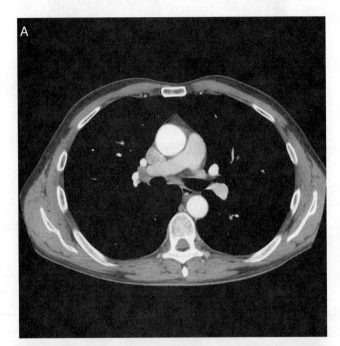

A

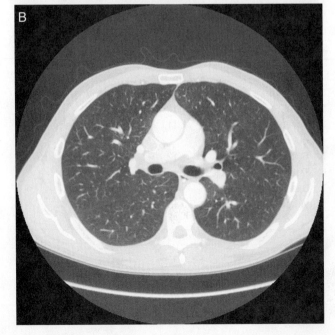

B

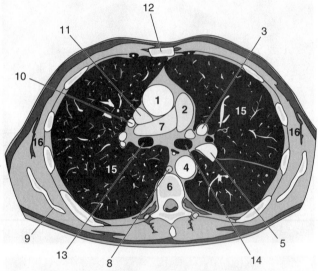

1. Ascending aorta
2. Main pulmonary a.
3. Left superior pulmonary v.
4. Descending aorta
5. Left pulmonary a.,
    descending branch
6. Vertebra
7. Right pulmonary a.
8. Azygos v.

9. Right scapula
10. Right upper
    pulmonary vv.
11. Superior vena cava
12. Sternum
13. Right main bronchus
14. Left main bronchus
15. Lung
16. Serratus anterior m.

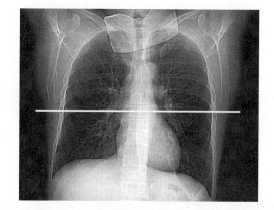

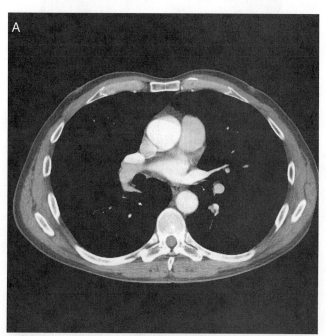

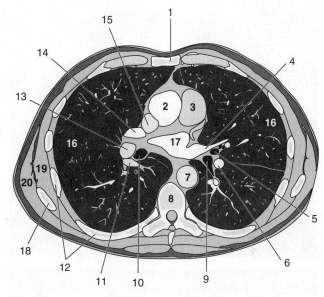

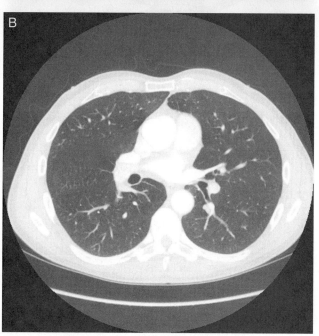

1. Sternum
2. Ascending aorta
3. Main pulmonary a.
4. Left superior pulmonary v.
5. Left upper lobe bronchus
6. Left lower lobe pulmonary a.
7. Descending aorta
8. Vertebra
9. Left lower lobe bronchus
10. Right bronchus intermedius
11. Right lower lobe segmental a.
12. Rib
13. Right interlobar pulmonary a.
14. Right superior pulmonary v.
15. Superior vena cava
16. Lung
17. Left atrium
18. Scapula
19. Serratus anterior m.
20. Latissimus dorsi m.

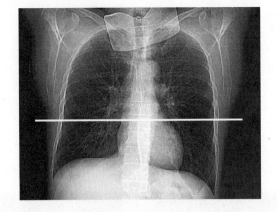

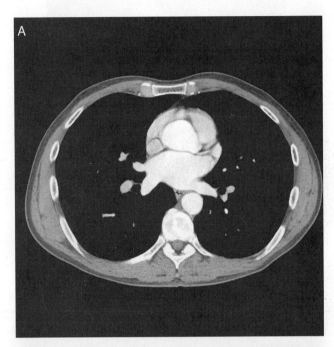

A

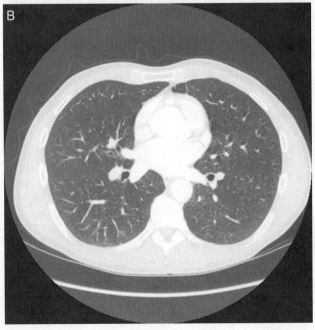

B

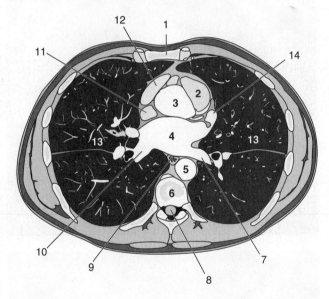

1. Sternum
2. Main pulmonary a.
3. Ascending aorta
4. Left atrium
5. Decending aorta
6. Vertebra
7. Left inferior pulmonary v.
8. Thecal sac containing spinal cord
9. Esophagus
10. Right inferior pulmonary v.
11. Superior vena cava
12. Right atrial appendage
13. Lung

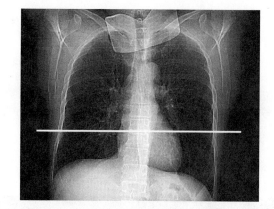

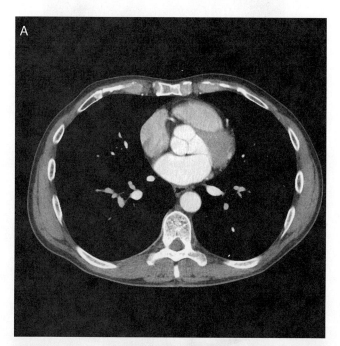

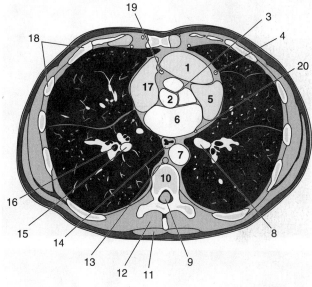

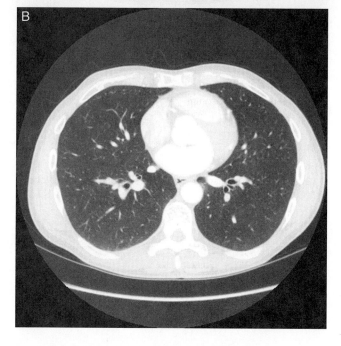

1. Right ventricle
2. Aortic root
3. Aortic valve
4. Left anterior descending a.
5. Left ventricle
6. Left atrium
7. Descending aorta
8. Left inferior pulmonary v.
9. Thecal sac
10. Vertebra
11. Trapezius m.
12. Erector spinae m.
13. Azygos v.
14. Esophagus
15. Right inferior pulmonary v.
16. Right lower lobe segmental bronchus
17. Right atrium
18. Ribs
19. Right coronary a.
20. Left circumflex coronary a.

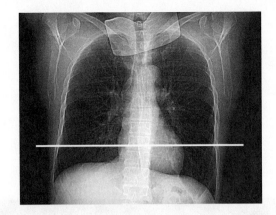

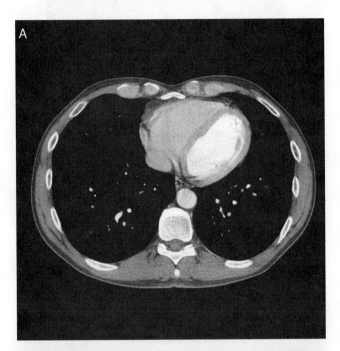

A

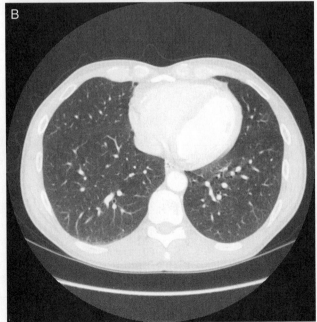

B

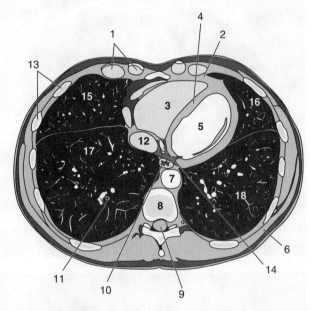

1. Costal cartilage
2. Pericardium
3. Right ventricle
4. Interventricular septum
5. Left ventricle
6. Latissimus dorsi m.
7. Aorta
8. Vertebra
9. Thecal sac with spinal cord
10. Esophagus
11. Pulmonary vessels
12. Inferior vena cava
13. Ribs
14. Coronary sinus
15. Lung, right middle lobe
16. Lung, lingula
17. Lung, right lower lobe
18. Lung, left lower lobe

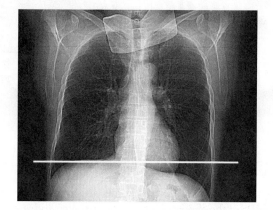

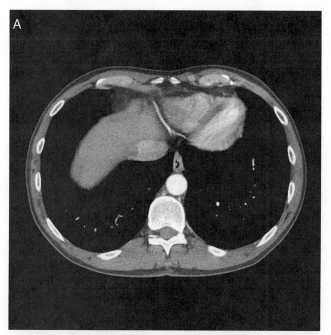

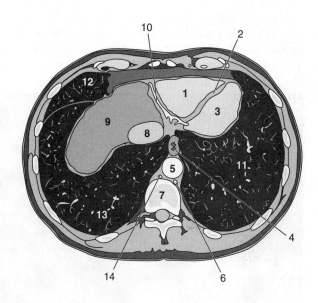

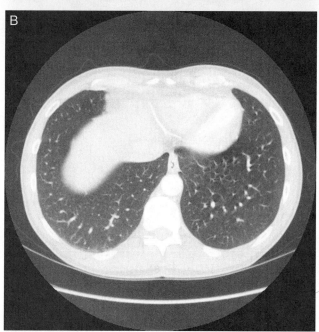

1. Right ventricle
2. Interventricular septum
3. Left ventricle
4. Esophagus
5. Aorta
6. Hemiazygos v.
7. Vertebra
8. Inferior vena cava
9. Liver
10. Right coronary a.
11. Lung, left lower lobe
12. Lung, right middle lobe
13. Lung, right lower lobe
14. Azygos v.

Chapter 17

ABDOMINOPELVIC ANATOMY

ABDOMEN/PELVIS

To include the entire liver and other abdominal organs, routine studies of the abdomen must include the costodiaphragmatic recesses of the lungs, which extend quite far caudally, laterally, and dorsally. Most indications require the administration of both oral and intravenous contrast media. Injection parameters vary according to the indication. The study that included the images below was initiated 70 seconds after the IV administration of 120 mL of contrast medium and therefore shows the contrast enhancement of both arteries and veins.

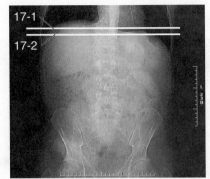

17-1
17-2

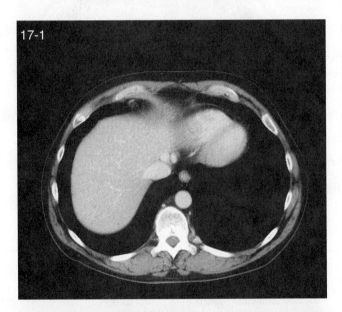

17-1

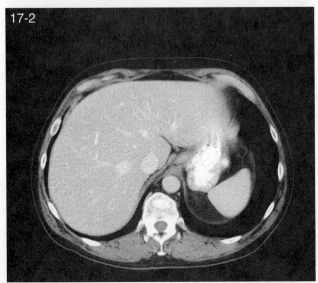

17-2

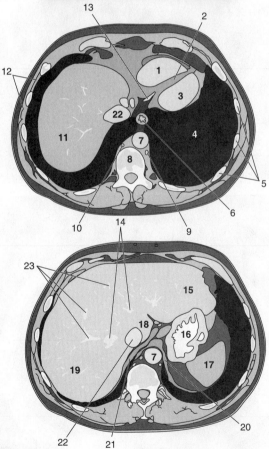

1. Right ventricle	13. Coronary v.
2. Intraventricular septum	14. Portal v., branches
3. Left ventricle	15. Liver, left lobe
4. Left lung	16. Stomach (barium-filled)
5. Ribs	17. Spleen
6. Esophagus	18. Liver, caudate lobe
7. Aorta	19. Liver, right lobe
8. Vertebra	20. Diaphragm, left crus
9. Hemiazygos v.	21. Diaphragm, right crus
10. Azygos v.	22. Inferior vena cava
11. Liver	23. Hepatic vv.
12. Intercostal mm.	

1. Falciform lig.
2. Left gastric a. and left gastric v.
3. Air in stomach
4. Stomach (barium-filled)
5. Spleen
6. Splenic a.
7. Left kidney
8. Left adrenal gland
9. Diaphragm
10. Dural sac and spinal cord
11. Aorta

12. Inferior vena cava
13. Portal v.
14. Liver
15. Spinal n.
16. Ribs
17. Transverse colon
18. Splenic v.
19. Left kidney, cortex
20. Left kidney, medulla
21. Vertebra
22. Right adrenal gland
23. Pancreas

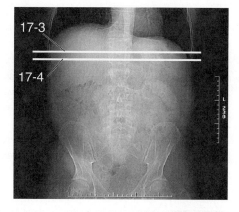

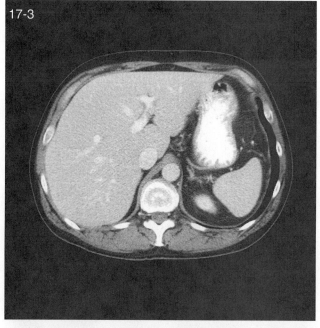

17-3

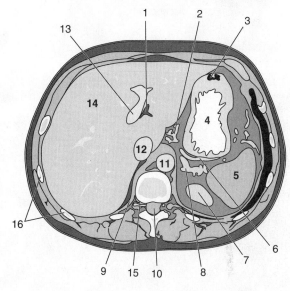

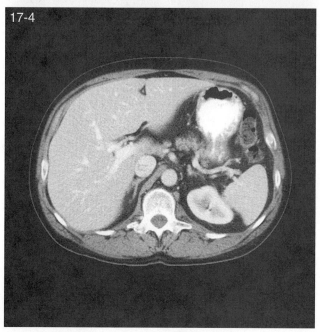

17-4

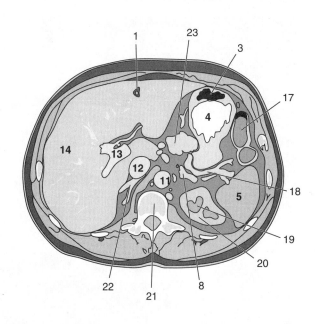

1. Hepatic a.
2. Duodenum
3. Stomach (barium-filled)
4. Colon, splenic flexure
5. Spleen
6. Pancreas
7. Left kidney
8. Celiac trunk
9. Aorta
10. Inferior vena cava
11. Portal v.
12. Liver
13. Vertebra
14. Dural sac and spinal cord
15. Rectus abdominis m.
16. Splenic v.
17. Pancreas. head
18. Portal v., confluence
19. Jejunum
20. Superior mesenteric a.
21. Left renal v.
22. Right kidney
23. Psoas m.
24. Erector spinae m.
25. Gall bladder

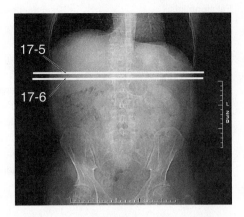

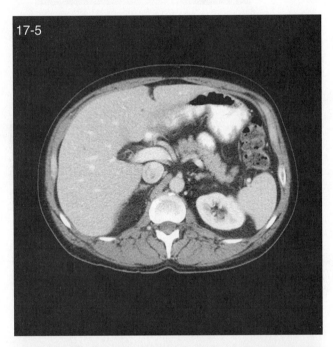

17-5

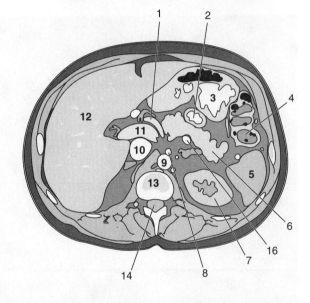

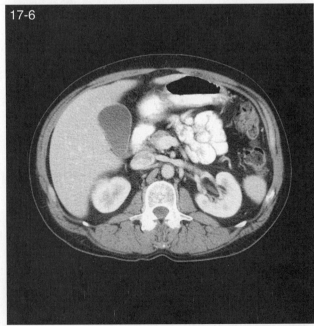

17-6

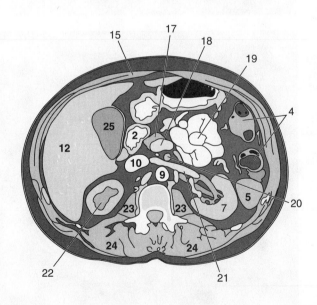

1. Pancreas
2. Superior mesenteric v.
3. Superior mesenteric a.
4. Jejunum/ileum
5. Descending colon
6. Left kidney
7. Right kidney

8. Duodenum
9. Aorta
10. Inferior vena cava
11. Transverse colon
12. Liver
13. Mesenteric vessels

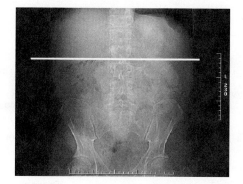

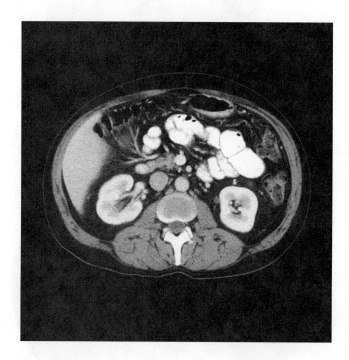

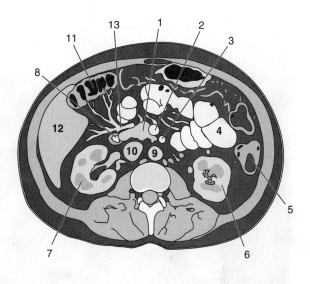

1. Mesenteric vessels
2. Jejunum/ileum
   Abdominal wall:
   3. External oblique m.
   4. Internal oblique m.
   5. Transverse m.
6. Left ureter
7. Inferior mesenteric a.
8. Aorta
9. Inferior vena cava
10. Left kidney
11. Right kidney
12. Fascia
13. Ascending colon
14. Psoas m.
15. Descending colon
16. Erector spinae m.
17. Quadratus lumborum m.

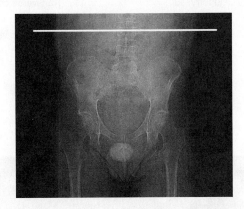

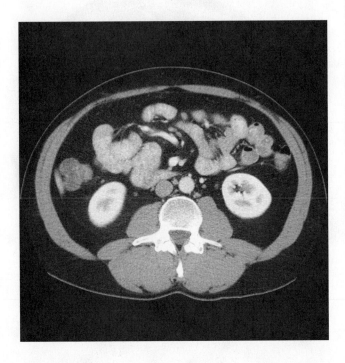

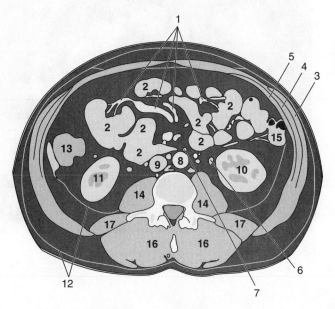

1. Mesenteric vessels
2. Jejunum/ileum
3. Left ureter
4. Psoas m.
5. Inferior vena cava
6. Ascending colon
7. Vertebra
8. Rectus abdomini s m.
9. Common iliac aa.
10. Cecum
11. Left common iliac a.
12. Iliacus m.
13. Left common iliac v.
14. Right common iliac a.
15. Right common iliac v.
16. Ilium
17. Erector spinae m.
18. Descending colon
19. Quadratus lumborum m.
20. Gluteus medius m.

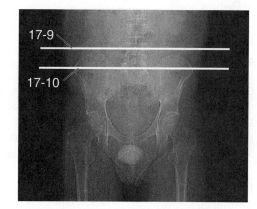

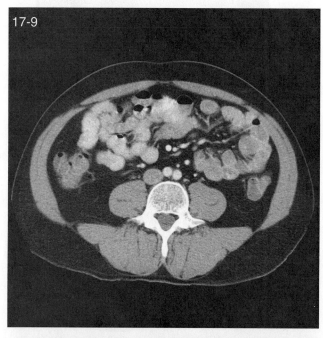

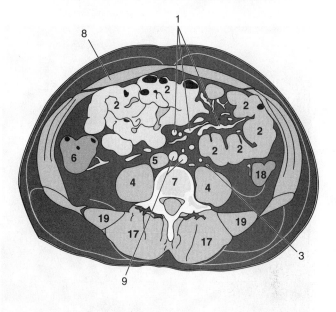

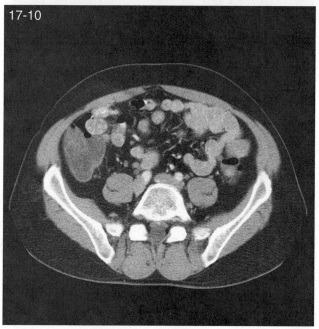

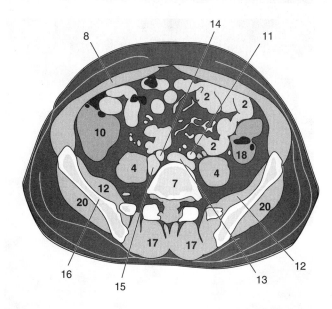

Male Pelvis

1. Mesenteric vessels
2. External iliac aa.
3. Gluteus minimus m.
4. Gluteus medius m.
5. Gluteus maximus m.
6. Sacrum
7. Internal iliac aa.
8. Right common iliac v.
9. Fascia
10. Rectus abdominis m.
11. Ilium

12. Bladder
13. Sigmoid colon
14. Piriformis m.
15. Left external iliac a.
16. Left external iliac v.
17. Right external iliac a.
18. Right external iliac v.
19. Left common iliac v.
20. Iliacus m.
21. Psoas m.
22. Ileum

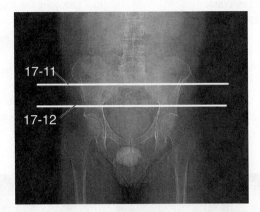

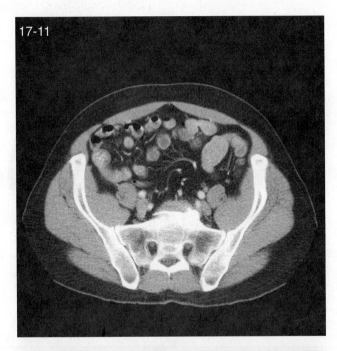

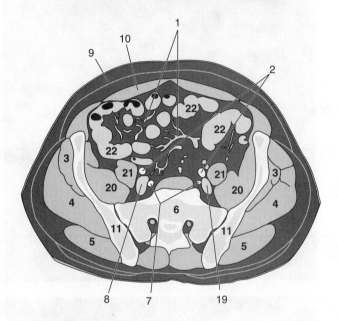

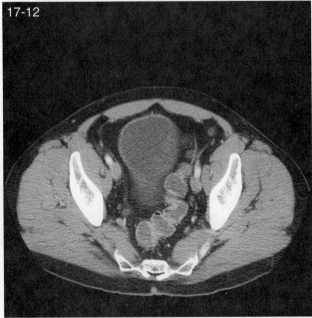

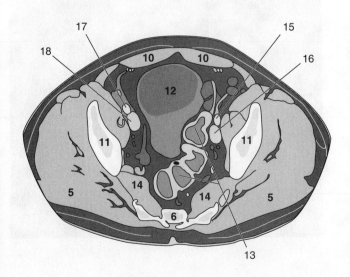

1. Bladder
2. Left external iliac a.
3. Left external iliac v.
4. Obturator internus m.
5. Seminal vesicles
6. Rectum
7. Coccyx
8. Ischium
9. Femoral head
10. Pubis
11. Right external iliac a.
12. Right external iliac v.
13. Rectus abdominis m.
14. Quadriceps femoris m.
15. Prostate gland
16. Iliopsoas m.
17. Sartorius m.
18. Femur
19. Gluteus maximus m.
20. Gluteus minimus m.
21. Gluteus medius m.
22. Tensor fascia lata m.

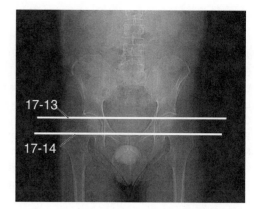

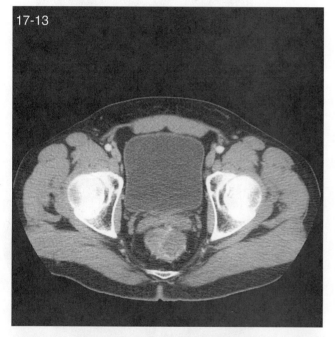

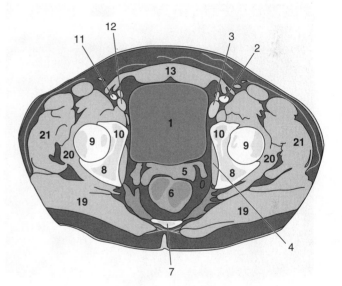

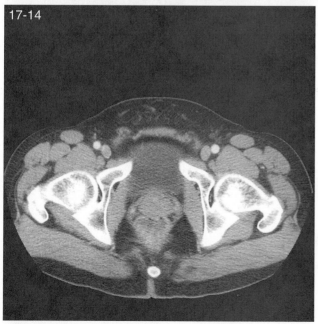

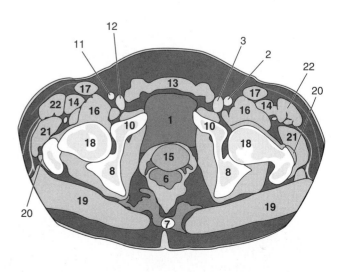

1. Penis
2. Spermatic cords
3. Left femoral a.
4. Left femoral v.
5. Obturator externus m.
6. Rectum
7. Right femoral a.
8. Right femoral v.
9. Bulb of penis with posterior urethra
10. Levator ani
11. Pubis
12. Femur
13. Adductor brevis m.
14. Gluteus maximus m.
15. Iliopsoas m.
16. Tensor fascia lata m.
    Quadriceps femoris m.:
    17. Vastis lateralis
    18. Rectus femoris
19. Sartorius m.
20. Ischium

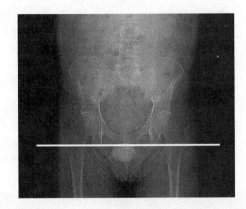

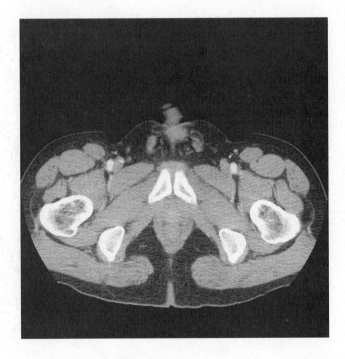

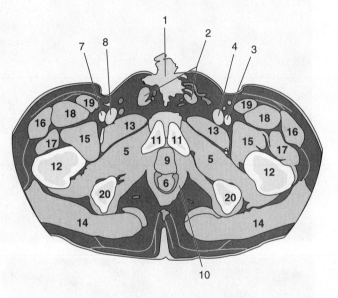

Female Pelvis

1. Bladder
2. Sigmoid colon
3. Left external iliac a.
4. Left external iliac v.
5. Gluteus minimus m.
6. Gluteus medius m.
7. Left ovary
8. Uterus (with IUD present)
9. Ilium
10. Gluteus maximus m.
11. Sacrum
12. Piriformis m.
13. Rectum
14. Right ovary

15. Iliacus m.
16. Right external iliac a.
17. Right external iliac v.
18. Rectus abdominis m.
19. Pubis
20. Femoral head
21. Vagina
22. Coccyx
23. Obturator internus m.
24. Iliopsoas m.
25. Sartorius m.
26. Tensor fascia lata m.
27. Ischium
28. Quadraceps femoris: rectus femoris

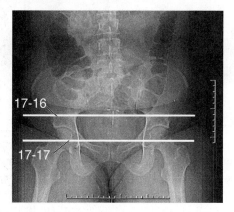

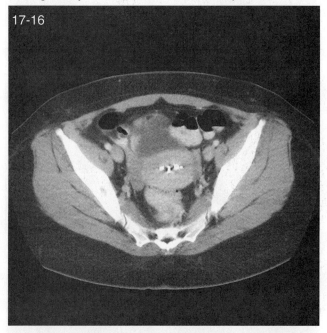

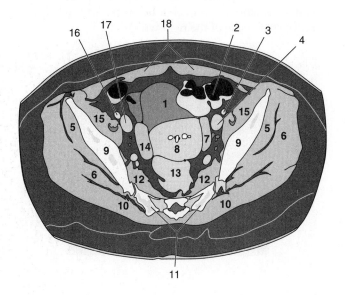

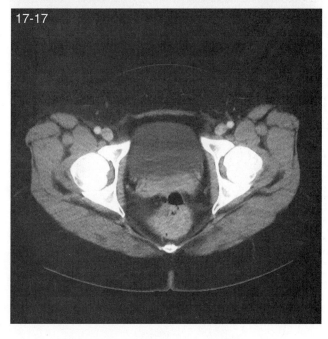

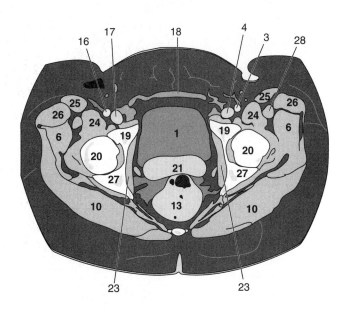

WRIST (RIGHT)

Proper positioning and appropriate annotation of the elbow, wrist, forearm, and hand can be challenging. Confusion as to whether an extremity is the right or left may occur when the patient's arm is positioned over the head. Therefore, it is common practice for the technologist to include a radiopaque marker to aid in identification of the scan orientation. In the scout below notice the BB placed on the ulnar side of the right wrist.

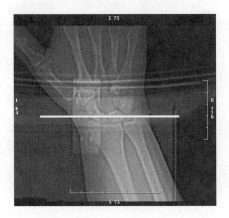

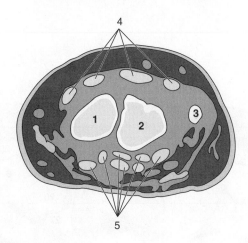

1. Scaphoid
2. Lunate
3. Ulna, styloid process
4. Extensor tendons
5. Flexor tendons

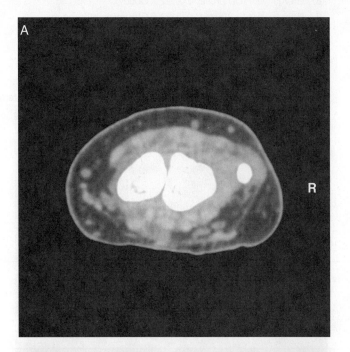

A

R

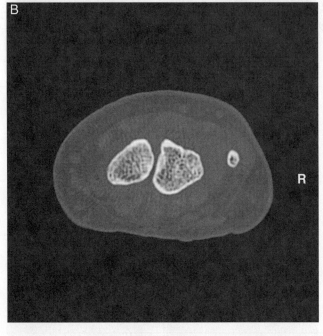

B

R

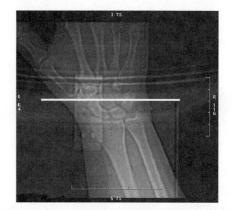

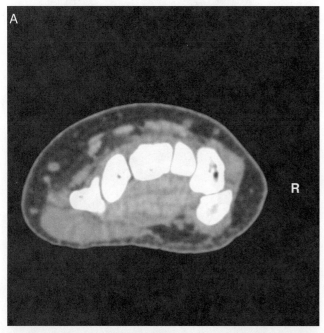

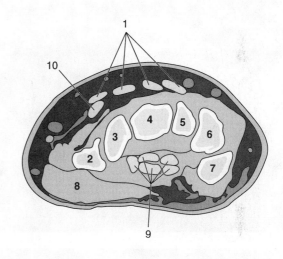

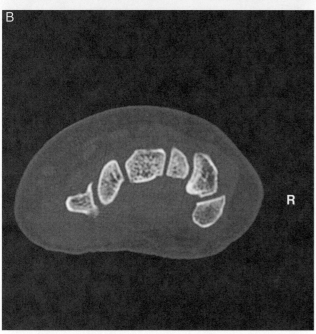

1. Extensor tendons
2. Trapezium
3. Scaphoid
4. Capitate
5. Hamate
6. Triquetrum
7. Pisiform
8. Abductor pollicis brevis and opponens pollicis mm.
9. Flexor digitorum superficialis and flexor digitorum profundus tendons
10. Radial a./v.

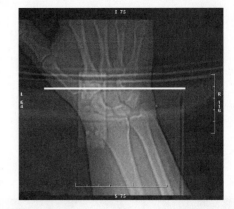

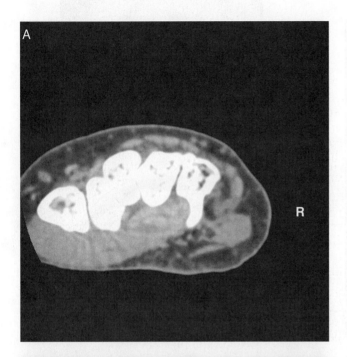

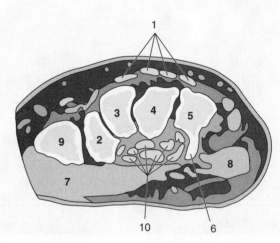

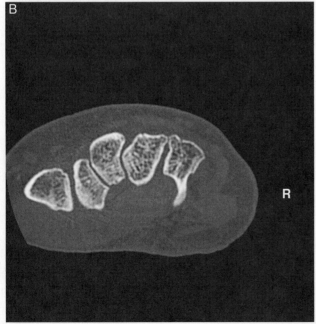

1. Extensor tendons
2. Trapezium
3. Trapezoid
4. Capitate
5. Hamate
6. Hamate, hook
7. Abductor pollicis brevis and opponens pollicis mm.
8. Abductor digiti minimi and opponens minimi mm.
9. First metacarpal
10. Flexor tendons

HIP (LEFT)

In the past, CT examination of the hips of postsurgical patients has been quite limited; the metal of the hip prosthesis caused extensive artifacts that markedly degraded images. Improvements in the design of CT systems now allow successful imaging of the total joint prosthesis and the soft tissues around them. Therefore, CT is now frequently used in the preoperative planning of revision arthroplasty.

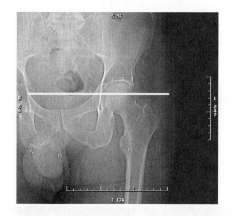

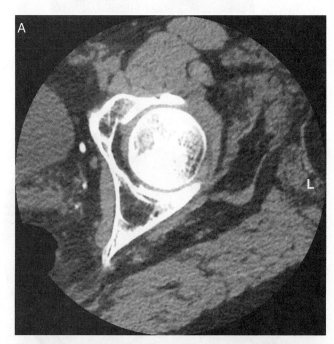

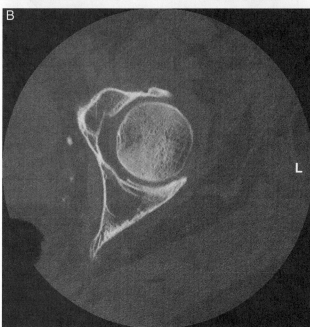

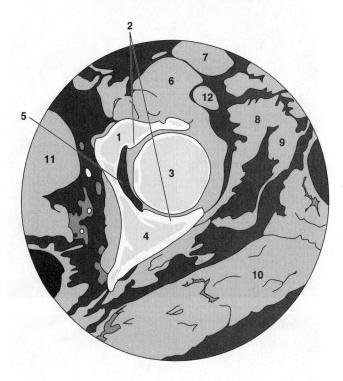

1. Acetabulum (anterior column)
2. Acetabulum
3. Femoral head
4. Acetabulum (posterior column)
5. Hip joint
6. Iliopsoas m.
7. Sartorius m.
8. Gluteus minimus m.
9. Gluteus medius m.
10. Gluteus maximus m.
11. Bladder
12. Rectus femoris m.

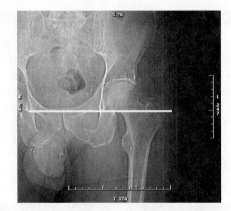

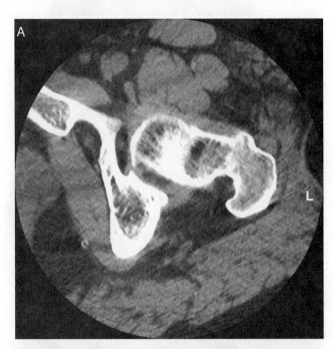

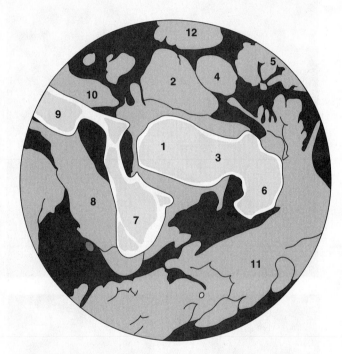

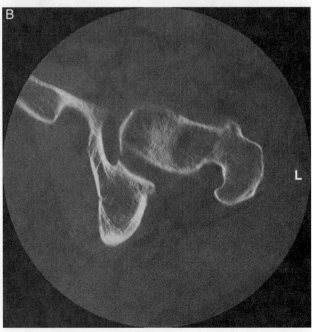

1. Femoral head
2. Iliopsoas m.
3. Femoral neck
4. Rectus femoris m.
5. Tensor fascia lata m.
6. Greater trochanter
7. Ischium/Ischial tuberosity
8. Obturator internus m.
9. Pubis
10. Pectineus m.
11. Gluteus maximus m.
12. Sartorius m.

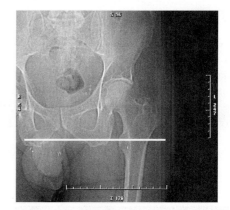

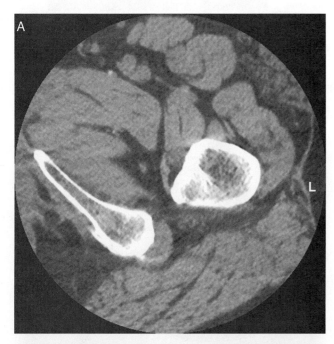

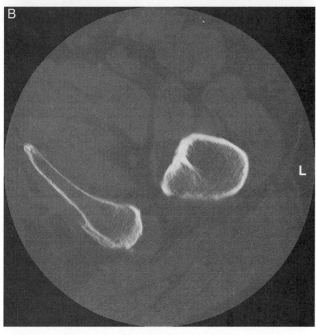

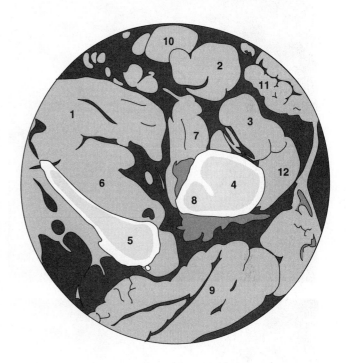

1. Adductor brevis m.
2. Rectus femoris m.
3. Vastus intermedius m.
4. Femur
5. Pubis, inferior ramus
6. Obturator externus m.
7. Iliopsoas m.
8. Femur, lesser trochanter
9. Gluteus maximus m.
10. Sartorius m.
11. Tensor fascia lata m.
12. Vastus lateralis m.

KNEE (LEFT)

Most CT examinations of the knee extend from the distal femur to beyond the tibial plateau, although like all musculoskeletal examinations, protocols are tailored to each patient and the specific clinical situation. Although both knees are included in the scan field of view, the display field of view is targeted to each knee separately.

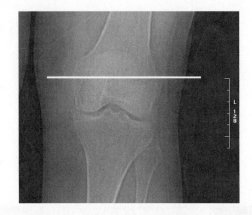

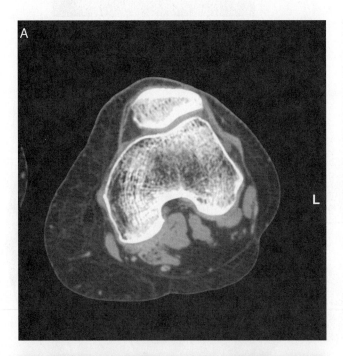

A

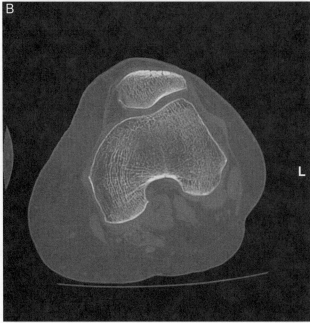

B

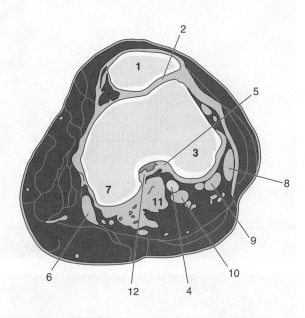

1. Patella
2. Patellofemoral joint
3. Lateral femoral condyle
4. Popliteal a.
5. Anterior cruciate lig.
6. Sartorius m.
7. Medial femoral condyle
8. Biceps femoris m.
9. Plantaris m.
10. Popliteal v.
11. Gastrocnemius m.
12. Posterior cruciate lig.

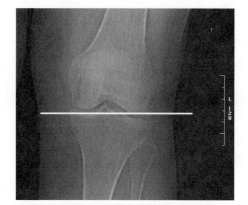

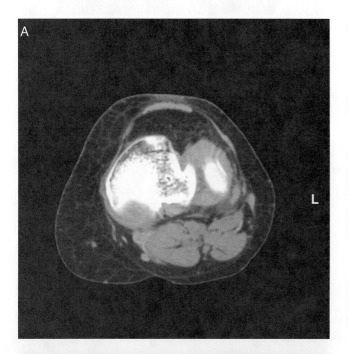

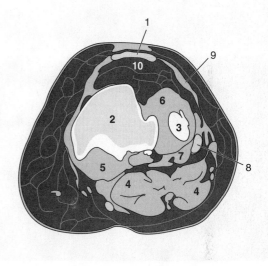

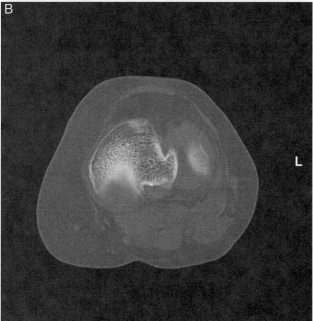

1. Patella tendon
2. Medial tibial plateau
3. Intercondylar eminence (tibial spine)
4. Gastrocnemius m.
5. Popliteus m.
6. Lateral meniscus
7. Plantaris m.
8. Biceps femoris m./tendon
9. Lateral patellar retinaculum
10. Hoffa's fat pad

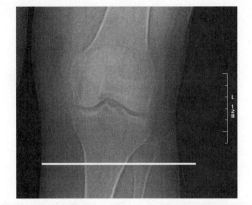

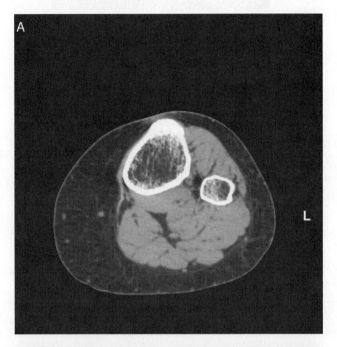

A

L

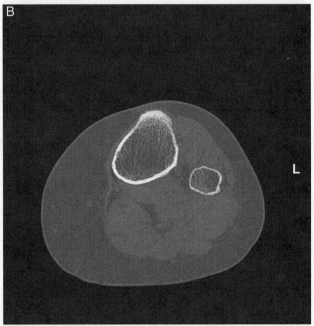

B

L

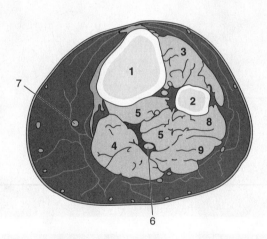

7

1

3

2

5

8

5

4

6

9

1. Tibia
2. Fibula
3. Tibialis anterior m.
4. Medial gastrocnemius m.
5. Popliteus m.
6. Posterior tibial a.
7. Saphenous v.
8. Soleus m.
9. Lateral gastrocnemius m.

FOOT

CT data acquisition of the foot and ankle can be obtained in a number of different imaging planes. The choice of plane depends on which aspect is of primary concern. For examinations of the foot, patients are most often positioned supine with legs flat on the table. Taping the feet together or using a foot holder will help to prevent motion during scanning.

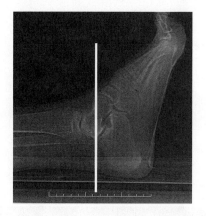

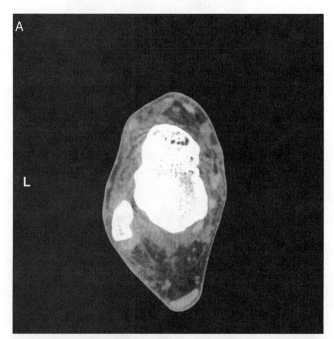

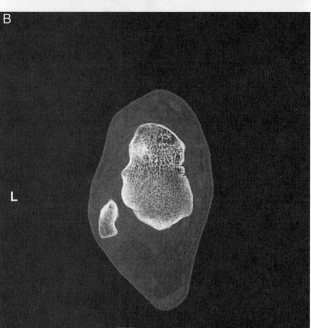

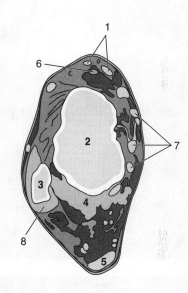

1. Anterior ankle tendons
2. Talus
3. Fibula, lateral malleolus
4. Flexor hallucis longus mm.
5. Achilles tendon
6. Anterior tibial a.
7. Medial ankle tendons
8. Peroneal tendons

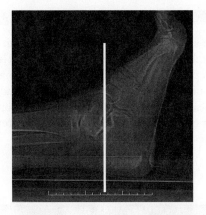

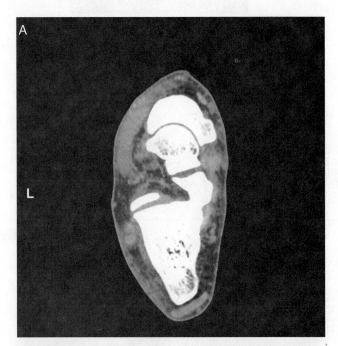

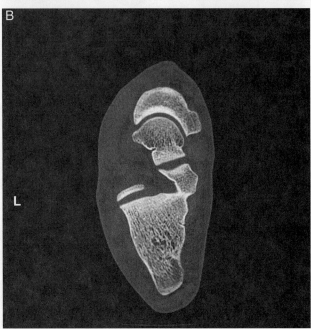

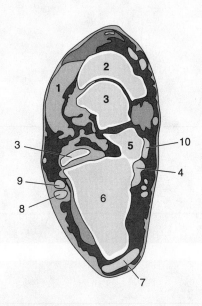

1. Extensor digitorum m.
2. Navicular
3. Talus
4. Flexor hallucis longus tendon
5. Calcaneous sustentaculum
6. Calcaneous
7. Achilles tendon
8. Peroneus longus tendon
9. Peroneus brevis tendon
10. Flexor digitorum tendon

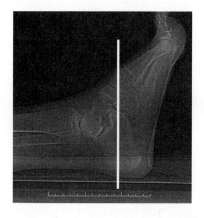

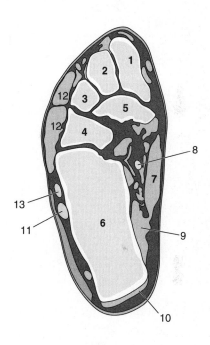

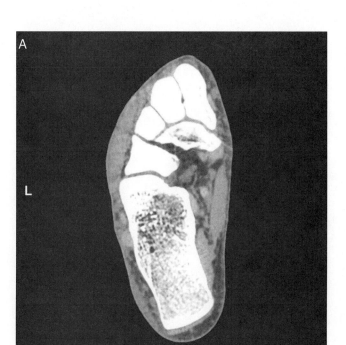

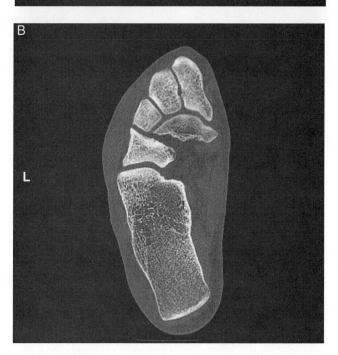

1. Cuneiform, intermedial (1st)
2. Cuneiform, intermedial (2nd)
3. Cuneiform, lateral (3rd)
4. Cuboid
5. Navicular
6. Calcaneous
7. Quadratus plantae m.
8. Posterior tibial a. branches
9. Quadratus plantae m.
10. Achilles tendon (insertion)
11. Peroneus longus tendon
12. Extensor digitorum brevis m.
13. Peroneus brevis tendon

Section IV

IMAGING PROCEDURES and PROTOCOLS

CHAPTER 19 • Neurologic Imaging Procedures

CHAPTER 20 • Thoracic Imaging Procedures

CHAPTER 21 • Abdomen and Pelvis Imaging Procedures

CHAPTER 22 • Musculoskeletal Imaging Procedures

CHAPTER 23 • Interventional CT and CT Fluoroscopy

CHAPTER 24 • PET/CT Fusion Imaging

INTRODUCTION

Each imaging facility has its own, often unique, set of examination protocols. For any given CT examination, the protocol will vary according the individual requirement of the imaging site. Factors that influence a specific site's protocol parameters include the type of equipment available (e.g., 64-slice versus 16-slice), the setting (e.g., inpatient versus outpatient), and the particular preferences of the radiologists in charge. Like all fields of medicine, CT is constantly evolving so it follows that examination protocols constantly undergo re-evaluation and refinement. A cookbook approach to CT scanning is impractical as it cannot possibly account for all possible variables. The protocols presented in this section are intended as examples of just a few of the many possible variations in current practice. There has been no attempt to survey institutions to determine the most prevalent protocols; protocols included here should not be considered either the most common or the best. They are simply one or two options among many. Many other protocol options can be found on the World Wide Web, posted by both equipment manufacturers and various university hospitals. The protocols in this text are in a tabular format to facilitate easy reference. When possible, the protocols include parameter variations for a 16- and a 64-detector system. Again, these are intended be illustrative, providing the reader an idea of the parameters most likely to be adjusted when switching from one type of detector configuration to another. Unless otherwise noted, protocols that include intravenous contrast enhancement use a 300 concentration, low-osmolality agent.

CT imaging increasingly relies on the integration of a variety of knowledge and skills. The first three sections of this text provide information on physics, patient care, and cross-sectional anatomy necessary to understand and carry out CT examination protocols. Hence, this section is intended to be a culmination of the sections that precede it. Within most categories of the examination protocols, one or two topics have been selected for expository writing. These essays are included to demonstrate the interdependency of the information provided in previous sections and to encourage the reader to assemble the knowledge gained thus far into a cohesive whole. Readers will notice that these essays provide information that is not strictly necessary to know to perform a high-quality examination. However, both new and seasoned CT technologists will appreciate the "extra" information, such as the signs and symptoms of various diseases and conditions, as these are so often observed in clinical practice.

ROUTINE SCANNING PROCEDURES

Although in actual practice there are exceptions to every rule, some standards of practice are assumed. We start with a discussion of these assumptions.

In all routine studies, one or two reference images (called "scouts" by some manufacturers) are acquired before scanning. The optimal reference image includes all areas to be scanned and therefore ensures that the anatomy to be imaged is within the range of the scanner (see Chapter 5).

Regardless of the type of scanner used, it is imperative that the operator input the correct directional instructions before scanning. This procedure requires indicating whether the patient is placed head or feet first into the gantry and whether he or she is lying supine, prone, or in the decubitus position. If the operator accurately enters this information into the system, the software correctly annotates the image as to left-right, anterior-posterior, and superior-inferior orientation.

After the scout image is obtained, the operator selects the location of cross-sectional slices. Scan parameters such as mAs, kVp, display field of view, and reconstruction algorithm(s) are selected. Most often, a preprogrammed group of scan parameters is selected so that the technologist must make only minor modifications to suit the particular patient or clinical indication.

It is important to correctly annotate the image as to whether contrast material is administered. All CT systems allow a notation concerning the use of contrast agents. Often, the notation +C is inputted after the introduction of contrast medium.

Routine procedure for some CT examinations includes scanning without contrast material, then repeating the study with intravenous contrast enhancement. Some protocols call for repeating the study at different phases of contrast enhancement. Whenever possible, the repeat scans should be taken at the same location as the unenhanced images.

A history should be taken for all patients. For examinations that require contrast enhancement, the history must include allergies as well as any renal complications (see Chapter 11).

Careful breathing instructions should be given to all patients undergoing body scanning. Some manufacturers suggest that technologists use a coaching procedure to increase the length of breath-hold for a helical study. This coaching requires the patient to take several deep breaths before taking one final breath and holding it for the maximum possible time, then exhaling slowly.

After completing a CT study, it is standard procedure to include a scout image that is cross-referenced by lines. These lines represent the location of each cross-sectional image. It is also typical to include patient data at the beginning or end of each examination. Data must then be stored in some fashion. The practice of transferring images to film is dwindling, but by no means has disappeared. When picture, archive, and communication systems (PACS) are used, images must be transmitted to the appropriate radiologist's workstation (Chapter 9). This information may also be included in a facility's examination protocols.

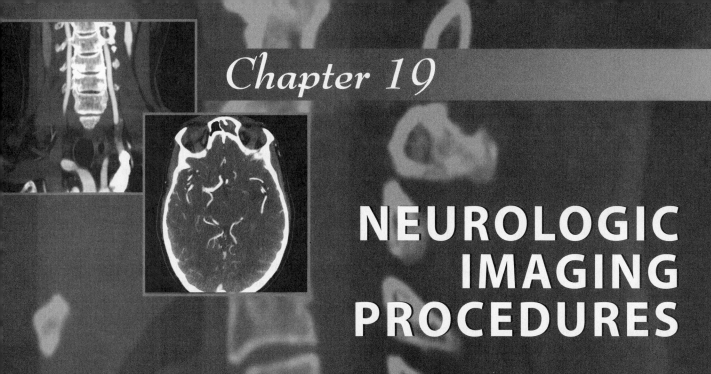

Chapter 19

NEUROLOGIC IMAGING PROCEDURES

Key Terms: supraorbital meatal line • glabellomeatal line • intracranial hemorrhage • Valsalva maneuver • split bolus • CT venography • thrombolytic therapy • completed or established stroke • cerebrovascular accident • stroke in evolution • progressive stroke • ischemic • hemorrhagic • thrombotic • embolic • subarachnoid hemorrhagic stroke • arteriovenous malformations • hypotensive stroke • transient ischemic attack (TIA) • atrial fibrillation • tissue plasminogen activator (t-PA) • penumbra • infarction • CT brain perfusion • rCBF • rCBV • MTT • central volume principle • basal ganglia • CVRC

GENERAL IMAGING METHODS FOR THE HEAD

The patient's head is positioned in the head holder for most protocols of the head. Depending on the design of the head holder, it can sometimes also be used for neck protocols. When the head holder is not used, a molded sponge is placed directly on the scan table and the patient's head is positioned within the sponge. In all cases, the patient should be made as comfortable as possible and immobilized as effectively as possible to prevent motion artifact on the images. This is often accomplished by placing small wedge sponges on either side of the patient's head. In most cases it is not necessary to ask the patient to suspend breathing for CT studies of the head or neck. Anatomy displayed in cross-sectional slices will look slightly different depending on the angulation used. The slice angle is determined by the position of the patient's head (i.e., moving the chin up or down) and the angle of the gantry. It was once common to program the cross-sectional slices of the brain to be parallel to the orbitomeatal line; however, more recent practice favors using the supraorbital meatal line (also called the glabellomeatal line) to reduce radiation exposure to the lens of the eye. Figure 19-1 illustrates lines used for positioning. A disadvantage of many multidetector CT systems is that they do not allow the gantry to be tilted when in helical mode. Therefore, axial (step-and-shoot) techniques are often used for routine brain imaging.

BOX 19–1   Key Concept

Recent practice favors programming slices of the brain parallel to the supraorbital meatal line (rather than the orbital meatal line) to reduce radiation exposure to the lens of the eye.

Changing the image plane from axial to coronal may provide additional information. There are two methods of achieving a coronal position for head scanning. One is to place the patient prone on the scanning table and ask the patient to extend the chin forward. An alternative approach is to place the patient supine and ask him to drop his head back as far as possible. This position usually requires a specialized head holder. In either position, the slice plane will be coronal. If the patient cannot extend the neck fully, the

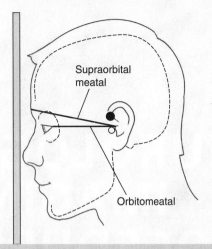

Supraorbital
meatal

Orbitomeatal

FIGURE 19-1 The basic localization points and planes used in CT positioning.

gantry may be angled to obtain a more coronal plane. The image obtained in either the prone or the supine coronal position is essentially the same. Obviously the images are flipped inferior-superior. The preferred position involves several factors, including patient comfort, radiologist preference, and the effect of gravity on anatomic structures (e.g., will fluid settle inferiorly or superiorly?).

Imaging the posterior fossa of the brain is a challenge in CT scanning. Because of the great difference in beam attenuation ability between the dense bone of the skull and the much less dense tissue of the brain, streak artifacts are common. This inherent limitation may be managed by decreasing slice thickness when scanning the posterior fossa and increasing the kVp setting.

BOX 19–2   Key Concept

Because of the dense bone of the skull, beam-hardening artifact is common in the posterior fossa.

Modern multislice CT scanners allow studies of the head to be routinely acquired with thinner slices than in the past–1.25 mm thickness is typical. These thin slices help to reduce beam-hardening artifacts. Images are often merged into thicker slices for viewing.

In examinations of the head, the helical CT mode is used mainly for the purpose of generating three-dimensional reformations or to minimize motion-related artifacts. In general, routine head studies are done using an axial mode, and CT angiography (CTA) studies of the head and neck are done using a helical mode.

Cross-sectional slices of the brain are viewed in multiple window settings. Standard window settings include soft-tissue (brain) 160/40 (approximate window width/window level) for slices in the posterior fossa, 100/30 for slices above; bone (particularly on trauma or postoperative patients) 2500/400; blood 200/60.

Narrow window widths are used to demonstrate the brain, as there is only a small difference in attenuation between the gray matter and the white matter (Chapter 4). Table 19-1 presents values of x-ray attenuation on unenhanced cranial CT. The slightly higher attenuation of the gray matter of the brain compared with white matter may be a result of both a lower gray matter water content and a higher blood volume.[1] Recall that on the Hounsfield scale zero refers to pure water; the value of cerebrospinal fluid (CSF) is slightly above that of water.

CT is the most frequently used initial examination for imaging of intracranial hemorrhage (ICH). The appearance of an ICH will change with the passage of time. This is because the red blood cells within the hemorrhage begin to deteriorate within several hours after leaving the vasculature. These changes are complex and depend on many factors, such as whether the patient is anemic or whether, and to what degree, blood has mixed with CSF. As a general rule, ICH will appear hyperdense to normal brain tissue for approximately 3 days, after which it will gradually decrease in density. This density loss begins at the periphery of the hematoma. As density diminishes, portions of the hematoma become isodense to brain tissue. This progressive density loss continues until the entire hematoma finally becomes hypodense to brain tissue. Although greatly simplified, ICH can be generally expected to appear hyperdense (i.e., white on the image) from onset to 3 days; from 4 to 10 days it is likely to contain a hyperdense center surrounded by concentric areas of hyperdense and hypodense tissue; from 11 days to 6 months it is likely to contain an isodense center surrounded by areas of hypodense tissue; by 6 months the ICH will be hypodense to brain[2] (Fig. 19-2). It is not the role of the technologist to interpret images. However, it is important that technologists recognize certain potentially critical pathologic changes so that when present, they can be brought to the attention of a radiologist. Although most patients with an ICH are seen through the emergency department where images are reviewed by radiologists and reported on quickly, some patients, particularly those with less acute presentations (e.g., headache) may arrive in the CT department as outpatients. In these situations, the technologist can play a vital role by bringing the

TABLE 19-1   X-ray Attenuation in Cranial CT (in Hounsfield Units)

Gray matter	35–45
White matter	20–30
Cerebrospinal fluid	4–8
Circulating blood	40–50
Clotted blood	60–110
Tissue calcification	80–150
Fat	–60 to –70
Air	–1000

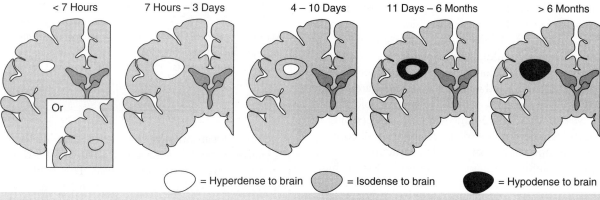

| < 7 Hours | 7 Hours – 3 Days | 4 – 10 Days | 11 Days – 6 Months | > 6 Months |

= Hyperdense to brain   = Isodense to brain   = Hypodense to brain

FIGURE 19-2 A simplified schematic of the evolution of intracranial hemorrhage as it appears on CT.

scan to the radiologist's attention so that these patients receive prompt medical attention.

CT is the primary imaging modality for emergent indications such as trauma and acute changes in neurologic status. For most applications concerning structural imaging of the brain and skull base, nonenhanced CT is usually adequate. IV contrast administration is indicated for infection and neoplasm, but in practice this is not frequently performed because those indications most often prompt an MRI, obviating the need for enhanced CT. However, in some situations MRI is contraindicated (e.g., patient with pacemakers) or unavailable, leaving enhanced CT the best diagnostic option.

BOX 19–3   Key Concept

It is not the role of the technologist to interpret images. However, it is important that technologists recognize certain potentially critical pathologic changes so that when present, they can be brought to the attention of a radiologist.

NECK PROTOCOLS

Routine scanning of the neck is typically performed with the patient supine and the neck slightly extended. It is most often performed in the helical mode. To reduce artifacts that degrade images in the lower neck, the patient should be instructed to lower the shoulders as much as possible. In some institutions images of the neck are acquired while the patient performs a modified Valsalva maneuver. This maneuver requires the patient to blow the cheeks out. This technique helps to distend the pyriform sinuses. Another technique that has been used to evaluate the aryepiglottic folds and pyriform sinuses is to ask the patient to pronounce a prolonged "e" during scanning.

Unless contraindicated, IV contrast media is used when scanning the neck. The goals in CT scanning of the neck are to allow sufficient time after contrast administration for mucosa, lymph nodes, and pathologic tissue to enhance, yet acquire images while the

vasculature remains opacified.[3] Scanning too early after the contrast media injection could result in certain types of neoplastic and inflammatory processes going undetected. However, by delaying scan acquisition the injected contrast agent will no longer opacify the vasculature. One strategy for addressing these contradictory goals is a contrast injection technique referred to as a split bolus. The total contrast dose is split, often in half. The first dose is given and a delay of about 2 minutes is observed. This allows time for structures that are slower to enhance to be opacified. The delay is followed by a second bolus containing the remainder of the contrast; scanning is initiated soon after the second injection is complete, using this second injection to more fully opacify the vessels. The split bolus injection technique is also frequently used for maxillofacial studies in which contrast media is indicated.

BOX 19–4   Key Concept

Unless contraindicated, IV contrast media is used when scanning the neck. The goals in CT scanning of the neck are to allow sufficient time after contrast administration for mucosa, lymph nodes, and pathologic tissue to enhance, yet acquire images while the vasculature remains opacified.

CTA OF THE HEAD AND NECK

Advances in multidetector CT systems and image post-processing techniques have expanded the role that CT plays in the evaluation of cervicocranial vascular disease. Although cerebral catheter angiography or digital subtraction angiography (both performed in the interventional radiology department) are still generally regarded as the gold standard for the imaging of cerebrovascular disorders, those techniques are time-consuming and are associated with a small, but significant, rate of permanent neurologic complications.[4] CT angiography has the advantages of being noninvasive and widely available. The time-saving nature of CTA over traditional angiography is particularly important in the case of patients suspected of suffering an acute stroke in which treatment decisions must be made quickly (a more detailed discussion of stroke begins at the end of this page). In addition, cerebral CTA can be combined with brain perfusion imaging to assess the viability of brain parenchyma and its vascular supply. Cerebral and carotid CTA techniques provide important information about vessel walls; three-dimensional postprocessing of the image data depicts the spatial relationship of complex vascular lesions to the surrounding structures, providing valuable information for the surgeon. Rapid, high-resolution scans are taken while contrast is in the arterial enhancement phase. The goals of CTA for cervicocranial vascular evaluation can be summarized as follows: 1) to accurately measure stenosis of the carotid and vertebral arteries and their branches, 2) to evaluate the circle of Willis for completeness using three-dimensional reformations of cerebral vasculature in relation to other structures, and 3) to detect other vascular lesions, such as dissections or occlusions. A modification of CTA, called CT venography (CTV) is used for the depiction of venous anatomy. Scan parameters are quite similar to CTA, except images are acquired while contrast is in the venous enhancement phase.

SPINE PROTOCOLS

Compared with conventional radiography, CT examinations of the spine produce images with inherently high soft tissue contrast. This contrast permits the visualization of structures such as the intervertebral disks, ligaments, and muscle, as well as bone detail. Visualization of intradural structures is improved by the intrathecal administration of water-soluble contrast material (Chapter 12). CT examinations are performed after myelography to enhance or clarify myelographic findings of intradural and extradural abnormalities. MRI provides even higher soft tissue sensitivity than CT, and in certain circumstances, it is the modality of choice for imaging the spine (e.g., multiple sclerosis, hydromyelia, syringomyelia). For some conditions, such as spinal stenosis, MRI is equivalent to CT. In some situations, CT is considered superior to MRI, such as in the evaluation of bony abnormalities of the spine.

Scans of the spine are often obtained after intrathecal contrast material is given for a fluoroscopic myelography study. Intrathecal contrast medium may be helpful for the diagnosis of degenerative disk disease and other disk diseases, such as extradural neoplasm. Most reports suggest a delay of 1 to 3 hours between the intrathecal injection and scanning. This delay allows the contrast material to dilute. If the scans are performed while the contrast material is too dense, intradural structures may be masked. Rolling the patient once or twice before scanning is recommended to mix the contrast material that may have settled since the myelogram.

BOX 19–5   Key Concept

When CT is performed after intrathecal contrast administration for fluoroscopic myelography, a delay of 1 to 3 hours between the contrast injection and scanning is recommended. This delay allows the contrast material to become sufficiently dilute.

Proper localization is essential in scanning the spine. All studies should include scout images in both anteroposterior (AP) and lateral projections. The scouts will permit vertebral levels to be readily counted and classified to ensure that scans are taken at the appropriate levels. When scanning the lumbar spine, it is important to note whether the patient has a sixth lumbar vertebra (an anatomic variant) that requires additional scans.

SPECIFIC NEUROLOGIC PROTOCOLS

Concepts learned in previous chapters can be applied to scanning the head, neck, and spine. Neurologic CT protocols are often designed to meets the needs of a specific structure or organ (i.e., circle of Willis) or to adapt to a particular clinical indication (i.e., suspected spinal arteriovenous malformation). Many factors must be considered in the development of a scanning protocol. The following detailed discussion of stroke and CT brain perfusion is presented here to provide the reader with a broader understanding of the many issues that may be taken into consideration in the design of CT protocols. Examples of various protocols are provided at the end of the chapter.

A Profile of Stroke

Introduction

The American Heart Association reports that cerebrovascular disorders such as ischemic and hemorrhagic strokes constitute the third most frequent cause of death in North America. Equally alarming, stroke is the leading cause of long-term disability. Approximately 20% to 30% of stroke victims do not survive, and 55% of stroke survivors have a disability.[5] Despite the significant advances in the treatment of stroke in recent years, cerebrovascular disorders continue to pose a considerable challenge to acute neurovascular management.

Therapeutic options, such as thrombolytic therapy, can limit the extent of brain injury and improve outcome after stroke when administered to patients who fall within narrow clinical guidelines. Many of these therapies are only effective if given early after the stroke has begun, hence the criticality of emergent imaging. However, these therapies are expensive and may result in potentially life-threatening complications, drawbacks that make it crucial that each case be assessed by its individual risk-benefit ratio. Most important, the location and extent of the ischemic lesion, combined with the severity of the blood flow reduction, are the main factors that predict outcome in the treatment of stroke.[6] These factors demand an assessment of cerebral blood circulation to determine whether a conservative or a more aggressive therapy is needed in the early stage of stroke.

To adequately explain cerebrovascular disorders it is necessary to begin with an analysis of the basic physiologic processes that result in the origin and development of stroke. This review will define common terms, list symptoms, and present risk factors. In the following section we discuss CT perfusion, a newer diagnostic option in the assessment of acute stroke.

Overview

Although the brain receives approximately 25% of the body's oxygen supply, the brain lacks the capacity for its storage. Brain cells require a constant supply of oxygen to maintain health and functionality. Blood provides this continuous supply through two main arterial systems: 1) the carotid arteries and 2) the basilar artery, formed by the vertebral arteries. These systems are connected in a unique way. They terminate in the circle of Willis, a vascular structure located on the floor of the cranial cavity. The circle of Willis loops around the brainstem, above the pons, giving off the major vessels supplying the brain. In general, it provides collateral blood supply to the brain for multiple arteries; however, it may not be completely interconnected in some patients, and of course, it does not help in supplying blood if the vascular deficit is distal to the circle of Willis.

A reduction of blood flow for even a short period of time can be disastrous and is the primary cause of a stroke. A completed, or established, stroke is the preferred medical term used to describe an acute episode of interrupted blood flow to the brain that lasts longer than 24 hours. Most completed strokes reach a maximal neurologic deficit within an hour of onset.[7] Terms used to describe stroke in the medical field include cerebrovascular accident (CVA) and apoplexy, which literally means, "struck with violence" or "being thunderstruck." These older terms are no longer favored because they imply a random, unpredictable, or uncertain nature to the condition.

A stroke in evolution, or progressive stroke, describes a time-limited event in which the neurologic deficits occur in a progressive pattern. In cases when the carotid artery distribution is affected, there is little chance it will progress beyond 24 hours. However, disruption involving vertebrobasilar distribution may continue to progress for up to 72 hours.[8]

Types of Stroke

Stroke may be divided into two main categories: ischemic, caused by a blockage in an artery, and hemorrhagic, caused by a tear in the artery's wall that produces bleeding in the brain. A third less-prevalent type is hypotensive, which occurs as a result of blood pressure that is too low.

Ischemic Stroke   Ischemic strokes are by far the most common, accounting for 80% of all strokes. Ischemia is defined as a deficiency of oxygen in vital tissues. Two main types of ischemic stroke exist: 1) thrombotic, caused from a blood clot or a fatty deposit within one of the brain's arteries; and 2) embolic, resulting from a traveling particle that forms elsewhere and is too large to pass through small vessels and eventually lodges in a smaller artery. In addition to the two main types, a less acute form of ischemic stroke exists. This form is referred to as a lacunar stroke.

Thrombotic Stroke   Thrombotic strokes occur when a clot that forms as the result of atherosclerosis blocks an artery that supplies blood to the brain. This condition is progressive and can be summarized as follows:

- Arterial walls slowly thicken, harden, and narrow (creating a stenosis) until blood flow is reduced.
- The abnormal arteries become vulnerable to injury, initiating an inflammatory response. It is hypothesized that this response plays a significant role in the evolution of stroke.
- The immune system reacts to the arterial injuries by releasing white blood cells at the site, specifically neutrophils and macrophages.
- Macrophages digest foreign debris, turning them into foamy cells that attach to the smooth muscle cells of the blood vessels, causing a buildup of these cells.
- Sensing further harm, the immune system releases factors called cytokines, which attract more white blood cells and perpetuate the entire cycle.
- These processes impede blood flow.
- To make matters worse, the injured inner walls of vessels fail to produce enough nitric oxide, a substance critical for maintaining blood vessel elasticity. Without adequate nitric oxide, arteries become calcified and lose elasticity.
- Hardened and rigid arteries are even more susceptible to injury. If they tear, a thrombus (clot) may form.
- If that happens, a thrombus could completely block the already narrowed artery, preventing oxygen from reaching a part of the brain, and stroke occurs.

Common focal sites of cerebrovascular atherosclerosis include the proximal common carotid artery, the origin of the internal carotid artery, the carotid siphon, and the proximal middle cerebral and vertebral arteries (Figs. 19-3, 19-4).

Embolic Stroke   An embolic stroke is caused when an artery in the brain is suddenly blocked by embolic material, which is usually a thrombus that developed elsewhere in the body. The embolus travels within the cervicocranial arteries until it becomes wedged in an artery in the brain. If the embolic material lodges for very long, the resulting reduced blood flow, or hypoperfusion, results in an infarct. This infarct may become hemorrhagic when the embolus moves, or fragments, and reperfusion occurs.

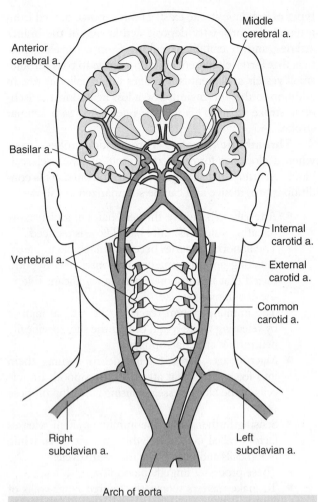

FIGURE 19-3   Branches of the aortic arch (anterior view).

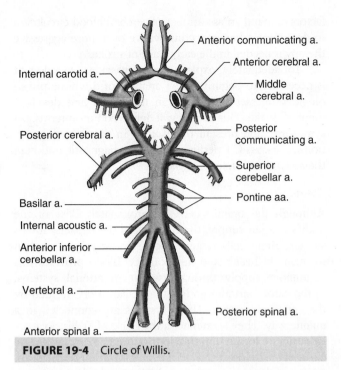

FIGURE 19-4   Circle of Willis.

The clinical findings depend on the location of the brain artery affected.

Emboli account for about 60% of strokes and may result from the following conditions:

- Atrial fibrillation, an abnormal rhythm (rapid quivering beat) in the atrium of the heart. The irregular beat may cause some blood to remain in the heart chamber where it forms clots, which then can break off and travel to the brain as emboli. Blood clots originally formed as a result of atrial fibrillation comprise approximately 15% of embolic strokes.
- At the site of artificial heart valves or as a result of heart valve disorders.
- After a heart attack or in association with heart failure, as a result of areas of the ventricles that do not move properly, allowing blood to stagnate and clot.
- From fat particles, tumor cells, or air bubbles that travel through the bloodstream. This type of emboli is rare.

Lacunar Stroke   Small arteries, such as those that supply the deep cerebral white matter, are also susceptible to atherosclerotic changes. A lacunar stroke occurs when one of these small arteries is blocked. In these deep parts of the brain, no other blood vessels exist that can help supply blood to that region. Therefore, a blockage results in tissue death in that area. The word lacuna describes a small, hollow cavity or pit. After a lacunar stroke, the tiny infarcts that result have been described as hollowed out—thus the name lacunar.

Lacunar infarcts are a series of very tiny ischemic strokes. Symptoms present in the patient as clumsiness, weakness, and emotional variability. Lacunar stroke accounts for 25% of strokes and can sometimes serve as a warning sign that a major stroke may be imminent.

Hemorrhagic Stroke   Rupture of a blood vessel in the brain causes leakage of blood into the brain parenchyma, CSF spaces around the brain, or both. Approximately 20% of strokes occur from hemorrhage. Hemorrhagic strokes are classified by how and where they occur.

BOX 19–6   Key Concept

Rupture of a blood vessel in the brain causes leakage of blood into the brain parenchyma, CSF spaces around the brain, or both.

Intracerebral Hemorrhage   Intracerebral hemorrhagic strokes occur within the brain parenchyma itself, and a hematoma often results. These strokes account for more than half of hemorrhagic strokes. Most often, they result from hypertension, which exerts excessive pressure on arterial walls already damaged by atherosclerosis. Heart attack patients who have been given drugs either to break up blood clots or to "thin blood" to reduce the likelihood of developing clots have a slightly elevated risk of this type of stroke.

Subarachnoid Hemorrhage   Subarachnoid hemorrhagic strokes occur when there is bleeding into the subarachnoid spaces and the CSF spaces. These strokes are usually caused by the rupture of an aneurysm.

Arteriovenous Malformation   Arteriovenous malformations (AVMs) are composed of tangles of arteries and arterialized veins. There is brain tissue interposed between the vessels, but it is usually abnormal and often scarred from previous tiny hemorrhages. The patient may not have been aware of these tiny hemorrhages or may have experienced them as bad headaches.

Normally, blood enters brain tissue through major cerebral arteries, and then passes through smaller arterioles and subsequently into the capillary bed. It is at the capillary level that the exchange of oxygen and glucose in brain cells occurs. A drop in pressure usually occurs as the blood travels from the arteries to the veins. The blood, depleted of oxygen, then enters the venous system to continue its systemic circulation.

When an AVM exists, blood is shunted directly from the arterial system to the venous system. This shunting allows oxygenated blood to enter the veins. In AVMs, the flow is high and the pressure is elevated within the veins. The elevated pressure can cause the vessels to rupture, resulting in a hemorrhagic stroke.

Hypotensive Stroke   Although rare, blood pressure that is too low can reduce oxygen supply to the brain enough to cause a stroke. Systemic hypoperfusion results when blood flow to the brain is lowered to a level too severe to be compensated by cerebral autoregulation mechanisms. These hypotensive episodes can be caused by cardiac pump failure, a major bleeding episode that causes a global decrease in cerebral blood flow, an overwhelming infection, or although rarely, from surgical anesthesia or overtreated high blood pressure. Hypotensive episodes cause infarction in the border zones between the major cerebral arteries, sometimes referred to as a watershed infarction, as well as widespread bilateral cerebral dysfunction. The primary areas of damage are within the circle of Willis between the anterior and middle cerebral arteries, and between the middle and posterior cerebral arteries in the parieto-occipital regions of the cerebral hemispheres[6] (Fig. 19-4).

Symptoms of Stroke

Transient Ischemic Attacks   A transient ischemic attack (TIA) is a reversible episode of focal neurologic dysfunction that typically lasts anywhere from a few minutes to a few hours. Attacks are usually caused by tiny emboli that lodge in an artery and then quickly break up and dissolve, with no residual damage.

TIAs are a significant indicator of stroke risk. Approximately 5% of patients who experience TIAs go on to suffer a stroke within a month. Without treatment, one-third of these patients will experience strokes within 5 years. Because of the relationship between atherosclerosis, coronary artery disease, and stroke, TIAs are also warning signs for a heart attack.

The clinical presentation of TIAs varies slightly depending on whether the carotid or basilar artery is involved.

Symptoms of TIAs in the Carotid Arteries   The carotid arteries are the more common sites of TIAs. The carotid arteries supply blood to the retinal artery. Emboli here cause symptoms originating in either the retina or the cerebral hemisphere. Reduction of oxygen to the eye results in a visual effect often described as a "shade being pulled down." Poor night vision is another manifestation of carotid artery TIA. When the cerebral hemisphere is affected, the patient may experience problems with speech, partial and temporary paralysis, tingling, and numbness, typically on one side of the body.

Symptoms of TIAs in the Basilar Artery   When TIAs result from occlusion of the basilar artery, both hemispheres of the brain may be affected. Therefore, symptoms often occur on both sides of the body and include the following:

- Temporarily dim, gray, blurry, or lost vision in both eyes
- Tingling or numbness in the mouth, cheeks, or gums
- Headache in the back of the head
- Dizziness
- Nausea and vomiting
- Difficulty swallowing
- Inability to speak clearly
- Weakness in the arm and legs, sometimes causing a sudden fall

Symptoms of a Major Ischemic Stroke   The onset of symptoms in a major ischemic stroke may vary, depending on the source. If the stroke is caused by a large embolus that has traveled to and lodged in an artery in the brain, the onset is sudden. Headache and seizures can occur within seconds of the blockage. If the stroke results from a thrombosis that has formed in a narrowed artery, symptoms manifest more gradually, during minutes to hours. On rare occasions the onset can progress from days to weeks.

The symptoms of a major ischemic stroke can be extremely variable. Early symptoms can be identical to those of a TIA, because the clot may block a branch of the carotid or basilar arteries. However, unlike a TIA, the symptoms do not resolve. A thrombosis on one side of the brain usually affects the opposite side of the body, with possible unilateral weakness, loss of feeling on one side of the face or in an arm or leg, or blindness in one eye. If the left hemisphere of the brain is affected, speech problems often occur. (In some patients, mostly those who are left-handed, a clot on the right side of the brain can affect speech.) Other symptoms may include an inability to express thoughts verbally or understand spoken words. The victim may experience major seizures and possibly coma.

Symptoms of Hemorrhagic Stroke   The symptoms of hemorrhagic stroke depend, to some extent, on where and how the hemorrhage occurs. Symptoms from cerebral hemorrhage usually begin very suddenly and evolve over the course of several hours. They include headache, nausea and vomiting, and altered mental state. A subarachnoid hemorrhage may produce warning signs from the leaky blood vessel a few days to a month before the aneurysm fully develops and ruptures. Warning signs may include abrupt headaches, nausea and vomiting, and sensitivity to light. When the aneurysm ruptures, the stroke victim may experience a terrible headache; neck stiffness; vomiting; an altered state of consciousness; eyes that become fixed in one direction or a loss of vision; or stupor, rigidity, and even coma.

Symptoms of Hypertensive Stroke   Symptoms resulting from hypertensive stroke are loss of vision, decreased alertness, and weakness that affects predominantly the shoulder, hand, and thigh.

Silent Brain Infarctions   As many as 31% of elderly patients experience silent brain infarctions.[7] These are small strokes that cause no apparent symptoms but are major contributors to changes in mental status in the elderly. Smokers and individuals with hypertension are at particular risk.

Stroke Risk Factors

Hypertension   Hypertension contributes to 70% of all strokes. It is estimated that controlling blood pressure could prevent nearly half of all strokes.

Homocysteine and Vitamin B Deficiencies   Abnormally high blood levels of the amino acid homocysteine, which occur with deficiencies of vitamin B_6, B_{12}, and folic acid, have been linked to an increased risk of coronary artery disease and stroke. Some experts believe that homocysteine is a major risk factor for stroke, second only to hypertension.[9,10]

Cholesterol and Other Lipids   It is well accepted than an unhealthy cholesterol balance plays a major role in atherosclerosis and consequent heart disease. However, the role cholesterol plays in stroke is less clear.

Atrial Fibrillation   Atrial fibrillation is a disorder of heart rate and rhythm in which the atria are stimulated to contract in a very rapid or disorganized manner rather than in an organized one. For individuals suffering from atrial fibrillation, their risk of stroke increases sixfold. By the age of 70, 10% of adults have this disorder.

Heart Disease   A diseased heart increases the risk of stroke. In fact, people with heart problems have more than twice the risk of stroke compared with people whose hearts work normally.[5] Heart disease and stroke are interconnected for many reasons. Chief among them is that the two disorders share common risk factors, including hypertension and diabetes.

Diabetes Mellitus   Diabetes is a strong risk factor for ischemic stroke, perhaps because of often associated factors such as obesity, high cholesterol levels, and hypertension. Diabetes does not appear to increase the risk of hemorrhagic stroke.

Migraine   Migraine sufferers, both men and women, have an increased risk for stroke, particularly before age 50. However, it is important to note that many people have migraines, and their risk is still low–2.7% for women and 4.6% for men, according to one study.[11] In both men and women with a history of migraines, the increased risk diminished with age.

Other Medical Conditions   A number of other medical conditions may contribute to the risk of stroke. These include sleep apnea, the presence of antibodies called antiphospholipids, and sickle cell anemia. Pregnancy also carries a very small risk, mostly in women with pregnancy-related hypertension and women delivering via cesarean section.

Heredity   An individual's genetic makeup may be responsible for many of the processes leading to stroke. Studies indicate that a family history of stroke, particularly on the paternal side, is a strong risk factor.

Smoking   People who smoke a pack of cigarettes daily are at almost 2.5 times the risk of stroke than that of nonsmokers. The nicotine and carbon monoxide in cigarette smoke damage the cardiovascular system in many ways. The risk is proportional to the dose, that is, the heavier the smoking, the higher the risk. In addition, birth control pills and smoking have a synergistic risk effect. Thus, women who take birth control pills and smoke significantly increase their risk of stroke. Quitting smoking significantly reduces the risk of stroke.

Obesity   Obesity is associated with stroke, most likely because being overweight reflects the presence of other risk factors, including insulin resistance and diabetes, hypertension, and unhealthy cholesterol levels. How a person carries extra weight also influences the risk of stroke. Weight that is centered around the abdomen (i.e., "apple shape") has a greater association with stroke than weight distributed around the hips (i.e., "pear shape").

Alcohol and Drug Abuse Heavy alcohol use is associated with a higher risk of both ischemic and hemorrhagic stroke. However, studies have indicated that moderate alcohol use does not increase an individual's risk of stroke and may even lower the risk of ischemic stroke.[12]

Intravenous drug abuse carries a high risk of stroke from cerebral embolism. Cocaine and methamphetamine are major factors in the incidence of stroke in young adults. Steroids used for bodybuilding also increase stroke risk.

Diagnosis and Treatment of Stroke

Although a detailed review of the many issues and options surrounding the treatment of stroke is beyond the scope of this text, it is worthwhile to touch on advances made in the past decade that have increased the importance of CT imaging in the diagnosis and treatment of stroke.

In June 1996, the U.S. Food and Drug Administration (FDA) approved a treatment for acute ischemic stroke. The treatment, known as tissue plasminogen activator (t-PA), was the first of its kind and revolutionized the way the medical community can respond to treating the 80% of stroke patients who experience ischemic strokes. t-PA is the only FDA-approved treatment for acute ischemic stroke. One dose of t-PA is required to treat an acute stroke patient at an average cost of approximately $2,000 per dose. Despite the high cost, the treatment has been shown to reduce disability, leading to an overall cost savings in hospital, nursing home, and rehabilitation care expenses.

To be effective, t-PA must be administered within 3 hours of the first signs of stroke. This means that the stroke victim must be transported to the hospital, diagnosed, and administered the t-PA treatment before the 3-hour window has expired. Unfortunately, only a small percentage of patients who suffer a stroke reach the hospital in time to be considered for the t-PA treatment.[13]

BOX 19-7   Key Concept

To be effective t-PA must be administered within 3 hours of the first signs of stroke. This means that the stroke victim must be transported to the hospital, diagnosed, and administered the t-PA treatment before the 3-hour window has expired.

The target of t-PA therapy is the tissue known as the penumbra. After an acute ischemic stroke, areas of tissue death (infarction) occur because of a local lack of oxygen. The penumbra is ischemic tissue that (without successful intervention) is destined for infarction, but is not yet irreversibly injured. It is the penumbra that may be salvageable with the administration of t-PA. The fully infarcted tissue will not

benefit from reperfusion after t-PA and may be at increased risk of hemorrhage. However, if reperfusion of the penumbra occurs expeditiously, this tissue will recover and the patient improves. This is why the timing of t-PA therapy is so critical. Stroke experts commonly refer to the sense of urgency in stroke treatment with the expression "time is brain."

Published guidelines recommend that the time between arriving at the emergency room to actual treatment should be 60 minutes or less.[14] During this hour, various tests must be performed, including a neurologic examination, blood tests, and a CT scan of the head to determine whether hemorrhage has occurred and contraindicates t-PA.

BOX 19-8   Key Concept

Evidence of intracranial hemorrhage on pretreatment noncontrast head CT contraindicates t-PA therapy.

Even assuming that all the appropriate diagnostic testing can be accomplished in an hour, this leaves only 2 hours for recognition of the symptoms of stroke and transportation to the appropriate emergency room.

Fast diagnosis of both the presence and type of stroke is critical in saving lives and reducing the likelihood of severe disability. Patients must be carefully selected because the treatment itself can cause bleeding that can be lethal if the stroke is hemorrhagic in origin. Criteria that exclude patients from receiving t-PA are included in Table 19-2.

Although MRI of the head can also be used to evaluate stroke patients for possible thrombolytic therapy, CT is used more frequently. This is because the imaging tool must be used quickly, and CT is much more available than MRI. In addition, noncontrast CT is regarded as more practical because the imaging time is shorter, it is better tolerated by many patients, there are no contraindications as may occur for MRI, and all relevant information is provided with only one imaging sequence. A noncontrast CT of the brain is routinely performed to differentiate ischemic stroke from hemorrhagic stroke, to assess the state of cerebral circulation and tissue, and, secondarily, to assess the underlying disease.

BOX 19-9   Key Concept

A noncontrast CT of the brain is routinely performed to differentiate ischemic stroke from hemorrhagic stroke, to assess the state of cerebral circulation and tissue, and, secondarily, to assess the underlying disease.

An unenhanced CT is an effective tool in determining the presence of intracranial bleeding and therefore well meets the first goal of imaging. However, in the first 6 hours after onset of an ischemic stroke, an unenhanced

Table 19-2   Contraindications to t-PA[13]

Evidence of intracranial hemorrhage on pretreatment noncontrast head CT

Clinical presentation suggestive of subarachnoid hemorrhage, even with normal CT

CT shows multilobar infarction (hypodensity greater than one-third cerebral hemisphere)

History of intracranial hemorrhage

Uncontrolled hypertension: At the time treatment should begin, systolic pressure remains > 185 mm Hg or diastolic pressure remains > 110 mm Hg despite repeated measurements
 Known arteriovenous malformation, neoplasm, or aneurysm

Witnessed seizure at stroke onset

Active internal bleeding or acute trauma (fracture)

Acute bleeding diathesis, including but not limited to:
 Platelet count < 100,000/mm³
 Heparin received within 48 hours, resulting in an activated partial thromboplastin time (aPTT) that is greater than upper limit of normal for laboratory
 Current use of anticoagulant (e.g., warfarin sodium) that has produced an elevated international normalized ratio (INR) > 1.7 or prothrombin time (PT) > 15 seconds

Within 3 months of intracranial or intraspinal surgery, serious head trauma, or previous stroke

Arterial puncture at a noncompressible site within past 7 days

CT will remain normal in about one-third of patients because the ischemia does not reach the critical level of structural integrity. Studies such as CT perfusion and CT angiography are sometimes done in addition to the noncontrast CT scan to address the other goal of imaging, to assess the state of the cerebral circulation and tissue. CT perfusion techniques measure cerebral blood flow, whereas CT angiography of the carotid arteries and vessels of the circle of Willis can demonstrate stenosis or occlusion of extracranial and intracranial arteries.

CT Brain Perfusion Scans

Various attempts have been made to establish a CT method to allow qualitative and quantitative evaluation of cerebral perfusion. CT perfusion provides this information by calculating regional blood flow (rCBF) and regional blood volume (rCBV) and mean transit time (MTT). Perfusion studies are obtained by monitoring the passage of iodinated contrast through the cerebral vasculature. Attractive characteristics of this approach are the widespread availability of CT scanners, their high image quality, and relatively low costs. In addition, simply extending the routine CT examination eliminates time-consuming transport of patients between CT and MR scanners that serves to further delay treatment.

BOX 19–10   Key Concept

Perfusion studies are obtained by monitoring the passage of iodinated contrast through the cerebral vasculature.

CT perfusion software that interfaces with helical scanners can meet the clinical needs for evaluation of acute and subacute stroke. Such applications produce a quantitative measure of regional hemodynamics by demonstrating blood flow in each pixel of the cerebral parenchyma that is imaged. The technique is based on the central volume principle, which states that cerebral blood volume can be calculated as the product of the total cerebral blood flow and the time needed for the cerebral blood passage: CBF = CBV/MTT. A workstation equipped with commercially available perfusion software can perform these complex calculations quickly. The goal in performing perfusion studies for patients with acute stroke is to distinguish infarcted tissue from the penumbra.

Technical Factors

The most common technique associated with CT perfusion scanning is based on the first pass of a contrast bolus through the brain tissue. With this technique a 50-mL IV bolus of a nonionic low osmolality contrast is injected at 4 to 5 mL/s. A helical scanner is used to produce a dynamic set of images at a single location. A 5-second scan delay is used; slices are typically 5 mm thick. Typical scan durations are in the range of 40 to 45 seconds.

The slices are produced by repeatedly scanning the same region at the same table position, a technique some manufacturers refer to as the cine mode. Multislice scanners allow several z position slices to be scanned simultaneously. Scans are typically acquired at 5-mm sections to lessen beam-hardening artifacts, and then reformatted into 10-mm-thick sections for viewing to improve the signal-to-noise ratio.

The brain perfusion protocol begins with an unenhanced scan of the whole brain. Although the level for scanning the enhanced portion of the study may be selected at the time of examination based on the unenhanced CT findings, a transverse slice through the level of the basal ganglia (Fig. 19-5) contains territories supplied by the anterior, middle, and posterior cerebral arteries, thus offering the opportunity to interrogate each of the major vascular regions.

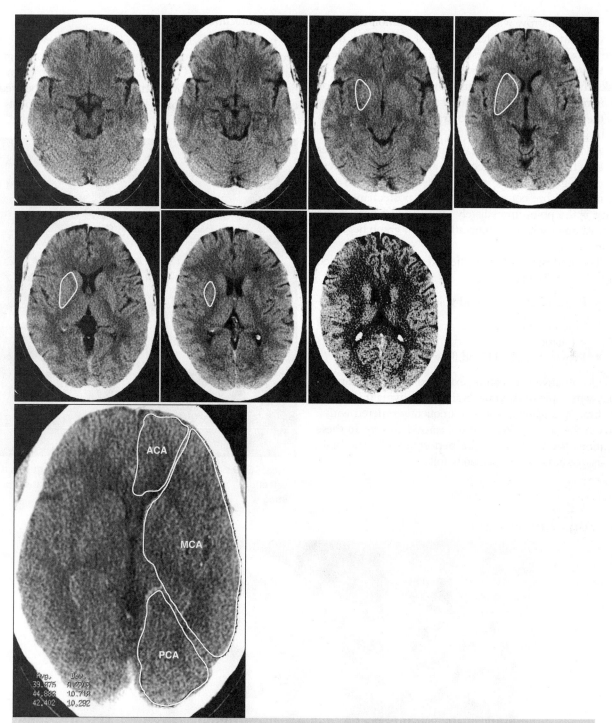

FIGURE 19-5 The level of the basal ganglia contains territories supplied by the anterior (ACA), middle (MCA), and posterior cerebral arteries (PCA). Therefore, this is the level most frequently scanned for brain perfusion studies. The outlined areas on the upper two rows of images are the basal ganglia. Images courtesy of the University of Michigan Health System.

A major limiting factor of older helical scanners was the 10- to 20-mm maximum anatomic coverage. Often a second bolus of contrast was necessary so that the patient could be scanned at a different location, typically in a more cephalad direction above the lateral ventricles. However, as scanners with expanded multidetector arrays have become more prevalent, this is no longer an issue. For

example, a 64-slice scanner will allow 40 mm of anatomic coverage for the perfusion study.

The first step in postprocessing the acquired images using the perfusion software is to select a reference artery and a reference vein. The reference artery should be 1) seen in cross-section, 2) one of the first to enhance, 3) produce a curve with a high enhancement peak, or 4) produce a curve with a narrow width. The most common choice of reference artery is the anterior cerebral artery. The reference vein should be the largest venous structure available or one that produces an enhancement curve with the highest peak. The superior sagittal sinus is the vein most often used as the reference. An ROI is placed on the reference artery and the reference vein so that contrast-enhancement curves can be generated.

Analysis of the contrast enhancement curves guides the selection of preenhancement and postenhancement images (Fig. 19-6). The preenhancement image is that last image before contrast arrives. The postenhancement image is the point immediately after the first pass of the contrast bolus when the time-attenuation graph begins to flatten.

The perfusion software then generates color-coded maps demonstrating:

- Regional cerebral blood volume, or rCBV

- Blood mean transit time, or MTT, through cerebral capillaries
- Regional cerebral blood flow or rCBR

Quantitative data can be extracted from the maps by placing multiple ROIs in the brain parenchyma (Fig. 19-7).

Brain perfusion studies are frequently ordered with a CTA of the circle of Willis or the carotid arteries. In these situations the CTA should be performed first; the brain perfusion study can immediately follow.

Clinical Indications

CT perfusion is most frequently ordered in the evaluation of acute stroke. It is also ordered for vasospasm and tumor grading. In addition, the CT perfusion technique can be modified to determine cerebrovascular reserve and can be used in conjunction with temporary balloon occlusion protocols.

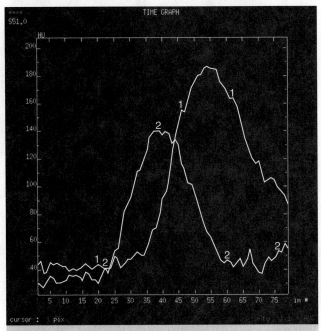

FIGURE 19-6 The contrast enhancement curves guides the selection of preenhancement and postenhancement images.

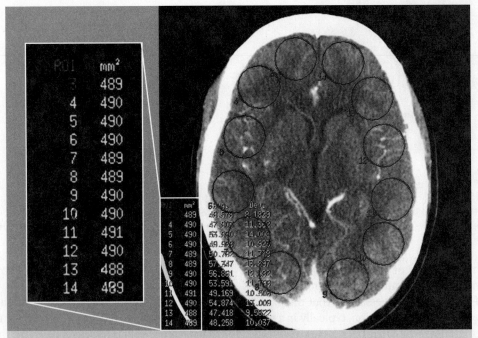

FIGURE 19-7 Quantitative data can be extracted from the maps by placing multiple ROIs in the brain parenchyma.

BOX 19-11   Key Concept

CT perfusion is most frequently ordered in the evaluation of acute stroke, but is also ordered for vasospasm or tumor grading. With some modification CT perfusion can also be used to determine cerebrovascular reserve during temporary balloon occlusion protocols.

CT Perfusion to Determine Cerebrovascular Reserve   CT brain perfusion studies can be used to evaluate patients with chronic cerebral ischemia related to underlying vascular stenosis.[15] In these situations, CT perfusion is used to determine cerebrovascular reserve capacity (CVRC). CVRC describes how far cerebral perfusion can increase from a baseline value after undergoing stimulation. It is essentially a "stress test" for the brain. Stimulation is provided through the intravenous administration of a drug such as acetazolamide (Diamox; Wyeth, Marietta, PA).

To evaluate CVRC a routine perfusion CT is performed. The patient is then given the acetazolamide, and the perfusion CT is repeated 20 minutes later with a second contrast injection. Pre and post acetazolamide scans should be acquired at the same anatomic level. ROIs on the resulting perfusion color maps should be placed in the same positions on pre and post acetazolamide scans. An allergy to sulfa drugs is a contraindication for acetazolamide. Acetazolamide is associated with certain side effects (e.g., weakness, numbness, bronchospasm); therefore, the patient should be monitored for at least 30 minutes after its administration.

CT Perfusion in Conjunction With Temporary Balloon Occlusion   Balloon occlusion is a treatment option for some patients with aneurysm or intracranial or head and neck tumors. Before permanent occlusion is performed a temporary test occlusion is performed in the angiography suite to determine whether the patient can tolerate permanent occlusion. However, some patients who pass the temporary balloon occlusion test may still not tolerate permanent occlusion.[16] Performing perfusion CT in conjunction with the temporary balloon occlusion test can help to identify these patients. The procedure is summarized as follows:

1. Patient undergoes angiography and balloon occlusion. Patients who pass the clinical portion of the examination are brought to the CT suite with the balloon in place.
2. A routine unenhanced head CT is performed.
3. The balloon is inflated by the neurointerventionalist and perfusion CT is performed.
4. The balloon is deflated and perfusion CT is repeated with a second contrast injection.

Summary

Dynamic perfusion CT imaging is a fast and effective means of determining cerebral perfusion. Combined with unenhanced CT and CT angiography, it provides a means for prompt assessment of vascular anatomy and regional hemodynamics. CT perfusion is a valuable tool in the assessment of patients with acute stroke but can also be used for other cerebrovascular disease.

CHAPTER SUMMARY

CT is instrumental in the diagnosis of neurologic abnormality or the evaluation of injury to the head, sinuses, temporal bone, neck, and spine. The introduction of multislice CT realized the advantages of wider scanning range, shorter scanning time, and finer z axis resolution, all useful factors in neuroradiologic diagnosis. CT is the primary imaging modality for emergent indications such as trauma and acute changes in neurologic status, including ischemia and intracranial hemorrhage. CTA has become an attractive alternative to digital subtraction angiography for rapid evaluation of the cervical and cerebral vasculature. CT also provides an accurate display of the anatomy and pathology of the spine. The value of CT with intrathecal contrast medium injection is well accepted, and the use of CT as a supplemental study after routine fluoroscopic myelography is widely used in spine evaluation.

REVIEW QUESTIONS

1. When performing a CT study of the brain, what effect will moving the patient's chin up or down have?
2. Describe how a patient can be positioned so that data can be acquired of the head in the coronal plane.
3. Describe the appearance of intracranial hemorrhage on the CT image.
4. Why might the split bolus method of contrast administration be used for CT studies of the neck? Describe the technique.
5. CT scans of the spine are often performed after a myelogram. What special considerations must be given for the intrathecal contrast material?
6. Explain why CT plays such a crucial role in the assessment and treatment of acute stroke.
7. What information do CT brain perfusion scans provide that is not available on unenhanced CT of the brain?

REFERENCES

1. von Kummer R. Imaging the cerebral parenchyma in ischemic stroke. In: Latchaw RE, Kucharczyk J, Moseeley ME, eds. Imaging of the Nervous System: Diagnostic and Therapeutic Applications. Philadelphia: Elsevier Mosby, 2005:199.
2. Taber KH, Hayman LA, Diaz-Marchan PJ, Rauch RA. Imaging intracranial hemorrhage and its etiologies. In: Latchaw RE, Kucharczyk J, Moseeley ME, eds. Imaging of the Nervous System: Diagnostic and Therapeutic Applications. Philadelphia: Elsevier Mosby, 2005:560–4.
3. Tanenbaum LN. Impact of computed tomography advances on clinical neuroimaging. In: Latchaw RE, Kucharczyk J

J, Moseeley ME, eds. Imaging of the Nervous System: Diagnostic and Therapeutic Applications. Philadelphia: Elsevier Mosby, 2005:40.

4. Gandhi D. Computed tomography and magnetic resonance angiography in cervicocranial vascular disease. J Neuroophthalmol 2004;24:306–14.

5. American Heart Association. 2008 Heart and Stroke Statistical Update. Dallas: American Heart Association, 2008. Available at: http://www.americanheart.org/presenter. jhtml?identifier=1200026. Accessed September 5, 2008.

6. The NINDS t-PA Stroke Study Group. Generalized efficacy of t-PA for acute stroke. Subgroup analysis of the NINDS t-PA Stroke Trial. Stroke 1997;28:2119–25.

7. Goetz CG, Pappert EJ. Textbook of Clinical Neurology. 1st Ed. Philadelphia: WB Saunders, 1999:373, 917.

8. Millikan CH, McDowell FH. Treatment of progressing stroke. Stroke 1981;12:397–409.

9. Nygard O, Nordrehaug JE, Refsum H, Ueland PM, Farstad M, Vollset SE. Plasma homocysteine levels and mortality in patients with coronary artery disease. N Engl J Med 1997;337:230–6.

10. Graham IM, Daly LE, Refsum HM, et al. Plasma homocysteine as a risk factor for vascular disease. The European Concerted Action Project. JAMA 1997;277:1775–81.

11. Etminan M, Takkouche B, Isorna FC, Samji A. Risk of ischaemic stroke in people with migraine: systematic review and meta-analysis of observational studies. BMJ 2005;330:63.

12. Reynolds K, Lewis B, Nolen JD, Kinney GL, Sathya B, He J. Alcohol consumption and risk of stroke: a meta-analysis. JAMA 2003;289:579–88.

13. Meadows M. Brain Attack: a look at stroke prevention and treatment. FDA Consumer Magazine. March–April 2005. Available at http://www.fda.gov/fdac/features/2005/205_ stroke.html. Accessed May 2008.

14. Marler JR, Jones PW, Emr E, eds. Setting new directions for stroke care: proceedings of a national symposium on rapid identification and treatment of acute stroke. Circulation 2005; 112(Suppl):IV-111–20.

15. Hoeffner EG, Case I, Jain R, et al. Cerebral perfusion CT: technique and clinical applications. Radiology 2004;231: 632–44.

16. Mathis JM, Barr JD, Jungreis CA, et al. Temporary balloon occlusion of the internal carotid artery: experience in 500 cases. AJNR Am J Neuroradiol 1995;16:749–54.

NEUROLOGIC PROTOCOLS

Head
Examples of clinical indications: Without contrast: intracranial hemorrhage, early infarction, dementia, hydrocephalus, cerebral trauma
Without and with contrast: Mass, lesion, arteriovenous malformation, metastasis, aneurysm, for symptoms of headache, seizure
Scouts: AP and lateral
Scan type: Axial
Scan plane: Transverse
Start location: Just below skull base
End location: Just above vertex
IV contrast: (if contrast is ordered) 100 mL at 1.0 mL/s. Scan delay = 5 minutes
Oral contrast: None
Reference angle: Angle gantry parallel to supraorbital meatal line (avoid lens of eyes)
DFOV: ~23 cm
SFOV: Head
Algorithm: Standard
Window settings: 140 ww/40 wl posterior fossa; 90 ww/35 wl vertex

	16-Detector Protocol	64-Detector Protocol
Gantry rotation time	2.0 s	1.0 s
Acquisition (detector width × number of detector rows = coverage)	0.625 mm × 16 = 10 mm	0.625 mm × 32 = 20 mm
Reconstruction (slice thickness/interval)	5.0 mm/5 mm (2 images per rotation)	5.0 mm/5 mm (4 images per rotation)
kVp/mA (posterior fossa)	140/150	140/330
kVp/mA (vertex)	120/150	120/330

Reconstruction 2:		
Algorithm: Bone		
Window setting: 4000 ww/400 wl		
DFOV: ~23		
Slice thickness/interval	2.5 mm/2.5 mm	2.5 mm/2.5 mm

Skull Base (Posterior Fossa)
Examples of clinical indications: Posterior fossa and brainstem tumors, hemorrhages, AVM, dural sinus, thrombosis
Scouts: AP and lateral
Scan type: Axial
Scan plane: Transverse (coronal images may also be of benefit)
Start location: Foramen magnum
End location: Through petrous ridges
IV contrast: (if contrast is ordered) 100 mL at 1.0 mL/s. Scan delay = when all contrast is administered
Oral contrast: None
Reference angle: Angle gantry parallel to infraorbital meatal line
DFOV: ~23 cm
SFOV: Head

(Continued)

Skull Base (Posterior Fossa) *(Continued)*		
Algorithm: Standard		
Window settings: 140 ww/40 wl		
	16-Detector Protocol	64-Detector Protocol
Gantry rotation time	2.0 s	1.0 s
Acquisition (detector width × number of detector rows = coverage)	0.625 mm × 16 = 10 mm	0.625 mm × 32 = 20 mm
Reconstruction (slice thickness/interval)	1.25 mm/1.25 mm (8 images per rotation)	1.25 mm/1.25 mm (16 images per rotation)
kVp/mA	140/170	140/340
Reconstruction 2:		
Algorithm: Bone		
DFOV: 18–20		
Window settings: 4000 ww/400 wl		
Slice thickness/interval	1.25 mm/1.25 mm	1.25 mm/1.25 mm

Temporal Bones		
Examples of clinical indications: Without contrast: cholesteatoma, inflammatory disease, fractures, evaluate implants With contrast: IAC tumor, hearing loss, acoustic neuroma, Schwannoma		
GROUP 1.		
Scouts: AP and lateral		
Scan type: Axial		
Scan plane: Transverse		
Start location: Just below the mastoid process		
End location: Just above petrous ridge (include entire mastoid, internal auditory canal, and external auditory canal)		
IV contrast: (if contrast is ordered) 100 mL at 1.0 mL/s. Scan delay = when all contrast is administered		
Oral contrast: None		
Reference angle: Angle gantry parallel to infraorbital meatal line (be sure patient's head is straight and not rotated in the head holder)		
DFOV: ~9.6 cm (center RAS coordinates for right side ~R35)		
SFOV: Head		
Algorithm: Bone		
Window settings: 4000 ww/ 400 wl		
	16-Detector Protocol	64-Detector Protocol
Gantry rotation time	1.0 s	1.0 s
Acquisition (detector width × number of detector rows = coverage)	0.625 mm × 16 = 10 mm	0.625 mm × 32 = 20 mm
Reconstruction (slice thickness/interval)	0.625 mm/0.625 mm (16 images per rotation)	0.625 mm/0.625 mm (32 images per rotation)
kVp/mA	140/170	140/170
Reconstruction 2:		
Algorithm: Bone		
Window setting: 4000 ww/400 wl		
DFOV: ~9.6 cm (center RAS coordinates for right side ~L35)		
Slice thickness	0.625 mm/0.625 mm	0.625 mm/0.625 mm

Reconstruction 3:		
Algorithm: Standard		
Window setting: 140 ww/40 wl		
DFOV: ~18 (include both sides)		
Slice thickness	2.5 mm/2.5 mm	2.5 mm/2.5 mm

GROUP 2.		
Scout: Lateral		
Scan type: Axial		
Scan plane: Coronal		
Start location: Just anterior to the temporomandibular joint		
End location: Just posterior to the mastoid (include entire mastoid, internal auditory canal, and external auditory canal)		
Reference angle: Angle gantry perpendicular to the infraorbital meatal line		
DFOV: ~9.6 cm (center RAS coordinates for right side ~R35)		
SFOV: Head		
Algorithm: Bone		
Window settings: 4000 ww/400 wl		
	16-Detector Protocol	64-Detector Protocol
Gantry rotation time	1.0 s	1.0 s
Acquisition (detector width × number of detector rows) = coverage	0.625 mm × 16 = 10 mm	0.625 mm × 32 = 20 mm
Reconstruction (slice thickness/interval)	1.25 mm/1.25 mm (8 images per rotation)	1.25 mm/1.25 mm (16 images per rotation)
kVp/mA	140/200	140/200

Reconstruction 2:		
Algorithm: Bone		
Window setting: 4000 ww/400 wl		
DFOV: 9.6 cm (center RAS coordinates for left side ~L35)		
Slice thickness/interval	1.25 mm/1.25 mm	1.25 mm/1.25 mm

Sinus Screen
Sinus screening is intended as an inexpensive, accurate, and low radiation dose method for confirming the presence of inflammatory sinonasal disease. If confirmed and the patient will then have endoscopic sinus surgery, the coronal images provide a "road map" for the surgeon.
Examples of clinical indications: Recurrent or chronic sinusitis
Scout: Lateral
Scan type: Axial
Scan plane: Coronal
Start location: Mid sella
End location: Through frontal sinus
IV contrast: None
Oral contrast: None
Reference angle: Angle gantry perpendicular to the orbital meatal line
DFOV: 16 cm

(Continued)

Sinus Screen *(Continued)*		
SFOV: Head		
Algorithm: Standard		
Window settings: 350 ww/50 wl		
	16-Detector Protocol	64-Detector Protocol
Scan Type	Helical	Axial
Gantry rotation time	1.0 s	1.0 s
Acquisition (detector width × number of detector rows) = coverage	0.625 mm × 16 = 10 mm	0.625 mm × 32 = 20 mm
Reconstruction (slice thickness/interval)	2.5 mm/2.5 mm (4 images per rotation)	2.5 mm/2.5 mm (8 images per rotation)
kVp/mA	120/150	120/150
Reconstruction 2:		
Algorithm: Bone		
Window setting: 4000 ww/400 wl		
DFOV: ~23		
Slice thickness/interval	2.5 mm/2.5 mm	2.5 mm/2.5 mm

Trauma Facial Bones		
Examples of clinical indications: Characterization of facial fractures and soft tissue injury		
Scouts: AP and lateral		
Scan type: Helical		
Scan plane: Transverse		
Start location: Just below mandible		
End location: Just above frontal sinus		
IV contrast: None		
Oral contrast: None		
Reference angle: Angle gantry parallel to infraorbital meatal line		
DFOV: 18 cm		
SFOV: Head		
Algorithm: Standard		
Window settings: 350 ww/50 wl		
	16-Detector Protocol	64-Detector Protocol
Gantry rotation time	0.8 s	0.8 s
Acquisition (detector width × number of detector rows = coverage	0.625 mm × 16 = 10 mm	0.625 mm × 32 = 20 mm
Reconstruction (slice thickness/interval)	1.25 mm/0.625	1.25 mm/0.625
Pitch	0.562	0.531
kVp/mA	120/250	140/250
Reconstruction 2:		
Algorithm: Bone		
Window setting: 4000 ww/400 wl		
DFOV: 18		
Slice thickness/interval	1.25 mm/0.625 mm	1.25 mm/0.625 mm

Reformations:
Coronal reformations using both standard and bone algorithm image data
Window setting: 140 ww/40 wl (standard algorithm); 4000 ww/400 wl (bone algorithm)
DFOV: ~18
Thickness/spacing: 1.2 mm/0.6 mm

Orbits

Examples of clinical indications: Without contrast: trauma, foreign body
With contrast: intraorbital masses, thyroid ophthalmopathy, inflammation, infection

GROUP 1.

Scouts: AP and lateral

Scan type: Axial

Scan plane: Transverse

Start location: Just below orbital floor

End location: Just above orbital roof

IV contrast (if contrast is ordered): 100 mL at 1.0 mL/s. Split bolus—two 50-mL injections. Two-minute delay between injections; scans initiated once second injection is complete.

Oral contrast: None

Reference angle: Angle gantry parallel to infraorbital meatal line

DFOV: 16 cm

SFOV: Head

Algorithm: Soft

Window settings: 350 ww/50 wl

	16-Detector Protocol	64-Detector Protocol
Gantry rotation time	1.0 s	1.0 s
Acquisition (detector width × number of detector rows) = coverage	0.625 mm × 16 = 10 mm	0.625 mm × 32 = 20 mm
Reconstruction (slice thickness/interval)	2.5 mm/2.5 mm (4 images per rotation)	2.5 mm/2.5 mm (8 images per rotation)
kVp/mA	120/200	120/200

Reconstruction 2:

Algorithm: Bone		
Window setting: 4000 ww/400 wl		
DFOV: 16 cm		
Slice thickness/interval	2.5 mm/2.5 mm	2.5 mm/2.5 mm

GROUP 2.

Scout: Lateral

Scan type: Axial

Scan plane: Coronal

Start location: Mid sphenoid sinus

End location: Anterior frontal sinus

Reference angle: Angle gantry perpendicular to the infraorbital meatal line

DFOV: 16

SFOV: Head

Algorithm: Soft

Window settings: 350 ww/50 wl

(Continued)

Orbits *(Continued)*		
	16-Detector Protocol	64-Detector Protocol
Gantry rotation time	1.0 s	1.0 s
Acquisition (detector width × number of detector rows) = coverage	0.625 mm × 16 = 10 mm	0.625 mm × 32 = 20 mm
Reconstruction (slice thickness/interval)	2.5 mm/2.5 mm (4 images per rotation)	2.5 mm/2.5 mm (8 images per rotation)
kVp/mA	140/200	140/200
Reconstruction 2:		
Algorithm: Bone		
Window setting: 4000 ww/400 wl		
DFOV: 16		
Slice thickness/interval	2.5 mm/2.5 mm	2.5 mm/2.5mm

Sella		
Examples of clinical indications: Pituitary mass, microadenoma, and parasellar masses		
GROUP 1.		
Scouts: AP and lateral		
Scan type: Axial		
Scan plane: Transverse		
Start location: Just below sellar floor		
End location: Through dorsum sellae		
IV contrast: 150 mL at 1.0 mL/s. Scan delay = 75 seconds		
Oral contrast: None		
Reference angle: Angle gantry parallel to infraorbital meatal line		
DFOV: 14 cm		
SFOV: Head		
Algorithm: Soft		
Window settings: 350 ww/50 wl		
	16-Detector Protocol	64-Detector Protocol
Gantry rotation time	2.0 s	1.0 s
Acquisition (detector width × number of detector rows) = coverage	0.625 mm × 16 = 10 mm	0.625 mm × 32 = 20 mm
Reconstruction (slice thickness/interval)	1.25 mm/1.25 (8 images per rotation)	1.25 mm/1.25 mm (16 images per rotation)
kVp/mA	140/140	140/280
Reconstruction 2:		
Algorithm: Bone		
Window setting: 4000 ww/400 wl		
DFOV: 12 cm		
Slice thickness/interval	1.25 mm/1.25 mm	1.25 mm/1.25 mm
GROUP 2.		
Scout: Lateral		
Scan type: Axial		
Scan plane: Coronal		

Start location: Anterior clinoid		
End location: Through dorsum sellae		
Reference angle: Angle gantry perpendicular to the infraorbital meatal line		
DFOV: 12		
SFOV: Head		
Algorithm: soft		
Window settings: 350 ww/50 wl		
	16-Detector Protocol	64-Detector Protocol
Gantry rotation time	2.0 s	1.0 s
Acquisition (detector width × number of detector rows) = coverage	0.625 mm × 16 = 10 mm	0.625 mm × 32 = 20 mm
Reconstruction (slice thickness/interval)	1.25 mm/1.25 mm (8 images per rotation)	1.25 mm/1.25 mm (16 images per rotation)
kVp/mA	140/140	140/280
Reconstruction 2:		
Algorithm: Bone		
Window setting: 4000 ww/400 wl		
DFOV: 12		
Slice thickness/interval	1.25 mm/1.25 mm	1.25 mm/1.25 mm

Brain Perfusion

Examples of clinical indications: Acute stroke, vasospasm, to determine cerebrovascular reserve, in conjunction with temporary balloon occlusion

Group 1. Noncontrast Head Refer to Table 14-2 (If a brain perfusion is ordered with a circle of Willis (CoW), or a CoW/carotid study, scan the CoW or CoW/carotid first, then perform the brain perfusion examination.)		
Group 2. Contrast Scan		
Scan type: Cine (table increment = 0)		
Scan plane: Transverse		
Slice location: Center at the level of the basal ganglia		
IV contrast: 50 mL (370 concentration) at 4.0 mL/s; 20 mL saline flush at 4.0 mL/s. Scan delay = 5 seconds		
Reference angle: Same gantry tilt and RAS coordinates as the noncontrast portion		
DFOV: 25		
SFOV: Head		
Algorithm: Standard		
Window settings: 90 ww/35 wl		
	16-Detector Protocol	64-Detector Protocol
Gantry rotation time	1.0 s	1.0 s
Acquisition (detector width × number of detector rows) = coverage	1.25 mm × 16 = 20 mm	0.625 mm × 64 = 40 mm
Scan time (continuous scanning at the same table position)	50 s	50 s
Reconstruction (slice thickness/interval/rotation) *image reconstructed for each 0.5 s of tube travel	5.0 mm/5.0 mm/0.5 s (8 images per rotation)	5.0 mm/5.0 mm/0.5 s (16 images per rotation)
kVp/mA	80/200	80/200

(Continued)

Brain Perfusion   *(Continued)*

Group 3. 2nd Contrast Scan With Diamox (when ordered)
Diamox is administered by IV injection.   20 minutes after Diamox injection, scan is repeated. All parameters remain the same as group 2, including injection of another 50 mL of 370 concentration iodinated contrast media.
After group 3 scans are complete, patient is escorted to the recovery area, where he or she will be monitored for 30 minutes. Page the neuroradiologist if patient exhibits any unexpected signs or symptoms, especially those indicative of a stroke.

CTA—Circle of Willis
Examples of clinical indications: Locate cerebral aneurysm or AVM in patients with SAH/ICH
Group 1. Noncontrast Head   Refer to Table 14-2
Group 2. Arterial Phase Scan
Scan type: Helical
Scan plane: Transverse
Start location: Just above the frontal sinuses
End location: Just below the skull base
IV contrast: 60 mL (370 concentration) at 4.0 mL/s. 20 mL saline at 4.0 mL/s. Scan delay = from timing bolus (use carotid artery at approximately level of C4 for ROI)
Oral contrast: None
Reference angle: No gantry tilt
DFOV: 25 cm
SFOV: Head
Algorithm: Standard
Window settings: 140 ww/40 wl posterior fossa; 90 ww/35 wl vertex

	16-Detector Protocol	64-Detector Protocol
Gantry rotation time	0.5 s	0.5 s
Acquisition (detector width × number of detector rows) = coverage	1.25 mm × 16 = 20 mm	0.625 mm × 64 = 40 mm
Reconstruction (slice thickness/interval	1.25 mm/0.625	1.25 mm/0.625
Pitch	0.938	0.984
kVp/mA	120/500	120/500

Reformations: Coronal and Sagittal
Window setting: 140 ww/40 wl
DFOV: ~18
Slice thickness/spacing: 2.0 mm/2.0 mm
Render mode: MIP

CTA—Circle of Willis/Carotid
Examples of clinical indications: Acute stroke, carotid atherostenosis, carotid dissections
Group 1. Noncontrast Head   Refer to Table 14-2
Group 2. Arterial Phase Scan
Scan type: Helical
Scan plane: Transverse
Start location: Just below the aortic arch
End location: Just above the frontal sinus

IV contrast: 80 mL (370 concentration) at 4.0 mL/s; 40 mL saline at 4.0 mL/s, Scan delay = from timing bolus (use carotid artery at approximately level of C4 for ROI)		
Oral contrast: None		
Reference angle: No gantry tilt		
DFOV: 25 cm		
SFOV: Large body		
Algorithm: Standard		
Window settings: 250 ww/30 wl—through foramen magnum; 140 ww/40 wl—through base of skull; 90 ww/35 wl—through vertex		
	16-Detector Protocol	64-Detector Protocol
Gantry rotation time	0.5 s	0.5 s
Acquisition (detector width × number of detector rows) = coverage	1.25 mm × 16 = 20 mm	0.625 mm × 64 = 40 mm
Reconstruction (slice thickness/interval)	1.25 mm/0.625 mm	1.25 mm/0.625
Pitch	0.938	0.984
kVp/mA	120/500	120/500
Reconstruction 2: For C-spine evaluation (only needed if history includes trauma)		
Algorithm: Bone		
Window setting: 4000 ww/400 wl		
DFOV: ~13		
Slice thickness/interval	2.5 mm/1.25 mm	2.5 mm/1.25 mm
Reformations: Coronal and Sagittal for both CoW and Carotids		
Window setting: 800 ww/200 wl		
DFOV: ~20		
Slice thickness/spacing: 2.0 mm/2.0 mm		
Render mode: MIP		

CTV—Cranial Venography		
Examples of clinical indications: Evaluation of cerebral venous disorders, dural sinus thrombosis		
Scouts: AP and lateral		
Scan type: Helical		
Scan plane: Transverse		
Start location: Just below the skull base		
End location: Just above the vertex		
IV contrast: 100 mL at 4.0 mL/s. Scan delay = 30 seconds (16-detector)/45 seconds (64-detector)		
Oral contrast: None		
Reference angle: No gantry tilt		
DFOV: 25 cm		
SFOV: Head		
Algorithm: Standard		
Window settings: 350 ww/40 wl		
	16-Detector Protocol	64-Detector Protocol
Gantry rotation time	0.5 s	0.5 s
Acquisition (detector width × number of detector rows) = coverage	0.625 mm × 16 = 10 mm	0.625 mm × 64 = 40 mm

(Continued)

CTV—Cranial Venography *(Continued)*		
Reconstruction (slice thickness/interval)	1.25 mm/0.625 mm	1.25 mm/0.625 mm
Pitch	0.562	0.531
kVp/mA	120/300	120/300
Reconstruction 2:		
Algorithm: Standard		
Window setting: 350 ww/40 wl		
DFOV: 25		
Slice thickness/interval	2.5 mm/1.25 mm	2.5 mm/1.25 mm
Reformations: Coronal and Sagittal		
Window setting: 800 ww/200 wl		
DFOV: 25		
Slice thickness/spacing: 2.0 mm/2.0 mm		
Render mode: MIP		

Neck (Soft Tissue)		
Examples of clinical indications: Neck mass, vascular abnormality		
(If patient has metal dental work, split scan into two groups and angle to reduce artifact)		
Scouts: AP and lateral		
Scan type: Helical		
Scan plane: Transverse		
Start location: Mid orbit		
End location: Clavicular heads		
IV contrast: 125 mL at 1.5 mL/s. Split bolus—1st injection 50 mL, 2-minute delay; 2nd injection 75 mL, scans initiated 25 seconds after the start of the second injection.		
Oral contrast: None		
Reference angle: Angle gantry parallel to hard palate		
DFOV: 18 cm		
SFOV: Large body		
Algorithm: Standard		
Window settings: 350 ww/50 wl		
	16-Detector Protocol	64-Detector Protocol
Gantry rotation time	0.8 s	0.8 s
Acquisition (detector width × number of detector rows) = coverage	0.625 mm × 16 = 10 mm	0.625 mm × 32 = 20 mm
Reconstruction (slice thickness/interval)	2.5 mm /1.25 mm	2.5 mm/1.25 mm
Pitch	0.562	0.531
kVp/auto mA	120/150–800	120/150–800
Reconstruction 2:		
Algorithm: Bone		
Window setting: 4000 ww/400 wl		
DFOV: 18 cm		
Slice thickness/interval	2.5 mm/1.25 mm	2.5 mm/1.25 mm

Reconstruction 3: From just below mandible to clavicular heads		
Algorithm: Bone		
Window setting: 4000 ww/400 wl		
DFOV: 30		
Slice thickness/interval	2.5 mm/1.25 mm	2.5 mm/1.25 mm

Cervical Spine		
Examples of clinical indications: Fracture, dislocation		
Scouts: AP and lateral		
Scan type: Helical		
Scan plane: Transverse		
Start location: Just above skull base		
End location: Mid T1 (include all cervical spine vertebrae, unless a level is specified)		
IV contrast: (only when requested by radiologist) 100 mL at 1.5 mL/s. Scan delay = when injection is complete		
Oral contrast: None		
Reference angle: No gantry tilt		
DFOV: ~13		
SFOV: Large body		
Algorithm: Standard		
Window settings: 350 ww/50 wl		
	16-Detector Protocol	64-Detector Protocol
Gantry rotation time	0.8 s	0.8 s
Acquisition (detector width × number of detector rows) = coverage	0.625 mm × 16 = 10 mm	0.625 mm × 32 = 20 mm
Reconstruction (slice thickness/interval)	2.50 mm/1.25 mm	2.50 mm/1.25 mm
Pitch	0.562	0.531
kVp/auto mA	140/125–325	140/125–325
Reconstruction 2:		
Algorithm: Bone		
Window setting: 4000 ww/400 wl		
DFOV: ~13 cm		
Slice thickness/interval	2.5 mm/1.25 mm	2.5 mm/1.25 mm
Reformations: Coronal and Sagittal		
Algorithm: Bone		
Window setting: 4000 ww/400 wl		
DFOV: Full		
Slice thickness/spacing	2.0 mm/2.0 mm	2.0 mm/2.0 mm
Render mode	Average	Average

Thoracic Spine		
Examples of clinical indications: Fracture, dislocation		
Scouts: AP and lateral		
Scan type: Helical		
Scan plane: Transverse		
Start location: Just above T1		
End location: Just below T12 (include all thoracic spine vertebrae, unless a level is specified)		
IV contrast: (only when requested by radiologist) 100 mL at 1.5 mL/s. Scan delay = when injection is complete		
Oral contrast: None		
Reference angle: No gantry tilt		
DFOV: ~16		
SFOV: Large body		
Algorithm: Standard		
Window settings: 350 ww/50 wl		
	16-Detector Protocol	64-Detector Protocol
Gantry rotation time	0.8 s	0.8 s
Acquisition (detector width × number of detector rows) = coverage	0.625 mm × 16 = 10 mm	0.625 mm × 32 = 20 mm
Slice thickness	2.50 mm/1.25 mm	2.50 mm/1.25 mm
Pitch	0.562	0.531
kVp/auto mA	140/100–350	140/100–350
Reconstruction 2:		
Algorithm: Bone		
Window setting: 4000 ww/400 wl		
DFOV: ~13 cm		
Slice thickness/interval	2.5 mm/1.25 mm	2.5 mm/1.25 mm
Reformations: Coronal and Sagittal		
Algorithm: Bone		
Window setting: 4000 ww/400 wl		
DFOV: Full		
Slice thickness/spacing	2.0 mm/2.0 mm	2.0 mm/2.0 mm
Render mode	Average	Average

Lumbar Spine
Examples of clinical indications: Fracture, dislocation
Scouts: AP and lateral
Scan type: Helical
Scan plane: Transverse
Start location: Just above L1
End location: Just below S1 (unless a level is specified by radiologist)
IV contrast: (only when requested by radiologist) 100 mL at 1.5 mL/s. Scan delay = when injection is complete
Oral contrast: None

Reference angle: No gantry tilt		
DFOV: 14–16		
SFOV: Large body		
Algorithm: Standard		
Window settings: 350 ww/50 wl		
	16-Detector Protocol	64-Detector Protocol
Gantry rotation time	0.8 s	0.8 s
Acquisition (detector width × number of detector rows) = coverage	0.625 mm × 16 = 10 mm	0.625 mm × 32 = 20 mm
Slice thickness	2.50 mm/1.25 mm	2.50 mm/1.25 mm
Pitch	0.562	0.531
kVp/auto mA	140/150–380	140/150–380
Reconstruction 2:		
Algorithm: Bone		
Window setting: 4000 ww/400 wl		
DFOV: ~13 cm		
Slice thickness/interval	2.5 mm/1.25 mm	2.5 mm/1.25 mm
Reformations: Coronal and Sagittal		
Algorithm: Bone		
Window setting: 4000 ww/400 wl		
DFOV: Full		
Slice Thickness/spacing	2.0 mm/2.0 mm	2.0 mm/2.0 mm
Render mode	Average	Average

CTA Spine
Examples of clinical indications: Localization of the shunt of spinal dural arteriovenous fistulas, spinal arteriovenous malformation, blunt trauma (suspected vascular injury)
Scouts: AP and lateral
Scan type: Helical
Scan plane: Transverse
Group 1. Arterial Phase
Start location: Skull base
End location: Sacrum (or levels specified by radiologist)
IV contrast: 120 mL (370 concentration) at 6 mL/s. Scan delay = bolus tracking; place ROI in the aorta just below diaphragm; manually trigger when enhancement value approaches 125 HU
Oral contrast: None
Reference angle: No gantry tilt
DFOV: 20
SFOV: Large body
Algorithm: Standard
Window settings: 350 ww/50 wl

(Continued)

CTA Spine *(Continued)*		
	16-Detector Protocol	64-Detector Protocol
Gantry rotation time	0.5 s	0.4 s
Detector coverage	1.25 mm × 16 = 20 mm	0.625 × 64 mm = 40
Slice thickness	1.25 mm/0.625	1.25 mm/0.625
Pitch	0.938	0.984
kVp/auto mA	140/100–750	140/100–750
GROUP 2. Delayed Scans		
Repeat parameters from group 1. Begin group 2 immediately after 1st group is complete.		
Reformations: Coronal and Sagittal		
Algorithm: Standard		
Window setting: 350 ww/50 wl		
DFOV: Full		
Slice thickness/spacing	2.0 mm/2.0 mm	2.0 mm/2.0 mm
Render mode	Average	Average

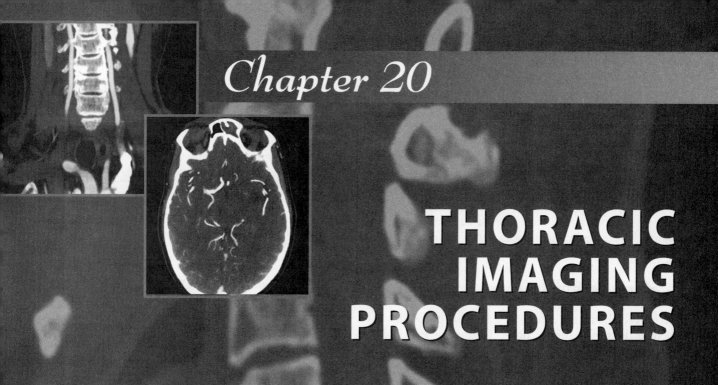

Chapter 20

THORACIC IMAGING PROCEDURES

Key Terms: HRCT • volumetric HRCT • thrombosis • embolism • systemic circulation • pulmonary circulation • CT venography • coronary circulation • atherosclerosis • ischemic heart disease • coronary artery disease • coronary artery bypass graft surgery • balloon angioplasty • coronary stenting • angioplasty • β-blockers • cardiac gating • R-R interval • prospective ECG gating • retrospective ECG gating • ECG-pulsed tube current modulation • calcium score

CT imaging of the chest presents unique challenges because of the continuous motion of the heart and vascular structures. Improvements in temporal and spatial resolution that have been realized as a result of multidetector-row CT (MDCT) have been particularly valuable in thoracic imaging. This technology allows the entire thorax to be scanned with thin sections during a single breath-hold, making consistent high-resolution imaging possible. Electrocardiographic (ECG) synchronization with MDCT is another valuable tool used to reduce cardiovascular motion artifact and improve image quality. Postprocessing techniques, such as three-dimensional (3D) and multiplanar reformations (MPR) can accurately display the pulmonary and coronary vasculature. These new, noninvasive CT imaging techniques can augment, and sometimes replace, the information provided from more invasive tests such as aortography, pulmonary angiography, and coronary angiography. Despite the enormous benefits presented by newer technologies, not all technical and diagnostic problems have been solved. We continue to struggle to find an ideal compromise between image quality, diagnostic accuracy, and patient radiation dose.

GENERAL THORACIC SCANNING METHODS

Most thoracic protocols are performed while the patient lies in a supine position on the scan table with the arms elevated above the head. In a few instances, primarily high-resolution CT protocols of the lungs, additional scans are obtained with the patient in the prone position. Using the shortest scan time possible helps to reduce artifacts created by respiratory motion. Whenever possible, scans of the chest should be acquired within a single breath-hold, as this will prevent misregistration that may be caused by uneven patient breathing between scans.

The thorax has the highest intrinsic natural contrast of any body part. The pulmonary vessels and ribs have significantly different attenuation values compared with the adjacent aerated lung. In most adults, the mediastinal vessels and lymph nodes are surrounded by enough fat to be easily identified. Because of this intrinsic natural contrast, intravenous (IV) iodinated contrast administration is not necessary for all thoracic indications. For example, scans done for the screening, detection, or exclusion of pulmonary nodules or primary lung diseases such as emphysema or fibrosis are typically done without

IV contrast administration. The use of IV contrast material is typically requested by the radiologist to differentiate vascular from nonvascular structures, particularly lymph nodes, to evaluate cardiovascular structures by seeing the inside of these structures, and to further characterize lesions by observing their pattern of enhancement.

The demarcation of the esophagus and the gastroesophageal junction can be improved by giving the patient an oral contrast agent, most often a barium suspension, shortly before beginning the scan, but is not necessary for most thoracic CT examinations.

CT OF THE AIRWAYS

Technical parameters used for CT imaging of the airways include the use of thin sections (1.25 mm or less), a fast acquisition that allows the entire lungs to be scanned during a single breath-hold, optimal spatial resolution, and the use of postprocessing techniques. Overlapping *z* axis image reconstruction of 50% is typical. Neither IV nor oral contrast media are routinely required; IV contrast may be used in cases of airway tumors.

BOX 20-1   Key Concept

Airway imaging is routinely performed at both inspiration and expiration.

Airway imaging is routinely performed at both inspiration and expiration. CT is generally accepted as the best imaging technique for assessment of disease of the central airways[1] and is most commonly used to look for narrowing that may occur in patients who have been intubated in the past. Applying postprocessing techniques, such as volume rendering, may be referred to as CT bronchography. Virtual bronchoscopy is accomplished with similar postprocessing techniques, but is different in that it offers an internal rendering of the tracheobronchial walls and lumen (see Chapter 8).

HIGH-RESOLUTION CT

High-resolution CT (HRCT) is used to evaluate the lung parenchyma in patients with known or suspected diffuse lung diseases such as fibrosis and emphysema. Like airway imaging, HRCT protocols use thin sections (1.5 mm or less), a fast acquisition to reduce motion artifact, and optimal spatial resolution. In addition to the thin sections, spatial resolution is optimized by the selection of an edge-enhancing algorithm (such as a bone algorithm) and a display field of view (DFOV) that is just large enough to include the lungs (Chapter 6). In some institutions, HRCT protocols are incremental, meaning images are obtained with an interval of 10 mm or more between slices and only approximately 10% of the lung parenchyma is scanned. This technique is intended to provide representative areas of lung disease. However, because evidence of some types of diffuse lung disease may not be uniform in distribution throughout the lung, this method of sampling may result in characteristic foci of the disease not being imaged.

BOX 20-2   Key Concept

HR CT of the chest is used for the assessment of lung parenchyma in patients with diffuse lung disease such as fibrosis and emphysema.

More recently, as MDCT scanners have become commonplace, the technique known as volumetric HRCT is replacing the HRCT axial protocols. Volumetric HRCT protocols use a helical mode to acquire images of the entire lung, rather than representative slices. Because these helical protocols cover the entire lung, they result in a more complete assessment of the lung. Lung nodules that could be missed between slices in incremental protocols are not missed with volumetric HRCT, and the central airways can be evaluated at the same time. In addition, they allow postprocessing techniques such as maximum (MIP) and minimum (MinIP) intensity projection reformation. Although there are clear advantages to the use of volumetric HRCT over an interspaced technique, the increased radiation exposure is a consideration. Many volumetric HRCT protocols decrease the tube current (mA) to reduce the radiation dose.[2]

BOX 20-3   Key Concept

Some HRCT protocols are designed so that only a representative 10% of the lung parenchyma is scanned. Other protocols, called volumetric HRCT, use a helical mode to acquire images of the entire lung.

Many HRCT protocols (both volumetric and axial) include more than one series of scans. In all patients there is a gradual increase in attenuation and vessel size from anterior to posterior lung regions owing to the effect of gravity on blood flow and gas volume. In addition, there can be atelectasis in the most dependent lung (i.e., the side touching the CT table) that can mimic or hide lung disease. An additional series of prone images can help to differentiate actual disease from what is not. Expiratory scans are used to look for areas of the lung that do not empty or get smaller, which indicates small airway disease. When the lungs are fully expanded the contrast between low-attenuation aerated air space and high-attenuation lung structure is maximized.[3] Therefore, HRCT protocols are routinely obtained at full inspiration. However, expiratory images are useful in many instances. For example, expiratory images better depict bronchiolitis and air trapping. The density gradient from the effects of gravity is more pronounced on expiratory images. For these reasons, HRCT protocols may include three series of scans: inspiratory supine, expiratory supine, and inspiratory prone. In volumetric protocols, only the inspiratory supine series is done in a helical mode. The additional images are done in the representative axial fashion to reduce the radiation exposure.

BOX 20–4   Key Concept

For HRCT studies prone images can help to differentiate actual disease from densities owing to the effects of gravity that mimic disease.

THORACIC CTA

The MDCT advantages of high temporal and spatial resolution are particularly well suited to accurately image the heart and thoracic vessels, and have resulted in many new scanning protocols. The following discussion of the use of MDCT in the diagnosis of pulmonary embolism explores many of the issues that must be addressed in CT angiography (CTA) examinations of the thorax. However, the detection of pulmonary embolism is just one of many indications for chest CTA.

CTA of Pulmonary Embolism

MDCT angiography has become an imaging mainstay in the diagnosis of pulmonary embolism (PE). MDCT scanners have energized this trend with improved image quality, thinner slices to promote enhanced postprocessing reconstruction, superb CT angiographic capability, and more rapid imaging to assist in scanning the dyspneic patient. CT pulmonary angiography is considered by many to be better than traditional catheter or invasive pulmonary angiography, which is limited in the number of projections and suffers from vessel overlap.

To assist the technologist in understanding the role of CT in the diagnosis of PE we start with a review of the basic medical terminology and anatomy relating to the pulmonary circulation. We then look briefly at the strengths and limitations of other common diagnostic options. Finally, we examine the specific parameters that make up a PE protocol.

Anatomy and Terminology Review

The formation, development, or existence of a clot within the vascular system is referred to as thrombosis. When thrombosis occurs during hemorrhage it may be a life-saving process. However, thrombosis can be life threatening when it occurs at other times. The danger is that the thrombus can occlude a vessel and stop the blood supply to an organ. If the thrombus detaches from its original site, it is referred to as an embolus. In addition to clotted blood, an embolus can be formed (albeit much less commonly) from fat, air, or tumor tissue.

The embolus is carried through the bloodstream and can ultimately occlude a vessel at a distance from its origin. For example, a thrombus that originated in a patient's leg veins after a hip fracture and long convalescence may travel up the inferior vena cava, through the right atrium, right ventricle, and pulmonary trunk into a pulmonary artery. There the embolus may partially or completely occlude the artery, resulting in symptoms such as chest pain or shortness of breath. Pulmonary embolism is a life-threatening condition.

Most pulmonary emboli are caused from thrombi originating in the lower extremities known as deep vein thrombosis (DVT). Pulmonary emboli can be caused by clots from the venous circulation, the right side of the heart, tumors that have invaded the circulatory system, or other sources such as amniotic fluid, air, fat, bone marrow, and foreign substances. Pulmonary emboli may arise within the body, or they may gain entrance from external forces, as sometimes occurs after a compound fracture. PE and DVT together are often referred to as venous thromboembolism.

Circulation   As the term circulation suggests, blood flow through vessels is arranged to form a circuit. The circular pattern of blood flow from the left ventricle of the heart through the blood vessels to all parts of the body and back to the right atrium is referred to as the systemic circulation. The left ventricle pumps blood into the ascending aorta. From there it flows into arteries that carry it into the various tissues and organs of the body. Within each structure blood moves from arteries to arterioles to capillaries. Here, the vital two-way exchange of substances occurs between blood and cells. Next, blood flows out of each organ by way of venules and then veins to drain eventually into the inferior or superior vena cava. These two great veins of the body return venous blood to the right atrium to complete the systemic circulation. But the blood has not quite come full circle back to its starting point, the left ventricle. To do this and start on its way again, it must first flow through another circuit, the pulmonary circulation. As depicted in Figure 20-1, venous blood moves from the right atrium to the right ventricle to the pulmonary artery to the lung and capillaries. Here, exchange of gases between blood and air occurs, which involves conversion of venous blood to arterial blood. This oxygenated blood then flows on through lung venules into four pulmonary veins and returns to the left atrium of the heart. From the left atrium it enters the left ventricle to be pumped again through the systemic circulation.

Pulmonary Artery   The pulmonary artery (Fig. 20-2) follows closely the subdivision of the bronchial tree. It arches over the right main bronchus and lies dorsal and slightly lateral to the bronchus. The artery decreases more rapidly in size than the bronchus it accompanies.

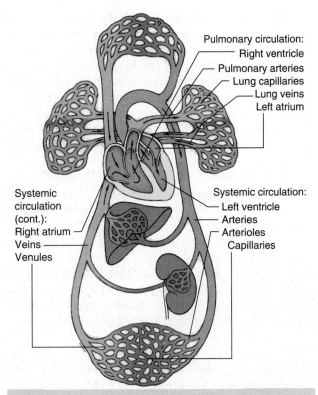

FIGURE 20-1 Relationship of systemic and pulmonary circulation.

By the time it reaches the secondary pulmonary lobule, it is approximately one-fourth to one-eighth the size of the alveolar duct. The pulmonary artery finally ends in a capillary network surrounding the alveolus. The pulmonary veins originate from the capillary network.

BOX 20–5   Key Concept

The pulmonary artery follows closely the subdivision of the bronchial tree, making it easy to identify on a cross-sectional image.

The main pulmonary artery divides into right and left pulmonary arteries. The right pulmonary artery passes under the aortic arch below the tracheal bifurcation and crosses in front of the right bronchus between its upper lobe and lower division branches. It divides into two branches, one going to the upper lobe, and one supplying the middle and lower lobes. Each of the branches of the subdivisions closely follows the corresponding branches of the bronchial tree, with the artery lying along the upper side of the bronchus most of the way. The left pulmonary artery is seen just below the aortic knob as it arches posteriorly into the left lung. The pulmonary artery forms the crescent-shaped shadow of the left hilum above the downward-curving left bronchus. The left pulmonary artery enters the hilum as

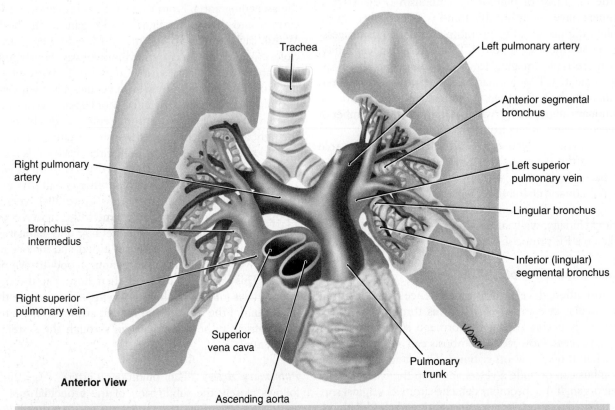

FIGURE 20-2 Relationship of pulmonary arteries, pulmonary veins, and tracheal bronchial tree. (Adapted from Agur AM, Dalley AF, eds. Grant's Atlas of Anatomy. 11th Ed. Philadelphia: Lippincott Williams & Wilkins, 2005;41, Figure 1.34.)

three branches. It then subdivides into upper and lower lobe arteries and then into the nine principal branches, five of which go to the upper lobe and four to the lower lobe following the corresponding bronchial branches.

When viewing the pulmonary artery and its divisions, as well as the adjacent bronchi, it is important to keep in mind some cross-sectional basics. According to the angle at which vessels and bronchi leave the hilum or return to it, CT scans will show them as round, oval, or elongated shapes. Vertical tubular structures will be cut as a round section; those with a gentle slant as oval; and those that lie almost horizontal will appear as long tubular branching structures (Fig. 20-3).

Other Diagnostic Options

PE is a relatively common condition. At least 100,000 cases of PE occur each year in the United States.[4] Untreated, PE is associated with a 30% death rate. It is the third most common cause of death in hospitalized patients. After diagnosis and treatment, the death rate drops dramatically. Compared with PE, DVT is less difficult to diagnose, and alone it very rarely causes death.[5]

Many patients with PE have no signs or symptoms. Others present with only nonspecific signs ranging from mild dyspnea to sudden massive chest pain. In addition, many clinical problems can simulate pulmonary embolism. These range from insignificant heartburn to life-threatening aortic dissection. It is well accepted that clinical judgment alone is unreliable in making the diagnosis of pulmonary embolism.[6-8] The timely and accurate diagnosis of acute PE is crucial to providing appropriate patient care and reducing mortality.

Ventilation-Perfusion Scanning Before the routine use of CTA, the nuclear medicine study ventilation-perfusion scans (or V̇Q scans) was the imaging study of choice in the diagnosis of PE. V̇Q studies do not directly visualize the emboli, but instead look for inequities of perfusion and ventilation. The use of V̇Q scanning in the diagnosis of PE is declining because of the high percentage (up to 73%) of studies performed in which the results are indeterminate.[8]

Pulmonary Angiography

Pulmonary angiography has long been considered the gold standard in the diagnosis of acute PE. However, it has several shortcomings. It is invasive and expensive, and has been associated with a small, but significant, risk of major complications. In addition, it is not universally available.

Using angiography as the gold standard implies it is 100% accurate. A number of researchers have challenged this assumption. Some studies have found that the safety of the examination and the accuracy of interpretation are highly dependent on the experience of the radiologist.[9,10]

Role of D-Dimer

A laboratory test known as D-dimer enzyme-linked immunosorbent assays (ELISA) can play a valuable role in the workup for possible PE. This inexpensive blood test can be used as a screening tool for suspected PE. If D-dimer values are within the normal range, there is a very low likelihood of PE.[11] Unfortunately, an abnormal D-dimer value does not confirm the presence of PE as many other causes may result in elevated D-dimer assays, including cancer, myocardial infarction, pneumonia, sepsis, and pregnancy. Therefore, this test is usually done with the understanding that an elevated value indicates the necessity for further diagnostic tests.

CTA

It is clear that a method less invasive than pulmonary angiography and more specific than V̇Q scanning to assess for thrombus in pulmonary arteries is a welcome advance. Helical CT offers direct visualization of the pulmonary vasculature and, as a substitute for V̇Q or angiography, plays a major role in the detection of both acute and chronic thromboembolic disease.

> **BOX 20-6   Key Concept**
>
> CT venography may be performed after imaging of the arterial system to assess for venous thrombosis within the pelvis and lower extremities.

In addition to imaging the pulmonary arterial system, CT venography (CTV) may be performed to assess for venous thrombosis within the pelvis and lower extremities. This is accomplished by obtaining a second scan series in a delayed venous phase (180 seconds after IV contrast injection) from the iliac crest through the knees. CTV is often able to detect venous thrombosis in the pelvis, which is typically obscured by bowel gas on ultrasonography.[12]

Advantages MDCT technology allows scans to be obtained much faster, allowing images to be obtained while iodinated contrast in the pulmonary arteries is at its peak.

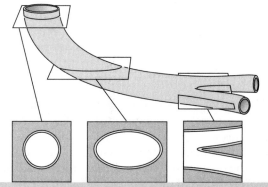

FIGURE 20-3 Hypothetical sloped tube cut at different degrees of inclination resulting in different shapes on cross-section.

A narrow slice can also be used to improve spatial resolution and visualization of small vessels. In addition, because the data are acquired as a volume rather than individual slices, slices can be reconstructed at overlapping intervals to further improve resolution. Another advantage of CT is that it is often helpful in establishing an alternative diagnosis in the absence of demonstrable PE. It can detect other abnormalities that may be contributing to the patient's symptoms such as congestive heart failure, pneumonia, interstitial lung disease, aortic dissection, malignancy, and pleural disease. Finally, using CT in the diagnosis of PE also appears to be cost-effective according to cost analysis of various diagnostic methods including $\dot{V}\dot{Q}$, ultrasonography, D-dimer assay, pulmonary angiography, and helical CT.[13]

Disadvantages MDCT in the diagnosis of PE has some limitations. Although larger emboli can still be diagnosed even in technically limited studies, the visualization of smaller arteries can be affected by problems with technique or suboptimal vessel opacification.

Breathing motion affects the peripheral (subsegmental) and smaller arteries more than the bigger central arteries, although the central and segmental arteries can still usually be evaluated even in studies limited by patient breathing. In most institutions PE scanning is performed in the caudal-to-cranial direction. Respiratory motion, which is greatest at the lung bases, can make interpretation difficult. Patient breathing creates more motion (and therefore artifact) at the diaphragm, but relatively little motion at the lung apices. Therefore, in cases in which the patient is unable to hold his or her breath for the entire scan, it is best to start the scan at the lung bases. Scanning in a caudal-to-cranial direction minimizes respiratory artifact.

BOX 20–7   Key Concept

CTA protocols to detect PE scan in a caudal-to-cranial direction to minimize respiratory artifact

---

Overt patient motion will create artifacts that can greatly degrade image quality. It is unlikely that a diagnostic examination can be produced in a patient unable to lie still for the length of time required to complete the test. Although newer scanners can often complete the arterial phase acquisition in just seconds, the patient must be able to lie still for that short time.

The need for contrast material can limit the use of helical CT. The most common contraindications for evaluating PE with helical CT are contrast material allergy and renal impairment.

As with all CT studies, radiation dose delivered requires careful consideration in developing protocols. For most patients, the risk-to-benefit ratio of using CT for diagnosing PE typically weighs heavily in favor of performing the study.[12] The decision to use CT for young or pregnant women, particularly those at low-to-moderate clinical suspicion, requires even greater scrutiny. During a typical CT pulmonary angiogram, the effective patient dose ranges from 4 to 8 mSv, with an absorbed breast dose of 21 mGy.[14] As a comparison, the absorbed breast dose during a screening mammogram is only 2.5 mGy.[14] However, the doses from CT protocols compare favorably with those of conventional angiography.[15,16] As in all CT examinations, the decision to perform a study on a pregnant patient belongs to the patient's physician in collaboration with the radiologist. The technologist's role is to identify patients who require additional scrutiny and to bring them to the attention of the radiologist.

BOX 20–8   Key Concept

The decision to use CTA for young or pregnant women requires careful scrutiny. The technologists role is to identify these patients and bring them to the attention of the radiologist.

Important Considerations New diagnostic methods are typically associated with a learning curve while staff becomes familiar with new protocols and radiologists become experienced in interpretation. This is certainly the case with using MDCT in the diagnosis of PE.

The most reliable sign of an acute embolus is a low-density filling defect projecting into the vessel lumen, outlined by contrast material (Fig. 20-4). This observation makes the dose, rate, and timing of contrast administration critical to the creation of diagnostic examinations. Because the time to maximal vascular opacification can vary with age, cardiac output, lung disease, and the position of the IV catheter, the quality of the examination is dependent on the experience of the technologist. Care must be taken so that maximal pulmonary vascular opacification coincides with image acquisition. In the hands of a qualified CT technologist knowledgeable in the techniques of bolus tracking and bolus triggering (Chapter 13), these obstacles are certainly surmountable.

BOX 20–9   Key Concept

The dose, rate, and timing of IV contrast administration are critical to the creation of diagnostic CTA examinations. Therefore, the quality of the examination is dependent on the experience of the technologist.

The use of a saline flush after the injection of the iodinated contrast is recommended for CTA pulmonary studies. This will eliminate beam-hardening artifacts from dense contrast media within the superior vena cava that may obscure small emboli in adjacent vessels, particularly in the right main and right upper lobe pulmonary arteries. In patients who are physically larger than average, a slightly wider slice thickness (2.0–2.5 versus 1.25 for small or average size patients) can be used to decrease quantum mottle.

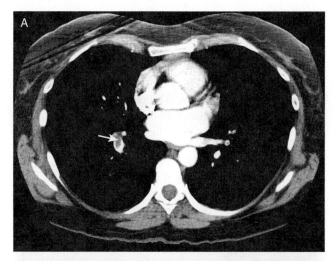

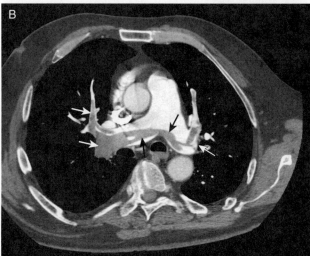

FIGURE 20-4   The most reliable sign of an acute embolus is a low-density filling defect into the vessel lumen, outlined by contrast material (arrow) as in image (A). Image (B) (different patient) shows extensive bilateral pulmonary artery filling defects with saddle embolism and multiple acute emboli extending into the bilateral upper lobe, middle lobe, and bilateral lower lobe pulmonary arteries. Images courtesy of the University of Michigan.

Although ECG gating can be used to reduce cardiac pulsation artifacts, this technique remains controversial when looking for PE because it requires a longer breath-hold and considerably increases radiation exposure.

Conclusion

MDCT is an excellent tool for assessing patients suspected of having PE. Quality examinations are dependent, to a large extent, on the skill and experience of the technologist. This offers excellent motivation for those working in CT to become familiar with PE protocols and the controversies that surround them. During the past decade data have accumulated comparing MDCT pulmonary angiography with other imaging methods. The result is a transition from the gold standard of conventional pulmonary angiography and VQ scanning to MDCT as the modality of choice for excluding PE.

CARDIAC CT

Introduction

For years coronary angiography provided the only method of imaging the coronary arteries. Although coronary angiography is a useful tool, it is invasive and is associated with a small–although not insignificant–risk of complications, including stroke, bleeding severe enough to require transfusion, vascular access complications, myocardial infarction, and even death. In addition, the procedure is associated with significant costs associated with personnel, equipment, and the additional costs related to the recovery time needed after arterial catheter removal, as well as the management of possible adverse events. For these reasons, coronary angiography is typically reserved for patients with serious symptoms and a high likelihood of having significant coronary artery disease, such as chest pain or after a stress test with positive findings. Advances in CT and magnetic resonance imaging technology (MRI) are changing established practices. Cardiac CT has emerged as a less-invasive imaging modality for the diagnosis of coronary artery disease (CAD) and is often used to avoid coronary angiography in low- and intermediate-risk patients, in particular. Continuous improvements in CT detector technology and in temporal (speed) and spatial (thin slices) resolution have resulted in clinical results with cardiac CT that are similar to those obtainable with conventional catheter coronary angiography.

Cardiovascular disease (CVD) is the leading cause of death in the United States, accounting for approximately 37% of deaths in 2003.[17] Coronary artery disease is responsible for the majority of these deaths, but also included are noncoronary cardiac diseases such as congenital heart disease and other forms of acquired heart disease (e.g., valvular disease, cardiomyopathies, tumors, and pericardial processes). Cardiac CT can provide not only anatomic information, but also functional information to aid in the diagnosis and treatment of CVD.

Our discussion of cardiac CT begins by reviewing the basic anatomy and physiology of the heart. The technologist's understanding of the structural anatomy and the path and timing of circulation is essential to the creation of high-quality cardiac CT images. From that foundation, we then consider the various technical aspects essential to performing high-quality cardiac CT examinations. Examples of specific cardiac CT protocols are included in tabular form at the end of this chapter.

Cardiac Anatomy

The cardiovascular system, which includes the heart, performs a vital pickup and delivery service for the body.

Blood cells pick up oxygen and nutrients from the respiratory and digestive systems and deliver them to cells. From the cells, blood picks up metabolic wastes and delivers them to excretory organs. Blood picks up hormones from endocrine glands and delivers them to their target cells. Directly or indirectly, the circulatory system contributes to every function of every cell and every function of the body as a whole.

The human heart is a four-chambered muscular organ with a size and shape roughly equivalent to a person's closed fist. Lying in the mediastinum, approximately two-thirds of its mass is left of midline. The lower border of the heart lies on the diaphragm, pointing toward the left to form a blunt point known as the apex. The upper border of the heart, or base, lies just below the second rib (Fig. 20-5).

Coverings

The heart is enclosed in a loose-fitting, double-layered sac called the pericardium. The outer layer is made of a tough white fibrous tissue known as the parietal layer. The inner, or visceral, layer of the pericardium is composed of a smooth, moist, serous membrane. This visceral layer closely envelops the heart and is also called the epicardium. Between the two layers is the pericardial space, which contains a small amount of fluid that serves to lubricate the constantly rubbing surfaces (Fig. 20-6).

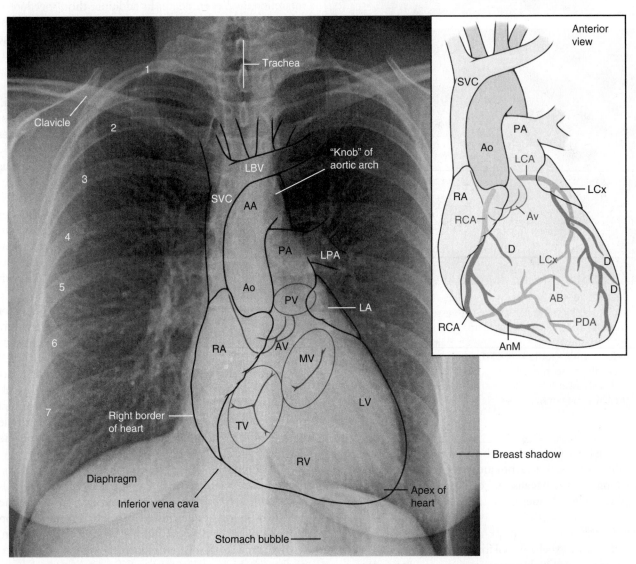

LBV = left brachiocephalic v.	LA = left atrium	PA = pulmonary a.	AV = aortic valve	LCx = left circumflex a.
RA = right atrium	SVC = superior vena cava	TV = tricuspid valve	AB = atrial branch	PDA = posterior descending branch
RV = right ventricle	AA = ascending aorta	MV = mitral valve	AnM = acute marginal branch	D = diagonal branches
LV = left ventricle	Ao = aorta	PV = pulmonary valve	RCA = right coronary a.	

FIGURE 20-5   The location of the heart in the thorax. Approximately two-thirds of the heart lies left of midline. The lower border of the heart lies on the diaphragm, pointing to the left in what is known as the apex. The upper border of the heart is called the base and lies just below the second rib.

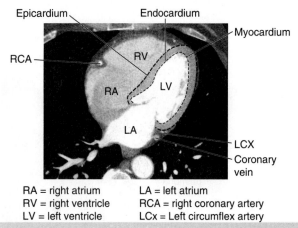

RA = right atrium   LA = left atrium
RV = right ventricle   RCA = right coronary artery
LV = left ventricle   LCx = Left circumflex artery

FIGURE 20-8 The layers of the heart are identified by arrows on the cross-sectional CT slice. Image courtesy of the University of Michigan.

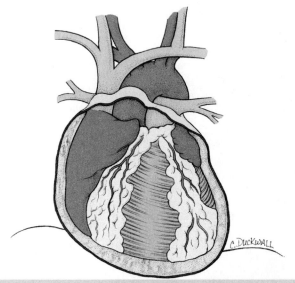

FIGURE 20-6 The heart is enclosed in a loose-fitting, double-layered sac called the pericardium.

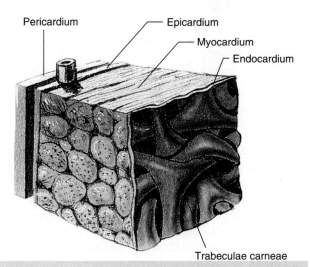

FIGURE 20-7 A section of the heart, enclosed in the pericardial sac. The majority of the heart is muscle, or myocardium. The outer covering is the epidcardium, and the inner lining is the endocardium.

The heart also consists of distinct layers of tissue (Fig. 20-7). The majority of the wall is composed of cardiac muscle, or myocardium. The outer covering of the myocardium is the epicardium (which is the inner section of the pericardium); the inner lining of the myocardium is the endocardium (Fig. 20-8).

Cavities

The interior of the heart is divided into four chambers, two upper and two lower. The upper cavities are called atria; these collect blood as it comes into the heart. The lower cavities are the ventricles, responsible for pumping blood out of the heart (Fig. 20-9). Because of their heavy pumping burden, the ventricles are considerably larger and thicker walled than the atria. Furthermore, the left ventricle has particularly thick walls because of the higher force required to pump blood through all the vessels of the body, except to and from the lungs, whereas the right ventricle sends blood only to the lungs.

Valves and Openings

Heart valves limit the flow of blood to only one direction. They lie at the exit of each of the four heart chambers. When open, the four heart valves ensure that blood flows freely in a forward direction. When closed, the valves prevent blood from flowing backward to its previous location. When heart valves open and close, they make the familiar "lub-DUB" (or "DUP") sound. The first sound is made by the tricuspid and mitral valves (i.e., the atrioventricular valves) closing at the beginning of systole (when the heart contracts and pumps blood out of the heart). The second sound is made by the aortic and pulmonary valves closing at the beginning of diastole (when the heart relaxes and fills with blood).

Each valve either consists of two or three folds of thin tissue (Fig. 20-10). The two atrioventricular valves are the tricuspid and mitral valves. The appropriately named tricuspid valve has three folds and is in the right side of the heart, between the right atrium and the right ventricle. The mitral valve has only two flaps and is therefore also called the bicuspid valve. It is in the left side of the heart, between the left atrium and left ventricle. The pulmonary and aortic valves are semilunar valves, consisting of half-moon–shaped flaps. The pulmonary valve is in the right side of the heart, between the right ventricle and the entrance to the pulmonary artery that carries blood to the lungs. The aortic valve is in the left side of the heart, between the left ventricle and the entrance to the aorta.

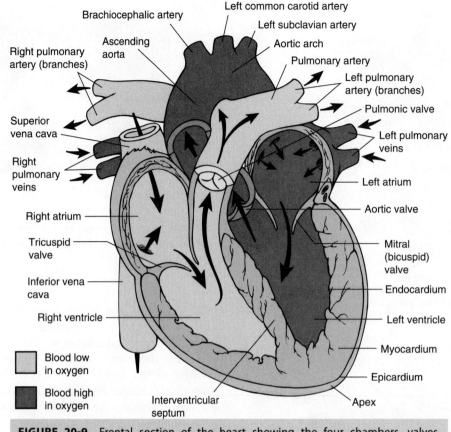

Left common carotid artery
Left subclavian artery
Brachiocephalic artery
Ascending aorta
Aortic arch
Pulmonary artery
Right pulmonary artery (branches)
Left pulmonary artery (branches)
Pulmonic valve
Superior vena cava
Left pulmonary veins
Right pulmonary veins
Left atrium
Right atrium
Aortic valve
Tricuspid valve
Mitral (bicuspid) valve
Inferior vena cava
Endocardium
Right ventricle
Left ventricle
Myocardium
☐ Blood low in oxygen
Epicardium
■ Blood high in oxygen
Interventricular septum
Apex

FIGURE 20-9 Frontal section of the heart showing the four chambers, valves, openings, and major vessels. Arrows indicate the direction of blood flow.

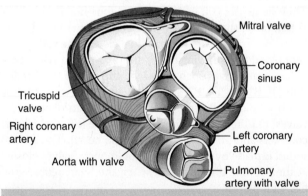

Mitral valve
Coronary sinus
Tricuspid valve
Right coronary artery
Left coronary artery
Aorta with valve
Pulmonary artery with valve

FIGURE 20-10 There are four valves located in the heart. Each valve contains either two or three folds of thin tissue (leaflets). When closed, the valve prevents blood from flowing backward to its previous location. When open, the valve allows blood to flow freely forward.

Circulation

The circuitous route of blood flow through vessels was described earlier in this chapter in the discussion of CT pulmonary angiography. Technologists should remain familiar with the pattern of blood flow that makes up both the systemic circulation and the pulmonary circulation as these play an important role in CTA of the heart.

Coronary Circulation Like all other cells in the body, the myocardial cells that make up the heart tissues must also be supplied with nutrients and oxygen and be freed of waste products. Coronary circulation refers to the movement of blood through the tissues of the heart. Blood is carried to the heart by the two coronary arteries and their branches. Cardiac veins remove deoxygenated blood and waste products.

BOX 20–10   Key Concept

Like all other cells in the body, the myocardial cells that make up the heart tissues must also be supplied with nutrients and oxygen. Coronary circulation refers to the movement of blood through the tissues of the heart.

The major vessels of the coronary circulation are the left main coronary artery (LM), which divides into the left anterior descending (LAD) and circumflex (LCX) branches, and the right coronary artery (RCA). In about 10% of the general population, an artery arises from the LM between the LAD and LCX. This artery is called the ramus intermedius and is considered a normal variant.

The left and right coronary arteries originate at the base (or ascending) portion of the aorta (Fig. 20-11).

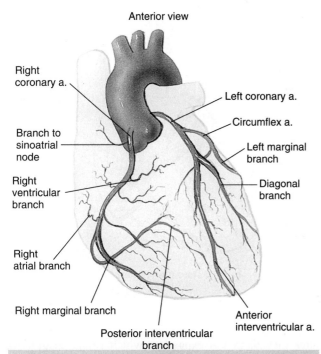

Anterior view

Right coronary a.

Branch to sinoatrial node

Right ventricular branch

Right atrial branch

Right marginal branch

Posterior interventricular branch

Left coronary a.

Circumflex a.

Left marginal branch

Diagonal branch

Anterior interventricular a.

FIGURE 20-11 The heart itself is supplied with blood by the two coronary arteries and their branches.

TABLE 20-1 Branches of the Coronary Arteries

Left coronary artery (LCA)	Right coronary artery (RCA)
Left anterior descending (LAD)	Conus
Septals	Acute marginal
Diagonals	SA nodes
Left circumflex artery (LCX)	AV nodes
Obtuse marginal	Posterior descending artery (PDA)
Marginals	Posterior lateral artery (PLA)
Ramus intermedius	

AV = atrioventricular; SA = sinoatrial.

These major coronary vessels lie on the epicardial surface of the heart and function as distribution vessels. Additional arteries branch off from the major coronary vessels and penetrate the myocardium to supply it with blood. The branches of the coronary arteries are listed in Table 20-1.

Most of the blood supplied by the coronary arteries is returned to the right atrium via the coronary sinus. Branches of the coronary sinus include the great cardiac vein (also called the left coronary vein), middle cardiac vein, and small cardiac vein (Fig. 20-12).

Coronary Artery Grafts and Stents

The buildup of fat and cholesterol plaque is called atherosclerosis. When plaque builds up in the coronary arteries a partial or total blockage results and the heart muscle does not get an adequate blood supply. This is referred to as ischemic heart disease or coronary artery disease (CAD). CAD is one of the leading causes of death in western societies. According to the American Heart Association, CAD is the single leading killer of American men and women.[18]

BOX 20–11 Key Concept

Technologists should be familiar with the basics of coronary artery bypass graft (CABG) surgery because it is a common indication for CT imaging, both in evaluating patients for possible CABG surgery and for assessing graft patency after the surgery is performed.

Coronary artery bypass graft surgery ([CABG], commonly pronounced "cabbage") is typically recommended when there is disease of the left main coronary artery or in three or more vessels, or if nonsurgical management has failed.[19] Technologists should be familiar with the basics of this procedure because it is a common indication for CT imaging, both in evaluating patients for possible CABG surgery and for assessing graft patency after the surgery is performed. Arteries or veins taken from elsewhere in the patient's body are grafted from the aorta to the coronary arteries to bypass atherosclerotic narrowings and improve the blood supply to the coronary circulation supplying the myocardium. The terms "single," "double," "triple," or "quadruple bypass" refer to the number of coronary arteries bypassed in the procedure. The arteries or veins used for the graft can be taken from different areas of the body (Fig. 20-13). The choice is highly surgeon-dependent. A common choice is the left internal mammary artery (LIMA), also referred to as the left internal thoracic artery (LITA), which is grafted to the LAD (Fig. 20-14). Another frequent choice is to use the saphenous vein from the leg (Fig. 20-15). Less frequently used is the radial artery from the forearm or the right internal mammary artery (RIMA), also called the right internal thoracic artery (RITA). Vessels used for grafts are redundant, which means that the body can compensate for their removal. Grafts may occlude in the months to years after bypass surgery is performed. A graft is considered patent (open) if there is flow through the graft without any significant graft stenosis (>70% diameter).

Balloon angiography and coronary stenting are less invasive than is CABG and are options for some patients. Angioplasty is a technique that is used to dilate an area of arterial blockage using a catheter with a small, inflatable, sausage-shaped balloon at its tip. However, angioplasty has some shortcomings. First, the opening created by angioplasty is not very smooth. This is because areas of stenosis are typically made up of both atheroma, which

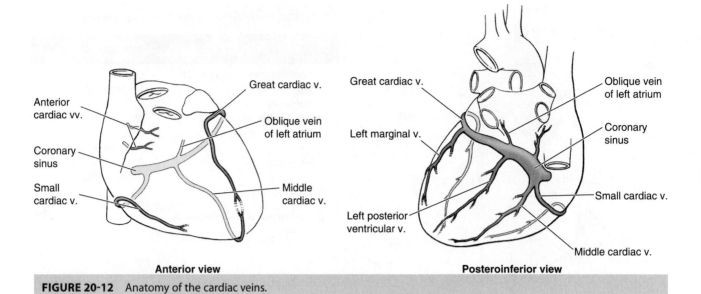

FIGURE 20-12   Anatomy of the cardiac veins.

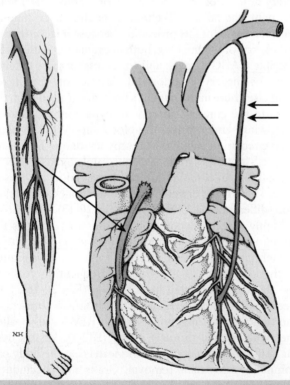

FIGURE 20-13   Common choices of vessels for coronary artery bypass grafting include the saphenous vein of the leg (single arrow), the LIMA from the inside of the chest wall (double arrow), and the radial artery of the forearm (not pictured).

is soft, and plaque, which is hard. The balloon may not be able to evenly expand areas with uneven degrees of hardness. Second, some of the areas compressed by the balloon will bounce back shortly after expansion. In addition, material within the expanded channel can proliferate

after the channel is expanded, which results in gradual restenosis of the vessel.

Coronary artery stents were designed to overcome some of the shortcomings of angioplasty. A common type of stent is made of self-expanding, stainless steel mesh. It is mounted on a balloon catheter in a collapsed form (Fig. 20-16). When the balloon is inflated, the stent expands and pushes against the inner wall of the coronary artery. In many cases, the stent is coated with a pharmacologic agent that is known to interfere with the process of restenosis. These stents are called drug-eluting stents, although they are often referred to as "coated" or "medicated" stents. Compared with angioplasty alone, stents open the disease segment into a rounder, bigger, and smoother opening and reduce the chance of restenosis. However, stents cannot be used in all situations. For instance, stents are difficult to place in arteries that have extreme bends and cannot be used in very small vessels. Like coronary grafts, technologists should recognize coronary stents because they are a common finding on CT images (Fig. 20-17). When doing a CT calcium score (discussed later), stents should be recognized so that they are not included in the images measured, as they will artificially increase the score.

BOX 20–12   Key Concept

Like coronary grafts, technologists should recognize coronary stents because they are a common finding in CT images.

Technique

General-purpose CT protocols can often be used in imaging of abdominal, thoracic, and cerebral vessels in which image quality is not substantially influenced by cardiac

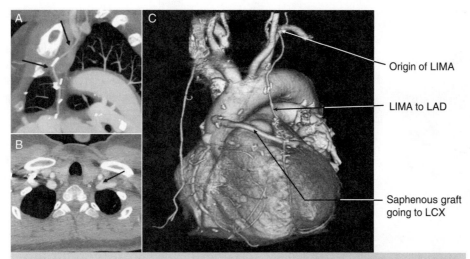

FIGURE 20-14 Image (A) is an axial demonstrating the origin of the LIMA graft from the left subclavian artery to the LAD coronary artery (LAD; arrow). Image (B) is a curved reformatted image of the graft (arrows). Image (C) is a three-dimensional reformation of the same graft. Images courtesy of the University of Michigan. (LCX = left circumflex artery.)

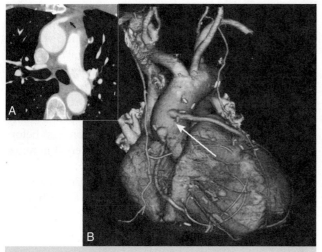

FIGURE 20-15 Image (A) is an axial image demonstrating the origin of the saphenous graft to the left circumflex artery. Image (B) is three-dimensional reformatted image demonstrating the graft. Images courtesy of the University of Michigan.

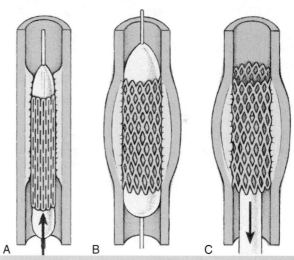

FIGURE 20-16 A common type of coronary stent is made from stainless steel mesh. (A) Balloon catheter positions the stent at the site of arterial stenosis, (B) inflation of the balloon dilates the artery and expands the stent, and (C) the balloon is collapsed and withdrawn, leaving the expanded stent in position.

motion or vessel pulsation. However, for studies of the heart and coronary arteries, dedicated cardiac CT acquisition techniques are needed to produce images free of motion artifact. In addition, care must be taken with the delivery of contrast medium to ensure optimal enhancement of the targeted structure and the surrounding tissues. Visualization of the coronary arteries, a major application of cardiac CT, is difficult because the coronary arteries are of relatively small caliber, are often tortuous in shape, and are subject to constant, often rapid, heart motion.

These challenges can be largely overcome by advances in MDCT technology that have improved both spatial and temporal resolution. Additionally, two other strategies are used to decrease cardiac motion artifacts. First, the patient's heart rate can be temporarily lowered by the administration of β-blockers (pronounced beta-blockers). Second, a technique called cardiac gating attempts to use only those images acquired during periods of lowest cardiac motion.

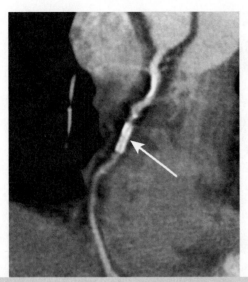

FIGURE 20-17 Visualization of a right coronary artery stent (arrow) on a curved MPR image. Image courtesy of the University of Michigan.

BOX 20–13 Key Concept

To reduce motion artifact on cardiac CTA images a patient's heart rate can be temporarily lowered by the administration of β-blockers.

BOX 20–14 Key Concept

In addition to pharmacologic heart rate control, a technique called cardiac gating attempts to use only those images acquired during periods of the lowest cardiac motion.

Pharmacologic Heart Rate Control

Essentially the CT scanner is a fast camera, but as fast as state-of-the-art scanners are, they cannot take a motion-free picture when the heart is beating too fast. Therefore, many institutions use β-blockers as part of their cardiac CT protocols. β-Blockers are used to lower the heart rate to less than 65 to 70 beats per minute (bpm) and to make the rhythm more regular.[20] Future improvements in scanner technology that further increase temporal resolution (i.e., increased scanner speed) may make the need for β-blockers less important, if not entirely obsolete.

To avoid complications, guidelines should be followed when β-blockers are considered. Protocols can include oral, intravenous (IV), or a combination of oral and IV administration.[20] Although metoprolol tartrate (brand name Lopressor) is probably the most commonly used β-blocker for cardiac CT studies, other options include acebutolol, atenolol, betaxolol, bisoprolol, and esmolol. The effects of an oral dose are seen within 1 hour of administration.

The peak effect of IV-push metoprolol occurs between 5 and 10 minutes after administration.[20] Contraindications are sinus bradycardia, which is defined as a heart rate less than 60 bpm; systolic blood pressure of less than 100 mm Hg; allergy to the medication or its constituents; decompensated cardiac failure; presence of asthma treated with β-agonist inhaler; active bronchospasm; and second- or third-degree atrioventricular block.[20] The decision to give β-blockers and the dosage to be given should be made by a physician and is beyond the scope of the CT technologist. The following administration protocols are provided as a frame of reference only to allow the technologist to better assist the radiologist.

BOX 20–15 Key Concept

The decision to give blockers and the dosage to be given should be made by a physician, nurse practitioner, or physician's assistant.

There is a substantial variation in protocols for β-blocker administration among institutions and in the literature.[20–23] At least one institution recommends that outpatients already on β-blockers double the morning dose on the day of the scan.[21] In this same institution patients receive a prescription for 10 mg of oral metoprolol from the referring physician to be taken 1 hour before the scheduled CT examination. Otherwise, patients are told to arrive 1 hour before the scan, and if their heart rate is more than 65 bpm, they are given 10 mg of metoprolol orally. If the patient's heart rate is more than 65 bpm just before scanning, 5 mg of metoprolol is given IV every 3 minutes, with a maximum of 25 mg.

Thoracic radiologists from the University of Michigan outline the following protocol for β-blocker administration.

1. Once all contraindications have been excluded, beginning 1 hour before scan time, the patient is given one oral dose of 50 mg of metoprolol. The patient is monitored, and the heart rate is checked every 15 minutes. If the heart rate remains greater than 65 bpm or if it is irregular and greater than 60 bpm, further assessment is done to determine whether the patient can be given an IV dose of β-blocker.
2. If further investigation deems the use of an IV β-blocker appropriate, the patient is initially given a 2.5-mg dose of IV metoprolol for 1 minute. If after 5 minutes the heart rate is greater than 65 bpm, a second dose of 2.5 mg of metoprolol is given. If the heart rate continues to remain elevated, up to two additional doses of 5 mg each of metoprolol can be given IV; each dose is given over 1 minute, with a 5-minute interval between doses. The patient's blood pressure and heart rate are checked before each dose is administered. The maximum total dose of metoprolol

given is 15 mg IV, with the sequence being 2.5, 2.5, 5, and 5 mg at 5-minute intervals.

3. After the CT examination, patients who received metoprolol are observed for 30 minutes. If the patient has bronchospasm, two puffs of an albuterol inhaler are given from a 17-gram inhaler canister. If the patient's heart rate drops to less than 45 bpm, the administration of atropine is considered. If the patient does not respond to the atropine and continues to have a low heart rate, resuscitative measures and administration of IV β-agonists such as dopamine or epinephrine may become necessary.

The University of Michigan guidelines are outlined in Table 20-2.

A regular heart rate of less than 65 bpm is particularly important when the structures of interest are small, such as the coronary arteries. When imaging larger cardiac structures, heart rate is less of an issue, although a slower, regular heart rate is still preferred.

Pharmacologic Vasodilatation

Most institutions also give patients nitroglycerin sublingually before coronary CT examinations.[21,22] The intention is to dilate vessels to improve visualization. In addition, nitroglycerin administration may help to prevent coronary spasm that can mimic stenosis on the CT image and therefore be a potential source of misdiagnosis. If used, short-acting nitroglycerin is given immediately before

TABLE 20-2 β-Blocker Administration Protocol[20]

Protocol	Parameter(s)	Action(s)
Assess whether β-blocker is necessary	If pulse is <65 bpm and regular or if pulse is <60 bpm and irregular	A β-blocker is **not** given.
	If pulse is >65 bpm or if pulse is >60 bpm and irregular	Screen for contraindications to giving a β-blocker.
Screen for contraindications to β-blockers	If any of the following conditions exist:	A β-blocker is **not** given.
	Heart rate <60 bpm	
	Systolic blood pressure <100 mm Hg	
	Decompensated cardiac failure	
	Allergy to β-blocker	
	Asthma or COPD with β₂-agonist inhaler use	
	Active bronchospasm	
	Second- or third-degree atrioventricular block	
	If the above conditions are absent	Oral metoprolol is given.
Administer metoprolol	If giving **oral** metoprolol,	One 50-mg dose of metoprolol is given orally, and patient is monitored for 1 hour, during which heart rate is checked every 15 minutes. If heart rate remains elevated, perform practice breath-hold. If heart rate still remains elevated, give IV metoprolol.
	If giving **IV** metoprolol,	Two 2.5-mg doses of metoprolol are given 5 minutes apart; then, two doses of 5 mg each are given 5 minutes apart. Total maximum dose 15 mg. Blood pressure and heart rate are checked before each IV dose.
Administer postprocedure care	If only one dose of oral metoprolol is given	No monitoring is necessary, and the patient can leave the department after study completion.
	If IV metoprolol is given	The patient is observed for 30 minutes.
	If heart rate drops to <45 bpm	Consideration is given to administering atropine.
	If bronchospasm occurs	A β-agonist inhaler is given.

bpm = beats per minute, COPD = chronic obstructive pulmonary disease

scan initiation. As either a spray or a tablet, a dose of 0.3 to 0.4 mg is commonly used.

ECG Gating

To minimize cardiac motion artifact, most cardiac CT protocols use images acquired during the point of the cardiac cycle with the least cardiac motion. Most often this point is during end-diastole, but may also be at end-systole.[24,25] In other words, just before or just after the left ventricle is fully contracted. However, different structures may be most still at slightly different phases of the cardiac cycle. For example, because the right coronary artery is farther from the center of the left ventricle than is the left coronary artery, there is variation between the two.[26] In addition, the precise point of minimal motion is patient- and heart-rate–dependent. For example, any change in heart rate or rhythm can alter the heart chamber size and subsequently change the location of the target structure in axial or three-dimensional (3-D) images, even if the individual axial image is not blurred. The most diagnostic studies are created when all of these factors are considered.

BOX 20–16   Key Concept

Prospective ECG gating attempts to identify the areas of lowest cardiac motion and acquire images only in those portions of the cardiac cycle. These methods use a signal, usually derived from the R wave of the patients ECG, to trigger image acquisition.

The two techniques that attempt to minimize cardiac motion in the study by selecting (or acquiring) images during cardiac segments with relatively slow cardiac motion are called prospective ECG triggering and retrospective ECG gating. Prospective ECG gating, also known as sequential or cine-mode scanning, seeks to identify the areas of lowest cardiac motion and acquire images only in those portions of the cardiac cycle, which minimizes radiation exposure. Retrospective gating methods acquire images throughout the cardiac cycle while the patient's ECG is recorded. Images are later reconstructed to create image sets at any desired phase of the cardiac cycle.

To understand either method of ECG gating, a rudimentary understanding of the ECG tracing is needed. The ECG provides a profile of the heart's electrical activity with time. Each heartbeat in a normally functioning heart exhibits a similar characteristic pattern consisting of five waves referred to as P, Q, R, S, and T (Fig. 20-18). The distance between two R waves represents one complete cardiac cycle and is sometimes referred to as the R-R interval. Hence, a scan that covers the entire heartbeat (a continuous acquisition) might be referred to as covering 100% of the R-R interval.

Prospective ECG gating methods use a signal, usually derived from the R wave of the patient's ECG, to trigger image acquisition. A delay between the R wave and scan initiation can be selected by the technologist. Using this trigger, and the preprogrammed delay, a scan is acquired during a finite portion of the R-R interval (Fig. 20-19). The table then moves to the next position, and the procedure is repeated until the entire area of interest is covered. This is sometimes referred to as a step-and-shoot system to differentiate it from helical CT techniques. Because scan acquisition is synchronized with the patient's heart rate, the total time of the examination may vary considerably from one patient to the next.

BOX 20–17   Key Concept

The primary advantage of the prospective gating method over the retrospective method is the dramatic reduction in radiation dose to the patient.

The primary advantage of this method over the retrospective method is the dramatic reduction in radiation dose to the patient. This reduction is attributable to the intermittent nature of the scan acquisition. Reducing the radiation dose is particularly important if cardiac studies are to be used as a screening examination for patients who have not yet exhibited clear cardiac symptoms but have risks associated with cardiac disease. Disadvantages

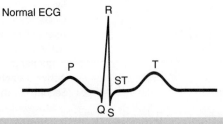

FIGURE 20-18 A normally functioning heart exhibits a similar characteristic pattern consisting of five waves referred to as P, Q, R, S, and T, constituting the electrocardiogram (ECG).

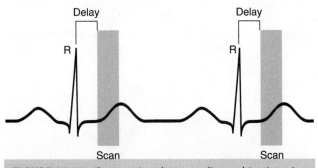

FIGURE 20-19 Prospective electrocardiographic triggering methods use a signal, usually derived from the R wave of the patient's electrocardiogram, to trigger image acquisition at a predefined point within the cardiac cycle. Thereafter, the table moves to the next position, and the procedure is repeated until the entire area of interest is covered.

of prospective methods are that this type of gating is very sensitive to cardiac motion artifacts and image misregistration.[27] This is particularly true in patients with irregular heartbeats.

> **BOX 20-18 Key Concept**
>
> Retrospective ECG gating methods acquire helical data throughout the cardiac cycle. Images are then reconstructed in specified portions of the cardiac cycle.

Retrospective ECG gating methods acquire helical data throughout the cardiac cycle. Using the ECG tracings that are acquired with the scan acquisition, images are reconstructed in specified portions of the cardiac cycle (Fig. 20-20). As a general rule, image reconstruction is performed at 60% to 65% of the cardiac cycle.[27] However, reconstructions are often created from other segments of the cardiac cycle and compared to determine which data set demonstrates the least cardiac motion. The axial image reconstructions are often referred to as the "source images" because these images are used to create 3-D and other image models. Because the retrospective method uses a helical technique, it is possible to combine multiple image sets from different phases in the cardiac cycle to produce a cine loop (i.e., a dynamic image set that resembles a video image). This type of image manipulation is sometime called four-dimensional imaging of the heart. The primary disadvantage of the retrospective ECG-gated method is the relatively high radiation dose to the patient. For example, the effective radiation dose with coronary angiography by 64-slice MDCT is estimated by one researcher to be approximately 11 to 22 mSv.[28] By comparison, a diagnostic coronary catheterization exposes the patient to a radiation

dose of about 5.6 mSv.[29] Although it can be argued that this dose represents an acceptable risk in the symptomatic patient, most researchers worry that it is too high a dose to use the examination as a screening tool for asymptomatic patients. To address this concern, manufacturers have developed methods that automatically decrease the tube current during the systolic phase of the ECG tracing. Hence, the higher tube current is only used during the diastolic phase of the cardiac cycle, the time when images are most likely to be reconstructed. This technique is called ECG-pulsed tube current modulation, or alternatively, ECG pulsing. Reducing the kilovoltage setting when scanning slim patients has also been suggested to decrease the radiation dose.[30]

> **BOX 20-19 Key Concept**
>
> To address concern about the radiation dose from retrospective ECG gating methods manufacturers have developed methods that automatically decrease the tube current during the systolic phase of the ECG tracing. This technique is called ECG-pulsed tube current modulation.

With either method, the greatest challenge to obtaining diagnostic images is heart rate variation.[26] Changes in heart rate or rhythm can result in misregistration of the targeted anatomy. In addition, high heart rate variability and the presence of arrhythmia make the use of ECG-pulsed tube current modulation impossible. Therefore, the advantages of using β-blocker protocols to lower the heart rate not only improve image quality but can reduce the radiation dose to the patient and thus the associated cancer risk.

Contrast Administration

Most cardiac CT protocols require the intravenous administration of iodinated contrast agents. Standard screening for contraindications to the contrast agent (e.g., renal impairment, iodine allergy) is necessary. An intravenous line is placed using a large-lumen (20-gauge or larger) flexible cannula in a vein of sufficient diameter to accommodate a relatively high injection rate; typically the antecubital vein is used, preferably on the right side. Hand veins are not routinely used because they are usually too small and (less importantly) the delay time between injection and the start of the scan must be adjusted. A low-osmolar or isosmolar, nonionic agent with an iodine concentration between 300 and 400 mg/mL is injected, with an injection rate between 3 to 6 mL/s. With such rapid injection rates, technologists must be particularly vigilant in guarding against contrast extravasation. The volume of contrast agent used per examination varies from 70 to 150 mL, depending on the scan protocol, scanner type, and the patient's weight.

In all areas of CT, exact protocols for optimal contrast administration are controversial. Cardiac CT is

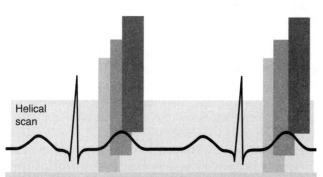

Helical scan

FIGURE 20-20 For retrospective electrocardiographic gating, an MDCT spiral scan is acquired throughout the cardiac cycle (represented by the blue-shaded area). Images are then reconstructed at the portion of the cardiac cycle estimated to have the least motion. Data sets from different segments can be created and evaluated to determine the portion with the least motion. The yellow-shaded area represents the first reconstructed data set, whereas the pink and green areas represent additional reconstructed data sets.

no exception; techniques for contrast use in this arena continue to evolve. Target enhancement is typically in the range of 200 to 300 HU.[31] However, the target range may vary somewhat depending on the specific indication.

The rapid evolution of MDCT scanning systems has not changed the need for the accurate timing of contrast injection and scan initiation. The contrast agent must flow from the IV site to the area of interest, so no matter how fast the image data can be acquired, the delay must be appropriate. Attempts to use a set time (for instance, 20 seconds when the area of interest is the coronary arteries) for all patients have been unsuccessful. This is because many patient-specific characteristics affect arterial enhancement. Among these factors are the patient's weight; ejection fraction (i.e., the fraction of blood pumped out of the ventricle with each heartbeat); and the presence of pulmonary disease. Therefore, the delay time used must be patient-specific (Chapter 13).

The optimal time to start image acquisition can be calculated for each patient using either a timing bolus or bolus tracking (Chapter 13). The timing bolus method consists of a single, low-dose slice repeated every 1 to 2 seconds after the injection of 10 to 20 mL of contrast material delivered at the same rate as will be used during the diagnostic scan. A region of interest (ROI) is placed, and a time-density curve is calculated that will predict the time to peak opacification (Fig. 20-21). The location of the monitoring slices and the placement of the ROI is dependent on the specific cardiac anatomy being investigated. For instance, the monitoring slice and subsequent ROI is placed in the ascending aorta for studies of the coronary arteries, whereas with pulmonary vein imaging, contrast enhancement is timed to the left atrium.

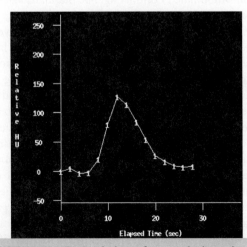

FIGURE 20-21 Timing bolus software calculates the delay between the start of the contrast injection and when the contrast peaks in the ascending aorta. Image courtesy of the University of Michigan.

The bolus tracking method does not require a separate injection. Instead, a series of low-dose monitoring scans begin shortly after the start of the injection; when the contrast density increases to a specific cutoff (usually approximately 150 HU), image acquisition is triggered. As with the timing bolus, the location of the monitoring slice is dependent on the specific cardiac examination.

Contrast injection is immediately followed by a saline solution bolus (often referred to as a "saline chaser"). There are a number of reasons for this practice. One is to make use of the otherwise wasted contrast material present in the IV tubing and in the arm vein of the patient during imaging. Using all of the contrast material allows for the reduction in the total dose of contrast loaded into the syringe. In addition, a saline chaser allows for more homogeneous opacification throughout the examination, that is, a more uniform HU from the top of the aorta to the base of the heart. Finally, a saline chaser reduces streak artifacts over the superior vena cava that result from the dense contrast material (Fig. 20-22). A saline chaser can also reduce inhomogeneities that occur, particularly in the superior vena cava and right atrium, when enhanced and nonenhanced blood meet.

Breath-hold

It is very important that the patient suspend respiration during scan acquisition. Breathing during the scan will result in motion artifact. Careful breath-hold instructions should be given to the patient before the scan begins. It is often helpful to have the patient practice holding his or her breath in moderate inspiration.

Technical aspects of cardiac CT are summarized in a step-by-step manner in Table 20-3.

CT Coronary Calcium Screening

Atherosclerosis is a build-up of fat, plaque, and other substances, including calcium. Coronary artery calcification is a marker of coronary artery disease (CAD). Patients with CAD may exhibit no symptoms of the disease; in many patients myocardial infarction is the first sign of CAD. The goal of CT for calcium scoring is to determine the location and extent of calcified plaque in the coronary arteries. This is a helpful diagnostic tool; by measuring the amount of calcium that builds up in the coronary artery CT can be used to predict the likelihood of subsequent cardiovascular events in people with no symptoms. It is frequently performed as a screening study for patients with risk factors for CAD but no clinical symptoms. The amount of calcification on cardiac CT is expressed as a calcium score. A negative examination shows no calcification within the coronary arteries and suggests that atherosclerotic plaque is minimal and that the chance of CAD developing during the next 2 to 5 years is low. A positive test means that CAD is present, regardless of whether or not the patient is experiencing any symptoms (Table 20-4). Different methods of scoring are used. The

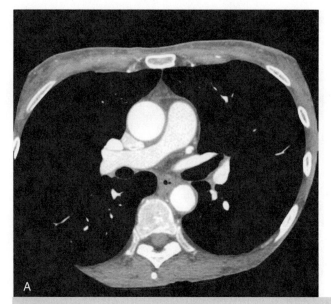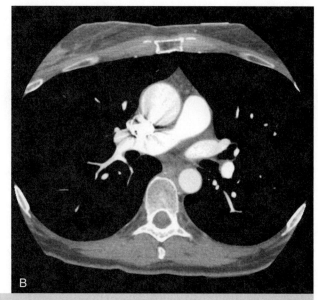

FIGURE 20-22   A. The use of a saline solution bolus immediately after the injection of an iodinated contrast material can reduce streak artifacts common over the superior vena cava. **B.** Artifacts seen in an image taken without a saline solutions bolus. Images courtesy of the University of Michigan.

TABLE 20-3   Cardiac CT Imaging: A Summary of the Steps

Patient Preparation

Have patient arrive at least 1 hour before scheduled examination.

Patient should refrain from ingesting caffeine for 12 hours before study.

Obtain patient history, with particular attention to contraindications to iodinated contrast agents, β-blockers, or nitroglycerin.

Explain the procedure to the patient, including the importance of breath-hold. If a contrast agent will be used, describe the sensations the patient may experience after injection.

For contrast-enhanced protocols, place an IV line in the antecubital vein (right arm preferred) using a flexible cannula no smaller than 20 gauge (18 gauge is preferred).

Connect ECG leads. Noise-free tracing requires a good contact between the lead and the patient's skin. If necessary, shave the skin over the lead site.

Work with the patient to position arms so they are straight and do not impede the flow of contrast material.

Assess heart rate. Consult with the radiologist regarding the administration of β-blockers if the heart rate is over 65 bpm. Patients with cardiac arrhythmias require special consideration.

If ordered by the radiologist, administer nitroglycerin just before scanning.

Scanning

Dual-injector heads are loaded with saline and iodinated contrast material.

Transit (delay) time is determined either by the timing bolus method or bolus tracking method.

Iodinated agent is injected: 70–150 mL at 4–6 mL/s, followed by 40 mL of saline solution.

Scan data are acquired using MDCT with thin collimation, fast gantry rotation, and imaging that is synchronized to the patient's heartbeat.

Post Scan

Patients who have received no β-blockers may leave.

Patients who have received a β-blocker are observed for 30 minutes to ensure their heart rate returns to normal.

Images are reconstructed per specific protocol.

ECG = electrocardiogram.

TABLE 20-4   CT Calcium Scoring[32]

Calcium Score	Presence of Plaque
0	No evidence of plaque
1–10	Minimal plaque
11–100	Mild plaque
101–400	Moderate plaque
More than 400	Extensive plaque

initial method, referred to as the Agatston Score, was designed for use with electron beam CT (EBCT) protocols. Because MDCT protocols use different scan parameters the original Agatston quantification method is of limited value for MDCT. Another calcium quantification method called the calcium volume score (or volume equivalent) is based on calcium area and plaque density or volume. This was developed to provide a reproducible measurement of calcium scoring. However, there are limitations to the calcium volume score method as well. Image attenuation values can vary by scanner and patient body size, resulting in calcium score differences that do not reflect actual calcium within the coronary artery. A third method of calcium quantification was developed to be an absolute calcium mass measurement and is performed in a manner similar to bone mineral density assessment. A standard calibration phantom is used that contains rods of various known calcium concentrations (Fig. 20-23). This phantom is positioned beneath the patient so that the length of the phantom covers the expected length of the heart. The patient is scanned and data from the calibration phantom are used in an algorithm to adjust for variations in attenuation caused by patient size and scanner (Fig. 20-24).

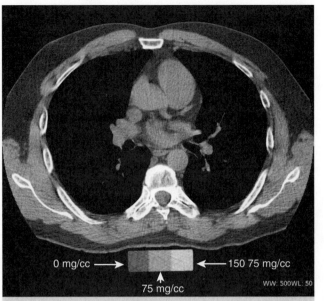

0 mg/cc ⟶   ⟵ 150 75 mg/cc

75 mg/cc

WW: 500 WL: 50

FIGURE 20-24 This transverse CT slice shows a cross-section of the patient's thorax and a three-sample calibration phantom under the thorax. Each sample is labeled according to its calcium hydroxyapatite concentration. Calcium hydroxyapatite is closely equivalent to actual human bone in composition. Image courtesy of the University of Michigan.

BOX 20-20   Key Concept

The amount of calcification on cardiac CT is expressed as a calcium score.

Until the introduction of MDCT with its associated subsecond scan time, coronary CT was performed exclusively with electron beam CT (EBCT) (Chapter 2). A four-detector-row CT with a 0.5-second gantry rotation time is the minimal requirement for a coronary calcium measurement.[33] Because coronary calcium measurement is applied mainly as a screening examination to asymptomatic patients, the radiation dose is of particular concern. Imaging of coronary calcifications is typically performed using a low-dose technique without contrast enhancement. The scan time is as short as possible to avoid artifacts from cardiac motion and breathing. Either a prospective or retrospective cardiac gating acquisition technique is used. The patient is supine and the scan extends from the midlevel of the left pulmonary artery down to the diaphragm. MDCT scanners are able to cover this 10- to 15-cm range in a single breath-hold.

BOX 20-21   Key Concept

Because the coronary calcium measurement is done mainly as a screening examination to asymptomatic patients, the radiation dose is of particular concern.

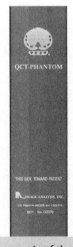

QCT PHANTOM

THIS SIDE TOWARD PATIENT

IMAGE ANALYSIS, INC.
U.S. Patent #4,985,906 and 4,922,915
SER. NO. G2070

FIGURE 20-23 The long axis of the calibration phantom is placed on and parallel to the long axis of the scanning table, under the patient's torso. Photo courtesy of Image Analysis, Inc.

A major criticism of CT coronary calcium scoring is the lack of a standardization regarding image acquisition techniques and with regard to the methods used for quantitative coronary calcification scoring.

CHAPTER SUMMARY

Advances in MDCT scanners have resulted in the ability to acquire information previously unavailable with CT. These advances have been particularly valuable in thoracic imaging, mitigating imaging problems that result from the continuous motion of the heart and vascular structures.

Cardiac imaging is one of the most exciting of the new applications made possible by MDCT. However, cardiac protocols are some of the least forgiving; technologists must be committed to producing optimal studies. Either examinations are done well or they are of little or no value. For these reasons, cardiac studies are considered by many technologists to be among the most challenging to perform. A familiarity with cardiac anatomy along with attention to the details of patient preparation and the careful administration of contrast material with the precise timing of contrast delivery are essential tools for the technologist.

REVIEW QUESTIONS

1. Describe how the development of MDCT scanners has improved thoracic imaging.
2. Why do HRCT protocols often contain more than one scan series? What type of HRCT protocols use helical mode and what type use standard axial mode? Why?
3. Why do PE protocols typically scan in the caudal-to-cranial direction? Why might a delayed venous phase scan from iliac crest through the knees be added to the protocol?
4. Why is the quality of CTA examinations particularly dependent on the skill of the technologist?
5. Describe the two basic methods used for CT cardiac gating. What are the advantages and disadvantages of each method?

REFERENCES

1. Grenier PA, Beigelman-Aubry C, Fetita C, Martin-Bouyer Y. Multi-detector-row CT of the airways. In: Schoepf UJ, ed. Multidetector-Row CT of the Thorax. Berlin: Springer, 2004:75.
2. Nishino M, Boiselle PM, Copeland JF, Raptopoulos V, Hatabu H. Value of volumetric data acquisition in expiratory high-resolution tomography. J Comput Assist Tomogr 2004;28:209–14.
3. Kauczor HU. MDCT in diffuse lung disease. In: Schoepf UJ, ed. Multidetector-Row CT of the Thorax. Berlin: Springer, 2004:85–7.
4. What is pulmonary embolism? Available at: http://www.nhlbi.nih.gov/health/dci/Diseases/pe/pe_what.html. Accessed June 2008.
5. Carson JL, Kelley MA, Duff A, et al. The clinical course of pulmonary embolism. N Engl J Med 1992;326:1240–5.
6. Stein PD, Henry JW. Prevalence of acute pulmonary embolism among patients in a general hospital and at autopsy. Chest 1995;108:978–81.
7. Rubinstein I, Murray D, Hoffstein V. Fatal pulmonary emboli in hospitalized patients. An autopsy study. Arch Intern Med 1988;148:1425–6.
8. The PIOPED Investigators. Value of the ventilation/perfusion scan in acute pulmonary embolism. Results of the prospective investigation of pulmonary embolism diagnosis (PIOPED). JAMA 1990;263:2753–9.
9. Stein PD, Athanasoulis C, Alavi A, et al. Complication and validity of pulmonary angiography in acute pulmonary embolism. Circulation 1992;85:462–8.
10. Baile EM, King GG, Muller NL, et al. Spiral computed tomography is comparable to angiography for the diagnosis of pulmonary embolism. Am J Respir Crit Care Med 2000;161:1010–5.
11. Abcarian PW, Sweet JD, Watabe JT, Yoon HC. Role of quantitative D-dimer assay in determining the need for CT angiography of acute pulmonary embolism. AJR Am J Roentgenol 2004;182:1377–81.
12. Kavanaugh JJ, Lake DR, Costello P. Pulmonary embolism imaging with MDCT. In: Saini S, Rubin GD, Kalra MK, eds. MDCT: A Practical Approach. Milan: Springer, 2006: 123–30.
13. van Erkel AR, Pattynama PM. Cost-effective diagnostic algorithms in pulmonary embolism: an updated analysis. Acad Radiol 1998;5(Suppl):s321–7.
14. Wiest PW, Locken JA, Heintz PH, Mettler FA Jr. CT scanning: a major source of radiation exposure. Semin Ultrasound CT MR 2002;23:402–10.
15. Huda W. When a pregnant patient has a suspected pulmonary embolism, what are the typical embryo doses from a chest CT and a ventilation/perfusion study? Pediatr Radiol 2005;35:452–3.
16. Winer-Muram HT, Boone JM, Brown HL, Jennings SG, Mabie WC, Lombardo GT. Pulmonary embolism in pregnant patients: fetal radiation dose with helical CT. Radiology 2002;224:487–92.
17. National Heart Lung and Blood Institute. Chapter 4: Disease Statistics (NHLBI Web site). In: NHLBI Factbook 2005: Web Version. Available at: http://www.nhlbi.nih.gov/about/factbook/chapter4.htmnumber of4_2. Accessed September 5, 2008.
18. Thom T, Haase N, Rosamond W, et al. Heart disease and stroke statistics–2006 update: a report from the American Heart Association Statistics Committee and Stroke Statistics Subcommittee. Circulation 2006;113:e85–151.
19. Medline Plus Web site. Medical Encyclopedia: Heart bypass surgery web page. Available at: http://www.nlm.nih.gov/medlineplus/print/ency/article/002946.htm. Accessed September 5, 2008.
20. Pannu HK, Alvarez W Jr, Fishman EK. Beta-blockers for cardiac CT: a primer for the radiologist. AJR Am J Roentgenol 2006;186(Suppl):S341–5.
21. Sandrasegaran K, Teague SD, Dohrman J. 64-slice CT coronary angiography. Poster presentation presented at Annual RSNA Meeting; November 28, 2006; Chicago, IL.
22. Schoenhagen P, Stillman AE. Halliburton SS, White RD. Cardiac CT Made Easy: An Introduction to Cardiovascular

Multidetector Computed Tomography. London: Informa Healthcare, 2006:117–8.

23. Budoff M. Interpreting CT angiography: three-dimensional reconstruction techniques. In: Budoff M, Shinbane J, Achenback S, Raggi P, Rumberger J, eds. Cardiac CT Imaging: Diagnosis of Cardiovascular Disease. London: Springer-Verlag, 2006:46.

24. Schoenhagen P, Stillman AE. Halliburton SS, White RD. Cardiac CT Made Easy: An Introduction to Cardiovascular Multidetector Computed Tomography. London: Informa Healthcare, 2006:102.

25. Gerber TC, Breen JF, Kuzo RS, et al, for the Mayo Foundation for Medical Education and Research. Computed tomographic angiography of the coronary arteries: techniques and applications. Semin Ultrasound CT MR 2006;27:42–55.

26. Mao S, Shinbane J. Methodology for image acquisition. In: Budoff M, Shinbane J, Achenback S, Raggi P, Rumberger J, eds. Cardiac CT Imaging: Diagnosis of Cardiovascular Disease. London: Springer-Verlag, 2006:19–21.

27. Woodard PK, Bhalla S, Javidan-Nejad C, Gutierrez FR. Non-coronary cardiac CT imaging. Semin Ultrasound CT MR 2006;27:56–75.

28. Hoffmann U, Ferencik M, Cury RC, Pena AJ. Coronary CT angiography. J Nucl Med 2006;47:797–806.

29. Coles DR, Smail MA, Negus IS, et al. Comparison of radiation doses from multislice computed tomography coronary angiography and conventional diagnostic angiography. J Am Coll Cardiol 2006;47:1840–5.

30. Abada HT, Larchez C, Daoud B, Sigal-Cinqualbre A, Paul JF. MDCT of the coronary arteries: feasibility of low-dose CT with ECG-pulsed tube current modulation to reduce radiation dose. AJRAm J Roentgenol 2006;186(Suppl):S387–90.

31. Jacobs JE. How to do coronary CT angiography: a radiologist's perspective. In: Contrast Use in CTA Applications. Appl Radiol [online supplement] 2005;34(Suppl 12):34–40. Available at: http://www.ctisus.org/cta_web/12_05/pdfs/AR_12-05_CTA_Jacobs.pdf. Accessed September 5, 2008.

32. Cardiac CT for calcium scoring. Available at: http://www.radiologyinfo.org/en/info.cfm?pg=ct_calscoring&bhcp=1. Accessed June 2008.

33. Becker CR. Plaque characterization–computed tomography. In: Higgins CB, de Roos A, eds. MRI and CT of the Cardiovascular System. Philadelphia: Lippincott Williams & Wilkins, 2006:377.

THORACIC PROTOCOLS

Routine Chest		
Examples of clinical indications: Infection, mass, empyema, evaluation of abnormalities discovered on chest radiographs, evaluation of known or suspected congenital thoracic anomalies, evaluation of trauma		
Scouts: AP and lateral		
Scan type: Helical		
Start location: Just above lung apices		
End location: Just below costophrenic angles (note: for known or suspected lung cancer, end just below adrenal glands)		
Breath-hold: Inspiration		
IV contrast: 80 mL at 3.0 mL/s. 50 mL saline flush. Scan delay = 35 seconds		
Oral contrast: None (note: for known or suspected lung cancer, give 16 oz barium sulfate just before examination)		
DFOV: ~38 cm (optimize for individual)		
SFOV: Large body		
Algorithm: Standard		
Window settings: 350 ww/50 wl (soft tissue); 1500 ww/−700 wl (lung)		
	16-Detector Protocol	64-Detector Protocol
Gantry rotation time	0.8 s	0.8 s
Acquisition (detector width × number of detector rows = detector coverage)	16 × 1.25 = 20 mm	64 × 0.625 = 40 mm
Reconstruction (slice thickness/interval)	2.5 mm/1.25	2.5 mm/1.25
Pitch	1.375	1.375
kVp	120	120
mA	Auto: min 100/max 150 (noise index 15)	Auto: min 100/max 150 (noise index 15)

Lung Nodule		
Examples of clinical indications: Evaluate suspected lung nodule		
Scouts: AP and lateral		
Scan type: Helical		
Start location: Just above lung apices		
End location: Just below costophrenic angles		
Breath-hold: Inspiration		
IV contrast: None		
Oral contrast: None		
DFOV: ~38 cm (optimize for individual)		
SFOV: Large body		
Algorithm: Standard		
Window settings: 350 ww/50 wl (soft tissue); 1500 ww/−700 wl (lung)		
	16-Detector Protocol	64-Detector Protocol
Gantry rotation time	0.5 s	0.5 s
Acquisition (detector width × number of detector rows = detector coverage)	16 × 1.25 = 20 mm	64 × 0.625 = 40 mm
Reconstruction (slice thickness/interval)	2.5 mm/2.0 mm	2.5 mm/2.0
Pitch	1.375	1.375

(Continued)

Lung Nodule *(Continued)*		
kVp	120	120
mA	80–160 (depending on patient size)	80–160 (depending on patient size)
Reconstruction 2:		
Algorithm: Standard		
Slice thickness/interval	1.25 mm/0.625 mm	1.25 mm/0625

High-Resolution Chest CT		
Examples of clinical indications: Asbestos exposure, inhalation injury, interstitial disease, diffuse pulmonary disease, suspected bronchiectasis, suspected small airway disease		
Scouts: AP and lateral		
Group 1. Supine Inspiration		
Scan type: Helical		
Start location: Just above lung apices		
End location: Just below costophrenic angles		
IV contrast: None		
Oral contrast: None		
Breath-hold: Inspiration		
DFOV: ~38 cm (optimize for individual)		
SFOV: Large body		
Algorithm: Bone		
Window settings: 1500 ww/−700 wl (lung)		
	16-Detector Protocol	64-Detector Protocol
Gantry rotation time	Small: 0.5 s	Small: 0.5 s
	Medium: 0.5 s	Medium: 0.5 s
	Large: 0.6 s	Large: 0.6 s
Acquisition (detector width × number of detector rows = detector coverage)	16 × 0.625 = 10 mm	32 × 0625 mm = 20
Reconstruction (slice thickness/interval)	1.25 mm/1.25 mm	1.25 mm/1.25 mm
Pitch	1.375	1.375
kVp	140	140
mA	Small: 150	Small: 150
	Medium: 300	Medium: 300
	Large: 375	Large: 375
Reconstruction 2:		
Algorithm: Bone		
Slice thickness/interval	1.25 mm/10 mm	1.25 mm/10 mm
Group 2. Supine Expiration		
Scan type: Axial		
Start location: Just above lung apices		
End location: Just below costophrenic angles		
Breath-hold: Expiration		
DFOV: ~38 cm (optimize for individual)		

SFOV: Large body		
Algorithm: Bone		
Window settings: 1500 ww/−700 wl (lung)		
	16-Detector Protocol	64-Detector Protocol
Gantry rotation time	1.0 s	1.0 s
Acquisition (detector width × number of detector rows = detector coverage)	1 × 1.25 = 1.25 mm	2 × 0.625 mm = 1.25 mm
Reconstruction (slice thickness/interval)	1.25 mm/20 mm	1.25 mm/20 mm
kVp/mA	140/220	140/220
Group 3. Prone Inspiration		
Scouts: PA and lateral		
Scan type: Axial		
Start location: Carina		
End location: Just below costophrenic angles		
Breath-hold: Inspiration		
DFOV: ~38 cm (optimize for individual)		
SFOV: Large body		
Algorithm: Bone		
Window settings: 1500 ww/−700 wl (lung)		
	16-Detector Protocol	64-Detector Protocol
Gantry rotation time	1.0 s	1.0 s
Acquisition (detector width × number of detector rows = detector coverage)	1 × 1.25 = 1.25 mm	2 × 0.625 mm = 1.25 mm
Reconstruction (slice thickness/interval)	1.25 mm/20 mm	1.25 mm/20 mm
kVp/mA	140/220	140/220

Tracheobronchial		
Scan patient with arms at side.		
Examples of clinical indications: Suspected congenital tracheobronchial anomalies, assessment of tracheal narrowing, detection or confirmation of tracheomalacia, suspected foreign body aspiration		
Group 1. Supine Inspiration		
Scouts: AP and lateral		
Scan type: Helical		
Start location: 7 cm below the carina		
End location: 1 cm above the epiglottis		
IV contrast: None		
Oral contrast: None		
Breath-hold: Inspiration		
DFOV: 22 cm		
SFOV: Large body		
Algorithm: Standard		
Window settings: 350 ww/50 wl (soft tissue); 1500 ww/−700 wl (lung)		
	16-Detector Protocol	64-Detector Protocol
Gantry rotation time	0.8 s	0.8 s

(Continued)

Tracheobronchial *(Continued)*		
Acquisition (detector width × number of detector rows = detector coverage)	16 × 0.625 = 10 mm	64 × 0.625 = 40 mm
Reconstruction (slice thickness/interval)	1.25 mm/0.625 mm	1.25 mm/0.625 mm
Pitch	1.375	1.375
kVp/mA	120/150	120/150

GROUP 2. Supine Expiration
Scan type: Helical
Start location: 7 cm below the carina
End location: 1 cm above the epiglottis Use the same start/end location and RAS coordinates as group 1
Breath-hold: Expiration
DFOV: 22 cm
SFOV: Large body
Algorithm: Standard

	16-Detector Protocol	64-Detector Protocol
Gantry rotation time	0.8 s	0.8 s
Acquisition (detector width × number of detector rows = detector coverage)	16 × 0.625 = 10 mm	64 × 0.625 = 40 mm
Reconstruction (slice thickness/interval)	1.25 mm/0.625 mm	1.25 mm/0.625
Pitch	1.375	1.375
kVp/mA	120/150	120/150

Chest Abdomen
Examples of clinical indications: Infection, mass, evaluation of trauma
GROUP 1. Venous Scan of Chest
Scouts: AP and lateral
Scan type: Helical
Start location: Just above lung apices
End location: Just below costophrenic angles
IV contrast: 125 mL at 3.0 mL/s. 50 mL saline flush. Scan delay = 35 seconds
Oral contrast: 900 mL, 1 hour before scan
Breath-hold: Inspiration
DFOV: ~38 (optimize for individual)
SFOV: Large body
Algorithm: Standard
Window settings: 350 ww/50 wl (soft tissue); 1500 ww/−700 wl (lung)

	16-Detector Protocol	64-Detector Protocol
Gantry rotation time	0.8 s	0.8 s
Acquisition (detector width × number of detector rows = detector coverage)	16 × 1.25 = 20 mm	64 × 0.625 = 40 mm
Reconstruction (slice thickness/interval)	2.5 mm/1.25 mm	2.5 mm/1.25 mm
Pitch	1.375	1.375
kVp	120	120
mA	Auto: min 100/max 150 (noise index 15)	Auto: min 100/max 150 (noise index 15)

Group 2. Venous Scan of Abdomen		
Begin 65 seconds after the start of the contrast injection		
Scan type: Helical		
Start location: Just above diaphragm		
End location: 1 cm below iliac crest		
Breath-hold: Inspiration		
DFOV: ~38 (optimize for individual)		
SFOV: Large body		
Algorithm: Standard		
	16-Detector Protocol	64-Detector Protocol
Gantry rotation time	0.8 s	0.8 s
Acquisition (detector width × number of detector rows = detector coverage)	16 × 1.25 = 20 mm	64 × 0.625 = 40 mm
Reconstruction (slice thickness/interval)	5.0 mm/5.0 mm	5.0 mm/5.0 mm
Pitch	1.375	1.375
kVp/mA	120/320	120/320

CTA—Chest for Pulmonary Embolism		
Examples of clinical indications: Suspected pulmonary embolism		
Scouts: AP and lateral (scouts should begin just above lung apices and extend to just below tibial plateau so that they can be used for both group 1 and group 2)		
Group 1. Arterial Scan		
Scan type: Helical		
Start location: Just below lowest hemidiaphragm		
End location: Lung apices (Scans are inferior to superior)		
IV contrast: 120 mL (370 concentration) total, split bolus; 70 mL at 4.0 mL/s. Scan delay = Smart Prep; set monitor location at the level of the main pulmonary artery, initiate the scan at first sight of contrast in the main pulmonary artery (~70 HU); 25-second pause after first 70-mL injection is complete, then 50 mL at 3 mL/s		
Oral contrast: None		
Breath-hold: Instruct patient to stop breathing (avoid deep inspiration)		
DFOV: ~38 (optimize for individual)		
SFOV: Large body		
Algorithm: Standard		
Window settings: 700 ww/180 wl (vascular)		
	16-Detector Protocol	64-Detector Protocol
Gantry rotation time	0.5 s	0.6 s
Acquisition (detector width × number of detector rows = detector coverage)	16 × 1.0 = 16 mm	64 × 0.625 = 40 mm
Reconstruction (slice thickness/interval)	1.25 mm/0.625 mm	1.25 mm/0.625 mm
Pitch	1.375	1.375
kVp/mA	120/500	120/500
Group 2. Lower Extremity Runoff Begin 180 seconds after the start of the contrast injection		
Scan type: Helical		
Start location: 2 cm below tibial plateau		
End location: Iliac crest (if patient has an inferior vena cava (IVC) filter, as seen on scout image, end 2 cm above the IVC filter)		

(Continued)

CTA—Chest for Pulmonary Embolism *(Continued)*		
Breath-hold: None		
DFOV: ~48 (optimize for individual)		
SFOV: Large body		
Algorithm: Standard		
	16-Detector Protocol	64-Detector Protocol
Gantry rotation time	0.8 s	0.8 s
Acquisition (detector width × number of detector rows = detector coverage)	16 × 1.0 = 16 mm	32 × 0.625 = 20 mm
Reconstruction (slice thickness/interval)	5.0 mm/7.5 mm	5.0 mm/7.5 mm
Pitch	1.375	1.375
kVp/mA	120/190	120/190

Cardiac Calcium Scoring (Gated)		
Position patient on the Cardiac CA score phantom. Do not use breast shields.		
Examples of clinical indications: Assessment of risk in asymptomatic individuals who have one or more risk factors for CAD; evaluation of patients presenting with equivocal symptoms of CAD; follow-up of patients undergoing therapy		
Scouts: AP and lateral		
Scan type: Cine		
Start location: 1 cm below carina		
End location: Just below heart apex		
Breath-hold: Inspiration		
IV contrast: None		
Oral contrast: None		
DFOV: 25		
SFOV: Large body		
Algorithm: Standard		
Window settings: 350 ww/50 wl		
	16-Detector Protocol	64-Detector Protocol
Gantry rotation time	0.4-s segment	0.35-s segment
Acquisition (detector width × number of detector rows = detector coverage)	16 × 1.25 = 20 mm	64 × 0.625 = 40 mm
Reconstruction (slice thickness/interval)	2.5 mm/2.5 mm	2.5 mm/2.5 mm
kVp/mA (small patient)	120/250–300	120/250–300
kVp/mA (medium patient)	120/350–400	120/350–400
kVp/mA (large to extra large patient)	120/450–550	120/450–550
Reconstruction 2:		
Algorithm: Standard		
DFOV: Optimize (include entire chest)		
Slice thickness/interval	2.5 mm/20 mm	2.5 mm/40 mm
Gating Information:		
Center R-peak %	75%	75%
Time between images	50 ms	50 ms
Image per R-R interval	3	3

CTA—Chest Aorta (Gated)

Examples of clinical indications: Blunt trauma, aortic dissection, aneurysm rupture, atherosclerotic occlusive disease, congenital vascular anomalies

GROUP 1. Unenhanced Scan

Scouts: AP and lateral

Scan type: Helical

Start location: 2 cm above aortic arch

End location: 2 cm below celiac artery

IV contrast: None

Oral contrast: None

Breath-hold: Inspiration

DFOV: ~38 (optimize for individual)

SFOV: Large body

Algorithm: Standard

Window settings: 350 ww/50 wl (soft tissue)

	16-Detector Protocol	64-Detector Protocol
Gantry rotation time	0.8 s	0.8 s
Acquisition (detector width × number of detector rows = detector coverage)	16 × 1.25 = 20 mm	64 × 0.625 = 40 mm
Reconstruction (slice thickness/interval)	5.0 mm/5.0 mm	5.0 mm/5.0 mm
Pitch	1.375	1.375
kVp/mA	100/150 (pt < 165 lbs) 120/150 (pt > 165 lbs)	100/150 (pt < 165 lbs) 120/150 (pt > 165 lbs)

GROUP 2. Gated Arterial Scan

Scan type: Cardiac helical

Scouts: AP and lateral

Start location: Just above lung apices

End location: 2 cm below celiac artery

IV contrast: 100 mL (370 concentration) at 4.0 mL/s; 20 mL saline at 4.0 mL/s. Scan delay = from timing bolus (use descending aorta at level of carina for ROI); add 3 seconds to peak for 16-detector, add 6 seconds to peak for 64-detector

Oral contrast: None

Breath-hold: Inspiration (hyperventilation)

DFOV: 25

SFOV: Large body

Algorithm: Standard

Window settings: 700 ww/180 wl (vascular)

	16-Detector Protocol	64-Detector Protocol
Gantry rotation time	0.4 s	0.35 s
Acquisition (detector width × number of detector rows = detector coverage)	16 × 1.25 = 20 mm	64 × 0.625 = 40 mm
Reconstruction (slice thickness/interval)	1.25 mm/1.25 mm	1.25 mm/1.25 mm
Pitch	Determined by patient's heart rate	Determined by patient's heart rate
kVp	100 (pt < 165 lbs) 120 (pt > 165 lbs)	100 (pt < 165 lbs) 120 (pt > 165 lbs)
ECG-modulated mA Small patient min/max	100–500	100–500
ECG-modulated mA Medium patient min/max	120–600	120–600
ECG-modulated mA Large patient min/max	140–700	140–700

CTA—Heart General		
Patient on 2 L of oxygen.		
Examples of clinical indications: Follow-up after CABG		
Scouts: AP and lateral		
GROUP 1. Unenhanced Scan		
Scan type: Helical		
Start location: Just above clavicular heads		
End location: 2 cm below heart apex		
IV contrast: None		
Oral contrast: None		
Breath-hold: Inspiration (hyperventilation)		
DFOV: ~38 (optimize; include entire chest)		
SFOV: Large body		
Algorithm: Standard		
Window settings: 350 ww/50 wl (soft tissue)		
	16-Detector Protocol	64-Detector Protocol
Gantry rotation time	0.4 s	0.35 s
Acquisition (detector width × number of detector rows = detector coverage)	16 × 1.25 = 20 mm	64 × 0.625 = 40 mm
Reconstruction (slice thickness/interval)	2.5 mm/1.25	2.5 mm/1.25 mm
Pitch	1.375	1.375
kVp/mA	120/150	120/150
GROUP 2. Gated Arterial Scan		
Scouts: AP and lateral		
Scan type: Cardiac helical		
Start location: Just above clavicular heads		
End location: 2 cm below heart apex		
IV contrast: 80 mL (IOCM) at 5.0 mL/s, 20 mL at 3.5 mL/s; 50 mL saline at 5.0 mL/s (if patient weight ≥ 210 lbs, use 120 mL 370 concentration contrast agent). Scan delay = from timing bolus (use aortic root at level of LMA for ROI); add 3 seconds to peak for 16-dectector/add 6 seconds to peak for 64-detector		
Oral contrast: None		
Breath-hold: Inspiration (hyperventilation)		
DFOV: 25		
SFOV: (dependent on patient size) Cardiac S, M, L		
Algorithm: Standard		
Cardiac filters: C1, C2, or C3 (by body habitus)		
Window settings: 700 ww/180 wl (vascular)		
	16-Detector Protocol	64-Detector Protocol Cardiac Helical
Gantry rotation time	0.4 s	0.35-s segment
Acquisition (detector width × number of detector rows = detector coverage)	16 × 0.625 mm = 10	64 × 0.625 = 40 mm
Reconstruction (slice thickness/interval)	0.625 mm/0.625 mm	0.625 mm/0.625 mm
Pitch/speed	Determined by patient's heart rate	Determined by patient's heart rate
kVp/mA	120/800	120/800

Phase Reconstructions:
DFOV: 25
Start location: Just above left atrial appendage
End location: Just below heart apex
40–50% by 5%, using 0.625-mm slice thickness
70–80 by 5% using 0.625-mm slice thickness
0–95% by 5% using 1.25-mm slice thickness

CTA—Coronary
Patient on 2L of oxygen. Do not use breast shield for the calcium score series, but use it for the rest of the examination. If patient is status post-CABG (from history or if sternal wires are seen on scout), skip the cardiac score series.
Examples of clinical indications: Suspected coronary artery disease (patients with nonspecific complaints or ambiguous stress tests), suspected coronary anomalies
Scouts: AP and lateral
GROUP 1. Cardiac Score (unenhanced)
Scan type: Cine
Start location: 1 cm below carina
End location: Just below heart apex
IV contrast: None
Oral contrast: None
Breath-hold: Inspiration (hyperventilation)
DFOV: 25
SFOV: Large body
Algorithm: Standard
Window settings: 350 ww/50 wl (soft tissue)

	16-Detector Protocol	64-Detector Protocol
Gantry rotation time	0.4 s	0.35 s
Acquisition (detector width × number of detector rows = detector coverage)	$16 \times 1.25 = 20$ mm	$64 \times 0.625 = 40$ mm
Reconstruction (slice thickness/interval)	2.5 mm/2.5 mm	2.5 mm/2.5 mm
kVp/mA	120/350	120/500

GROUP 2. Gated Arterial Scan
Scouts: AP and lateral
Scan type: Cardiac helical
Start location: Just above clavicular heads
End location: 2 cm below heart apex
IV contrast: 60 mL (IOCM) at 5.0 mL/s, 20 mL at 3.5 mL/s (if patient weight is ≥ 210 lbs, use 370 concentration of LOCM); 50 mL saline at 5.0 mL/s. Scan delay = from timing bolus (use aortic root at level of LMA for ROI); add 6 seconds to peak
Oral contrast: None
Breath-hold: Inspiration (hyperventilation)
DFOV: 25
SFOV: (dependent on patient size) Cardiac S, M, L
Algorithm: Standard
Cardiac filters: C1, C2, or C3 (by body habitus)
Window settings: 700 ww/180 wl (vascular)

(Continued)

CTA—Coronary   *(Continued)*

	16-Dectector Protocol Cardiac Helical	64-Detector Protocol Cardiac Helical
Gantry rotation time	0.4 s	0.35-s segment
Acquisition (detector width × number of detector rows = detector coverage)	16 × 0.625 = 10	64 × 0.625 = 40 mm
Reconstruction (slice thickness/interval)	0.625 mm/0.625 mm	0.625 mm/0.625 mm
Pitch	Determined by patient's heart rate	Determined by patient's heart rate
kVp/mA	120/800	120/800

Phase Reconstructions:

DFOV: 25
Start location: Just above left atrial appendage End location: Just below heart apex
40–50% by 5%, using 0.625-mm slice thickness
70–80 by 5% using 0.625-mm slice thickness
0–95% by 5% using 1.25-mm slice thickness

CTA—Pulmonary Veins (Gated)

Examples of clinical indications: Radiofrequency catheter ablation (RFCA) of the pulmonary veins and posterior left atrium can be used to treat atrial fibrillation. CTA of the pulmonary veins can provide anatomic information for RFCA, including the number, location, and angulation of pulmonary veins and their branches, and left atrial volume.

Scouts: AP and lateral

Scan type: Cardiac helical

Start location: Just above lung apices

End location: 2 cm below celiac artery

IV contrast: 100 mL (use 370 concentration if patient is > 210 lbs) at 4.0 mL/s; 50 mL saline at 4.0 mL/s. Scan delay = from timing bolus (use left atrium for ROI)

Oral contrast: None

Breath-hold: Inspiration (hyperventilation)

DFOV: 25

SFOV: Large body

Algorithm: Standard

Cardiac filters: C1, C2, or C3 (special bowtie filter for cardiac applications)

Window settings: 700 ww/180 wl (vascular)

	16-Detector Protocol	64-Detector Protocol
Gantry rotation time	0.4 s	0.35 s
Acquisition (detector width × number of detector rows = detector coverage)	16 × 1.25 = 20 mm	64 × 0.625 = 40 mm
Reconstruction (slice thickness/interval)	1.25 mm/1.25 mm	1.25 mm/1.25 mm
Pitch	Determined by patient's heart rate	Determined by patient's heart rate
kVp	100 (pt < 165 lbs) 120 (pt > 165 lbs)	100 (pt < 165 lbs) 120 (pt > 165 lbs)
ECG-modulated mA Small patient min/max	100–500	100–500

ECG-modulated mA Medium patient min/max	120–600	120–600
ECG-modulated mA Large patient min/max	250–700	250–700
Reconstruction 2:		
Algorithm: Standard		
DFOV: Optimize (include full chest)		
Center R-peak delay: 75%		
Slice thickness/interval: 1.25 mm/1.25 mm		
Phase Reconstructions:		
DFOV: 25		
Start location: Just above left atrial appendage		
End location: Just below heart apex		
0–95% by 5% using 1.25-mm slice thickness		

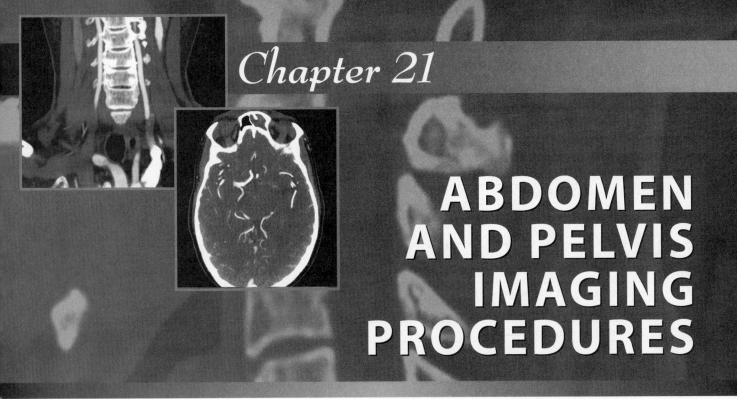

Chapter 21

ABDOMEN AND PELVIS IMAGING PROCEDURES

Key Terms: fatty infiltration of the liver
• hemangioma • hepatic arterial phase
• portal venous phase • corticomedullary phase
• nephrogram phase • excretory phase
• incidentalomas • adrenal adenoma • intracellular lipid content • contrast washout • vermiform appendix • focused appendiceal CT
• kidney stones • renal stones • renal calculi • nephrolithiasis • urolithiasis
• hydronephrosis • renal colic

GENERAL ABDOMINOPELVIC SCANNING METHODS

CT evaluation of the abdomen and pelvis requires greater attention to patient preparation than CT evaluation of any other area of the body. Most CT scans of the abdomen require the administration of an oral contrast agent to demonstrate the intestinal lumen and to distend the gastrointestinal tract. The use of oral contrast material is imperative to differentiate a fluid-filled loop of bowel from a mass or an abnormal fluid collection. Either a dilute barium suspension or a dilute water-soluble agent may be used with equal effectiveness (Chapter 12). In general, the greater the volume of oral contrast material, the better the bowel opacification. Although a volume of at least 600 mL is desired, patient compliance may be a limiting factor. Patients should be given only clear liquids for at least 2 hours before scanning to ensure that food in the stomach is not mistaken for pathologic tissue.

Air and water are excellent as low-attenuation contrast agents. Air or carbon dioxide is frequently used to insufflate the colon for CT colonography, producing a very high negative contrast. Water or a low Hounsfield units (HU) oral barium sulfate suspension (e.g., VoLumen, Bracco Diagnostics) is sometimes used in place of positive contrast agents. These low HU agents will not obscure mucosal surfaces or superimpose abdominal vessels on postprocessed images. The latter is important in CT angiography (CTA) of the abdomen and pelvis (Chapter 12). The use of a low HU oral contrast has an added advantage in that it does not mask radiopaque stones in the common bile duct or urinary tract. Few institutions routinely administer rectal contrast material. When it is used, the most common indication is for colon cancer staging. The bladder is best appreciated on CT when filled with urine or contrast agent. The vagina is seen in cross section as a flattened ellipse of soft tissue between the bladder and rectum. An inserted tampon will outline the cavity of the vagina with air density and is useful in identification of the vaginal canal.

BOX 21–1   Key Concept

In general, for abdominopelvic CT the greater the volume of oral contrast material, the better the bowel opacification. Although a volume of at least 600 mL is desired, patient compliance may be a limiting factor.

BOX 21–2   Key Concept

The bladder is best appreciated on CT when filled with urine or contrast agent.

Intravenous contrast agents improve the quality of studies of the abdomen and pelvis by opacifying blood vessels, increasing the CT density of vascular abdominal organs, and improving image contrast between lesions and normal structures. The appropriate timing, rate, and dose of the IV contrast agent are essential. For most examinations of the body, image acquisition must be completed before IV contrast medium reaches the equilibrium phase (Chapter 13). Modern scanners can accomplish this; as a result precontrast scans are now seldom obtained for routine abdomen studies, but may be used for specific indications (e.g., diagnosis of fatty infiltration or other alteration of parenchymal attenuation). Multiphasic imaging is frequently used for specialized studies of the pancreas, liver, and kidney as well as in many abdominal CTA protocols. The factors that should be considered in determining appropriate injection protocols for these studies are the same as for other areas of the body, namely contrast medium injection duration, contrast arrival time, and scan duration (Chapter 12).

BOX 21-3   Key Concept

Multiphasic imaging is frequently used for specialized studies of the pancreas, liver, and kidney as well as in many abdominal CTA protocols.

CT of the abdomen and pelvis is used for the evaluation of virtually all organs and most vessels. Radiologists systematically examine each organ and structure imaged (Table 21-1).[1] In any given slice, much more information is present than can be displayed by any single window width and level setting. A routine soft-tissue window setting (window width approximately 450; window level approximately 50) will adequately display most abdominal anatomy. However, the liver may also be examined using "liver windows" that are narrower (window width approximately 150; window level approximately 70) and intended to improve the visibility of subtle liver lesions. The lung bases are contained in slices of the upper abdomen and must be viewed using lung windows (window width approximately 1500; window level approximately −600). Bone windows (window width approximately 2000; window level approximately 600) may help to reveal abnormalities of the bones.

The display field of view (DFOV) should be just large enough to include the skin surface over the key areas of the body (frequently portions of the arms placed over the head of the patient are cut off to avoid requiring an excessively large DFOV). If previous studies are available, it is generally advisable to use the same DFOV, unless a change in patient condition (e.g., large weight

TABLE 21-1   Examples of Structures and Abnormalities Examined on CT Studies of the Abdomen and Pelvis

Organ/Structure	Characteristics or Abnormality Examined
Lung bases	Nodules, infiltrates, scars, pleural effusions, atelectasis
Liver	Size, homogeneous parenchymal attenuation, uniform enhancement, portal veins, hepatic veins, hepatic arteries
Biliary tree and gallbladder	Visible bile ducts, biliary ductal dimension, wall thickness, presence and distention of the gallbladder, low-density stones, high-density stones
Spleen	Size (normal up to 14 cm), inhomogeneous enhancement early, homogeneous enhancement late, splenules, splenic vein, splenic artery
Adrenal	Y or V shape, limb thickness less than 1 cm, no convex margins
Pancreas	Size and position, head, neck, body, tail, visible pancreatic duct, patent splenic vein, lucent peripancreatic fat
Kidneys	Size 9 to 13 cm in adults, symmetric enhancement, calyces and pelvis and ureter, position and orientation
Lymph nodes	Retroperitoneum, mesentery, omentum, porta hepatic, pelvis
Blood vessels	Aorta, inferior vena cava, celiac axis, superior and inferior mesenteric arteries, renal arteries, renal veins, splenic vein, superior mesenteric vein, portal vein, gonadal veins
Stomach	Position, distention, wall thickness, fold thickness
Duodenum and small bowel	Position, distention, wall thickness, surrounding fat, mesentery
Colon and rectum	Position, distention, wall thickness, luminal contents, diverticula
Uterus and ovaries	Size, position, appropriate for age and phase of the menstrual cycle, masses
Prostate and seminal vesicles	Size, calcifications
Bladder	Distention, wall thickness, luminal contents
Bones	Degenerative changes, metastatic disease, mineralization

Adapted from Brant WE. Introduction to CT of the Abdomen and Pelvis. In: Webb WR, Brant WE, Major NM, ed. Fundamentals of Body CT. 3rd Ed. Philadelphia: Saunders, 2006:169–70.

gain) necessitates adjustment. Using the same DFOV as the previous study allows easy visual comparison of any changes in size of lesions or structures when both studies are displayed side by side on PACS monitors or film viewboxes.

Although landmarks easily visible on the scout images are often used to guide technologists as to where cross-sectional slices should begin and end, technologists must verify that the anatomy of interest has indeed been scanned. For instance, scans of the abdomen often begin at the base of the lungs and terminate at the iliac crest. However, if cross-sectional images that contain the iliac crest still contain sections of the liver, scanning must be extended until the entire liver has been imaged. Similarly, scanning should not start or stop in the middle of obvious abnormality.

BOX 21-4   Key Concept

In any given slice, much more information is present than can be displayed by a single window width and level setting. Therefore, images are often reviewed in two or more window settings.

Most protocols of the abdomen and pelvis are performed while the patient lies in a supine position on the scan table with the arms elevated above the head. In a few instances changing the patient position and obtaining additional slices can provide added information. Such is the case when initial scans fail to differentiate the margins of the pancreas from the duodenum. In this situation, the patient is often given additional oral contrast material and additional slices are obtained with the patient lying in a right decubitus position.

BOX 21-5   Key Concept

For abdominopelvic scanning, patients are asked to hold their breath during data acquisition to reduce movement and decrease motion artifacts. Patient movement during scanning will cause anatomic structures to be displaced, distorted, or blurred.

Patients are asked to hold their breath during scan acquisition to reduce movement and decrease motion artifacts. Patient movement during scanning will cause anatomic structures to be displaced, distorted, or blurred. The speed of MDCT scanners has reduced, but not eliminated, artifacts caused by cardiac motion, vessel pulsation, and bowel peristalsis.

There is a wide range in the number of protocols used at different institutions for CT of the abdomen and pelvis, from just 2 to more than 40. Protocols can be of a general nature (e.g., routine abdomen and pelvis), or they can be designed to address a particular clinical question or to evaluate a specific abdominal or pelvic

organ (e.g., suspected appendicitis, renal mass). At some institutions scans are routinely checked by a radiologist while the patient is still on the scan table. At others, scans are not reviewed before the patient leaves the department. The advantage of the latter approach is improved patient throughput; however, a possible disadvantage is that patients may need to return for additional imaging because of suboptimal techniques or to clarify a finding seen on routine scans. A third option is that only certain examinations (such as adrenal studies) are checked by the radiologist before the patient leaves the department. These are most commonly examinations when the protocol may be modified on the fly or intervention may be called for. In these institutions technologists are often encouraged to carefully review images and call a radiologist whenever they suspect abnormal results.

ORGAN-SPECIFIC CONSIDERATIONS

Liver

The normal CT attenuation of the liver in unenhanced studies varies among individuals and ranges from 38 to 70 HU. In healthy subjects the attenuation of the liver is at least 10 HU greater than that of the spleen. Fatty infiltration of the liver is one of the most common abnormalities diagnosed by liver CT and can result from a variety of causes including alcoholism, obesity, diabetes, chemotherapy, corticosteroid therapy, hyperalimentation (i.e., total parental nutrition–intravenous feeding), and malnutrition. Fatty infiltration reduces the CT attenuation of the involved liver. With fatty infiltration, the liver is at least 10 HU lower than that of the spleen. Although it is most commonly a diffuse process (hence the lower attenuation is seen throughout the liver), fatty infiltration can also be focal and inhomogeneous. In the latter case it can be difficult to differentiate from tumorous mass. Fatty infiltrate (either diffuse or focal) is most accurately assessed on noncontrast CT. Many operators include a region of interest (ROI) measurement of the liver and of the spleen. A spleen measurement that is more than 10 HU higher than that of the liver indicates fatty infiltrate of the liver (Fig. 21-1).

Another common finding in the liver is a cavernous hemangioma. These benign tumors are often discovered incidentally during hepatic imaging by ultrasonography, CT, or magnetic resonance (MR). Although in the majority of cases hemangiomas are solitary, some patients have multiple lesions. Most hemangiomas have a characteristic appearance on CT. On unenhanced CT hemangiomas appear as a well-defined hypodense mass of the same density as other blood-filled spaces, such as the inferior vena cava. After IV contrast administration the lesion shows progressive pooling of contrast in rounded or oval blood-filled spaces at the lesion periphery. In most cases, with further delay the lesion fills in slowly from the periphery, eventually becoming uniformly enhanced. Occasional lesions may not fill in completely, likely because of central thrombosis (Fig. 21-2).

> **BOX 21–6 Key Concept**
>
> Fatty infiltration of the liver results in lower than normal attenuation of the liver and an abnormal attenuation difference between the liver and spleen. This is most accurately assessed on noncontrast CT. Many operators include an ROI of the liver and of the spleen. When the liver measurement is at least 10 HU lower than that of the spleen, fatty infiltrate of the liver is indicated.

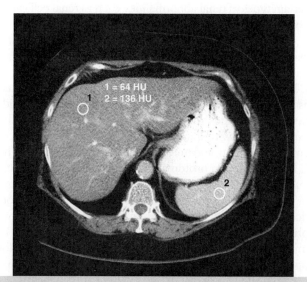

FIGURE 21-1 A ROI measurement is placed within the liver and spleen. If the spleen measures 10 HU or more than the liver, fatty infiltrate of the liver is indicated.

> **BOX 21–7 Key Concept**
>
> Most liver hemangiomas have a characteristic appearance on CT. On unenhanced CT hemangiomas appear as a well-defined hypodense mass. After IV contrast administration the lesion shows progressive "filling-in" enhancement from the periphery. Eventually the lesion becomes uniformly enhanced.

Because the liver derives approximately 25% of its blood supply from the hepatic artery and the remaining 75% from the portal vein, there are several phases of enhancement after the intravenous (IV) administration of a bolus of contrast material. The first is the hepatic arterial phase typically occurring 15 to 25 seconds after the contrast bolus, followed by the portal venous phase, which begins at 60 to 70 seconds after contrast injection. Based on contrast circulation, the hepatic arterial phase can be further divided (Chapter 13). The equilibrium phase, sometimes called the late or delayed phase, occurs several minutes after injection.

For routine abdominal CT or as part of a chest, abdomen, and pelvic study, the liver is most often scanned just once, during the portal venous phase. However, for some indications scanning in more than one enhancement phase may improve the examination's sensitivity.[2] Some tumors are supplied by an abnormal number of external blood vessels (i.e., hypervascular tumors). Because of this increased blood supply these tumors will display more intense enhancement after an IV contrast injection; these are often described as hyperenhancing. Tumors that are hyperenhancing relative to surrounding liver tissue are best detected during the late arterial phase. Liver metastases tend to be hypervascular in cases of primary tumors of the thyroid or pancreatic islet cells, carcinoid tumors, renal cell carcinoma, some breast tumors,

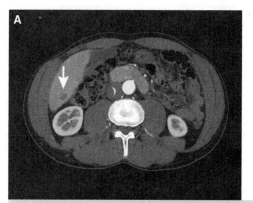 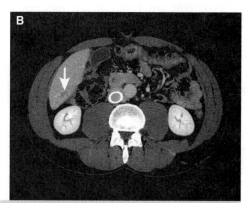

FIGURE 21-2 A. Hemangiomas (arrows) have a characteristic appearance on CT, appearing as a well-defined hypodense mass of the same density as other blood-filled spaces. **B.** After IV contrast administration, the lesion shows progressive filling in enhancement from the periphery; eventually, most lesions become uniformly enhanced (not shown). Images courtesy of the University of Michigan Health Systems.

and melanoma.[2] When these are suspected, dual-phase imaging is often beneficial. However, the majority of liver metastases are hypovascular and develop from primary tumors of the colon and rectum, pancreas, lung, urothelium, prostate, and most gynecologic malignancies. When these conditions are suspected images are typically acquired in a single (portal venous) phase.

BOX 21–8 Key Concept

For routine abdominal CT the liver is most often scanned just once, during the portal venous phase. However, for some indications (e.g., hypervascular liver lesions or hepatic vascular anatomy), scanning in more than one enhancement phase improves the examination's sensitivity.

Pancreas

CT is the imaging method of choice for evaluation of the pancreas for most indications and provides more reliable overall data than methods such as ultrasound, plain film radiography, and contrast examination of the gastrointestinal tract.

The pancreas differs in size, shape, and location depending on the individual patient. In general, the pancreas is located between the areas of the twelfth thoracic vertebra (superiorly) and the second lumbar vertebra (inferiorly). A technique that includes the use of thin slices and IV contrast enhancement improves the likelihood of visualizing the main pancreatic duct. In a jaundiced patient, noncontrast scans through the area of the common bile duct may allow visualization of common bile duct calculi. Water or low-attenuation oral contrast agents are preferred because dense contrast may obscure small stones. When initial scans fail to differentiate the margins of the pancreas from the duodenum, the patient is often given additional oral contrast material and additional slices are obtained with the patient lying in a right decubitus positions.

Multiphasic protocols are common for pancreatic indications. Most commonly, data acquisition is timed to coincide with the late arterial phase (approximately 35 to 40 seconds after a bolus injection) and the portal venous phase (approximately 65 to 70 seconds after a bolus injection). Because the exact timing of these phases is patient-dependent, bolus-tracking software is often used (Chapter 13).

Kidneys and Ureters

Most renal abnormalities are best seen on CT after IV contrast medium administration. Unenhanced CT is generally reserved to demonstrate calcifications and calculi that may be obscured by contrast agent (discussed in detail later in this chapter) or it is used as a baseline for attenuation measurements when enhancement is calculated as a feature of renal mass characterization. MDCT is the current modality of choice for renal evaluation.[3]

BOX 21–9 Key Concept

Unenhanced CT of the kidneys and ureters is generally reserved to demonstrate calcifications and calculi that may be obscured by a contrast agent.

When the examination is performed to evaluate a renal mass, scans are typically taken before the contrast bolus and at one or more phases after IV contrast administration. The corticomedullary phase typically occurs approximately 30 to 70 seconds after the contrast bolus; the nephrogram phase is seen from 80 to 120 seconds after the contrast bolus; the excretory phase begins about 3 minutes after injection and can last 15 minutes or longer. Two-dimensional and three-dimensional reformations may be helpful in defining certain types of renal abnormalities, such as renal cell carcinoma and ureteropelvic junction (UPJ) obstruction.

CT urography (CTU) is a relatively new imaging examination designed to provide a comprehensive evaluation of the upper and lower urinary tract. Many different CTU protocols are currently being used. CTU is defined as a diagnostic examination optimized for imaging the kidneys, ureters, and bladder. The examination involves the use of MDCT with thin-slice imaging, IV administration of contrast medium, and imaging in the excretory phase.[4] The CTU examination protocol is often tailored to the clinical question. Protocols may include only the excretory phase, or may contain as many as four phases (unenhanced, corticomedullary, nephrographic, and excretory). Excretory phase imaging for CTU studies can range from 3 to 16 minutes after injection. Longer delays are beneficial for opacification of the distal ureters. Contrast administration is accomplished using one of two different approaches; a single-bolus injection or a split-bolus injection. A single-bolus injection administers 100 to 150 mL of LOCM injected at a rate of 2 to 3 mL/s; scans are typically obtained in the nephrographic phase to assess the renal parenchyma and in the excretory phase to assess the urinary tract mucosa. Protocols for split-bolus injections vary somewhat, but all divide the contrast media dose into two bolus injections with a delay of 2 to 15 minutes between injections; the patient is scanned once after the second injection, reducing the radiation dose; at this point, the contrast material injected first is providing excretory phase opacification and the contrast material injected second is providing renal parenchymal enhancement. The goal of the split bolus is to image a combined nephrographic-excretory phase.

Other techniques that may be used during CTU to optimize the visualization of the urinary tract include the use of abdominal compression bands, intravenous saline hydration (approximately 250 mL of 0.9% [normal] saline), and low-dose furosemide (Lasix) injection.

Multiphase CTU imaging is associated with a relatively high radiation dose. The benefits of the examination must be carefully weighed against the risks on a patient-by-patient basis. The split-bolus technique has been gaining in popularity because by combining two phases, the radiation dose is reduced.

PROTOCOL DEVELOPMENT FOR SPECIFIC ABDOMINOPELVIC APPLICATIONS

Concepts learned in previous chapters can be applied to scanning the abdomen and pelvis. The following detailed discussions of three specific applications will provide the reader with a broader understanding of how protocols are developed to meet the needs of a specific organ or clinical indication.

CT of the Adrenal Glands

CT has become the modality of choice in the detection and characterization of adrenal masses.[5-7] This utilization can be traced to two major developments. First, because CT is so frequently used in the diagnosis of abdominal symptoms and disorders, it often uncovers unsuspected adrenal masses. In fact, because the CT studies are often ordered as a result of unrelated symptoms and the adrenal masses are found incidentally, researchers have coined the term *incidentalomas* to describe them.[8] Second, CT has gained widespread acceptance as the technique of choice for differentiating adrenal adenomas (benign adrenal masses) from metastases.[6-11]

The characterization of adrenal masses is accomplished by assessing their attenuation values and by evaluating the degree of iodinated contrast that is washed out of the mass on delayed imaging.[5-11] Because accurate characterization often requires an adjustment in the scan protocol, CT technologists should be familiar with current information. An astute technologist can save a patient the time, money, and the radiation exposure of a repeat examination by identifying an incidentaloma and tailoring the study to provide the radiologist with the data necessary to characterize the mass as benign or malignant.

BOX 21-10   Key Concept

Determining whether an adrenal mass is benign or malignant is accomplished by assessing its attenuation values and by evaluating the degree of iodinated contrast that is washed out of the mass on delayed imaging. An astute technologist can save a patient the time, money, and the radiation exposure of a repeat examination by identifying an incidentaloma and tailoring the study to provide the radiologist with the data necessary to characterize the mass as benign or malignant.

We begin by reviewing the basic anatomy and physiology of the adrenal gland. Common adrenal gland disorders are defined. This background material is followed by a look at literature that outlines the role of CT in the detection and characterization of adrenal abnormalities.

Anatomy and Physiology of the Adrenal Gland

The adrenal glands are part of the endocrine system. The endocrine system is a group of specialized organs and body tissues that produce, store, and secrete chemical substances known as hormones. As the body's chemical messengers, hormones transfer information and instructions from one set of cells to another. Endocrine glands do not have ducts to transport their product. (Unlike the endocrine glands, exocrine glands such as the mammary and salivary glands possess ducts to carry their secretory product to a surface.) The word *endocrine* is derived from the Greek terms *endo*, meaning "within," and *krine*, meaning "to separate or secrete." Endocrine glands produce hormones that are secreted directly into the blood and are then carried throughout the body, where they influence only those cells that have receptor sites for that hormone.

The adrenal glands are complex endocrine organs named for their location, which is adjacent to the kidneys (thus the name *ad-renal*). They are also occasionally referred to as suprarenal glands (*supra* means "above"). Located at the top of each kidney, they are triangular, and a normal gland weighs about 5 g (Fig. 21-3). On a cross-sectional image adrenal glands have a characteristic Y, V, or T shape (Fig. 21-4). Encased in a connective tissue capsule and usually partially buried in an island of fat, the adrenal glands, like the kidneys, are retroperitoneal; that is, they lie posterior to the peritoneum.

The outer portion of the gland is called the cortex, and the inner substance the medulla. Although the adrenal cortex and adrenal medulla are structurally one organ, they function as two separate glands. The cortex and medulla of the adrenal gland, like the anterior and posterior lobes of the pituitary, develop from different embryonic tissues and secrete different hormones. The adrenal cortex is essential to life, but the medulla may be removed with no life-threatening effects.[12] The hypothalamus of the brain influences both portions of the adrenal gland.

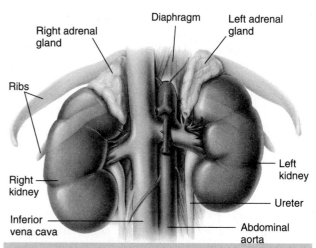

FIGURE 21-3 The triangular-shaped adrenal glands are located at the top of both kidneys.

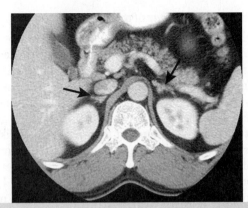

FIGURE 21-4 On a cross-sectional image, the adrenal gland has a characteristic Y, V, or T shape.

Adrenal Cortex Three different zones or layers of cells make up the adrenal cortex. Each region produces a different group or type of hormone.[13] Chemically, all the cortical hormones are steroid derivatives. That is, molecularly, they all contain the four-ring structure of the sterol nucleus. Mineralocorticoids are secreted by the outermost region of the adrenal cortex. As their name suggests, mineralocorticoids play an important part in regulating mineral salt (electrolyte) metabolism. Glucocorticoids are secreted by the middle region of the adrenal cortex. Their main function is to affect the metabolism in diverse ways. They decrease inflammation and increase resistance to stress. The innermost zone of the adrenal cortex, the zona reticularis, secretes gonadocorticoids, or sex hormones. Male hormones (androgens) and female hormones (estrogens) are secreted in both sexes by the adrenal cortex, but their effect is usually masked by the hormones from the testes and ovaries. Tumors of the adrenal cortex that secrete large amounts of androgens are known as virilizing tumors because they produce masculinizing effects in the patient.

Adrenal Medulla The adrenal medulla secretes two catecholamines, about 80% epinephrine and 20% norepinephrine.[14] Catecholamines is the general name for the group of compounds that mediate signaling in the sympathetic nervous system. These hormones affect smooth muscle, cardiac muscle, and glands the same way that sympathetic stimulation does; they serve to increase and prolong sympathetic effects. Increased epinephrine secretion by the adrenal medulla is one of the body's first responses to stress.

Adrenal Gland Disorders

The adrenal glands can have congenital defects, and they can be damaged by infections and destructive tumors. Although rare, the adrenal cortex can also be invaded by acute bacterial disease such as septicemia owing to meningococcus, which can result in failure of the cortex followed by shock and death (Waterhouse-Friderichsen syndrome).[15] In addition, chronic infection of the cortex by the tuberculosis bacillus or a fungal infection such as histoplasmosis can cause adrenal deficiency. Cancer may metastasize to the adrenal glands, although it rarely produces severe adrenal insufficiency.[15]

Primary adrenal masses can be divided into two categories based on whether they hypersecrete a hormone.[5] Hyperfunctioning adrenal masses produce a hormone that results in an endocrine imbalance. Examples of hyperfunctioning adrenal masses are pheochromocytomas, aldosteronomas, and those that power Cushing syndrome. Nonfunctioning adrenal masses cause enlargement of the adrenal gland but no significant increased hormone production. Adrenal adenomas are the most common primary nonfunctioning adrenal tumors.[5]

Diseases that result in hyperfunctioning of the adrenal gland can originate from either the adrenal medulla or the adrenal cortex. Pheochromocytoma is a neoplasm of the adrenal medulla. Most often they are unilateral and benign, but in about 10% of cases they are bilateral and in about 10% of cases they are malignant.[16] These tumors secrete hormones that can cause heart palpitations and hypertension. Hyperfunctioning tumors of the adrenal cortex can result in overproduction of cortisol (Cushing syndrome), androgens (hyperandrogenism), or aldosterone (Conn syndrome or primary hyperaldosteronism). In 15% to 25% of cases of Cushing syndrome, the cause is a primary adrenal neoplasm, usually a benign adenoma.[17] The overproduction of androgens can be caused by adrenocortical tumor, adrenal adenoma, or adrenal carcinoma.[18] Conn syndrome is a result of an adrenal adenoma in about 80% of patients, and adrenal gland hyperplasia (diffuse overgrowth without a dominant mass) in 20%.[5] The underlying reasons for the development of an adenoma or hyperplasia are not known.

Characterization of Adrenal Masses

Adrenal masses are common.[19] It is estimated that in up to 5% of patients undergoing abdominal CT such an incidentaloma is discovered.[20] The majority of these masses are benign, clinically silent lesions producing no endocrine abnormality. It has been reported that benign adrenal cortical adenomas are 60 times more common than primary adrenal cortical carcinomas.[21] However, even in oncology patients, most adrenal masses are adenomas rather than metastasis.[22] In cases in which the patient has a history of cancer, particularly cancer of the lung, metastasis to the adrenal gland indicates advanced disease that is not amenable to surgical resection and potential cure.[5] Therefore, differentiating an adrenal mass as benign or malignant is especially critical in the oncology patient, because they are more likely to have an adrenal metastasis than is a nononcology patient, and because it will greatly affect treatment and prognosis.

Although the vast majority of adrenal incidentalomas are benign, the consequences of misidentifying the uncommon malignant adrenal mass are dire. Therefore, every adrenal mass warrants follow-up for characterization. In the past, this characterization was accomplished primarily through repeated follow-up CT scan to assess for size change or fine-needle aspiration (FNA) biopsy of the adrenal mass. Although quite accurate, biopsy is by nature somewhat invasive and has some associated risks. Ideally, FNA biopsy would be performed only on those masses that had a high likelihood of malignancy.

Specialized imaging protocols attempt to characterize lesions of the adrenal gland. The goals of imaging are to reduce the number of unnecessary biopsies, the number of follow-up studies needed for an accurate diagnosis, and the cost of care.

BOX 21–11   Key Concept

Specialized adrenal imaging protocols attempt to characterize lesions of the adrenal gland. The goals of imaging are to reduce the number of unnecessary biopsies, the number of follow-up studies needed for an accurate diagnosis, and the cost of care.

There are certain general imaging findings that can help in differentiating benign adrenal lesions from malignant ones. Larger lesions have a greater likelihood of being malignant. In particular, lesions greater than 4 cm in diameter are more likely to be either a metastasis or a primary adrenal carcinoma than are smaller lesions.[5] Adenomas most often grow slowly, so lesions that change in size quickly may be malignant. The shape of the adrenal mass can also be a helpful indicator of malignancy. Adenomas tend to have smooth margins

and a homogeneous density, but metastases are more often heterogeneous and have an irregular shape. Unfortunately, although these characteristics are useful indicators in differentiating a benign from a malignant mass, they are not specific enough to be used alone in making a diagnosis.

However, two unique features of adenomas on CT can be used to differentiate adenomas from malignant lesions with a high degree of accuracy. One is based on an anatomic (histologic) trait, and the second is physiologic in nature. The variance in intracellular lipid (fat) content between adenomas and malignant adrenal masses reflects the anatomic difference. The way each type of mass responds to iodinated contrast enhancement is indicative of the physiologic difference.

Intracellular Lipid Content   On CT, fat has characteristically low attenuation properties, ranging from approximately −100 to −50 HU. Hence, the amount of intracellular lipid (fat molecules) a mass contains affects its CT appearance; masses with a higher fat content are reflected as areas of lower attenuation (darker) on the CT image. This fact is useful because malignant adrenal masses contain very little lipid within their cellular cytoplasm. Conversely, most adenomas contain an abundance of intracytoplasmic fat. Korobkin et al.[23] performed a study that demonstrated a high correlation between adrenal fat content and low attenuation on CT. Because malignancies do not contain enough fat to be reflected in lower CT attenuation, it can be safely concluded that any homogeneous adrenal mass that measures less than 10 HU on unenhanced CT is benign. However, the converse cannot be made. That is, lesions measuring greater than 10 HU on unenhanced CT cannot automatically be assumed to be malignant. Although 70% of adenomas

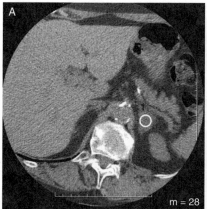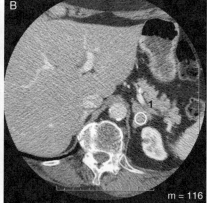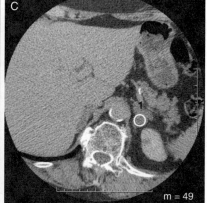

FIGURE 21-5 This series of scans illustrates how adrenal masses may be characterized using contrast medium washout. **A.** Unenhanced image, in which the adrenal mass measures 28 HU. **B.** Initial enhanced image, in which the mass measures 116 HU. **C.** Image taken after a delay of 15 minutes, in which the mass measures 44 HU. Washout = (116 – 44) / 116 – 28) = 0.81 (or 81% washout). Because this is greater than 60%, the measurement indicates the adrenal mass is benign. Images courtesy of the University of Michigan Health Systems.

possess an abundance of intercellular lipid, approximately 30% do not. In other words, adenomas can be classified as lipid-rich when they measure less than or equal to 10 HU, or as lipid-poor when they measure greater than or equal to 10 HU.[7]

BOX 21-12   Key Concept

Any homogenous adrenal mass that measures less than 10 HU on unenhanced CT is benign; no adjustment to the scan protocol is necessary.

Two issues created the need for an additional CT imaging strategy. The first, of course, is the fact that on unenhanced CT alone, an incidentaloma that is greater than or equal to 10 HU cannot be accurately characterized, because it could represent either a malignant mass or a lipid-poor adenoma. The second factor is that most CT examinations of the body are performed with contrast enhancement; therefore, an unenhanced image of the adrenal gland may not be immediately available. Often, an enlarged adrenal gland is first noticed on an enhanced CT study. In this situation, the ability to characterize the adrenal mass from the enhanced study could save the patient a return visit for an unenhanced examination.

Contrast Washout   The second imaging parameter to differentiate adenomas from metastases relies on physiologic differences in perfusion. Adenomas enhance rapidly with intravenous contrast media, and the agent washes out rapidly. Metastases also enhance quickly but retain the contrast longer. This difference in washout of iodinated contrast can be exploited to further differentiate benign from malignant adrenal lesions (Fig. 21-5).

Typically, contrast-enhanced CT is performed in the portal venous phase of enhancement, approximately 60 seconds from the start of the bolus injection of iodinated contrast material. Although this phase is useful for detecting most abnormalities of the liver and pancreas, it is of no use in the characterization of adrenal incidentalomas, because at 60 seconds after injection, adenomas may have the same attenuation values as malignant adrenal masses (i.e., typically both enhance similarly). However, if additional images are taken from 5 to 15 minutes after the contrast injection, differences in washout of the contrast agent can be assessed. Several studies have investigated the use of delayed CT to characterized adrenal lesions.[7,10,11,19]

The degree of washout can be calculated using either of two simple formulas.* The first formula assumes that unenhanced, enhanced (at portal venous phase), and

15-minute-delayed images are available. If these images are all available, an ROI is placed on the adrenal mass and an HU measurement is taken on each set of images. The washout can then be calculated as follows:

$$\frac{\text{Enhanced} - \text{Delayed}}{\text{Enhanced} - \text{Unenhanced}} \times 100 = \% \text{ washout}$$

To illustrate, an ROI is placed on the adrenal mass; unenhanced = 28 HU; enhanced = 116 HU; 15-minute delayed = 44 HU. Therefore,

$$\frac{116 - 44}{116 - 28} \times 100 = 81\%$$

The second formula is designed for situations in which unenhanced images are not available and is called the relative washout. It is calculated as follows:

$$\frac{\text{Enhanced} - \text{Delayed}}{\text{Enhanced}} \times 100 = \% \text{ relative washout}$$

Using the above example:

$$\frac{116 - 44}{116} \times 100 = 62\% \text{ relative washout}$$

A washout of greater than 60% is specific for adenoma, and a washout less than 60% indicates malignancy. When a relative washout value is used, the threshold is 40%.[9] Hence, a relative washout value that is equal or greater to 40% is specific for adenomas and, when relative washout is less than 40%, malignancy is likely. When washout or relative washout values obtained using CT indicate that an adrenal mass has a high likelihood of malignancy, biopsy is often used to confirm the diagnosis.

Using CT imaging guidelines has made a significant impact on the number of biopsies performed on adrenal masses. At the University of Michigan, an imaging protocol was established for the characterization of incidentalomas. Before the implementation of these guidelines, 40% to 57% of adrenal masses biopsied were adenomas. After the imaging protocols were applied, only 12% of biopsied adrenal masses were adenomas.[24]

Summary

The adrenal gland is a frequent site of a clinically silent mass. The incidental discovery of an unsuspected adrenal mass has increased in past years, correlating to the increased use of body CT. The majority of incidentalomas are benign. Although the possibility of malignancy is small, the risk necessitates that each adrenal mass be evaluated further. Biopsy can provide a definitive diagnosis, but biopsy is somewhat invasive and is associated with a small but real risk of complications. These circumstances have

---

*The formulas are given and explained here, but adrenal mass calculations are widely available on the World Wide Web.

prompted the search for a noninvasive imaging procedure that can accurately characterize adrenal masses as either benign or malignant. Two traits of adenomas, one anatomic and one physiologic, have allowed CT to be used to differentiate adenomas from malignant lesions with a high degree of accuracy. A homogeneous adrenal mass with an associated attenuation number on unenhanced CT of less than 10 HU is considered lipid-rich and can confidently be identified as an adenoma. To rule out malignancy in a mass whose attenuation value is greater than 10 HU, another aspect must be considered, that of contrast washout. This trait is examined by comparing the attenuation value of the mass just after contrast enhancement with the attenuation value of the mass 15 minutes after contrast has been injected. In this way, lipid-poor adenomas can be distinguished from nonadenomas. A percentage washout threshold value of greater than or equal to 60% or a relative percentage washout threshold of greater than or equal to 40% is specific for adenoma.

Technologists play an important role in the identification and characterization of adrenal masses, as they are often the first to discover an incidentaloma. A technologist who is aware of the issues surrounding the characterization of adrenal mass can bring an incidentaloma to the attention of the radiologist. Small adjustments such as the addition of delayed images may save the patient the time, expense, and the additional radiation exposure of a repeat examination.

CT in the Diagnosis of Acute Appendicitis

The usefulness of CT in the diagnosis of acute appendicitis has been reported as far back as 1985.[25] Only in the last 15 years, however, with advances such as helical scanning and MDCT technology has appendiceal CT emerged as the dominant imaging method for the evaluation of adults with suspected appendicitis.[26-28] This section begins by reviewing the basic anatomy and physiology of the appendix; the origin and development of appendicitis are then explored. This background material is followed by a look at recent literature outlining the role CT plays in the detection of acute appendicitis.

Anatomy and Function of Appendix

The appendix is a small, tubelike structure projecting from the cecum (Fig. 21-6). It is often referred to as the vermiform appendix; the adjective *vermiform* literally means wormlike. The appendix can vary in length from less than 1 cm to greater than 30 cm, although the majority fall between 6 and 9 cm.[29] The base of the appendix is fixed to the cecum, whereas the remainder of the appendix is free. This fact accounts for its variable location; the tip can be found in a retrocecal, pelvic, subcecal, preileal, or right pericolic position (Fig. 21-7). McBurney's point is the name given to the point that is one third of the distance from the right anterior superior iliac spine to the

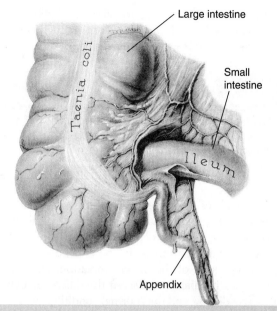

FIGURE 21-6 The appendix is a finger-sized structure found at the base of the cecum, arising proximal to the ileocecal valve.

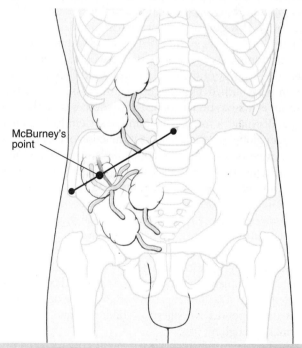

FIGURE 21-7 Variable locations of the normal appendix.

umbilicus. Patients with acute appendicitis often, but not always, have tenderness at this point.

The variable position of the appendix is important because it contributes to the diverse clinical presentation of acute appendicitis. This variation in positioning also makes the appendix more challenging to locate on cross-sectional images. In addition, appendiceal absence, duplication, and diverticula have all been described. These findings further complicate the task of identifying disease. Such considerations will be explored later.

BOX 21-13   Key Concept

The variable position of the appendix is important because it contributes to the diverse clinical presentation of acute appendicitis. This variation in positioning also makes the appendix more challenging to locate on cross-sectional images.

The wall of the appendix is composed of all tissue layers typical of the intestine, but the wall is thicker and contains a concentration of lymphoid tissue. Similar to the tonsils, the lymphatic tissue in the appendix is typically in a constant state of chronic inflammation. This scenario often makes it difficult to discern the difference between pathologic disease and the "normal condition."[30]

For many years, it was believed that the appendix had no function in modern humans. It was thought to be vestigial, that is, serving an important function in our evolutionary ancestors, but diminishing in importance or becoming useless as the species evolved. (Other examples of vestiges are the wings of the ostrich and the eyes of the blind cavefish.) This philosophy is apparent in a description by Romer and Parsons, authors of a standard text of comparative anatomy: "Its major importance would appear to be financial support of the surgical profession."[31] Some more recently published reports question the assumption that the appendix has no function. These sources state that the appendix plays a role in the immune system by secreting immunoglobulin.[29] Regardless of its function or lack thereof, there is consensus that the appendix is not essential and can be removed with no associated predisposition to sepsis or any other manifestation of immunocompromise.

The amount of lymphoid tissue in the appendix affects its size. Lymphoid tissue increases throughout puberty, remains steady for the next decade, and then begins a steady decrease with increasing age. After the age of 60, virtually no lymphoid tissue remains within the appendix, and complete obliteration of the appendiceal lumen is common.[29] This finding correlates with the observation that the appendix is longest in childhood and gradually shrinks throughout life.[30]

Incidence of Acute Appendicitis

Appendicitis is common; the lifetime occurrence is approximately 7%.[29,32] The peak occurrence of appendicitis is seen in patients between ages 10 and 40, with a mean age of 31 years and a median age of 22 years. It is slightly more common in males than in females, with a ratio of 1.14:1.[33] The standard for management of appendicitis is appendectomy.

It is not uncommon for surgeons to remove a healthy appendix in patients undergoing surgery for another disorder (e.g., Crohn's disease). These surgeries are referred to as incidental appendectomies. In the case of Crohn disease, this surgery is performed to avoid confusing the diagnosis later on, because the symptoms of Crohn disease can mimic those of appendicitis. With the rate of incidental appendectomies included, the lifetime rate of appendectomy is 12% for men and 25% for women.[29]

In children, appendicitis is the most common condition requiring emergency abdominal surgery.[34] Appendicitis is diagnosed in 1% to 8% of children who come to the emergency department for the evaluation of abdominal pain. However, this condition is rare in very young children (i.e., younger than 5 years of age).[33,34]

Prognosis

The mortality from appendicitis in the United States has steadily decreased from a rate of 9.9 per 100,000 in 1939 to 0.2 per 100,000 as of 1986.[29] The decrease in mortality is mainly attributed to advances in anesthesia, intravenous fluids, and the effectiveness of antibiotics. The principal factors associated with mortality are whether rupture occurs before surgical treatment and the age of the patient. The case-fatality rate of appendicitis jumps from less than 1% with no perforation to 5% or higher when perforation occurs.[26] The mortality rate of ruptured appendicitis in the elderly is approximately 15%, much higher than in younger age groups.[29]

Death is usually attributable to uncontrolled sepsis–peritonitis, intra-abdominal abscesses, or Gram-negative septicemia.

Morbidity rates parallel mortality rates; they are significantly increased by rupture of the appendix and affected to a lesser extent by old age. In one report, complications occurred in 3% of patients with nonperforated appendicitis and in 47% of patients who experienced perforation.[29]

Overall, the perforation rate is approximately 19%, and is significantly higher in elderly patients (44%) and small children (36%).[33] The accurate and timely diagnosis of acute appendicitis is important to minimize morbidity. Prompt surgical treatment may reduce the risk of appendix perforation.[26,32,34] Because prompt treatment is important, a margin of error in overdiagnosis is generally considered acceptable.[32] However, overdiagnosis must be weighed against the risks and expense associated with unnecessary surgery.

Etiology and Pathogenesis

The pathophysiology of appendicitis begins with obstruction of the narrow appendiceal lumen. Obstruction has multiple causes. Fecaliths are the most common cause of appendiceal obstruction.[29] Lymphoid hyperplasia (the proliferation of normal cells resembling lymph tissue) is another common cause and can be related to viral illnesses, including upper respiratory tract infection, mononucleosis, or gastroenteritis.[32] Less common causes are hardened barium from previous x-ray studies, tumors, vegetable and fruit seeds, and intestinal parasites.

A predictable series of events leads to the eventual rupture of the appendix. When the appendiceal lumen is obstructed, normal secretion by the appendiceal mucosa will rapidly produce distention. The capacity of the normal appendiceal lumen is only 0.1 mL.[29] Therefore, only a minimal amount of secretion behind an obstruction is sufficient to cause distention, which then stimulates the nerve endings of the viscera. This stimulation results in vague, dull, diffuse pain in the midabdomen or lower epigastric region. Peristalsis is also stimulated by the sudden distention, so that early in the course of appendicitis cramping may occur along with the visceral pain. Distention continues as a result of continuing mucosal secretions and rapid multiplication of bacteria residing in the appendix. This distention often causes reflex nausea and vomiting, and the abdominal pain becomes more severe. The inflammatory process soon expands to involve the adjacent peritoneum; involvement of this region produces the characteristic shift in pain to the right lower quadrant.

The mucosa of the appendix—like the rest of the gastrointestinal tract—is susceptible to bacterial invasion when impairment of blood supply occurs. Therefore, as progressive distention affects blood flow, tissue necrosis develops in areas with the poorest blood supply. As distention, bacterial invasion, compromise of vascular supply, and tissue death progress, perforation occurs. Perforation generally occurs just beyond the obstruction because that is the point at which intraluminal tension is typically the greatest.

However, this sequence is not inevitable. There have been reports of episodes of acute appendicitis spontaneously subsiding.[29] Many patients with acute appendicitis undergoing surgery report previous similar—but less severe—attacks of right lower quadrant pain. Pathologic examination of the appendices removed from these patients often reveals thickening and scarring, which suggests old, healed, acute inflammation.[35,36]

Clinical Presentations

The diagnosis of acute appendicitis remains problematic. Patients with the disease may present with a wide variety of clinical manifestations, and thus the diagnosis may elude even the most experienced clinicians.[37] The classic presentation of a patient with appendicitis is right lower quadrant pain, abdominal rigidity, and migration of pain from the periumbilical region to the right lower quadrant.[26] These findings occur in approximately 50% of patients.[37] Unusual presentations can occur when 1) the appendix is not in its normal location, 2) the patient is young or elderly, and 3) the patient is pregnant. No single clinical finding can effectively rule out or confirm the diagnosis of acute appendicitis. Diagnosis is particularly difficult in women of childbearing age because acute gynecologic conditions such as pelvic inflammatory disease may mimic signs of appendicitis.[26] Consequently, the false-negative appendectomy (i.e., removal of a normal appendix) rate has been reported to be as high as 47% in female patients who are between 10 and 39 years of age.[37] These difficulties contribute to the many malpractice claims related to the misdiagnosis of appendicitis.[38] The overall diagnostic accuracy rate achieved by the traditional history, physical examination, and laboratory tests has been approximately 80%.[37]

Abdominal pain is the most common symptom of appendicitis. Loss of appetite (anorexia) and nausea and vomiting are also common symptoms (Table 21-2). In a classic presentation, a patient with appendicitis reports symptoms that occur in a predicable sequence. This sequence starts as poorly localized periumbilical pain followed by nausea and vomiting, followed by migration

---

TABLE 21-2 Prevalence of Common Signs and Symptoms of Appendicitis[a]

Symptom	Frequency (%)
Abdominal pain	99–100
Anorexia	99
Right lower quadrant pain or tenderness	96
Nausea	90
Vomiting	75
Low-grade fever	67–69
Classic symptom sequence (vague periumbilical pain to anorexia/nausea/unsustained vomiting to migration of pain to right lower quadrant to low-grade fever)	50
Rebound tenderness	26
Right lower quadrant guarding	21

[a]Data from Old JL, Dussing RW, Yap W, Dirks J. Imaging for suspected appendicitis. Am Fam Physician 2005;71:71–8; Jaffe BM, Berger DH. Schwartz's Principles of Surgery, Part II: Special Considerations. The Appendix. 8th Ed. New York: McGraw Hill, 2005: Chapter 29; and Rhea JT, Halpern EF, Ptak T, Lawrason JN, Sacknoff R, Novelline RA. The status of appendiceal CT in an urban medical center 5 years after its introduction: experience with 753 patients. AJR Am J Roentgenol Am J Roentgenol 2005;184:1802–8.

of pain to the right lower quadrant. Again, although this is the most common pattern of symptoms, it occurs in only approximately half of patients who have appendicitis. Clinical examination may help confirm the diagnosis in atypical cases.

If the inflamed appendix lies in the typical anterior position, the classic right lower quadrant physical signs will be present (Table 21-3).[29] In these cases tenderness is often the most intense at or near McBurney's point. Direct rebound tenderness is usually present. Additionally, referred or indirect rebound tenderness is common. This type of pain is referred to as Rovsing's sign and indicates peritoneal irritation. Rovsing's sign is elicited when palpation in the left lower quadrant produces pain in the right lower quadrant. Increased pain with coughing (Dunphy's sign) is a less consistent finding, but this sign may also be present. It is common for patients who have appendicitis to prefer to lie supine—with knees drawn up—for comfort.

If the appendix is in a retrocecal position, the anterior abdominal findings are less pronounced, and tenderness may be more pronounced in the flank.[29] The posteriorly located appendix may lie near to the iliopsoas muscle, giving rise to the psoas sign, another indicator of appendicitis.[26] This test is performed by having the patient lie on his or her left side as the examiner slowly extends the right thigh, thus stretching the iliopsoas muscle. The test finding is positive if extension produces pain.

When the inflamed appendix hangs into the pelvis, abdominal findings may be entirely absent, and the diagnosis may be missed unless a digital examination of the rectum is performed. As the examining finger exerts pressure on the peritoneum of the cul-de-sac of Douglas, pain is felt in the suprapubic area as well as locally within the rectum.[29] Pain resulting from the internal rotation of the right thigh is called the obturator sign and is also an indicator that the diseased appendix resides in the pelvis.[26]

Differential Diagnosis

Although the signs and symptoms associated with acute appendicitis in its many presentations are well described, it must be remembered that an essentially identical clinical picture can result from a wide variety of other acute processes within or near the peritoneal cavity (Table 21-4).

Laboratory Tests

In general, laboratory tests such as the white blood cell (WBC) count, differential, and C-reactive protein (CRP) are only moderately helpful in confirming the diagnosis of appendicitis because many other conditions can produce the same abnormal laboratory results (i.e., laboratory tests have low specificity for appendicitis). The WBC count is elevated (greater than 10,000 per mm^3) in 70% to 90% of all cases of acute appendicitis.[39] Unfortunately, the WBC is elevated in up to 70% of patients with other causes of right lower quadrant pain.[32] Repeated WBC measurements during 4 to 8 hours may aid in the diagnosis as the WBC count often increases in acute appendicitis (except in cases of perforation, in which it may fall).[39] Similarly, an increase in the number of neutrophil leukocytes in the blood (i.e., neutrophilia) is present in the majority of appendicitis cases. CRP is a laboratory test that measures the concentration of a serum protein that indicates acute inflammation. The CRP is most likely to be elevated

---

TABLE 21-3   Common Signs of Acute Appendicitis[a]

Sign	Description
McBurney's sign	Localized right lower quadrant pain or guarding on palpation of the abdomen
Rovsing's sign	Pain in right lower quadrant with palpation of left lower quadrant
Dunphy's sign	Increased pain in the right lower quadrant with coughing
Hip flexion	Patient maintains hip flexion with knees drawn up for comfort
Psoas sign	Pain on hyperextension of right thigh
Obturator sign	Pain on internal rotation of right thigh

[a]Data from Old JL, Dussing RW, Yap W, Dirks J. Imaging for suspected appendicitis. Am Fam Physician 2005;71:71–8; Jaffe BM, Berger DH. Schwartz's Principles of Surgery, Part II: Special Considerations. The Appendix. 8th Ed. New York: McGraw Hill, 2005: Chapter 29; and Rhea JT, Halpern EF, Ptak T, Lawrason JN, Sacknoff R, Novelline RA. The status of appendiceal CT in an urban medical center 5 years after its introduction: experience with 753 patients. AJR Am J Roentgenol Am J Roentgenol 2005;184:1802–8.

TABLE 21-4   Diseases Most Commonly Mistaken for Appendicitis[a]

Pediatric Patients	Adult Patients
Abdominal pain of unknown origin	Abdominal pain of unknown origin
Mesenteric lymphadenitis	Gastroenteritis
Gastroenteritis	Diverticulitis
Meckel's diverticulitis	Gallbladder disease
Testicular torsion	Pancreatitis
Urinary tract infection	Urinary tract infection
	Bowel obstruction
	Pelvic inflammatory disease
	Ovarian cyst/cyst rupture
	Intra-abdominal tumors

[a]Data from Graffeo CS, Counselman FL. Appendicitis. Emerg Med Clin North Am 1996;14:653–71.

in appendicitis if symptoms are present for more than 12 hours.[39] An elevated CRP level combined with an elevated WBC count and neutrophilia is a good indicator of acute appendicitis. Therefore, if all three of these findings are absent, the chance of appendicitis is low.[32] In one study, researchers reported that only 4% of patients had normal laboratory test findings.[40]

In patients with appendicitis, a urinalysis may demonstrate changes such as mild pyuria, proteinuria, and hematuria. However, urinalysis is more effective in excluding urinary tract causes of abdominal pain than in diagnosing appendicitis.[32]

In summary, although abnormal laboratory tests are almost always present in patients who have appendicitis, clinicians typically do not place too much emphasis on the value of these tests: laboratory test findings can be normal in a small number of cases of appendicitis and abnormal test results have a low specificity for appendicitis.

Imaging Studies

As mentioned earlier, many diseases other than acute appendicitis may produce signs and symptoms indistinguishable from those of acute appendicitis. In situations for which a clear diagnosis of appendicitis cannot be made by the patient's history, physical examination, and laboratory evaluation, radiologic testing–particularly ultrasonography and CT–can be useful.

Plain radiographs of the abdomen are frequently obtained as part of the general evaluation of a patient with an acute abdomen, but they are rarely helpful in diagnosing acute appendicitis.[39] Barium enema is unreliable in the diagnosis of acute appendicitis and has been replaced by ultrasonography and CT.

Ultrasonography is inexpensive and widely available, does not require contrast agents, and poses no special risk to the fetus in pregnant patients. It is particularly well suited for evaluating right lower quadrant or pelvic pain in pediatric and female patients. However, the technique used to visualize the appendix, called graded compression sonography, is highly operator dependent.[26,29,32,41,42] Some of the difficulties with ultrasonography are related to the fact that a normal appendix must be identified to rule out acute appendicitis.[26] This is difficult in obese or very muscular patients or when there is an associated ileus that produces shadowing secondary to overlying gas-filled loops of bowel.[26,27,31] Accuracy of ultrasound also decreases with retrocecal or pelvic locations of the appendix. In addition, the following scenarios can occur: a false-positive scan can occur in the presence of periappendicitis from surrounding inflammation; a dilated fallopian tube can be mistaken for an inflamed appendix; or inspissated stool can mimic an appendicolith.[26,29] Finally, patients often complain of discomfort resulting from the transducer pressure during ultrasound evaluation. Despite these limitations, when institutions are comfortable with ultrasound for the evaluation of suspected appendicitis, ultrasonography continues to serve as the primary imaging study in children and in young or pregnant women.

CT is more accurate than ultrasonography; also, because it is not as dependent on the skill and experience of the operator, CT is more reproducible from hospital to hospital.[26] The diagnostic accuracy rate of CT for acute appendicitis is reported to range between 93% and 98%.[26,29,37,39,43] Findings on CT increased the certainty of diagnosis more than findings on ultrasonography.[44] Although ultrasonography is recommended as the initial imaging study in children, young women, and pregnant women, CT is most often recommended as the initial study in all other patients. In addition, CT is recommended for patients in whom sonographic evaluation is suboptimal or indeterminate, or for those patients in whom perforation is suspected.[26,39,44,45] Table 21-5 compares ultrasonography with CT for suspected appendicitis.

Common CT Findings in Acute Appendicitis   The most common CT findings in acute appendicitis are a dilated nonopacified appendix (Fig. 21-8), soft tissue stranding (inflammation) into adjacent periappendiceal fat

---

TABLE 21-5   Comparison of Ultrasonography and CT for Suspected Appendicitis[a]

Category	Ultrasonography	CT
Accuracy (%)	71–97	93–98
Advantages	Easily available, noninvasive, no radiation, rapid, no preparation needed, ability to diagnose other sources of pain (especially gynecologic disorders)	More accurate, better identification of phlegmon and abscess, may complement ultrasonography when results are suboptimal, better ability to detect normal appendix, better at determining alternative diagnosis (e.g., ureter stone, diverticulitis, and pancreatitis)
Disadvantages	Highly operator dependent, not as accurate as CT, difficult with large body habitus, cannot rule out appendicitis if appendix is not apparent	Radiation exposure, patient discomfort/risk if contrast media is used, more expensive than ultrasonography, not as good for gynecologic disorders

[a]Data from Old JL, Dussing RW, Yap W, Dirks J. Imaging for suspected appendicitis. Am Fam Physician 2005;71:71–8.

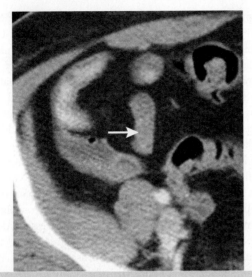

FIGURE 21-8 A common CT finding in acute appendicitis is a dilated nonopacified appendix (arrow). Image courtesy of the University of Michigan Health Systems.

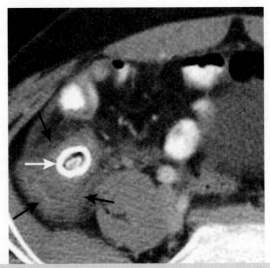

FIGURE 21-10 Appendicolith (white arrow) with surrounding inflammation (black arrows). Image courtesy of the University of Michigan Health Systems.

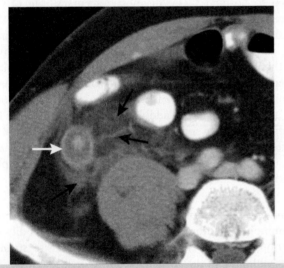

FIGURE 21-9 A thickened appendix (white arrow) surrounded by abnormal inflamed fat (black arrows) is shown. Image courtesy of the University of Michigan Health Systems.

BOX 21–14   Key Concept

There is considerable variation in appendicitis protocols; they may use different combinations of oral, rectal, IV, or no contrast material. Protocols also differ regarding the anatomic area to be included in the scan. For diagnosing appendicitis the reported accuracy of all protocol variations is high. These techniques may vary most in their rate of providing an alternative diagnosis when the appendix is found to be normal.

(Fig. 21-9), and appendicolith (Fig. 21-10).[46] When the appendix is not seen, appendicitis is typically excluded if other signs of appendicitis are absent.[47] In addition, CT scans are generally considered to be negative for appendicitis in the following scenarios: 1) the appendiceal lumen fills completely with oral or rectal contrast material or air; 2) the appendiceal lumen contains air and contrast material, and the appendix is less than or equal to 6 mm in maximum diameter; 3) the appendiceal wall is less than 2 mm thick; 4) no periappendiceal inflammation is present[47] (Figs. 21-11, 21-12).

Different investigators have suggested different combinations of CT findings to obtain a definitive diagnosis of appendicitis. For example, Wijetunga and colleagues[47] interpreted the CT scan as positive for appendicitis if three or more of the following criteria are present: 1) the appendix is greater than 6 mm in maximum diameter; 2) there is no contrast material in the appendiceal lumen; 3) inflammatory changes in the periappendiceal fat are present (e.g., fat stranding or phlegmon, extraluminal gas bubbles, fluid collection, or enlarged lymph nodes); 4) appendicoliths (one or more) are present; and 5) cecal wall thickening is present. Occasionally, patients with right lower quadrant pain will have CT images that show only one indication of appendicitis. In these situations, the radiologist may be uncertain as to whether appendicitis is present.[5] Other researchers have diagnosed appendicitis solely on the basis of the presence of an abnormal appearance of the appendix.[48,49]

Appendiceal CT Protocols

All current protocols incorporate the prospective acquisition of thin-section ($\leq$5 mm) images. Thin slices improve the z axis resolution by reducing partial volume averaging,

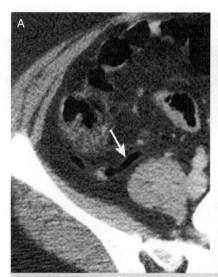
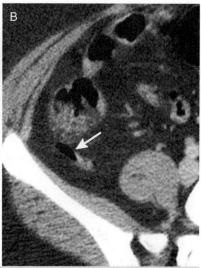

FIGURE 21-11 Normal air-filled appendix (arrow). Images courtesy of the University of Michigan Health Systems.

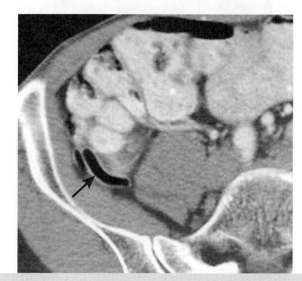

FIGURE 21-12 Appearance of a normal appendix (arrow) on a scan done with IV and oral contrast. Image courtesy of the University of Michigan Health Systems.

thereby improving the visualization of appendiceal abnormalities.[50] There is considerable variation in appendicitis protocols reported in the literature. The various procedures use different combinations of oral, rectal, IV, or no contrast materials (Table 21-6). Protocols also differ regarding the anatomic area to be included in the scan. It is interesting to note that regardless of the technique used, the reported accuracy in diagnosing appendicitis is high.[28,44] The various techniques differ in their rate of providing alternative diagnoses when the appendix is found to be normal. However, the related studies have also varied in the patient selection criteria and other important design criteria, so it is difficult to draw definite conclusions by simply comparing results. Consequently, debate still exists over the optimal appendicitis CT protocol.

Some investigators advocate a protocol that limits the scan area to the lower abdomen and upper pelvis.[47,51,52] This technique is referred to as focused appendiceal CT and has the advantage of reducing the patient's radiation exposure. The disadvantage of a focused technique is the potential for incomplete visualization or nonvisualization of the appendix. This is of particular concern because the appendix can vary considerably in length and position (Figs. 21-13, 21-14). In addition, limiting the scan area to the lower abdomen and upper pelvis may reduce the ability to provide alternative diagnoses when the appendix is normal.

Focused appendiceal CT protocols have been proposed with the range of contrast media choices seen in Table 21-6. When contrast is given orally, adequate opacification of ileocecal bowel may take 45 to 90 minutes. Rao et al.[51] have suggested a technique designed to reduce this wait time. In this protocol, a limited CT study of the right lower quadrant is performed after the rapid administration of rectal contrast material. A limitation of this scanning method is that some patients will require additional scanning of the proximal abdomen or the distal pelvis to identify disease not included in the initial scan range. In addition, other researchers express doubt that rectally administered contrast material provides sufficient added benefit to warrant its use.[47,53,54]

A CT protocol has also been advocated that includes the entire abdomen and pelvis but does not incorporate any contrast agents.[48,53] This examination can typically be performed in 10 minutes or less, does not expose the patient to the potential risks associated with intravenous iodinated contrast agents, and requires no bowel preparation. This technique is often favored in patients with

TABLE 21-6   Examples of Different CT Protocols for the Diagnosis of Acute Appendicitis

Researchers	Oral Contrast	Rectal Contrast	IV Contrast	Accuracy in Diagnosing Appendicitis (%)	Rate of Providing Alternative Diagnoses (%)
Raman et al.[19a]	Yes	No	Yes	97.6	66.2
Kamel et al..[22]	Yes	No	Yes	99	66
Peck et al.[24]	No	No	No	97.5	22
Funaki et al.[25]	Yes	No	No	95	54
Lane et al.[27]	No	No	No	97	35
Rao et al.[28]	No	Yes	No	98	62
Rao et al.[29]	Yes	Yes	Yes	98	80

[a]This study included various groups of patients examined with different techniques of intravenous (IV), oral, and rectal contrast agents. Figures reported are for the majority subset that included both IV and oral contrast agents.

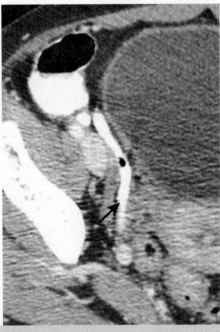

FIGURE 21-13 Contrast-filled appendix located in the pelvis. Image courtesy of the University of Michigan Health Systems.

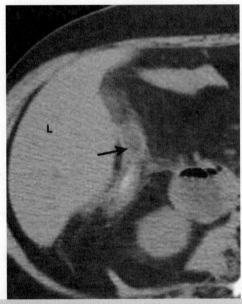

FIGURE 21-14 Unusual right upper quadrant location of an inflamed appendix indicated by arrow. (L = liver). Image courtesy of the University of Michigan Health Systems.

large body habitus, because diagnostic accuracy may be compromised in patients who have little abdominal and intrapelvic fat.[37]

Probably the most widespread CT approach is to scan the entire abdomen and pelvis with both intravenous and oral contrast material. Those who use this method believe that contrast-enhanced CT is essential to diagnose many of the other conditions that cause acute abdominal pain and may simulate appendicitis. Jacobs et al.[55] state, "… our study findings demonstrated that use of intravenous contrast material significantly improved the readers' ability to identify the inflamed appendix, to diagnose acute appendicitis, and to establish alternative diagnoses.… Finally, diagnosis of appendicitis may be missed with a focused

helical CT technique if the inflamed appendix lies outside the limited scanning field of view."

Opacification of the terminal ileum and cecum with oral contrast material has been advocated to avoid a false-positive result, a scenario in which fluid-filled terminal ileal loops are misdiagnosed as a distended, inflamed appendix.[37] The oral administration of up to 800 mL of contrast medium during a minimum of 1 hour before scanning enables the opacification of both the small bowel and right colon in most patients.[47] Water-soluble agents such as diatrizoate sodium (Hypaque, GE Healthcare) mixed with sorbitol (an osmotic laxative) tend to stimulate peristalsis and thus move through the small intestine more quickly than do barium suspensions.[47]

Conclusion

Although appendicitis is a common cause of acute abdominal pain, its diagnosis can be problematic because patients who have the disease may present with a wide variety of clinical manifestations and because a number of other clinical conditions can simulate appendicitis. CT has proved to be an important imaging tool that substantially improves diagnostic accuracy, particularly in patients with atypical clinical presentations. To date, various investigators have used the following CT protocols to diagnose appendicitis: without contrast material, with contrast material administered both orally and rectally, with rectal contrast material only, or with oral and intravenous contrast material.

CT in the Diagnosis of Urinary Tract Calculi

Introduction

Imaging plays an essential role in the diagnosis and initial management of urolithiasis. The imaging methods used have undergone considerable evolution in recent years. One major advance is the use of noncontrast helical computed tomography (NCHCT) in patients who are suspected of having renal colic. Here we review various aspects of the formation, diagnosis, and management of urolithiasis.

Terminology The terms *kidney stones, renal stones, renal calculi, nephrolithiasis,* and *urolithiasis* are often used interchangeably to refer to the gravel-like deposits that may appear in any part of the urinary system, from the kidney to the bladder. These deposits may be small or large, single or multiple. Sometimes they are barely bigger than a sugar granule, whereas in other cases they are so large that they fill the entire renal pelvis. The term *nephrolithiasis* is derived from the Greek *nephros* [kidney] and *lithos* [stone]. Urolithiasis is from the Greek term *ouron* (i.e., urine). The term *calculus* (plural, *calculi*) is the Latin word for pebble. Specifically, the term *renal calculi* is used to describe stones that are located in the kidney, whereas *ureterolithiasis* refers to stones that are in a ureter.

The passage of renal calculi from the kidney through the urinary tract is frequently accompanied by acute, usually severe, pain that is referred to as renal colic. Ureteral stones can sometimes cause ureteral obstruction resulting in dilatation, distention, and enlargement of the collection system in the kidney; these changes are collectively referred to as hydronephrosis. However, renal or bladder stones are not always painful and sometimes remain undetected for many years. In some cases, stones are discovered as an incidental finding when a patient undergoes ultrasound or x-ray examinations for unrelated conditions.

Epidemiology

The incidence of nephrolithiasis is slightly more than 1 case per 1000 patients per year and has been slowly increasing in recent decades.[56] The National Institutes of Health estimate that 10% of people in the United States will have a kidney stone at some point in their lives.[57] Kidney stones are most common in middle-aged people, with peak onset in the fourth decade of life. Urinary tract stones are three times more common in men than in women. Whites are affected more often than persons of Asian ethnicity, who are affected more often than blacks. In addition, urolithiasis occurs more frequently in hot, arid areas than in temperate regions.[56,58] This geographic propensity is thought to be linked to the likelihood of dehydration and consequent increased urine concentration that is an important factor influencing stone formation. Kidney stones tend to recur. Approximately 50% of patients with previous urinary calculi have a recurrence within 10 years.[58]

Causes

Unlike many other medical conditions such as diverticulitis, kidney stones are not a result of modern lifestyles. In fact, stone disease can be traced back to the earliest human records. Scientists have found evidence of kidney stones in a 7000-year-old Egyptian mummy.[57]

When there is no clear precipitating factor identified that can be linked to stone formation, the condition is referred to as idiopathic nephrolithiasis. Urinary tract infection and kidney disorders such as polycystic kidney disease are associated with stone formation. A number of metabolic diseases are associated with nephrolithiasis (e.g., hyperparathyroidism, hyperoxaluria). In general, the development of stones is related to decreased urine volume or increased excretion of stone-forming components such as calcium, oxalate, urate, cystine, xanthine, and phosphate. The stones form in the urine-collecting system of the kidney. For many patients, hereditary factors are important. A person with a family history of kidney stones is more likely to develop stones. Genetic factors may play a role in up to 45% of calcium stone cases.[59]

Normal urine is supersaturated with calcium oxalate, the primary constituent of most kidney stones. However, stones will not form unless there is one of a number of abnormalities such as overexcretion of stone constituents, a persistent imbalance in urinary pH, or an obstruction or infection in the urinary tract. In some cases, the underlying problem is simply poor fluid intake leading to concentrated urine.[60]

Although certain foods may promote stone formation in people who are susceptible, researchers do not believe that eating any specific food causes stones to form in people who are not susceptible.[57] Therefore, there are no specific dietary recommendations to prevent stone formation. However, once a stone has been analyzed, the patient's diet can be evaluated, and then changes can be recommended that will reduce the likelihood of recurrence.

Types of Stones Stone composition often provides clues to an underlying metabolic abnormality. There are four basic types of urinary stones: calcium salts, uric acid, magnesium ammonium phosphate (called struvite), and cystine (Table 21-7). These four types of renal calculi are associated with more than 20 different causes. A fifth type of stone is drug-induced. A number of medications can precipitate in urine causing stone formation. These include indinavir, guaifenesin, triamterene, silicate (overuse of antacids containing magnesium silicate), and sulfa drugs.

Calcium salt stones are the most common type of stone, accounting for approximately 75% of stone cases. They occur when there is too much calcium in the urine or blood. There are a variety of conditions that result in excessive urine calcium (hypercalciuria) or excessive blood calcium (hypercalcemia). Defective kidney function may allow too much calcium in the urine, or excessive calcium may be absorbed from the stomach and intestines. Some calcium stones are caused by an excess of a chemical called oxalate that is present in many foods such as spinach or chocolate. Oxalate binds easily with the calcium to form a stone. It is interesting to note that excessive dietary calcium is not thought to be a factor in stone formation, so calcium restriction is no longer recommended.[58]

Struvite stones form when the urinary tract is infected with certain bacteria that secrete specific enzymes. These bacteria, called urea-splitting bacteria, have the ability to precipitate a chemical reaction that results in the formation of struvite stones. Women are twice as likely to have struvite stones as are men.[59] Because struvite stones are almost always caused by urinary tract infections, they are often called "infection stones."

Uric acid stones most often form as a result of high concentrations of uric acid crystals, a condition known as hyperuricuria. These stones are associated with urine pH less than 5.5, high purine intake (e.g., organ meats, legumes, fish, meat extracts, gravies), or malignancy. Approximately 25% of patients who have a kidney stone composed of uric acid have gout.[61]

Cystine stones are found in patients with an inherited disorder that causes abnormal transport of the amino acids cystine, ornithine, lysine, and arginine in the kidney and gastrointestinal tract.

Presentation and Differential Diagnosis

It is estimated that 80% to 85% of urinary calculi will pass spontaneously.[61] There are several factors that influence the ability to pass a stone, including the person's size, prior stone passage, prostate enlargement, pregnancy, and the stone's size. A 4-mm stone has an 80% chance of passage, whereas a 5-mm stone has a 20% possibility of passage.[62]

In some situations, the presence of renal stones will be accompanied by considerable discomfort. Urolithiasis should always be considered in the differential diagnosis of abdominal pain.[58] The classic patient with renal colic is in excruciating unilateral flank or lower abdominal pain, pacing about and unable to lie still. The pain is not related to any precipitating event (such as trauma) and is not relieved by postural changes. This presentation is in contrast to a patient with peritoneal irritation who will typically remain as motionless as possible to minimize discomfort. Some patients with urolithiasis complain of nausea and vomiting that is caused by stimulation of the celiac plexus. Fever is not part of the presentation of uncomplicated nephrolithiasis. If fever is present, hydronephrosis with infection, pyonephrosis, or perinephric abscess should be suspected.[61]

The pain of renal colic often begins as vague flank pain. Patients will often ignore this early symptom until the pain advances into waves of severe pain. The symptoms the patient experiences will vary depending on the stone's location (Table 21-8). Typically, the pain tends to migrate caudally and medially as the stone works its way down the ureter.

It should be noted that the size of the stone does not necessarily predict the severity of the pain; a very tiny crystal with sharp edges can cause intense pain, whereas a larger round stone may not be as problematic.[59] If the stone is too large to pass easily, pain continues as the muscles in the wall of the tiny ureter try to squeeze the stone along into the bladder. As the stone moves down the ureter closer to the bladder, the patient may complain of urinary frequency or a burning sensation during urination.

TABLE 21-7 Types and Percentage Composition of Renal Stones[a]

Type	Percentage
Calcium salts	75
Calcium oxalate	
Calcium phosphate	
Calcium urate	
Struvite	15
Uric acid	6
Cystine	2
Drug-induced stones	2

[a]Adapted from Craig S. Renal calculi. eMedicine. http://www.emedicine.com/emerg/topic499.htm. Accessed July 28, 2008.

TABLE 21-8 Relationship of Stone Location to Symptom Presentation[58]

Stone Location	Common Symptoms
Kidney	Vague flank pain, hematuria
Proximal ureter	Flank pain, and upper abdominal pain
Middle section of ureter	Anterior abdominal pain, and flank pain
Distal ureter	Dysuria, urinary frequency, anterior abdominal pain, and flank pain

Many other conditions can cause symptoms similar to those of renal colic. In women, gynecologic conditions such as ovarian torsion, ovarian cyst, and ectopic pregnancy must be considered. In men, symptoms of testicular tumor, epididymitis, or prostatitis may mimic the symptoms of distal ureteral stones.[58] Other general causes of abdominal pain such as appendicitis, cholecystitis, diverticulitis, colitis, constipation, or hernia may present with similar discomfort. In patients older than 60 years with no prior history of stones, abdominal aortic aneurysm must be ruled out before the diagnosis of nephrolithiasis is pursued.[58,61] Finally, other urologic conditions, such as renal or ureteral tumors, must also be excluded.

Diagnosis

An organized diagnostic approach in the confirmation of urinary calculi is recommended because of the various presentations of renal colic and its broad differential diagnosis.[59]

The diagnosis of urinary tract calculi begins with a detailed medical history including whether there is a family history of calculi, the duration of symptoms, and the pattern of pain with time. Additionally, signs and symptoms of sepsis are sought. The physical examination, rather than confirming the diagnosis of urinary calculi, is often more valuable for ruling out nonurologic disease.

All patients suspected of having urinary calculi should have a urinalysis performed. Aside from the typical microhematuria, other important findings are the urine pH and the presence of crystals, which may also help identify the stone composition. Patients with uric acid stones usually present with acidic urine, whereas those with stone formation resulting from infection have an alkaline urine.[58] A urine culture should be routinely performed because identifying the presence of bacteria can affect the choice of therapy. A small amount of pus in the urine (pyuria) is often a response to irritation caused by a stone. If pyuria is not accompanied by the presence of bacteria, it is not generally thought to signify a coexistent urinary tract infection.

Diagnostic Imaging Although renal colic may be suspected based on the patient's medical history and physical examination findings, diagnostic imaging is essential to confirm the size and location of urinary tract calculi and assess obstruction. Several imaging modalities can be used; each has advantages and limitations (Table 21-9).

Noncontrast Helical CT NCHCT was first described in 1995 by Smith et al.[64] Since that time, NCHCT has gained widespread acceptance among radiologists, urologists, and emergency medicine physicians and has become the standard technique for evaluation of suspected renal colic.[65] The advantage of NCHCT compared with all other techniques is its diagnostic accuracy. More than 99% of stones–including those that are

TABLE 21-9 Imaging Modalities Used in the Diagnosis of Ureteral Calculi[58,63]

Modality	Sensitivity (%)	Specificity (%)	Advantages	Limitations
Ultrasonography	19	97	Accessible Inexpensive Safe Radiolucent stones in the kidney visible No radiation dose	Limited accuracy for renal stones Ureteral stones not seen Poor anatomic information Reproducibility of size measure ment limited Postprocedure fragmentation not readily appreciated Limited assessment of other conditions for an alternative diagnosis
Plain film radiography	45–59	71–77	Accessible Inexpensive Good reproducibility for size measurement Fragmentation readily assessed Good for follow-up of ureteral calculi	Radiation Bowel gas may limit visibility No information about caliceal anatomy or anatomy Radiolucent stones not seen Poor assessment of other condi tions for an alternative diagnosis
Intravenous urography (IVU)	64–87	92–94	Accessible Excellent anatomic definition	Radiation Use of contrast media Poor visualization of nongenitourinary conditions Delayed images required in high-grade obstruction

(Continued)

TABLE 21-9   Imaging Modalities Used in the Diagnosis of Ureteral Calculi[58,63]   *(Continued)*

Modality	Sensitivity (%)	Specificity (%)	Advantages	Limitations
Noncontrast helical CT	95–100	94–96	Very high diagnostic accuracy All stones visible (except stones composed of protease-inhibitor crystals) Caliceal anatomy may be reconstructed Provides indirect signs of the degree of obstruction Provides information on nongenitourinary conditions	Radiation dose higher than that of IVU Relatively expensive

radiolucent on plain film radiography–will be seen on NCHCT.[66] The exceptions are the rarely occurring pure matrix and protease-inhibitor medicine stones.[62]

NCHCT can be rapidly performed and interpreted and does not require the administration of intravenous contrast material. NCHCT also provides most of the information required for the immediate management of ureteral calculi. A plain frontal radiograph of the kidneys, ureters, and bladder (KUB) is frequently used for follow-up purposes. In addition to demonstrating the size and site of the stone, measurement of stone density can also be useful. Stones of greater than 1000 HU appear to respond less well to extracorporeal shock wave lithotripsy (ESWL).[67] Through a number of secondary CT signs, the presence of associated urinary tract obstruction can also be inferred from NCHCT.[62]

Renal stone CT examinations use continuous data acquisition from the top of the kidneys to the base of the bladder. Collimation is typically 2.5 mm to 3 mm. Thin slices allow identification of small stones that may be overlooked with thicker slices.

BOX 21-15   Key Concept

Renal stone protocols use a helical scan mode from the top of the kidneys to the base of the bladder and a slice thickness of 3 mm or less. Thin slices allow identification of small stones that may be overlooked with thicker slices.

The greatest drawback to the use of NCHCT is that it delivers a relatively high radiation dose, particularly to the gonads. Heneghan et al.[65] estimated the dose to the ovaries were 18 mGy with a single-detector row scanner and 23 mGy with a multidetector row scanner, which is considerably higher than the dose from a standard intravenous urogram series (2.5 mGy). This level of radiation exposure is of particular concern because many patients who have stone disease are young and have a tendency to experience repeat stone formation. Therefore, these patients have the potential of undergoing CT of the abdomen and pelvis many times during the course of their lives.

BOX 21-16   Key Concept

The greatest drawback to the use of CT in the diagnosis of urinary tract calculi is that it delivers a relatively high radiation dose, particularly to the gonads. This is of particular concern because many patients who have stone disease are young and have a tendency to experience repeat stone formation. Therefore, these patients have the potential of undergoing CT of the abdomen and pelvis many times during the course of their lives. Lower dose techniques can reduce the exposure but exposure can still be high if multiple examinations are obtained.

Because of the aforementioned concerns, researchers have looked at ways to reduce the radiation dose while maintaining the diagnostic accuracy that sets NCHCT apart.[65,68] The Heneghan study concluded, "In patients who weighed less than 200 lb (90 kg), unenhanced helical CT performed at a reduced tube current of 100 mA demonstrated a high accuracy when compared with the accuracy of the standard technique… This CT technique results in a concomitant decrease in radiation dose of 25% from multi-detector row CT and 42% for single-detector row CT. This technique has been incorporated into our routine protocol for detection of stones and, in our opinion, promises particular benefit to young patients who experience repeat stone formation."[65]

Conclusion

Urinary tract calculi are a common medical problem, occurring in approximately 10% of the population at some point in their lives. Stones can be composed of a variety of materials, although the most common consist of calcium salts. Many different causes of stone formation have been identified, although in many individual cases no clear cause of urinary tract calculi can be identified.

Although there is a classic presentation of urinary tract calculi, many other conditions can cause symptoms similar to kidney stones. Diagnosis requires a detailed medical history, physical examination, and urinalysis. In addition, diagnostic imaging is essential to uncover information about the urinary tract calculi.

The goal of modern imaging is to provide accurate information concerning the presence, size, and precise location of a renal or ureteral stone, and the likely presence or absence of obstruction, in addition to delineating the intracaliceal anatomy. Because of its many advantages, NCHCT is currently the imaging method of choice in the identification and evaluation of urinary tract calculi, although concerns about radiation dose exist.

CHAPTER SUMMARY

CT of the abdomen and pelvis is used for the evaluation of virtually all organs and most vessels. Most facilities use a number of protocols that can be either of a general nature or be designed to address a particular clinical question. Radiologists consider a wide range of factors when developing specific protocols. Although the technologist is not expected to possess the same depth of knowledge concerning these factors as a radiologist, it is imperative that they recognize, at least in a broad sense, the underlying issues that drive protocol decisions.

REVIEW QUESTIONS

1. List the reasons CT examinations of the abdomen and pelvis require greater attention to patient preparation than evaluation of any other area of the body.
2. List the various window settings at which images of the abdomen and pelvis might be displayed and the application of each.
3. When is the liver scanned just once? What phase of enhancement is chosen? When might a liver be scanned in more than one phase of contrast enhancement? Name three phases of liver enhancement and indicate the approximate delay necessary to acquire scan data in each.
4. Why must technologists be familiar with concepts surrounding the identification and characterization of adrenal masses?
5. The degree of adrenal contrast washout can be calculated by using either of two formulas. Explain the circumstances for which each of the formulas should be used.
6. Why is the identification of the appendix on cross-sectional slices sometimes difficult?
7. What can be done to reduce the radiation dose to the patient of a CT examination for the diagnosis of urinary tract calculi?

REFERENCES

1. Brant WE. Introduction to CT of the abdomen and pelvis. In: Webb WR, Brant WE, Major NM, eds. Fundamentals of Body CT. 3rd Ed. Philadelphia: Saunders, 2006:169–70.
2. Valette PJ, Pilleul F, Crombe-Ternamian A. Imaging benign and metastatic liver tumors with MDCT. In: Marchal G, Vogl TJ, Heiken JP, Rubin GD, eds. Multidetector-Row Computed Tomography, Scanning and Contrast Protocols. Milan, Italy: Springer, 2005:32.
3. Brant WE. Kidneys and ureters. In: Webb WR, Brant WE, Major NM, eds. Fundamentals of Body CT. 3rd Ed. Philadelphia: Saunders, 2006:275.
4. Van Der Molen AJ, Cowan NC, Mueller-Lisse UG, Nolte-Ernsting CC, Takahashi S, Cohan RH, CT Urography Working Group of the European Society of Urogenital Radiology (ESUR). CT urography: definition, indications and techniques. A guideline for clinical practice. Eur Radiol 2008;18:4–17.
5. Mayo-Smith WW, Boland GW, Noto RB, Lee MJ. State-of-the art adrenal imaging. Radiographics 2001;21:995–1012.
6. Blake MA, Krishnamoorthy SK, Boland GW, et al. Low-density pheochromocytoma on CT: a mimicker of adrenal adenoma. AJR Am J Roentgenol 2003;181:1663–8.
7. Pena CS, Boland GW, Hahn PF, Lee MJ, Mueller PR. Characterization of indeterminate (lipid-poor) adrenal masses: use of washout characteristics at contrast-enhanced CT. Radiology 2000;217:798–802.
8. Dunnick NR, Korobkin M. Imaging of adrenal incidentalomas: current status. AJR Am J Roentgenol 2002;179:559–68.
9. Caoili EM, Korobkin M, Francis IR, Cohan RH, Dunnick NR. Delayed enhanced CT of lipid-poor adrenal adenomas. AJR Am J Roentgenol 2000;175:1411–5.
10. Korobkin M, Brodeur FJ, Francis IR, Quint LE, Dunnick NR, Londy F. CT time-attenuation washout curves of adrenal adenomas and nonadenomas. AJR Am J Roentgenol 1998;170:747–52.
11. Szolar DH, Kammerhuber FH. Adrenal adenomas and nonadenomas: assessment of washout at delayed contrast-enhanced CT. Radiology 1998;207:369–75.
12. Seers Training Web site. U.S. National Cancer Institute's Surveillance, Epidemiology and End Results (SEER) Program. Available at: http://training.seer.cancer.gov/module_anatomy/unit6_3_endo_glnds3_adrenal.html. Accessed July 25, 2008.
13. Kemppainen RJ. Adrenal gland. In: AccessScience at McGraw-Hill. Available at: http://www.accessscience.com.proxy.lib.umich.edu, DOI 10.1036/1097-8542.011700. Accessed July 28, 2008.
14. Bowen R. Pathophysiology of the endocrine system. Available at: http://arbl.cvmbs.colostate.edu/hbooks/pathphys/endocrine/adrenal/index.html. Last updated: July 25, 2006. Accessed July 28, 2008.
15. Christy NP. Adrenal gland disorders. In: AccessScience at McGraw-Hill. Available at: http://www.accessscience.com.proxy.lib.umich.edu, DOI 10.1036/1097-8542.011800. Accessed July 28, 2008.
16. Bravo El, Gifford RW Jr. Current concepts. Pheochromocytoma: diagnosis, localization and management. N Engl J Med 1984;311:1298–303.
17. Kaye TB, Crapo L. The Cushing syndrome: an update of diagnostic tests. Ann Intern Med 1990;112:434–44.
18. Leung AK, Robson WL. Hirsutism. Int J Dermatol 1993;32:773–7.
19. Dunnick NR, Korobkin M, Francis I. Adrenal radiology: distinguishing benign from malignant masses. AJR Am J Roentgenol 1996;167:861–7.
20. Caoili EM, Korobkin M, Francis IR, et al. Adrenal masses: characterization with combined unenhanced and delayed enhanced CT. Radiology 2002;222:629–33.
21. Schteingart DE. Management approaches to adrenal incidentalomas. A view from Ann Arbor, Michigan. Endocrinol Metab Clin North Am 2000;29:127–39,ix–×.

22. Korobkin M, Francis IR, Kloos RT, Dunnick NR. The incidental adrenal mass. Radiol Clin North Am 1996;34:1037–54.

23. Korobkin M, Giordano TJ, Brodeur FJ, et al. Adrenal adenomas: relationship between histologic lipid and CT and MR findings. Radiology 1996;200:743–7.

24. Paulsen SD, Nghiem HV, Korobkin M, Caoili EM, Higgins EJ. Changing role of imaging-guided percutaneous biopsy of adrenal masses: evaluation of 50 adrenal biopsies. AJR Am J Roentgenol 2004;182:1033–7.

25. Gale ME, Birnbaum S, Gerzof SG, Sloan G, Johnson WC, Robbins AH. CT appearance of appendicitis and its local complications. J Comput Assist Tomogr 1985;9:34–7.

26. Old JL, Dusing RW, Yap W, Dirks J. Imaging for suspected appendicitis. Am Fam Physician 2005;71:71–8.

27. Rhea JT, Halpern EF, Ptak T, Lawrason JN, Sacknoff R, Novelline RA. The status of appendiceal CT in an urban medical center 5 years after its introduction: experience with 753 patients. AJR Am J Roentgenol 2005; 184:1802–8.

28. Daly CP, Cohan RH, Francis IR, Caoili EM, Ellis JH, Nan B. Incidence of acute appendicitis in patients with equivocal CT findings. AJR Am J Roentgenol 2005;184:1813–20.

29. Jaffe BM, Berger DH. Schwartz's Principles of Surgery. Part II: Special Considerations. The Appendix. New York: McGraw Hill, 2005; Chapter 29.

30. Fawcett DW, Raviola E. Bloom and Fawcett: A Textbook of Histology. New York: Chapman and Hall, 1994:636.

31. Romer AS, Parsons TS. The Vertebrate Body. 6th Ed. Philadelphia: WB Saunders, 1986:389.

32. Hardin DM Jr. Acute appendicitis: review and update. Am Fam Physician 1999;60:2027–34.

33. Korner H, Sondenaa K, Soreide JA, et al. Incidence of acute nonperforated and perforated appendicitis: age-specific and sex-specific analysis. World J Surg 1997;21:313–7.

34. Kwok MY, Kim MK, Gorelick MH. Evidence-based approach to the diagnosis of appendicitis in children. Pediatr Emerg Care 2004;20:690–8.

35. Butler C. Surgical pathology of acute appendicitis. Hum Pathol 1981;12:870–8.

36. Miranda R, Johnston AD, O'Leary JP. Incidental appendectomy: frequency of pathologic abnormalities. Am Surg 1980;46:355–7.

37. Birnbaum BA, Wilson SR. Appendicitis at the millennium. Radiology 2000;215:337–48.

38. Phillips RL Jr, Bartholomew LA, Dovey SM, Fryer GE Jr, Miyoshi TJ, Green LA. Learning from malpractice claims about negligent, adverse events in primary care in the United States. Qual Safety Health Care 2004;13:121–6.

39. Graffeo CS, Counselman FL. Appendicitis. Emerg Med Clin North Am 1996;14:653–71.

40. Sasso RD, Hanna EA, Moore DL. Leukocytic and neutrophilic counts in acute appendicitis. Am J Surg. 1970:120: 563–6.

41. Lee JH, Jeong YK, Park KB, Park JK, Jeong AK, Hwang JC. Operator-dependent techniques for graded compression sonography to detect the appendix and diagnose acute appendicitis. AJR Am J Roentgenol 2005;184:91–7.

42. Wise SW, Labuski MR, Kasales CJ, et al. Comparative assessment of CT and sonographic techniques for appendiceal imaging. AJR Am J Roentgenol 2001;176:933–41.

43. Raman SS, Lu DS, Kadell BM, Vodopich DJ, Sayre J, Cryer H. Accuracy of nonfocused helical CT for the diagnosis of acute appendicitis: a 5-year review. AJR Am J Roentgenol 2002; 178:1319–25.

44. Terasawa T, Blackmore CC, Bent S, Kohlwes RJ. Systematic review: computed tomography and ultrasonography to detect acute appendicitis in adults and adolescents. Ann Intern Med 2004;141:537–46.

45. Wilson EB, Cole JC, Nipper ML, Cooney DR, Smith RW. Computed tomography and ultrasonography in the diagnosis of appendicitis: when are they indicated? Arch Surg 2001;136:670–5.

46. Kamel IR, Goldberg SN, Keogan MT, Rosen MP, Raptopoulos V. Right lower quadrant pain and suspected appendicitis: nonfocused appendiceal CT–review of 100 cases. Radiology 2000;217:159–63.

47. Wijetunga R, Tan BS, Rouse JC, Bigg-Wither GW, Doust BD. Diagnostic accuracy of focused appendiceal CT in clinically equivocal cases of acute appendicitis. Radiology 2001; 221:747–53.

48. Peck J, Peck A, Peck C, Peck J. The clinical role of noncontrast helical computed tomography in the diagnosis of acute appendicitis. Am J Surg 2000;180:133–6.

49. Funaki B, Grosskreutz SR, Funaki CN. Using unenhanced helical CT with enteric contrast material for suspected appendicitis in patients treated at a community hospital. AJR Am J Roentgenol 1998;171:997–1001.

50. Weltman DI, Yu J, Krumenacker J, Huang S, Moh P. Diagnosis of acute appendicitis: comparison of 5- and 10-mm CT sections in the same patient. Radiology 2000;216:172–7.

51. Rao PM, Rhea JT, Novelline RA, Mostafavi AA, Lawrason JN, McCabe CJ. Helical CT combined with contrast material administered only through the colon for imaging of suspected appendicitis. AJR Am J Roentgenol 1997;169: 1275–80.

52. Rao PM, Rhea JT, Novelline RA, et al. Helical CT technique for the diagnosis of appendicitis: prospective evaluation of a focused appendix CT examination. Radiology 1997;202:139–44.

53. Lane MJ, Liu DM, Huynh MD, Jeffrey RB Jr, Mindelzun RE, Katz DS. Suspected acute appendicitis: nonenhanced helical CT in 300 consecutive patients. Radiology 1999;213:341–6.

54. Federle MP. Focused appendix CT technique: a commentary. Radiology 1997;202:20–1.

55. Jacobs JE, Birnbaum BA, Macari M, et al. Acute appendicitis: comparison of helical CT diagnosis focused technique with oral contrast material versus nonfocused technique with oral and intravenous contrast material. Radiology 2001;220: 683–90.

56. Bushinsky DA. Nephrolithiasis. J Am Soc Nephrol 1998;9: 917–24.

57. National Kidney and Urologic Diseases Information Clearinghouse webpage. Available at: http://kidney.niddk.nih.gov/kudiseases/pubs/stonesadults/index.htm. Accessed August 18, 2008.

58. Portis AJ, Sundaram CP. Diagnosis and initial management of kidney stones. Am Fam Physician 2001;63:1329–38.

59. University of Maryland Medicine: Kidney Stones. Available at: http://www.umm.edu/ency/article/00458.htm. Accessed August 18, 2008.

60. Scheinman SJ. New insights into causes and treatment of kidney stones. Hosp Pract (Minneap) 2000;35:49–63.
61. Craig S. Renal calculi. eMedicine. Available at: http://www.emedicine.com/emerg/topic499.htm. Accessed September 5, 2008.
62. Sandhu C, Anson KM, Patel U. Urinary tract stones–Part I: role of radiological imaging in diagnosis and treatment planning. Clin Radiol 2003;58:415–21.
63. MedicineNet.com. Renal Stone. Available at: http://www.medicinenet.com/script/main/art.asp?ArticleKey=8353&pf=3&track=qpadict Accessed September 5, 2008.
64. Smith RC, Rosenfield AT, Choe KA, et al. Acute flank pain: comparison of non-contrast-enhanced CT and intravenous urography. Radiology 1995;194:789–94.
65. Heneghan JP, McGuire KA, Leder RA, DeLong DM, Yoshizumi T, Nelson RC. Helical CT for nephrolithiasis and ureterolithiasis: comparison of conventional and reduced radiation-dose techniques. Radiology 2003;229:575–80.
66. Smith RC, Coll DM. Helical computed tomography in the diagnosis of ureteric colic. BJU Int 2000;86(Suppl 1):33–41.
67. Joseph P, Mandal AK, Singh SK, Mandal P, Sankhwar SN, Sharma SK. Computerized tomography attenuation value of renal calculus: can it predict successful fragmentation of the calculus by extracorporeal shock wave lithotripsy? A preliminary study. J Urol 2002;167:1968–71.
68. Spielmann AL, Heneghan JP, Lee LJ, Yoshizumi T, Nelson RC. Decreasing the radiation dose for renal stone CT: a feasibility study of single- and multidetector CT. AJR Am J Roentgenol 2002;178:1058–62.

ABDOMEN AND PELVIS PROTOCOLS

Routine Abdomen Pelvis
Protocol is the same for routine abdomen (no pelvis) except that the scan ends at the iliac crests (or lower, if necessary to include the entire liver)
Examples of clinical indications: Suspected abdominal mass, tumor staging, abscess
Scouts: AP and lateral
Scan type: Helical
Start location: Just above diaphragm
End location: Just below symphysis pubis
Breath-hold: Inspiration
IV contrast: 125 mL at 3.0 mL/s; 50 mL saline flush. Scan delay = 65 seconds
Oral contrast: 675 mL barium sulfate suspension (1.5 bottles Readi-Cat 2). An additional 225 mL (the remainder of the second bottle) given just before scanning.
DFOV: ~38 cm (optimize for individual)
SFOV: Large body
Algorithm: Standard
Window settings: 400 ww/50 wl (soft tissue)l; 150 ww/70 wl (liver—for slices that contain liver); 1500 ww/–700 wl (lung—for slices that contain lung)

	16-Detector Protocol	64-Detector Protocol
Gantry rotation time	0.8 s	0.8 s
Acquisition (detector width × number of detector rows = detector coverage)	16 × 1.25 = 20 mm	64 × 0.625 = 40 mm
Reconstruction (slice thickness/interval)	5 mm/5 mm	5 mm/5 mm
Pitch	1.375	1.375
kVp	120	120
mA	≥230	≥230

Abdomen Pelvis Aorta (Post Stent, Nongated)
3D reformations needed if surgery was sooner than 1 year.
Examples of clinical indications: Follow-up endovascular repair
Scouts: AP and lateral
Scan type: Helical
GROUP 1. Noncontrast Scan
Start location: 2 cm above celiac artery
End location: Just below the symphysis pubis
Breath-hold: Inspiration
IV contrast: None
Oral contrast: None
DFOV: ~38 cm (optimize for individual)
SFOV: Large body
Algorithm: Standard
Window settings: 350 ww/50 wl (soft tissue)

	16-Detector Protocol	64-Detector Protocol
Gantry rotation time	0.8 s	0.8 s

Acquisition (detector width × number of detector rows = detector coverage)	16 × 1.25 = 20 mm	64 × 0.625 = 40 mm
Reconstruction (slice thickness/interval)	5.0 mm/5.0 mm	5.0 mm/5.0 mm
Pitch	1.375	1.375
kVp	120	120
mA	200	200

GROUP 2. *Arterial Scan*

Start location: 2 cm above celiac artery

End location: Just below the symphysis pubis

Breath-hold: Inspiration

IV contrast: 125 mL (370 concentration) at 4 mL/s

Scan delay: Smart Prep; set monitor location at the level of the celiac artery

Oral contrast: None

DFOV: same as group 1

SFOV: Large body

Algorithm: Standard

Window settings: 350 ww/50 wl (soft tissue)

	16-Detector Protocol	64-Detector Protocol
Gantry rotation time	0.8 s	0.8 s
Acquisition (detector width × number of detector rows = detector coverage)	16 × 0.625 = 10 mm	64 × 0.625 = 40 mm
Reconstruction (slice thickness/interval)	2.5 mm/1.5 mm	0.625 mm/0.625 mm
Pitch	1.375	1.375
kVp	120	120
mA	400	500

GROUP 3. *Delayed Scan*

Start location: 2 cm above the stent

End location: 2 cm below the stent

Breath-hold: Inspiration

IV contrast: No additional IV contrast

Scan delay: 60 seconds

Oral contrast: None

DFOV: same as group 1

SFOV: Large body

Algorithm: Standard

Window settings: 350 ww/50 wl (soft tissue)

	16-Detector Protocol	64-Detector Protocol
Gantry rotation time	0.8 s	0.8 s
Acquisition (detector width × number of detector rows = detector coverage)	16 × 0.625 = 10 mm	64 × 0.625 = 40 mm
Reconstruction (slice thickness/interval)	2.5 mm/1.5 mm	0.625 mm/0.625 mm
Pitch	1.375	1.375
kVp	120	120
mA	400	500

(Continued)

Abdomen Pelvis Aorta (Post Stent, Nongated) *(Continued)*		
Reconstruction 2:		
Slice thickness/interval	None	2.5 mm/1.25 mm

Arterial Venous Liver		
Three-phase liver for suspected hemangioma; repeat group 2, 600 seconds after IV injection		
Examples of clinical indications: Evaluation of suspected hypervascular hepatic tumors, including hepatocellular carcinoma and metastases from carcinoid, islet cell carcinoma, thyroid carcinoma, renal cell carcinoma, breast carcinoma, melanoma, and sarcomas.		
Scouts: AP and lateral		
Scan type: Helical		
Group 1. Arterial Scan		
Start location: Just above diaphragm		
End location: At iliac crest (or through entire liver)		
Breath-hold: Inspiration		
IV contrast: 125 mL at 4 mL/s; 50 mL saline at 4.0 mL/s		
Scan delay: 35 seconds		
Oral contrast: VoLumen or water; 450 mL 30 minutes prior; 225 mL 10 minutes prior, 225 mL just before scan (in scan room)		
DFOV: ~38 cm (optimize for individual)		
SFOV: Large body		
Algorithm: Standard		
Window settings: 350 ww/50 wl (soft tissue); 150 ww/70 wl (liver)		
	16-Detector Protocol	64-Detector Protocol
Gantry rotation time	0.8 s	0.8 s
Acquisition (detector width × number of detector rows = detector coverage)	16 × 1.25 = 20 mm	64 × 0.625 = 40 mm
Reconstruction (slice thickness/interval)	5.0 mm/5.0 mm	5.0 mm/5.0 mm
Pitch	1.375	1.375
kVp	120	120
mA	400	500
Group 2. Venous Scan		
Start location: Just above diaphragm		
End location: At iliac crest (or through entire liver)		
Breath-hold: Inspiration		
IV contrast: No additional		
Scan delay: 65 seconds		
Oral contrast: No additional		
DFOV: same as group 1		
SFOV: Large body		
Algorithm: Standard		
Window settings: 350 ww/50 wl (soft tissue)		

	16-Detector Protocol	64-Detector Protocol
Gantry rotation time	0.8 s	0.8 s
Acquisition (detector width × number of detector rows = detector coverage)	16 × 0.625 = 10 mm	64 × 0.625 = 40 mm
Reconstruction (slice thickness/interval)	5.0 mm/5.0 mm	5.0 mm/5.0 mm
Pitch	1.375	1.375
kVp	120	120
mA	400	500
Reconstruction 2: Chest images only		
Algorithm: Standard		
Slice thickness/interval: 2.5 mm/1.25 mm		

Arterial Venous Pancreas
Examples of clinical indications: Pancreatitis, suspected tumors of the pancreas
Scouts: AP and lateral
Scan type: Helical
Group 1. Arterial Scan
Start location: Just above diaphragm
End location: At iliac crest
Breath-hold: Inspiration
IV contrast: 125 mL (370 concentration) at 4 mL/s; 50 mL saline at 4.0 mL/s
Scan delay: 40 seconds
Oral contrast: VoLumen or water; 450 mL 30 minutes prior; 225 mL 10 minutes prior, 225 mL just before scan (in scan room)
DFOV: ~38 cm (optimize for individual)
SFOV: Large body
Algorithm: Standard
Window settings: 350 ww/50 wl (soft tissue)

	16-Detector Protocol	64-Detector Protocol
Gantry rotation time	0.8 s	0.8 s
Acquisition (detector width × number of detector rows = detector coverage)	16 × 0.625 = 10 mm	64 × 0.625 = 40 mm
Reconstruction (slice thickness/interval)	0.625 mm/0.625 mm	0.625 mm/0.625 mm
Pitch	1.375	1.375
kVp	120	120
mA	400	500

Group 2. Venous Scan
Start location: Just above diaphragm
End location: At iliac crest
Breath-hold: Inspiration
IV contrast: No additional
Scan delay: 65 seconds
Oral contrast: No additional
DFOV: same as group 1

(Continued)

Arterial Venous Pancreas   *(Continued)*

SFOV: Large body

Algorithm: Standard

Window settings: 350 ww/50 wl (soft tissue)

	16-Detector Protocol	64-Detector Protocol
Gantry rotation time	0.8 s	0.8 s
Acquisition (detector width × number of detector rows = detector coverage)	16 × 0.625 = 10 mm	64 × 0.625 = 40 mm
Reconstruction (slice thickness/interval)	0.625 mm/0.625 mm	0.625 mm/0.625 mm
Pitch	1.375	1.375
kVp	120	120
mA	400	500

Reconstruction 2: Both groups

Algorithm: Standard

Slice thickness/interval: 2.5 mm/2.5 mm

Mesenteric

Examples of clinical indications: Ischemic bowel, bleeding, tumor resection

Scouts: AP and lateral

Scan type: Helical

Group 1. Arterial Scan

Start location: Just above diaphragm

End location: Just below symphysis pubis

Breath-hold: Inspiration

IV contrast: 125 mL (370 concentration) at 4 mL/s; 50 mL saline at 4.0 mL/s

Scan delay: Smart Prep; set monitor location at the level of the celiac artery

Oral contrast: VoLumen or water; 450 mL 60 minutes prior; 450 mL 30 minutes prior, 225 mL 20 minutes prior, 225 mL just before scan (in scan room)

DFOV: ~38 cm (optimize for individual)

SFOV: Large body

Algorithm: Standard

Window settings: 350 ww/50 wl (soft tissue)

	16-Detector Protocol	64-Detector Protocol
Gantry rotation time	0.8 s	0.8 s
Acquisition (detector width × number of detector rows = detector coverage)	16 × 1.25 = 20 mm	64 × 0.625 = 40 mm
Reconstruction (slice thickness/interval)	1.25 mm/0.8 mm	0.625 mm/0.625 mm
Pitch	1.375	1.375
kVp	120	120
mA	400	500

Group 2. Venous Scan

Start location: Just above diaphragm

End location: Just below symphysis pubis

Breath-hold: Inspiration

IV contrast: No additional		
Scan delay: 35 seconds		
Oral contrast: No additional		
DFOV: same as group 1		
SFOV: Large body		
Algorithm: Standard		
Window settings: 350 ww/50 wl (soft tissue)		
	16-Detector Protocol	64-Detector Protocol
Gantry rotation time	0.8 s	0.8 s
Acquisition (detector width × number of detector rows = detector coverage)	16 × 1.25 = 20 mm	64 × 0.625 = 40 mm
Reconstruction (slice thickness/interval)	1.25 mm/0.8 mm	0.625 mm/0.625 mm
Pitch	1.375	1.375
kVp	120	120
mA	400	500
Reconstruction 2: Both groups		
Algorithm: Standard		
Slice thickness/interval: 2.5 mm/2.5 mm		

Enterography		
Examples of clinical indications: Crohn disease, inflamed bowel		
Scouts: AP and lateral		
Scan type: Helical		
Start location: Just above diaphragm		
End location: Just below symphysis pubis		
Breath-hold: Inspiration		
IV contrast: 125 mL (370 concentration) at 4 mL/s; 50 mL saline at 4.0 mL/s		
Scan delay: 65 seconds		
Oral contrast: VoLumen or water; 450 mL 60 minutes prior; 450 mL 30 minutes prior, 225 mL 20 minutes prior, 225 mL just before scan (in scan room)		
DFOV: ~38 cm (optimize for individual)		
SFOV: Large body		
Algorithm: Standard		
Window settings: 350 ww/50 wl (soft tissue)		
	16-Detector Protocol	64-Detector Protocol
Gantry rotation time	0.8 s	0.8 s
Acquisition (detector width × number of detector rows = detector coverage)	16 × 1.25 = 20 mm	64 × 0.625 = 40 mm
Reconstruction (slice thickness/interval)	1.25 mm/0.8 mm	0.625 mm/0.625 mm
Pitch	1.375	1.375
kVp	120	120
mA	400	500
Reconstruction 2		
Algorithm: Standard		
Slice thickness/interval: 2.5 mm/2.5 mm		

Appendicitis/Diverticulitis		
Examples of clinical indications: Suspected appendicitis or diverticulitis		
Scouts: AP and lateral		
Scan type: Helical		
Start location: Just above diaphragm		
End location: Just below symphysis pubis		
Breath-hold: Inspiration		
IV contrast: 125 mL at 3 mL/s; 50 mL saline at 3.0 mL/s		
Scan delay: 65 seconds		
Oral contrast: 675 mL barium sulfate suspension (1.5 bottles Readi-Cat 2). An additional 225 mL (the remainder of the second bottle) given just before scanning		
DFOV: ~38 cm (optimize for individual)		
SFOV: Large body		
Algorithm: Standard		
Window settings: 350 ww/50 wl (soft tissue)		
	16-Detector Protocol	64-Detector Protocol
Gantry rotation time	0.8 s	0.8 s
Acquisition (detector width × number of detector rows = detector coverage)	16 × 1.25 = 20 mm	64 × 0.625 = 40 mm
Reconstruction (slice thickness/interval)	5.0 mm/5.0 mm	5.0 mm/5.0 mm
Pitch	1.375	1.375
kVp	120	120
mA	≥230	≥230
Reconstruction 2: 3 cm above the iliac crest through pelvis		
Algorithm: Standard		
Slice thickness/interval: 2.5 mm/1.25 mm		

Colonography		
Examples of clinical indications: Evaluation of colon after incomplete or unsuccessful colonoscopy		
Scouts: AP and lateral		
Scan type: Helical		
GROUP 1. Supine Scan		
Start location: Just above diaphragm		
End location: At lesser trochanters		
Breath-hold: Inspiration		
IV contrast: None		
Rectal contrast: Inflate colon with CO_2. (Check scout for air; if not sufficient, administer additional CO_2 and repeat scout.)		
DFOV: ~38 cm (optimize for individual)		
SFOV: Large body		
Algorithm: Standard		
Window settings: 350 ww/50 wl (soft tissue)		
	16-Detector Protocol	64-Detector Protocol
Gantry rotation time	0.8 s	0.8 s
Acquisition (detector width × number of detector rows = detector coverage)	16 × 1.25 = 20 mm	64 × 0.625 = 40 mm
Reconstruction (slice thickness/interval)	2.5 mm/1.25 mm	2.5 mm/1.25 mm

Pitch	1.375	1.375
kVp	120	120
mA	120	120
Group 2. Prone Scan		
All scan parameters remain the same as group 1		

Adrenal Mass (With Delay)

Examples of clinical indications: Characterization of known adrenal mass

Scouts: AP and lateral

Scan type: Helical

Group 1. Noncontrast Scan

Start location: Just above diaphragm

End location: Just below kidney

Breath-hold: Inspiration

IV contrast: None

Oral contrast: None

DFOV: ~25 cm

SFOV: Large body

Algorithm: Standard

Window settings: 350 ww/50 wl (soft tissue)

	16-Detector Protocol	64-Detector Protocol
Gantry rotation time	0.8 s	0.8 s
Acquisition (detector width × number of detector rows = detector coverage)	16 × 1.25 = 20 mm	64 × 0.625 = 40 mm
Reconstruction (slice thickness/interval)	2.5 mm/2.5 mm	2.5 mm/2.5 mm
Pitch	1.375	1.375
kVp	120	120
mA	≥230	≥230

Note: Place ROI on affected adrenal. If measure is 10 HU or less, end the examination. If greater than 10 HU continue with groups 2 and 3.

Group 2. Contrast-Enhanced Scan

Start location/End location: repeat group 1

Breath-hold: Inspiration

IV contrast: 150 mL at 3 mL/s; 50 mL saline at 3.0 mL/s

Scan delay: 60 seconds

Oral contrast: None

All scan parameters the same as group 1

Group 3. Delayed Scan

Start location/ End location: repeat group 1

Breath-hold: Inspiration

IV contrast: No additional

Scan delay: 15 minutes

Oral contrast: None

All scan parameters the same as group 1

Renal Mass		
Examples of clinical indications: Known or suspected renal mass		
Scouts: AP and lateral		
Scan type: Helical		
GROUP 1. Noncontrast Scan		
Start location: 2 cm above kidneys		
End location: 2 cm below kidneys		
Breath-hold: Inspiration		
IV contrast: None		
Oral contrast: None		
DFOV: ~38 cm (optimize for individual)		
SFOV: Large body		
Algorithm: Standard		
Window settings: 350 ww/50 wl (soft tissue)		
	16-Detector Protocol	64-Detector Protocol
Gantry rotation time	0.8 s	0.8 s
Acquisition (detector width × number of detector rows = detector coverage)	16 × 1.25 = 20 mm	64 × 0.625 = 40 mm
Reconstruction (slice thickness/interval)	2.5 mm/2.5 mm	2.5 mm/2.5 mm
Pitch	1.375	1.375
kVp	120	120
mA	400	400
GROUP 2. Delayed Scan		
Start location: Just above diaphragm		
End location: Just below symphysis pubis		
Breath-hold: Inspiration		
IV contrast: 100 mL at 3 mL/s; 50 mL saline at 3.0 mL/s		
Scan delay: 150 seconds		
Oral contrast: None		
All scan parameters the same as group 1		

Renal Stone
Examples of clinical indications: Known or suspected renal or ureteral calculi
Scouts: AP and lateral
Scan type: Helical
Start location: 2 cm above kidneys
End location: Symphysis pubis
Breath-hold: Inspiration
IV contrast: None
Oral contrast: None
DFOV: ~38 cm (optimize for individual)
SFOV: Large body
Algorithm: Standard
Window settings: 350 ww/50 wl (soft tissue)

	16-Detector Protocol	64-Detector Protocol
Gantry rotation time	0.8 s	0.8 s
Acquisition (detector width × number of detector rows = detector coverage)	16 × 1.25 = 20 mm	64 × 0.625 = 40 mm
Reconstruction (slice thickness/interval)	2.5 mm/2.5 mm	2.5 mm/2.5 mm
Pitch	1.375	1.375
kVp	120	120
mA		
160 lbs or less	140	140
Over 160 lbs	Match weight	Match weight
Reconstruction 2: True pelvis (top of sacroiliac joint to symphysis pubis)		
Algorithm: Standard		
Slice thickness/interval: 2.5 mm/2.5 mm		

CT Urogram

Begin running a 250 mL bag of 0.9% saline through IV when the patient first gets on the CT table.

Examples of clinical indications: Hematuria, known or suspected urothelial disease such as transitional cell carcinoma

Scouts: AP and lateral

Scan type: Helical

Group 1. Noncontrast Scan

Start location: 2 cm above kidneys

End location: Just below symphysis pubis

Breath-hold: Inspiration

IV contrast: None

Oral contrast: None

DFOV: ~38 cm (optimize for individual)

SFOV: Large body

Algorithm: Standard

Window settings: 350 ww/50 wl (soft tissue)

	16-Detector Protocol	64-Detector Protocol
Gantry rotation time	0.8 s	0.8 s
Acquisition (detector width × number of detector rows = detector coverage)	16 × 1.25 = 20 mm	64 × 0.625 = 40 mm
Reconstruction (slice thickness/interval)	5 mm/5 mm	5 mm/5 mm
Pitch	1.375	1.375
kVp	120	120
mA		
200 lbs or less	80	80
More than 200 lbs	200	200

Group 2. Excretory Scan

Start location: Just above diaphragm

End location: At iliac crest

Breath-hold: Inspiration

(Continued)

CT Urogram *(Continued)*		
IV contrast (split bolus): 75 mL at 3 mL/s; 20 mL saline at 3 mL/s		
Injection delay: 600 seconds, then 100 mL at 3 mL/s; 20 mL saline at 3 mL/s		
Scan delay: Scan begin 100 seconds after second contrast injection		
Oral contrast: None		
DFOV: Same as group 1		
SFOV: Large body		
Algorithm: Standard		
Window settings: 350 ww/50 wl (soft tissue)		
	16-Detector Protocol	64-Detector Protocol
Gantry rotation time	0.8 s	0.8 s
Acquisition (detector width × number of detector rows = detector coverage)	16 × 0.625 = 10 mm	64 × 0.625 = 40 mm
Reconstruction (slice thickness/interval)	0.625 mm/0.625 mm	0.625 mm/0.625 mm
Pitch	1.375	1.375
kVp	120	120
mA	400	500
Reconstruction 2: Both groups		
Algorithm: Standard		
Slice thickness/interval: 2.5 mm/2.5 mm		

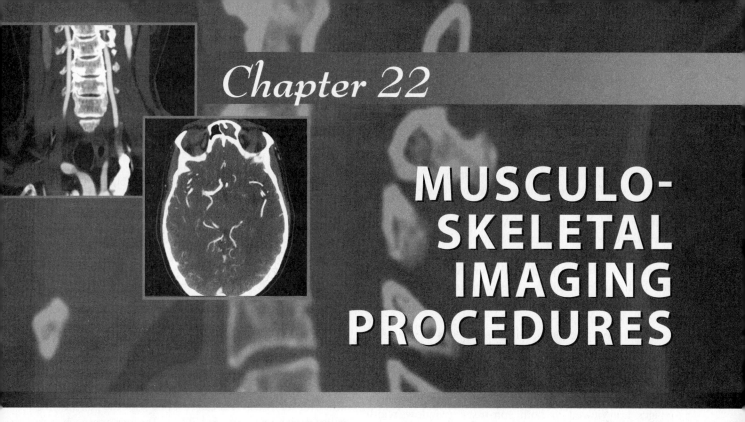

MUSCULO-SKELETAL IMAGING PROCEDURES

Key Terms: CT arthrography • double contrast technique • direct axial plane • oblique coronal plane

GENERAL MUSCULOSKELETAL SCANNING METHODS

Along with magnetic resonance imaging (MRI), CT is a major method for the evaluation of musculoskeletal anatomy and disease. CT is helpful in providing specific information about bone and other mineralized tissue. It is also a useful method of evaluating bone and soft tissue tumors. It adds details to information obtained with conventional radiography in cases of multiple fractures (e.g., in the pelvis). CT is also used to evaluate joints, especially after air or iodinated contrast material is injected into the joint.

CT of the musculoskeletal system offers several advantages: 1) display of cross-sectional anatomy and spatial relationships, 2) ability to image both sides of the body to permit comparison (particularly useful in evaluating asymmetry of joints), 3) ability to display bone and soft tissue components simultaneously, 4) excellent contrast sensitivity, and 5) ability to perform multiplanar and three-dimensional reformation retrospectively.

The development of multidetector row CT (MDCT) has allowed the acquisition of slices as thin as 0.5 mm, resulting in isotropic voxels (Chapter 6). This enables multiplanar reformation (MPR) images to be created in any plane with the same spatial resolution as the original sections. MDCT also allows extensive anatomic coverage, which is often necessary in the evaluation of patients with

musculoskeletal trauma. In these situations, scans of the skeleton can be combined with other CT studies. Such is often the case in the evaluation of pelvic trauma, which may include CT angiography (CTA) to look for vascular injury, as well as a CT cystogram to exclude bladder injury.

The techniques used to scan the musculoskeletal system are tailored to each patient and region being examined. Patients should be positioned carefully so that both sides are as symmetric as possible. The lower extremities are usually scanned with the patient supine and placed feet first into the scanner. The upper extremities are often scanned with the patient supine and placed head first into the scanner. Anteroposterior (AP) and lateral scout images are taken to localize the area of interest. In general, when scanning long bones, the plane of the CT section should be perpendicular to the long axis.

BOX 22–1 Key Concept

Protocols for scanning the musculoskeletal system are tailored to each patient. Intravenous contrast medium is not routinely administered for musculoskeletal trauma, but is valuable for other indications, such as the evaluation of infection or soft-tissue tumor. Most musculoskeletal protocols include multiplanar reformations.

Most musculoskeletal protocols include multiplanar reformations. If a fracture is seen on the cross-sectional images, three-dimensional reformations are often performed. Surgical planning is often aided by three-dimensional reformations.

The patient should be made as comfortable as possible with pillows and angle sponges so that inadvertent motion does not degrade the study. It is seldom necessary for a patient to hold their breath during image acquisition. Depending on the area and abnormality in question, there is wide variation in the positioning of the patient. For example, the ankles are usually scanned with the knees bent and the soles of the feet flat against the table and the gantry angled. However, this position is often modified so that the patient extends his legs straight out and the gantry is perpendicular to the lower leg.

Intravenous (IV) contrast medium is not routinely administered for musculoskeletal trauma, but is often valuable for other indications. IV contrast administration may be helpful in evaluating the vascularity of a tumor or in showing the relationship of major arteries or veins to musculoskeletal masses.

The reconstruction algorithm selected is based on the clinical application. In cases in which soft tissue or muscle imaging is of primary interest, a standard algorithm is used. If bone detail is needed, data are also reconstructed in a high-resolution (bone) algorithm. Musculoskeletal images are viewed in both soft-tissue (window width approximately 450; window level approximately 50) and bone (window width approximately 2000; window level approximately 600) window settings.

EXAMINATIONS WITH UNIQUE CHALLENGES

The general rules of scanning learned in previous chapters apply to musculoskeletal protocols. However, a few specific examinations are worth mentioning for their unique positioning challenges.

Wrist

CT examinations of the wrist are indicated for complex fractures involving the distal radius and ulna, scaphoid fracture, or other carpal fracture that are unclear on conventional x-ray images. CT may also be of value in the detection of subtle fractures.

BOX 22-2   Key Concept

It is often difficult to comfortably and stably position the patient for a CT examination of the wrist. Different approaches are used. Sometimes the patient is positioned with his arm over his head. Another approach is to have the patient sit or stand on the far side of the scanner and extend his arm into the scanner. A third, less favorable, approach is to scan the patient's wrist as it rests on his abdomen.

Stable positioning is the key to obtaining good image quality by avoiding motion artifacts. However, patient positioning of the wrist is at best awkward and, particularly in patients with other trauma-related injuries, can pose a significant obstacle to the study. Many different approaches are used. Probably the most common is to extend the patient's arm over the head. This can be done with the patient lying either supine or prone (Fig. 22-1). Another approach is to have the patient sit or stand at the far end of the CT scanner with his arm resting on the CT table (Fig. 22-2). If direct coronal imaging is desired, the patient's elbow is bent so that his arm is positioned parallel to the gantry. The patient is told to maintain the position while the table moves a short distance and is instructed to move his body along with the table. The patient is asked to look away from the gantry to minimize corneal radiation exposure. If the patient's hand cannot be positioned using one of these approaches, a third method is to position the patient supine on the table with his arm resting on the belly. Scans are obtained through both the wrist and the section of the abdomen on which it rests. In this situation tube current must be increased to at least 300 mAs so that image noise is sufficiently suppressed. Because of the radiation exposure to the patient's abdomen, this method is used only when other approaches have failed.

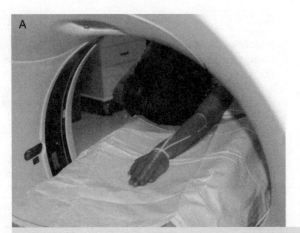 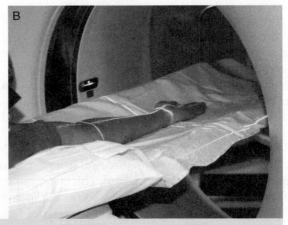

FIGURE 22-1   Patient positioning of the wrist is frequently awkward. One method has the patient lie on the scan table, either prone (A) or supine (B), and extend the affected arm over the head.

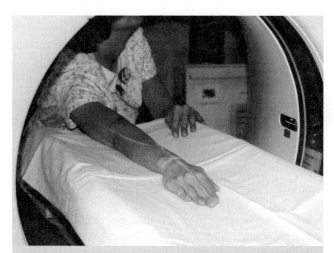

FIGURE 22-2   Another method of patient positioning for a CT examination of the wrist is to have the patient sit or stand at the far end of the CT scanner with his arm resting on the CT table.

Correctly annotating right/left, superior/inferior, and anterior/posterior on examinations of the hand, wrist, forearm, or elbow can be problematic. Recall that CT systems begin with the assumption that the patient is in the classic "anatomic position" (Chapter 1). This is characterized by an individual with his arms along his side with the palms of the hands facing forward. If the technologist inputs directional instructions that the patient is supine and head-first in the scanner, it assumes that the arms are down by the patient's side and annotates images with right/left, superior/inferior, and anterior/posterior accordingly. This annotation system is disrupted for the upper extremity when the patient is positioned so that the arm is raised over the head, or is positioned on the far end of the scanner with the arm extended. Scanner manufacturers vary in the suggested approach to this dilemma. Technologists should consult the specific scanner's operating instructions or contact the manufacturer's application consultant for the appropriate method of inputting directional instructions on these examinations. Fortunately, there is no difficulty in understanding the images with respect to anterior/posterior (volar/dorsal with respect to the hands and wrists) or superior/inferior (proximal/distal) regardless of labeling, although it is preferable that the labeling be correct. It is, however, crucial that the images correctly indicate which hand/wrist/elbow is the left one and which the right one, whether the extremities are imaged together or separately. One approach is to place small radiopaque markers (e.g., one for left and two for right) on the extremities at one edge of the scan range.

BOX 22–3   Key Concept

Special care must be taken when annotating examinations of the hand, wrist, forearm, or elbow.

Shoulder

Noncontrast CT is often requested for the evaluation of bony trauma. Thin slices are acquired in the axial plane beginning at the acromioclavicular joint and extending a few centimeters below the most inferior fracture line (determined by careful examination of the last few slices or asking a radiologist for assistance).

CT arthrography of the shoulder is useful for evaluation of the joint capsule and intracapsular structures and for finding loose bodies within the joint. CT arthrography can be performed either with a single or double contrast technique (0.5 to 3.0 mL of iodinated contrast material and approximately 10 mL of room air; Chapter 12). Thin axial slices begin at just above the acromioclavicular joint and end just below the glenoid fossa.

For either indication the patient is positioned supine on the CT table. The arm to be examined is downward alongside the body, the opposite arm is extended over the patient's head to reduce the x-ray beam absorption as much as possible (Fig. 22-3).

BOX 22–4   Key Concept

CT arthrography is useful for evaluation of the joint capsule and intracapsular structures and for finding loose bodies within the joint.

Knee

Although MRI is the primary modality for the evaluation of internal derangement of the knee, CT remains the modality of choice in certain situations, such as tibial plateau fractures. The primary indication of knee CT is to assess the degree and alignment of fracture fragments, particularly at the articular surfaces. Knee CT is also performed to assess the integrity of the bone around a prosthesis. The display field of view (DFOV) is focused on one knee only and must include the patella, both femoral condyles, and the

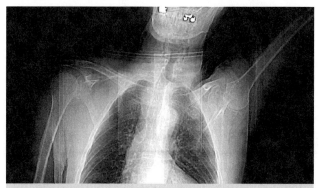

FIGURE 22-3   For a shoulder CT the patient is positioned supine on the CT table. As seen in this scout image, the arm to be examined is downward, and the opposite arm is extended over the patient's head to reduce the x-ray beam absorption as much as possible.

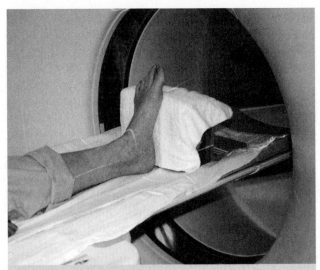

FIGURE 22-4 When the patient is positioned with the toes pointing straight up, data are acquired in the direct axial plane.

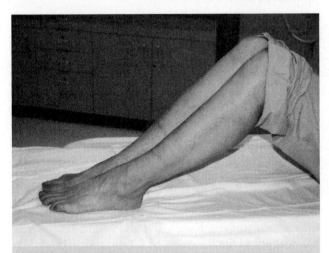

FIGURE 22-5 When the patient is positioned with knees bent, feet flat on the scan table, and the gantry is angled perpendicular to the subtalar joint, data are acquired directly in the oblique coronal plane.

proximal tibia through the fibular head. The patient typically lies supine on the scanner table with legs extended, knees side-by-side, and enters the scanner feet first. CT of the knee is sometimes performed immediately after an arthrogram of the knee in which iodinated contrast or air has been injected directly into the joint space.

Foot and Ankle

For CT of the ankle the DFOV should be large enough to include the hindfoot (talus and calcaneus), the midfoot (navicular, cuboid, and the three cuneiforms), and at least the proximal bases of all five metatarsals. For most patients, it is possible to scan both ankles simultaneously within a 22-cm DFOV, allowing a side-by-side comparison of the symptomatic ankle with the normal ankle. For CT of the foot, the DFOV should be enlarged to include the entire forefoot (metatarsals and phalanges) along with the hindfoot and midfoot.

CT data of the foot and ankle can be displayed in a number of different imaging planes. Some of these planes can be obtained directly by positioning the patient in a specific position, whereas other planes are best displayed by reformatting the data. The choice of which plane(s) to display depends on which joint is of primary concern.

For the foot, the axial plane is defined as the plane parallel to the plantar surface of the foot. This plane is acquired directly when the patient is positioned so that the toes are pointing straight up (Fig. 22-4). Data are collected directly in the oblique coronal plane when the patient is positioned with bent knees so that his feet lie flat on the scanning table. The gantry is then tilted, typically 20° to 30° (top of the gantry away from the patient) so the scan plane is perpendicular to the subtalar joint (Fig. 22-5).

CHAPTER SUMMARY

Although MRI is the primary imaging modalities for many musculoskeletal disorders, CT is the modality of choice in certain situations. Compared with MRI, MDCT with MPR is superior in the detection and evaluation of fractures. MDCT is also useful in the detection of fine calcification, which is particularly important in the diagnosis of cartilage- or bone-forming tumors and other abnormalities of bone formation. In other clinical situations CT and MRI examinations are complementary and both are performed to provide a comprehensive diagnosis.

REVIEW QUESTIONS

1. Explain why thin slices are important for most CT examinations of the musculoskeletal system.
2. Provide at least two examples of clinical indications in which intravenous contrast medium administration may be of value in musculoskeletal imaging.
3. Explain why correctly annotating CT studies of the elbow, forearm, wrist, or hand might be problematic.

MUSCULOSKELETAL PROTOCOLS

The protocols used to scan the musculoskeletal system are tailored to each patient and region being examined. The clinical indication for the examination will also affect scan parameters. Radiologists typically review each request for a musculoskeletal CT examination and adjust the protocol to be used to fit the circumstances. Included are some examples of musculoskeletal protocols. Oral contrast media is not indicated for musculoskeletal protocols. Unless specified by the radiologist, examinations are performed without intravenous contrast media, as well. Clinical indications that may necessitate IV contrast include infection or tumor. When IV contrast is ordered, 150 mL of LOCM is injected at 2 mL/s and scanning begins after 60 seconds. When IV contrast is ordered for studies of the upper extremity, inject in the nonsymptomatic arm, if possible.

Shoulder/Scapula		
Positioning: Patient supine, affected arm at side. Opposite arm above head.		
Scouts: AP and lateral		
Scan type: Helical		
Start location: Just above acromioclavicular joint		
End location: Just below scapular tip		
DFOV: ~25 cm (adjust to cover from skin surface to midline)		
SFOV: Large body		
Algorithm: Bone		
Window setting: 2000 ww/500 wl (bone)		
	16-Detector Protocol	64-Detector Protocol
Gantry rotation time	0.8 s	0.8 s
Acquisition (detector width × number of detector rows = detector coverage)	16 × 0.625 = 10 mm	32 × 0.625 = 20 mm
Reconstruction (slice thickness/interval)	1.25 mm/0.625 mm	1.25 mm/0.625 mm
Pitch	0.562	0.531
kVp/mA	140/300	140/300
Reconstruction 2:		
Algorithm: Standard		
Slice thickness/interval: 1.25 mm/0.625 mm		
Window setting: 350 ww/50 wl		
MPRs: Bone algorithm		
Slice thickness/interval: 2 mm/2 mm		
Planes: 　1. Oblique-axial (Fig. 22-6A) 　2. Oblique-sagittal (Fig. 22-6B) 　3. Oblique-coronal (Fig. 22-6C)		

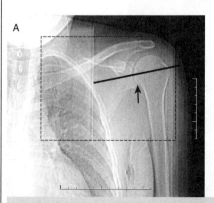
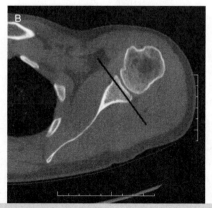
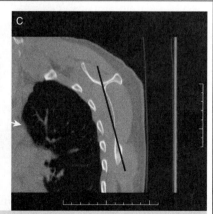

FIGURE 22-6   A. Oblique-axial MPR can be programmed from the scout image and should be perpendicular to the glenoid fossa (arrow). **B.** Oblique-sagittal MPR can be programmed from an axial image and should be parallel to the surface of the glenoid fossa. **C.** Oblique-coronal MPR can be programmed from an oblique-sagittal MPR image and should be along the body of the scapula.

Wrist		
Positioning: Patient prone, affected arm over head and extended; arm oblique. Alternative: Patient supine, arm at side.		
Scouts: AP and lateral		
Scan type: Helical		
Start location: Just proximal to distal radioulnar joint		
End location: At proximal metacarpals		
DFOV: ~10 cm (adjust to include skin surface)		
SFOV: Large body		
Algorithm: Bone plus		
Window setting: 2000 ww/500 wl (bone)		
	16-Detector Protocol	64-Detector Protocol
Gantry rotation time	0.8 s	0.8 s
Acquisition (detector width × number of detector rows = detector coverage)	16 × 0.625 = 10 mm	32 × 0.625 = 20 mm
Reconstruction (slice thickness/interval)	0.625 mm/0.3 mm	0.625 mm/0.3 mm
Pitch	0.562	0.531
kVp/mA	140/300	140/300
Reconstruction 2:		
Algorithm: Standard		
Slice thickness/interval: 0.625 mm/0.3 mm		
Window setting: 350 ww/50 wl		
MPRs: Bone plus algorithm		
Slice thickness/interval: 2 mm/2 mm		
Planes:		
1. Axial (Fig. 22-7A)		
2. Coronal (Fig. 22-7B)		
3. Sagittal (Fig. 22-7C)		
4. Oblique-sagittal (Fig. 22-7D)		

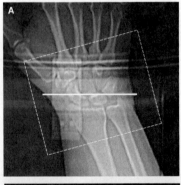
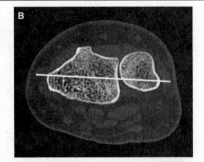
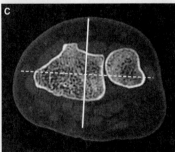
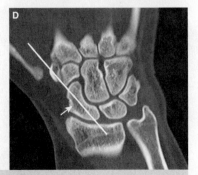

FIGURE 22-7   A. Axial MPR can be programmed from the scout image and should be perpendicular to the radius. **B.** Coronal MPR can be programmed from an axial image and should be centered at the distal radioulnar joint through the radial tuberosity. **C.** Sagittal MPR can be programmed from an axial image and should be perpendicular to the plane used in the coronal MPR. **D.** Oblique-sagittal MPR can be programmed from a coronal MRP image and should follow the long axis of the scaphoid (arrow).

Elbow		
Positioning: Patient prone, affected arm over head and extended; arm oblique. Alternative: Patient supine, arm at side.		
Scouts: AP and lateral		
Scan type: Helical		
Start location: Just above elbow joint		
End location: Just below radial tuberosity		
DFOV: ~15 cm (adjust to include skin surface)		
SFOV: Large body		
Algorithm: Bone plus		
Window setting: 2000 ww/500 wl (bone)		
	16-Detector Protocol	64-Detector Protocol
Gantry rotation time	0.8 s	0.8 s
Acquisition (detector width × number of detector rows = detector coverage)	16 × 0.625 = 10 mm	32 × 0.625 = 20 mm
Reconstruction (slice thickness/interval)	1.25 mm/0.625 mm	1.25 mm/0.625 mm
Pitch	0.562	0.531
kVp/mA	140/300	140/300
Reconstruction 2:		
Algorithm: Standard		
Slice thickness/interval: 1.25 mm/0.625 mm		
Window setting: 350 ww/50 wl		
MPRs: Bone algorithm		
Slice thickness/interval: 2 mm/2 mm		

Planes:
  1. Axial (Fig. 22-8A)
  2. Oblique-coronal (Fig. 22-8B)
  3. Oblique-sagittal (Fig. 22-8C)		

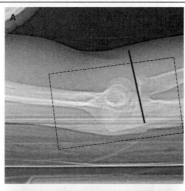
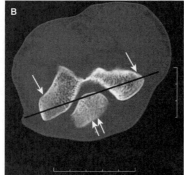
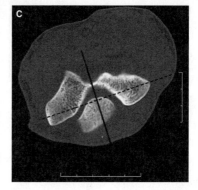

FIGURE 22-8   A. Axial MPR can be programmed from the scout, and should be parallel to the radial head. **B.** Oblique-coronal MPR can be programmed from an axial image at the level of the humeral epicondyles (arrows) and the olecranon (double arrow). **C.** Oblique-sagittal MPR can be programmed from an axial image and be perpendicular to the plane of the oblique-coronal MPR.

Hip/Proximal Femur

Positioning: Patient supine, legs flat on table (no cushion or wedge under knees).

Scouts: AP and lateral

Scan type: Helical

Start location: Just above sacroiliac joints

End location: Approximately 4 cm below lesser trochanters (include entire fracture if present)

DFOV: ~30 cm (adjust to include skin surface)

SFOV: Large body

Algorithm: Bone

Window setting: 2000 ww/500 wl (bone)

	16-Detector Protocol	64-Detector Protocol
Gantry rotation time	0.8 s	0.8 s
Acquisition (detector width × number of detector rows = detector coverage)	16 × 0.625 = 10 mm	32 × 0.625 = 20 mm
Reconstruction (slice thickness/interval)	1.25 mm/0.625 mm	1.25 mm/0.625 mm
Pitch	0.562	0.531
kVp/mA	140/400	140/400

Reconstruction 2:

Algorithm: Standard

Slice thickness/interval: 1.25 mm/0.625 mm

Window setting: 350 ww/50 wl

MPRs: Bone algorithm

Slice thickness/interval: 2 mm/2 mm

Planes:

    1. Axial (Fig. 22-9A)

    2. Coronal to femur (Fig. 22-9B)

    3. Sagittal to femur (Fig. 22-9C)

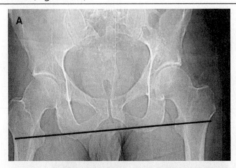

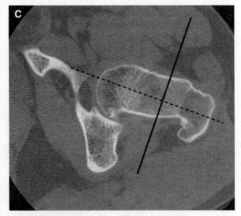

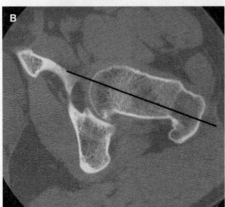

FIGURE 22-9 **A.** Axial MPR can be programmed from an AP scout. **B.** Coronal MPR can be programmed from an axial image and should follow the long axis of the femoral neck. **C.** Sagittal MPR can be programmed from an axial image and should be perpendicular to the coronal MPR plane.

Knee/Tibial Plateau		
Positioning: Patient supine, legs flat on table; tape feet together		
Scouts: AP and lateral		
Scan type: Helical		
Start location: Just above patella		
End location: Just below fibular head		
DFOV: ~20 cm (adjust to include skin surface; affected knee only)		
SFOV: Large body		
Algorithm: Bone plus		
Window setting: 2000 ww/500 wl (bone)		
	16-Detector Protocol	64-Detector Protocol
Gantry rotation time	0.8 s	0.8 s
Acquisition (detector width × number of detector rows = detector coverage)	16 × 0.625 = 10 mm	32 × 0.625 = 20 mm
Reconstruction (slice thickness/interval)	1.25 mm/0.625 mm	1.25 mm/0.625 mm
Pitch	0.562	0.531
kVp/mA	140/300	140/300
Reconstruction 2:		
Algorithm: Standard		
Slice thickness/interval: 1.25 mm/0.625 mm		
Window setting: 350 ww/50 wl		
MPRs: Bone algorithm		
Slice thickness/interval: 2 mm/2 mm		
Planes:		
1. Axial (Fig. 22-10A)		
2. Coronal (Fig. 22-10B)		
3. Sagittal (Fig. 22-10C)		

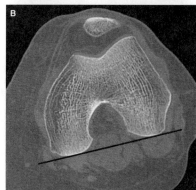
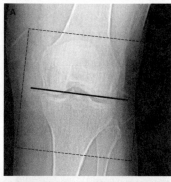
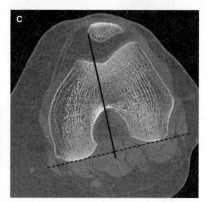

FIGURE 22-10   A. Axial MPR can be programmed from an AP scout and should be parallel to the tibial plateau. **B.** Coronal MPR can be programmed from an axial image and should be parallel to the femoral condyles. **C.** Sagittal MPR can be programmed from an axial image and should be perpendicular to the coronal MPR.

Ankle/Distal Tibia		
Positioning: Patient supine, legs flat on table. Use foot holder or tape feet together.		
Scouts: AP and lateral		
Scan type: Helical		
Start location: Just above tibial plafond (just above ankle joint)		
End location: Through calcaneus		
DFOV: ~16 cm (adjust to include skin surface)		
SFOV: Large body		
Algorithm: Bone plus		
Window setting: 2000 ww/500 wl (bone)		
	16-Detector Protocol	64-Detector Protocol
Gantry rotation time	0.8 s	0.8 s
Acquisition (detector width × number of detector rows = detector coverage)	16 × 0.625 = 10 mm	32 × 0.625 = 20 mm
Reconstruction (slice thickness/interval)	0.625 mm/0.3 mm	0.625 mm/0.3 mm
Pitch	0.562	0.531
kVp mA	140/200	140/200
Reconstruction 2:		
Algorithm: Standard		
Slice thickness/interval: 0.625 mm/0.3 mm		
Window setting: 350 ww/50 wl		
MPRs: Bone algorithm		
Slice thickness/interval: 2 mm/2 mm		
Planes:		
1. Axial (Fig. 22-11A)		
2. Coronal (Fig. 22-11B)		
3. Sagittal (Fig. 22-11C)		

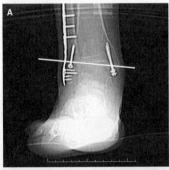

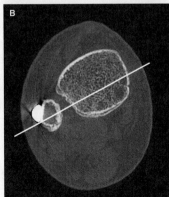

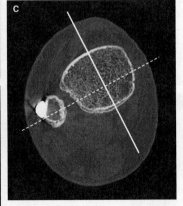

FIGURE 22-11   A. Axial MPR can be programmed from an AP scout parallel to the top of the talus. **B.** Coronal MPR can be programmed from an axial image at the level of the distal tibia. **C.** Sagittal MPR can be programmed from an axial image at the level of the distal tibia. They are perpendicular to the coronal MPR plane.

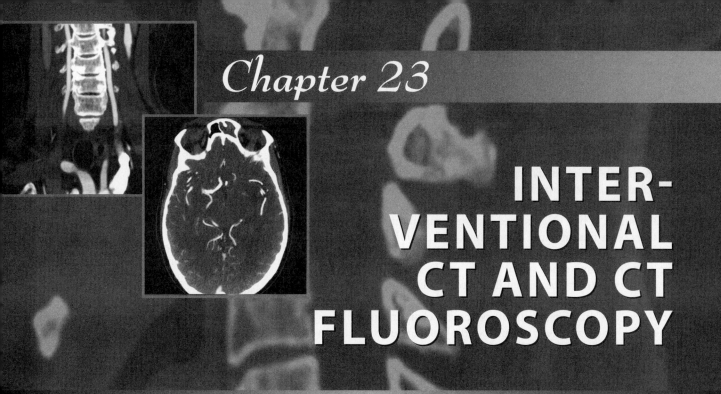

Chapter 23

INTER-VENTIONAL CT AND CT FLUOROSCOPY

Key Terms: percutaneous procedures • sequential CT • CT fluoroscopy • intermittent fluoroscopy • needle-holding devices

CT is a valuable tool for use in interventional procedures such as biopsies and abscess drainage. The use of CT to guide percutaneous procedures offers several advantages. High-resolution CT images provide precise three-dimensional localization of lesions. CT images permit the clinician to plan an access route to the lesion by showing the relationship of surrounding structures. Because the tip of the needle within the structure can be visualized and slice thickness can be as narrow as 0.5 mm, interventions can be performed on small structures. Because of the wide latitude of beam attenuation information gathered by CT, an extremely low-density material such as gas can be imaged as well as high-density material such as metal, bone, or synthetic catheters. The ability to accurately image high-density material allows the use of any type of instrument (i.e., needle, drainage tube, or other devices). In addition, contrast material can be injected when vascularity, an anatomic space, or an abnormal cavity need further delineation. Patients can be placed in a variety of positions to allow easier access to the lesion. Improving the accuracy of the procedure diminishes the associated risks.

IMAGING TECHNIQUES FOR CT-GUIDED INTERVENTIONS

> **BOX 23–1   Key Concept**
>
> Two different imaging techniques are used for CT-guided interventions: sequential CT and (CTF). Techniques to reduce radiation dose should be used with either method.

Two different imaging techniques are used for CT-guided interventions: sequential CT and CT fluoroscopy (CTF). Sequential CT has all of the advantages listed above, but it does have some drawbacks. The procedure can be lengthy because of the numerous single or helical CT images that are obtained. The process requires a scan acquisition, the needle placement, another scan acquisition, adjustment of the needle, another scan acquisition, and so forth until the needle is confirmed to be in the correct location. More important, the intermittent visualization prohibits the clinician from making the rapid adjustments that are possible with conventional fluoroscopy.

CTF capabilities are not standard on scanners; CTF must be purchased as an addition to a helical scanner. CTF allows for the near real-time capabilities of traditional fluoroscopy while maintaining the superior contrast resolution and three-dimensional anatomic display of CT. These benefits expand the ability to perform image-guided interventions in anatomically complex locations. Although there are concerns about the radiation dose delivered from either method, with CTF there is the additional concern about radiation exposure to the operator.[1-4] It is not uncommon for a single department to use both approaches, depending on the clinical problem. They can be used separately or in combination.

Techniques to reduce radiation dose should be used during interventions with either sequential CT or CTF. When sequential CT is used, the mAs should be set as low as possible. One study reported success in both catheter placement and percutaneous biopsy when parameters were reduced to 30 mAs (from the standard setting of 175 to 250 mAs).[5] When CTF is used it is very important that CTF exposure time and tube current (mA) be kept as low as possible. Dose rates, which can be high with the continuous (i.e., near real-time) mode of acquisition, can be minimized by exclusively using intermittent fluoroscopy.[3,6] In addition, personnel must take care to reduce their own radiation exposure. It is unacceptable to introduce the clinician's or assistant's hands into the CT beam. Needle-holding devices have been developed for CTF and have been shown to significantly reduce exposure to the hand.[7] Using a lead drape to cover the nonbiopsy region of the patient can significantly reduce scatter, protecting both the patient and the staff.

BOX 23-2   Key Concept

When using CTF it is unacceptable to enter the CT beam with the hands. Dose rates can be minimized by exclusively using intermittent fluoroscopy (rather than the real-time mode of image acquisition).

INDICATIONS FOR CT-GUIDED PROCEDURES

The indications for CT-guided procedures vary from institution to institution, depending on the preferences of the radiologists and on the equipment available. Some of the most common indications include the drainage of abscesses and pneumothoraces, punctures of abdominal and thoracic masses and lesions, percutaneous diskectomy of herniated disks, lumbar spine or pelvic interventions, percutaneous administration of chemotherapeutic agents, thermoablative procedures, and percutaneous vertebroplasty.[8]

The steps to each procedure will vary somewhat. CT-guided biopsies are perhaps the most common interventional procedure; understanding the basic steps involved can provide a framework for other CT-guided procedures.

CT-Guided Biopsies

In theory, the risk associated with needle biopsy increases as needle diameter increases. When a cutting needle is used the risk may be increased. However, the overall complication rate is small, approximately 2%. The primary complication of biopsy procedures is bleeding (often related to undetected coagulopathy).[9] Highly vascularized lesions increase this risk. A bleeding disorder is a contraindication to percutaneous biopsy. However, patients are often treated with blood products or medications to temporarily remedy the disorder so that the biopsy can be performed. The most common complication of CT-guided lung biopsy is the occurrence of a pneumothorax during or after the intervention.[8]

TABLE 23-1   Supplies for Biopsy and Drainage Procedures

Personal protective equipment: face shields, sterile gowns, sterile gloves, foot coverings

Sterile 4 × 4 gauze sponges

Sterile drape

Sterile needles (18, 20, 22 gauge)

Sterile syringes (assorted sizes)

Scalpel

Choice of Procedure Needles (usually selected before procedure based on route and indications)
   Spinal needles (18, 20, 22 gauge)
   Chiba (20, 22 gauge; 15, 20 cm)
   Cutting needles (such as Trucut) (14, 16, 18 gauge)
   Franseen (18, 20 gauge)
Automatic Core Biopsy System (biopsy gun)
   20 gauge; 9, 15, 21 cm
   18 gauge; 9, 15, 21 cm

Metallic skin markers

Skin marking pen

Betadine

1% lidocaine

Pigtail catheter (8, 10, 12, 14 French)

Fascial dilators (7–13 French)

Guide wires (0.35 inch)

Amplatz wire

Specimen tubes for laboratory studies

Aerobic and anaerobic culture tubes

Formalin or nonbacteriostatic saline

Stopcocks

Suture (nylon or Prolene)

Drainage bag and connecting tubing

Tape

Biopsy (using the sequential CT method) can be performed on any scanner without the purchase of additional computer software, but some supplies, such as specialized needles, are required (Table 23-1).

The purpose of CT-guided biopsy is to document neoplastic disease (primary, metastatic, or recurrent) or to differentiate neoplastic disease from other processes, such as inflammatory disease, postoperative changes, posttherapeutic changes, or normal structures. Therefore, the goal in a biopsy procedure is to obtain an adequate sample for laboratory evaluation with minimal trauma to surrounding tissues. The goal is achieved with accurate and expedient placement of the needle.

CT-guided biopsy is not a complicated procedure. It can be broken down into several basic steps.

1. The procedure is explained to the patient and written consent is obtained.
2. Appropriate laboratory values are obtained. Most laboratory evaluations include prothrombin time, partial thromboplastin time, and platelet count.
3. The scan is plotted. This process includes careful review of the patient's previous imaging studies to determine the optimal patient position, whether oral

or intravenous contrast medium is indicated, and the appropriate level for the biopsy.

4. A scan is performed through the selected area. An important consideration in scanning for a biopsy procedure is patient breathing. Clear instructions are essential so that each breath is as similar as possible. The breathing command should be given for each scan sequence. As the needle is placed, the patient is again asked to suspend breathing.

5. The best location for needle entry is selected. Ideally, the trajectory of the needle is planned to avoid penetration of uninvolved structures such as bowel and vascular structures. Once a location is selected a metallic marker is placed on the skin at or adjacent to the proposed skin entry site with the localizer light on the CT scanner.

6. The scan is repeated to confirm the suitability of the selected entry location.

7. With the distance measurement on the CT system, the distance from the marker on the patient's skin to the lesion is measured. This measure determines the optimal depth and angle for needle placement.

8. The patient's skin is prepared according to aseptic procedure guidelines. A sterile drape is applied, a local anesthetic (lidocaine 1%) is administered, and the biopsy needle is placed.

9. The scan is repeated (3- to 5-mm slice thickness is typical) at the needle location as well as one slice above and one slice below the expected needle location until the tip of the needle is visualized.

10. If the CT image confirms the correct location of the needle, a tissue sample is taken and prepared according to laboratory protocols.

11. A postprocedure scan is taken (typically at 5-mm slice thickness) to identify complications such as pneumothorax or hematoma.

CT-Guided Fluid Aspiration and Abscess Drainage

The features that make CT an excellent choice for guiding a needle biopsy are also beneficial in performing percutaneous abscess drainage.

Fluid collections that respond the most favorably to percutaneous abscess drainage are well-defined, unilocular, free-flowing, and accessible. Often, abscess drainage is performed under less favorable conditions (e.g., fluid collection is multiloculated, composed of necrotic tissue, or poorly defined) if the patient is a poor surgical candidate.

The needle placement technique duplicates that used in percutaneous biopsy. In general, the shortest, straightest access route to the collection is favored. However, care should be taken to avoid major vessels, bowel loops, and the pleural space. The fluid collection can be entered in one step with a drainage catheter or a needle. Alternatively, a needle can be place into the fluid collection, a guidewire advanced, and a catheter placed using exchange techniques. After the catheter is in place, the collection is aspirated as completely as possible. Catheters are usually left to gravity

drainage. When drainage is complete, the catheter is withdrawn gradually. For fluid collections in which only aspiration of a specimen is desired, this is accomplished through the targeting needle, which is subsequently withdrawn.

CHAPTER SUMMARY

CT is an excellent tool to guide interventional procedures because it allows for accurate visualization of needle placement, including puncture site and position within the tissues. Any scanner can be used to guide interventions in the sequential mode, although CT fluoroscopy requires add-on software. The radiation dose delivered to the patient during either method of CT-guided intervention is a concern. In addition, CTF has the potential for significant exposure to the staff. A wide range of interventions can be performed under CT guidance. The specific indication will influence the exact steps to be taken to perform the procedure.

REVIEW QUESTIONS

1. List the advantages of using CT to guide interventions. What are the drawbacks?

2. Compare sequential CT techniques to those of CTF. What are the specific advantages and disadvantages of each method?

3. Explain why breathing instructions to the patient are so critical during a CT-guided biopsy procedure.

REFERENCES

1. Krause ND, Haddad ZK, Winalski CS, Ready JE, Nawfel RD, Carrino JA. Musculoskeletal biopsies using computed tomography fluoroscopy. J Comput Assist Tomogr 2008; 32:458–62.

2. Neeman Z, Dromi SA, Sarin S, Wood BJ. CT fluoroscopy shielding: decreases in scattered radiation for the patient and operator. J Vasc Interv Radiol 2006;17:1999–2004.

3. Wagner AL. Selective lumbar nerve root blocks with CT fluoroscopic guidance: technique, results, procedure time, and radiation dose. AJNR Am J Neuroradiol 2004; 25:1592–4.

4. Tsalafoutas IA, Tsapaki V, Triantopoulou C, Gorantonaki A, Papailiou J. CT-guided interventional procedures without CT fluoroscopy assistance: patient effective dose and absorbed dose considerations. AJR Am J Roentgenol 2007;188:1479–84.

5. Lucey BC, Varghese JC, Hochberg A, Blake MA, Soto JA. CT-guided intervention with low radiation dose: feasibility and experience. AJR Am J Roentgenol 2007;188:1187–94.

6. Buls N, Pagés J, de Mey J, Osteaux M. Evaluation of patient and staff doses during various CT fluoroscopy guided interventions. Health Physics 2003;85:165–73.

7. Irie T, Kajitani M, Itai Y. CT fluoroscopy-guided intervention: marked reduction of scattered radiation dose to the physician's hand by use of a lead plate and an improved I-I device. J Vasc Interv Radiol 2001;12:1417–21.

8. Vogl TJ, Herzog C. Multislice CT: interventional CT. In: Marchal G, Vogl TJ, Heiken JP, Rubin GD, eds. Multidetector-Row Computed Tomography: Scanning and Contrast Protocols. Milan: Springer, 2005:101–2.

9. Picus D, Weyman PJ, Anderson DJ. Interventional computed tomography. In: Lee JKT, Sagel SS, Stanley RJ, eds. Computed Body Tomography. New York: Raven Press, 1989:94.

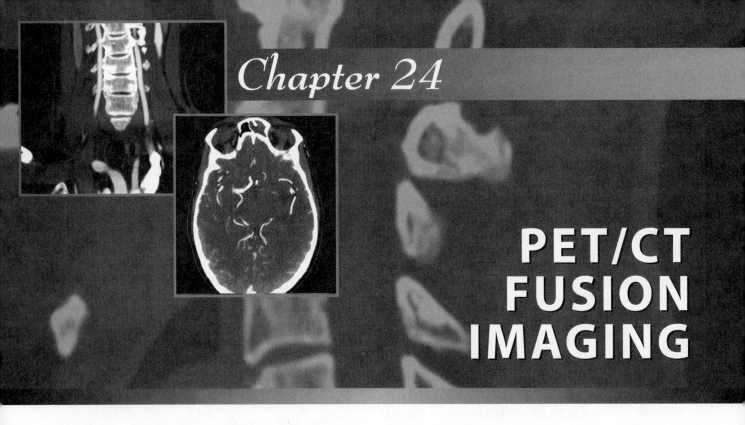

Chapter 24

PET/CT FUSION IMAGING

INTRODUCTION

CT provides exquisite anatomic detail that is essential in the diagnosing, staging, and restaging of cancer, as well as the planning and monitoring of cancer treatment. Anatomic imaging provided by CT and magnetic resonance imaging (MRI) has a high sensitivity for the detection of obvious structural disruption but is not as useful in characterizing these abnormalities as malignant or benign. Necrotic tissue, scar tissue, and inflammatory changes often cannot be differentiated from malignancy based on anatomic imaging alone. In addition, lymph nodes that are not enlarged but are harboring malignant cells cannot be identified as abnormal on traditional cross-sectional images. Because of these limitations to anatomic methods, researchers sought to develop imaging methods that can detect abnormal behavior of tissue. In a broad sense, molecular imaging can be defined as any methodology that investigates events at the molecular and cellular levels. The nuclear medicine community developed the molecular imaging method known as positron emission tomography (PET), which provides metabolic detail. Whereas CT provides structural information about the body, PET provides functional information regarding how the cells of the body operate. The introduction of the radiotracer fluorine-18 fluorodeoxyglucose (FDG) has played a key role in advancing PET.

BOX 24–1   Key Concept

Anatomic imaging provided by CT and MRI has a high sensitivity for the detection of obvious structural disruption but is not as useful in characterizing these abnormalities as malignant or benign.

Although either CT or PET can be used individually, it is often a combination of the modalities that provides the most complete diagnosis. Traditionally, such imaging has been performed at different times, in different places, and on different equipment. When the results of PET and CT scans are "fused" together, the combined images provide information on cancer location and metabolism (Fig. 24-1). However, even when the time difference between examinations is small, aligning images acquired on two different scanners is a complex problem. PET/CT scanners are composed of a multidetector CT scanner in conjunction with, but separate from, a PET scanner. During a study, the patient passes first through the CT scanner and then into the imaging field of the PET scanner. In PET/CT imaging, the strengths of the two modalities complement each other. This helps the reporting physician see the functional information provided by PET and localizes this more accurately with CT, which provides structural information about the body.

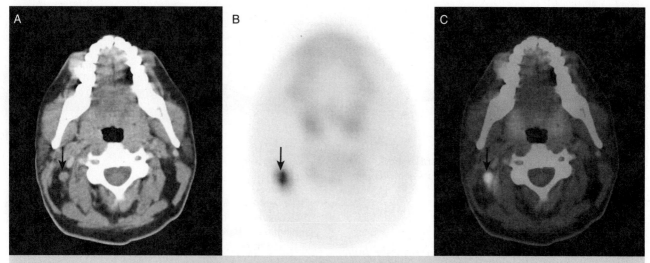

FIGURE 24-1   PET/CT fuses anatomic information in the form of CT data (A) and functional information in the form of PET data (B) so that these information sets can be viewed and interpreted together (C). Actual PET/CT images are always displayed in color. To view a color version of this image, please review the image bank found at http://thepoint.lww.com/RomansCT. Images courtesy of Dr. Saabry Osmany, Department of Nuclear Medicine and PET, Singapore General Hospital, Singapore.

BOX 24–2   Key Concept

Molecular imaging can be defined as any methodology that investigates events at the molecular and cellular levels.

The hybrid PET/CT scanners pose a staffing dilemma. The responsibilities of a PET/CT technologist combine the responsibilities of a nuclear medicine and CT technologist, yet technologists are very rarely trained in both modalities. Each discipline has a different set of requirements related to clinical procedures, radiation protection, and clinical history as a result of the nature of the ionizing radiation used. In addition to the PET/CT procedures, some imaging departments perform standard diagnostic CT scans on their PET/CT scanners. Currently, PET/CT technologists may have either a nuclear medicine or CT background. Once technologists get credentialed by either the ARRT (American Registry of Radiologic Technologists) or the NMTCB (Nuclear Medicine Technology Certification Board), they typically get experiential training at a facility that offers the technology. However, as PET/CT application broadens, organizations such as the ASRT (American Society of Radiologic Technology) and the SNMTS (Society of Nuclear Medicine Technologist Section) are developing a means to provide a more formalized educational approach for training technologists.

The field of nuclear medicine technology is beyond the scope of this text. However, the interested CT technologist can benefit from understanding at least the basics of PET/CT. Before one can recognize the unique features of this fused modality, one must first be acquainted with FDG-PET.

AN INTRODUCTION TO FDG-PET IMAGING

In recent years PET has emerged as an essential tool in the management of cancer patients. Such management involves both appropriate diagnosis and accurate staging. Staging refers to the process of determining the extent and distribution of disease. This crucial step greatly influences the choice of treatment.

A familiarity with the mechanism of FDG uptake is essential in recognizing the physiologic variants that are frequently encountered in PET imaging with FDG. To introduce FDG-PET we 1) briefly explain PET imaging, 2) discuss the normal physiologic variants related to FDG uptake, 3) examine benign and pathologic causes of increased FDG uptake, and 4) define the term standard uptake value (SUV) and discuss its importance in the interpretation of PET images.

How Does PET Work?

PET creates an image from the radiation given off when positrons (i.e., antimatter electrons) encounter electrons in the body. To do this, patients are given a radiopharmaceutical with a short half-life, made up of a radionuclide (in this case ^{18}F) linked to a pharmaceutical agent (deoxy-glucose; Fig. 24-2). The radionuclide emits positrons that encounter electrons in the body. They annihilate each other, producing high-energy photons (i.e., annihilation photons) that can be detected by the imaging device (Fig. 24-3). The pharmaceutical portion of the radiopharmaceutical (deoxy-glucose) allows localization that favor glycolysis.

PET is unique because it creates images of the body's physiologic functions, such as blood flow and metabolism.

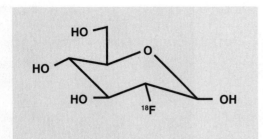

FIGURE 24-2 A diagram of the structure of ^{18}F-FDG, which consists of the radionuclide ^{18}F attached to a deoxygenated glucose molecule.

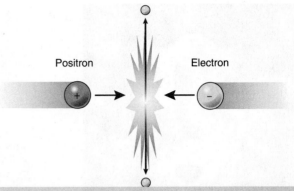

FIGURE 24-3 An illustration of the annihilation reaction that occurs when a positron encounters an electron. The annihilation photons travel at 180° from each other and are detected through the process of coincidence detection.

Most other imaging methods only demonstrate organ structure. Therefore, anatomic modalities are only capable of detecting disease when it distorts anatomy. In contrast, PET permits assessment of chemical and physiologic changes related to metabolism. This type of assessment is important because functional changes often predate structural changes in tissues. PET may therefore demonstrate pathologic changes long before they would be revealed by modalities like CT or MRI (Fig. 24-4).

PET uses unique radiopharmaceuticals different from those used in traditional nuclear medicine. PET radiopharmaceuticals can be labeled with isotopes that are basic biologic substrates. These isotopes mimic natural molecules such as sugars, water, proteins, and oxygen. As a result, PET is often capable of revealing more about the cellular-level metabolic status of a disease compared with the capabilities of other imaging modalities. Currently, the most commonly used PET radiopharmaceutical is ^{18}F-FDG.

Many normal tissues use glucose for energy. FDG is a glucose analog that is taken up by cells and then trapped intracellularly in the glycolytic pathway. Therefore, FDG uptake is basically a map of glucose metabolism. Increased glucose use is frequently associated with malignancies. Tumor imaging with FDG is based on the fact that malignant tumors often favor the glycolytic pathway for metabolism.[1] FDG is administered intravenously and is then transported into cells by glucose transporter proteins. To a certain extent, higher accumulations of FDG usually correlate with more aggressive tumors and a greater number of viable tumor cells.[1]

BOX 24–3   Key Concept

Tumor imaging with FDG is based on the fact that malignant tumors often favor the glycolytic pathway for metabolism.

FDG Imaging Pitfalls

Tumor cells, however, are not the only cells that exhibit an increased uptake of FDG.[2,3] Because FDG maps glucose metabolism, its distribution can be altered by any physical

activity. Normal physiologic accumulation of FDG occurs in the brain, muscles, salivary glands, myocardium, gastrointestinal tract, urinary tract, brown adipose tissue, thyroid gland, and gonadal tissues.[4,5] It is important to recognize and understand normal variants of FDG uptake and benign disease to avoid mistaking them with pathologic processes.

The timing of a patient's last meal before a PET study will have a considerable effect on the quantities of glucose and insulin in the circulation, thereby affecting FDG uptake. Similarly, the patient's state of hydration can alter the distribution of FDG in the body by altering the patient's excretion of the tracer. To avoid confounding results that may complicate imagine interpretations, patients are required to fast from 4 to 6 hours before their PET examinations. If the patient's blood sugar level is more than 200 mg/dL before the injection of FDG, this could limit the study's sensitivity.

BOX 24–4   Key Concept

The timing of a patient's last meal and level of hydration can affect the PET results. Patients are required to fast from 4 to 6 hours before their PET examinations. In addition, for insulin-dependent diabetic patients, the timing of an insulin injection may affect the PET results. Insulin should be given as far from the time of FDG injection as feasible.

Although all diabetic patients should control their blood sugar level with oral hypoglycemic medication or insulin, the timing of an insulin injection may affect the PET scan. An insulin injection close to the time of FDG administration induces diffusely increased uptake of FDG in the skeletal muscles.[6] Therefore, insulin should be given as far from the time of FDG injection as feasible.

Skeletal Muscles

Vigorous exercise in the days before the scan can cause intense uptake in the associated skeletal muscles. This

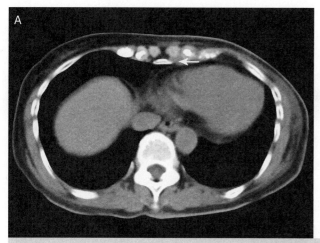
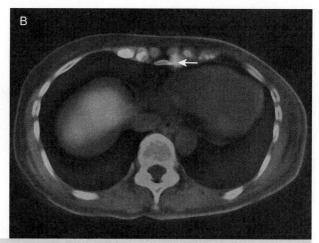

FIGURE 24-4 **A.** Image shows a normal-sized left internal mammary node seen on CT scan (arrow). **B.** Image is a PET/CT image of the same patient showing an intensely FDG-avid focus in the region of the left internal mammary node (arrow). Actual PET/CT images are always displayed in color. To view a color version of this image, please review the image bank found at http://thepoint.lww.com/RomansCT. Images courtesy of Dr. Saabry Osmany, Department of Nuclear Medicine and PET, Singapore General Hospital, Singapore.

may be related not only to the exercise activity, but also to stress-induced muscle tension (as is often seen in the trapezius and paraspinal muscles).[2] Hyperventilation may induce uptake in the diaphragm as well. Muscle uptake is typically symmetric and is therefore easy to differentiate from abnormal activity. However, occasionally the uptake can be focal and unilateral, which makes interpretation more difficult–particularly in patients who have head and neck cancer or lymphoma.

Head and Neck

Glucose is the source of energy in the brain; hence brain cortex tissue generally has an intense uptake. In the fasting state, the brain is known to account for as much as 20% of total-body glucose metabolism. FDG accumulation in the brain is fairly predictable. However, FDG uptake in some parts of the face and neck can be highly variable. Uptake of the salivary glands–including the parotid, submandibular, and sublingual glands–can range from mild to intense.[2] In addition, salivary gland uptake may be symmetric or asymmetric. Asymmetry in the salivary gland can be attributed to the patient's position or inflammatory changes after surgery or radiotherapy. Also, radiotherapy can decrease uptake on the irradiated side.

Fairly consistent low-to-moderate FDG uptake occurs in the tonsils and base of the tongue. Uptake in the normal thyroid typically ranges from no accumulation to mild uptake. However, it has been reported that increased uptake in the normal thyroid is seen in approximately 2% of scans of healthy individuals.[7]

The six muscles that control the movements of the eye (i.e., extraocular muscles), the muscles of the oral cavity, and the laryngeal muscles reveal varying degrees of FDG uptake.[2] A moderate amount of uptake is usually

seen in the anterior part of the floor of the mouth because of the genioglossus muscle, which prevents the tongue from falling back in supine patients. If a patient grinds his or her teeth or chews gum, the muscles of mastication may appear very prominent. Excessive talking after injection can cause prominent FDG uptake within the larynx. Laryngeal uptake is normally very subtle and appears in the form of an inverted V shape (Fig. 24-5).[2] [Note: PET/CT fusion images (rather than just PET images) have been included to provide anatomic landmarks.]

Thorax and Myocardium

Uptake by the heart muscle is highly variable, not only from one patient to another but even in the same patient imaged on different occasions.[8] To understand why this is true, it is helpful to look at the myocardium's sources of energy. Under normal aerobic conditions, 50% to 70% of total energy is obtained from the oxidation of fatty acids, with the rest being primarily obtained from carbohydrates (glucose and lactate). However, the percentage each energy source contributes is affected by many factors: nutrition, hormones, level of myocardial work, and level of myocardial blood flow. Particularly relevant to PET is that under fasting conditions, myocardial fatty acid metabolism is the predominant energy source. This scenario occurs because plasma insulin levels fall, resulting in increased decomposition of fat cells from adipose tissues and the subsequent increase of fatty acid levels in the plasma. More fatty acids are delivered to the myocardium, which decreases the myocardium's need for glucose metabolism. Conversely, after an individual eats, plasma insulin levels inhibits fat breakdown within adipose tissue; consequently, plasma fatty acid levels decrease, which in turn decreases myocardial fatty acid metabolism. As a consequence, glucose becomes a primary source of energy.

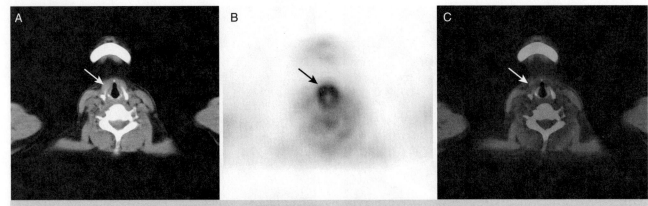

FIGURE 24-5 Normal vocal cords (arrows) on (A) CT, (B) PET, (C) PET/CT fusion images. Actual PET/CT images are always displayed in color. To view a color version of this image, please review the image bank found at http://thepoint.lww.com/RomansCT. Images courtesy of Dr. Saabry Osmany, Department of Nuclear Medicine and PET, Singapore General Hospital, Singapore.

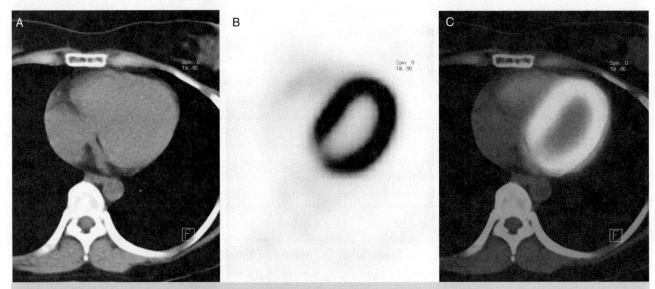

FIGURE 24-6 Image showing physiologic left ventricular on (A) CT, (B) PET, (C) PET/CT fusion images. Actual PET/CT images are always displayed in color. To view a color version of this image, please review the image bank found at http://thepoint.lww.com/RomansCT. Images courtesy of Dr. Saabry Osmany, Department of Nuclear Medicine and PET, Singapore General Hospital, Singapore.

However, despite patient fasting, many variations in uptake can be seen. These range from absent to very intense uptake within the left ventricle (Fig. 24-6). A less common observation is intense uptake within the right ventricle.[2]

Thymus

In children, thymus uptake is normal, appearing as an inverted shape.[5] In adults, increased FDG activity in the thymus after chemotherapy or radiotherapy is a normal variant. This phenomenon is called thymic rebound (Fig. 24-7).

Breast

FDG uptake in the breast varies. There is increased uptake in women who have dense breasts or in women who receive hormonal therapy.[9] Increased FDG activity is normally seen in the nipples. In addition, there is increased FDG uptake in the breasts of women who are lactating.[10]

Lung

Chronic obstructive pulmonary disease necessitates excessive contraction of accessory muscles for expiration. This results in increased intercostal uptake that can be misinterpreted as metastases to the ribs or as bone marrow uptake.[5] Hyperventilation may induce uptake in the diaphragm.[5]

Gastrointestinal Tract

It is unclear why FDG uptake occurs in the digestive tract.[5] Gastric activity has a characteristic J-shape within the left upper abdomen, and uptake can be either faint

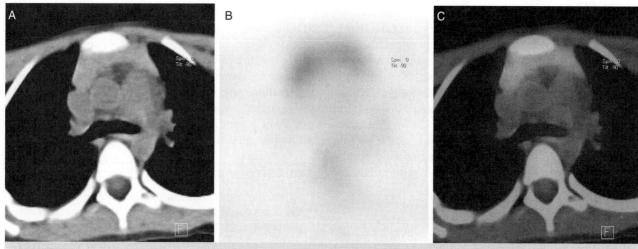

FIGURE 24-7 Image showing thymic rebound in a postchemotherapy patient on (A) CT, (B) PET, (C) PET/CT fusion images. Actual PET/CT images are always displayed in color. To view a color version of this image, please review the image bank found at http://thepoint.lww.com/RomansCT. Images courtesy of Dr. Saabry Osmany, Department of Nuclear Medicine and PET, Singapore General Hospital, Singapore.

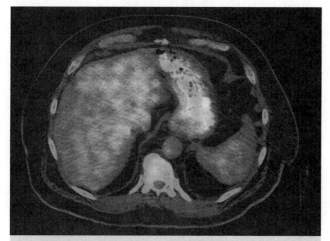

FIGURE 24-8 PET/CT image of normal stomach wall uptake. Actual PET/CT images are always displayed in color. To view a color version of this image, please review the image bank found at http://thepoint.lww.com/RomansCT. Image courtesy of Department of Radiology, University of Michigan Medical Center.

or intense (Fig. 24-8). FDG uptake is mostly seen in the large bowel and to a lesser extent in the small bowel and stomach.[5] Activity in the cecum is usually higher than that in the other colonic segments. Attempts to use laxatives, antimicrobials, smooth muscle relaxants, or glucagon to reduce bowel activity and therefore reduce uptake have met with variable success and are generally not recommended.[5] Uptake in the bowel can be seen as either faint or intense and in a diffuse pattern or concentrated in the right lower quadrant. Diffuse uptake in the bowel is often associated with normal findings at colonoscopy, whereas focal uptake may indicate inflammation.[11] There

is also a risk that high bowel activity in normal patients or in patients with inflammatory bowel disease may mask celiac, mesenteric, and iliac lymph node uptake. Focal colonic uptake should be further evaluated by colonoscopy.[5] Also, the patient's age affects the degree of uptake in the bowel, which further complicates interpretation; activity increases until approximately age 60, and thereafter bowel activity decreases.

Kidney and Lower Urinary Tract

Within the urinary tract, glucose behaves much differently than does FDG. Glucose is not excreted by the kidneys, but FDG is excreted by these organs. This scenario results in intense activity within the collecting system, ureters, and urinary bladder.[2] Hydration and the use of diuretics can reduce FDG activity in the kidneys and ureters and decrease the radiation dose to the genitourinary tract.[2,5] Abnormalities in organs that are in the vicinity of the bladder—such as the uterus, ovaries, or prostate—may be difficult to detect. Researchers have tried catheterization of the bladder to alleviate these diagnostic difficulties; however, in addition to the invasive nature of catheterization, this technique has created additional problems in interpretation.[12]

Reproductive System

Normal increase in endometrial FDG uptake occurs during ovulation and menstruation.[13] However, in postmenopausal patients, increased ovarian uptake is associated with malignancy.[13] To avoid possible misinterpretation, some authors have suggested performing FDG imaging within a week before, or a few days after, the menstrual flow phase.[2] Moderately intense testicular activity that declines with age is regarded as a normal variant.

Bone Marrow

The bone marrow has generally low FDG uptake that is mostly seen in vertebral bodies.[2,5] After chemotherapy, there is increased uptake as a result of bone marrow recovery that usually resolves 1 month after therapy.[14] Additionally, postchemotherapy patients who receive granulocyte colony-stimulating factors may also exhibit diffuse bone marrow hypermetabolism of FDG (Fig. 24-9). Bone fractures can show FDG uptake. If increased uptake persists beyond 3 months, infection or malignancy should be suspected.[15] In areas that have been treated with radiotherapy, FDG uptake decreases.

Although whole-body PET typically does not include areas distal to the mid-thigh or the upper extremities, it has been argued that FDG imaging may be useful for the evaluation of soft-tissue infection, osteomyelitis, knee and hip prostheses, or infection.[16] FDG uptake is expected in the bone marrow within the proximal part of the humeral and femoral bones. In addition, uptake in the sternoclavicular, acromioclavicular, and glenohumeral joints is normal. The degree of FDG accumulation in the joints is proportional with patient age. This scenario may be the result of chronic, often low-level, inflammatory processes that occur in aging joints.[5] FDG uptake can also be seen in the metaphyses of young patients.

Blood Vessels

FDG activity is seen in the aorta and other blood vessels. This finding correlates with age and most likely relates to atherosclerotic plaque inflammation.[17]

Miscellaneous

FDG accumulation in the axillae can occur normally if there is extravasation at the site of injection (Fig. 24-10).[18] Therefore, the injection should be performed in the arm opposite to the primary lesion. To avoid possible misinterpretation, any extravasation should be noted by the technologist performing the examination. FDG uptake can also be seen at the incision site after surgery and at ostomy or chest tube sites.[19]

BOX 24-5   Key Concept

To avoid possible misinterpretation, any extravasation of the radiopharmaceutical should be noted by the technologist performing the examination.

Benign Pathologies that Affect Uptake

It should be apparent from the preceding discussion that examinations using FDG are not tumor-specific searches. In addition to the several sites that have normal physiologic accumulation, FDG can accumulate in nonneoplastic pathologic conditions.[2] Abnormal uptake is associated with infections of either an acute or chronic nature, including infections of the soft tissue and bone as well as tuberculosis.[20,21] Increased uptake is often associated with inflammatory conditions such as Crohn's disease, granulomatous disease (e.g., sarcoidosis, tuberculosis), and autoimmune diseases such as Graves' disease.[22–24] Postoperative healing scars and postradiotherapy signs are other inflammatory-induced changes that can result in increased FDG uptake.[2]

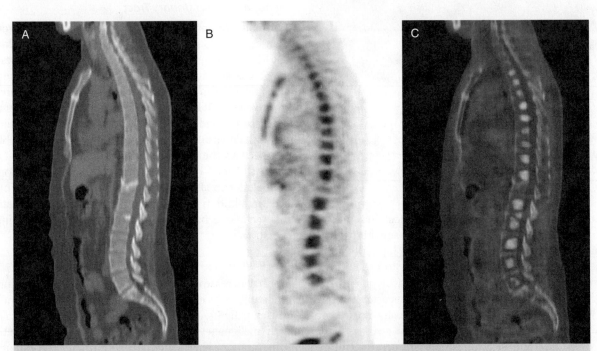

FIGURE 24-9   CT reformation of the spine (A) is used in conjunction with the PET image (B); the fusion image (C) displays diffuse bone marrow hypermetabolism secondary to granulocyte-colony stimulating factor administration. Actual PET/CT images are always displayed in color. To view a color version of this image, please review the image bank found at http://thepoint.lww.com/RomansCT. Images courtesy of Dr. Saabry Osmany, Department of Nuclear Medicine and PET, Singapore General Hospital, Singapore.

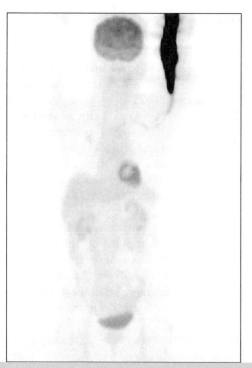

FIGURE 24-10 PET image (posterior view) showing extravasation of ^{18}F-FDG in the right arm secondary to subcutaneous injection. Image courtesy of Department of Radiology, University of Michigan Medical Center.

Standard Uptake Value (SUV)

Similar to the interpretation of other imaging studies, FDG-PET scans are interpreted mainly by qualitative means. That is, an area of abnormality is detected by comparison with background activity. However, along with FDG imaging, another method–one that is semiquantitative–can be useful in characterizing lesions as benign or malignant. This is particularly true when areas are judged to be equivocal by qualitative analysis alone. This other parameter is an index of glucose metabolism referred to as standard uptake value (SUV)–a measure of the relative uptake in tissues with an assigned numeric value. To obtain an SUV, the abnormality of interest is first identified on the PET scan. A region of interest (ROI) is then placed on the abnormality, and the activity (concentration of radioactivity) in becquerel (Bq) per milliliter is measured. The decay-corrected activity is then used to compute the SUV by the following formula:

$$SUV = \frac{\text{Radioactivity Concentration in ROI}}{\text{Injection Dose (Bq)/Patient Weight (g)}}$$

The SUV may change according to the time of image acquisition after FDG injection; therefore, the time of acquisition after FDG injection must be standardized for these values to be useful.[25] The accuracy of the patient's body weigh will also affect the SUV; some investigators

have advocated the use of lean body weight instead of total body weight.[26]

The SUV correlates well with the malignant potential of a lesion. Lesions with values greater than 2.5 have been shown to have a high likelihood of malignancy, whereas lesions with values less than 2 are usually benign. However, as different centers use different ways of acquiring and processing PET/CT studies, variability in SUV values can be seen among machines and centers. Certain PET image findings can indicate the approximate SUV of a lesion. As a rough guideline, the SUV of the liver should be in the range of 2 to 2.5, and the SUV of the mediastinal blood pool should be approximately 1.5 to 2.0. Therefore, a lesion in the chest with FDG uptake greater than that of the mediastinal blood pool is viewed with suspicion. Likewise, a lesion in the abdomen that has FDG uptake greater than that in the liver is also viewed with suspicion.

BOX 24–6   Key Concept

SUV is an index of glucose metabolism. The number represents the relative uptake of radionuclides in tissues.

PET/CT FUSION

FDG-PET is highly sensitive in detecting malignant lesions in tumors that are hyperglycemic. However, benign entities, such as infectious and inflammatory processes can be problematic because they also exhibit increased FDG uptake. Additionally, it is easy to see how normal physiologic accumulation of FDG can make clinical interpretation difficult. This scenario is further complicated given that PET provides only limited anatomic landmarks. Hence, even with knowledge of the normal distribution of FDG uptake, it is often difficult to confidently identify an area as normal or pathologic with PET alone. The technique of correlating CT images, which provide excellent anatomic landmarks, with PET images has been shown to improve diagnostic accuracy compared with PET alone.[27] However, correlating images from a CT study to a PET study can be difficult given that the position of the patient and the time interval between scans vary.

BOX 24–7   Key Concept

PET/CT or PET/MRI combines the benefits of anatomic information from CT and metabolic information from PET. Anatomic imaging provided by CT and MRI has a high sensitivity for the detection of obvious structural disruption but is not as useful in characterizing these abnormalities as malignant or benign.

To optimize the combined benefits of anatomic information from CT and metabolic information from PET, a combined PET/CT scanner was developed. With the combined PET/CT scanner, the patient undergoes a CT scan followed immediately by a PET scan during the same imaging session. This method provides more precise coregistration of the two modalities by addressing problems associated with repositioning and prolonged time between scanning methods.

In the field of nuclear medicine, attenuation is when photons are absorbed in the body (this should not be confused with the similar term beam attenuation frequently used in CT). In PET, loss of counts can occur because of attenuation, image artifacts, scatter and random image noise, image artifacts, and image distortion. Without attenuation correction, significant artifacts may occur. In a dedicated PET system, attenuation correction features are built into the process using a PET transmission scan. However, when PET/CT is used, data from the CT images can be used for attenuation correction of the PET emission data, eliminating the need for a separate, time-consuming transmission scan. Using the CT data for attenuation correction provides more accurate and efficient attenuation correction compared with a PET transmission scan.[28] The use of the CT scan for attenuation correction allows the data from the two imaging methods to be overlayed electronically and displayed on a workstation. The data can be simultaneously and interactively viewed as CT data, PET data, and superimposed CT and PET data in any percentage combination desired (e.g., 50% CT/50% PET data).

BOX 24–8   Key Concept

Like standard CT, decisions must be made before each specific PET/CT examination. These decisions include whether intravenous or oral contrast material is required, and whether the correlative CT portion of the examination is needed only for attenuation correction and localization, or whether more detailed anatomic CT information is needed.

Clinical Procedures for ¹⁸F-FDG PET/CT

Like standard CT, protocols for PET/CT continue to evolve as the technology improves. Also like standard CT, decisions must be made before each specific PET/CT examination as to whether intravenous or oral contrast material is required. In addition, radiologists must decide whether the CT portion of the examination is for attenuation correction and localization only, in which case scans are acquired at a lower dose (40 to 80 mAs is typical) or whether the full range of CT information is needed, in which case the mAs is similar to standard CT examinations. These decisions are based on the clinical questions posed and whether the patient already has undergone a recent, diagnostic CT. A typical PET/CT procedure consists of the following steps:

- A detailed medical history is obtained.
- The patient fasts for at least 6 hours before the scan.
- Oral contrast material is given, if indicated.
- The patient receives an intravenous injection of 370 to 555 MBq (10 to 15 mCi) of FDG.
- Approximately 30 to 60 minutes after the intravenous FDG injection the patient is placed on the examination table.
- The patient is positioned in the scanner in the same manner as for standard CT examinations (e.g., arms are raised for chest and abdomen studies, sponges are used to ensure the patient's comfort, immobilization devices are used when needed).
- Scouts are acquired and cross-sectional slices are planned.
- Intravenous contrast material is administered, if indicated. Injection protocols mimic those used in standard CT protocols of the same body part.
- The patient is given clear breathing instructions (shallow breathing is the most common). The patient is asked to breath in the same manner for both CT and PET portions of the examination. Motion correction such as respiratory gating is recommended when available.
- The CT scan is performed.
- Attenuation correction factors are generated from the CT data to be applied to the PET data.
- The PET scan is obtained as a series of acquisitions at overlapping bed positions. Acquisition parameters are usually facility and camera specific.
- Reconstruction of PET data occurs depending on facility protocol.
- Reconstructed PET and CT images are available for viewing on a workstation.
- Images should be checked before the patient leaves.
- Delayed or repeat images may be helpful in select cases.

CHAPTER SUMMARY

CT is an anatomic modality and has a high sensitivity for the detection of obvious structural disruption. However, functional changes often predate structural changes in tissues. To detect the abnormal behavior of tissues an imaging method that investigates events at a cellular level must be used. PET studies provide functional and metabolic detail and often demonstrate pathologic changes long before they would be revealed by anatomic modalities like CT. To optimize the combined benefits of metabolic information from PET and anatomic localization from CT, a combined PET/CT scanner was developed. With the combined PET/CT scanner, the patient undergoes a CT scan followed immediately by a PET scan during the same imaging session. The PET and CT images are then aligned. With PET/CT, areas of abnormal PET radiotracer uptake can be localized to specific anatomic structures (such as lymph nodes), aiding interpretation. Acquiring a CT at diagnostic CT settings can be convenient to the patient because a complete assessment of the anatomic status of disease can also be obtained in just one appointment. Combining the two modalities does, however, pose staffing challenges because it is rare that a technologist is trained in both modalities.

REVIEW QUESTIONS

1. Explain the difference between anatomic and functional imaging methods.
2. Why is it important for a patient to fast before a PET examination?
3. Explain why the CT portion of a PET/CT examination might be done at an mAs setting that would result in a noisy image.

REFERENCES

1. Brown RS, Leung JY, Fisher SJ, Frey KA, Ethier SP, Wahl RL. Intratumoral distribution of tritiated-FDG in breast carcinoma: correlation between Glut-1 expression and FDG uptake. J Nucl Med 1996;37:1042–7.
2. Abouzied MM, Crawford ES, Nabi HA. 18F-FDG imaging: pitfalls and artifacts. J Nucl Med Technol 2005;33:145–55.
3. Kostakoglu L, Hardoff R, Mirtcheva R, Goldsmith SJ. PET-CT fusion imaging in differentiating physiologic from pathologic FDG uptake. Radiographics 2004;24:1411–31.
4. Goerres GW, von Schulthess GK, Hany TF. Positron emission tomography and PET CT of the head and neck: FDG uptake in normal anatomy, in benign lesions, and in changes resulting from treatment. AJR Am J Roentgenol 2002;179:1337–43.
5. El-Haddad G, Alavi A, Mavi A, Bural G, Zhuang H. Normal variants in [18F]-fluorodeoxyglucose PET imaging. Radiol Clin North Am 2004;42:1063–81, viii.
6. Torizuka T, Clavo AC, Wahl RL. Effect of hyperglycemia on in vitro tumor uptake of tritiated FDG, thymidine, L-methionine and L-leucine. J Nucl Med 1997;38:382–6.
7. Kang KW, Kim SK, Kang HS, et al. Prevalence and risk of cancer of focal thyroid incidentaloma identified by 18F-fluorodeoxyglucose positron emission tomography for metastasis evaluation and cancer screening in healthy subjects. J Clin Endocrinol Metab 2003;88:4100–4.
8. Herrero P, Gropler RJ. Imaging of myocardial metabolism. J Nucl Cardiol 2005;12:345–58.
9. Vranjesevic D, Schiepers C, Silverman DH, et al. Relationship between 18F-FDG uptake and breast density in women with normal breast tissue. J Nucl Med 2003;44:1238–42.
10. Hicks RJ, Binns D, Stabin MG. Pattern of uptake and excretion of (18)F-FDG in the lactating breast. J Nucl Med 2001;42:1238–42.
11. Tatlidil R, Jadvar H, Bading JR, Conti PS. Incidental colonic fluorodeoxyglucose uptake: correlation with colonoscopic and histopathologic findings. Radiology 2002;224:783–7.
12. Vesselle HJ, Miraldi FD. FDG PET of the retroperitoneum: normal anatomy, variants, pathologic conditions, and strategies to avoid diagnostic pitfalls. Radiographics 1998;18:805–23.
13. Lerman H, Metser U, Grisaru D, Fishman A, Lievshitz G, Even-Sapir E. Normal and abnormal 18F-FDG endometrial and ovarian uptake in pre- and postmenopausal patients: assessment by PET/CT. J Nucl Med 2004;45:266–71.
14. Sugawara Y, Fisher SJ, Zasadny KR, Kison PV, Baker LH, Wahl RL. Preclinical and clinical studies of bone marrow uptake of fluorine-1-fluorodeoxyglucose with or without granulocyte colony-stimulating factor during chemotherapy. J Clin Oncol 1998;16:173–80.
15. Zhuang H, Sam JW, Chacko TK, et al. Rapid normalization of osseous FDG uptake following traumatic or surgical fractures. Eur J Nucl Med Mol Imaging 2003;30:1096–103.
16. Chacko TK, Zhuang H, Nakhoda KZ, Moussavian B, Alavi A. Applications of fluorodeoxyglucose positron emission tomography in the diagnosis of infection. Nucl Med Commun 2003;24:615–24.
17. Tatsumi M, Cohade C, Nakamoto Y, Wahl RL. Fluorodeoxyglucose uptake in the aortic wall at PET/CT: possible finding for active atherosclerosis. Radiology 2003;229:831–7.
18. Chiang SB, Rebenstock A, Guan L, Burns J, Alavi A, Zhuang H. Potential false-positive FDG PET imaging caused by subcutaneous radiotracer infiltration. Clin Nucl Med 2003;28:786–8.
19. Zhuang H, Cunnane ME, Ghesani NV, Mozley PD, Alavi A. Chest tube insertion as a potential source of false-positive FDG-positron emission tomographic results. Clin Nucl Med 2002;27:285–6.
20. Stumpe KD, Dazzi H, Schaffner A, von Schulthess GK. Infection imaging using whole-body FDG-PET. Eur J Nucl Med 2000;27:822–32.
21. Bakheet SM, Powe J, Ezzat A, Rostom A. F-18-FDG uptake in tuberculosis. Clin Nucl Med 1998;23:739–42.
22. Bicik I, Bauerfeind P, Breitbach T, von Schulthess GK, Fried M. Inflammatory bowel disease activity measured by positron-emission tomography. Lancet 1997;350:262.
23. Lewis PJ, Salama A. Uptake of fluorine-18-fluorodeoxyglucose in sarcoidosis. J Nucl Med 1994;35:1647–9.
24. Chen YK, Chen YL, Liao AC, Shen YY, Kao CH. Elevated 18F-FDG uptake in skeletal muscles and thymus: a clue for the diagnosis of Graves' disease. Nucl Med Commun 2004;25:115–21.
25. Coleman RE. Clinical PET in oncology. Clin Positron Imaging.1998;1:15–30.
26. Zasadny KR, Wahl RL. Standardized uptake values of normal tissues at PET with 2-[fluorine-18]-fluoro-2-deoxy-D-glucose: variations with body weight and a method for correction. Radiology 1993;189:847–50.
27. Kluetz PG, Meltzer CC, Villemagne VL, et al. Combined PET/CT imaging in oncology. Impact on patient management. Clin Positron Imaging 2000;3:223–30.
28. Townsend DW. Dual-modality imaging: combining anatomy and function. J Nucl Med 2008;49:938–55.

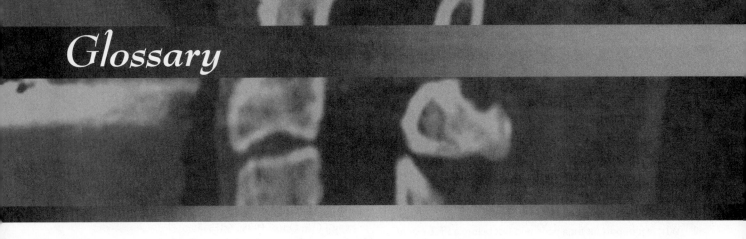

Glossary

Absorption efficiency: Number of photons absorbed by the detector; dependent on the physical properties of the detector face (e.g., thickness, material).

ACR CT accreditation phantom: A solid phantom that contains four modules and is constructed primarily from a water-equivalent material. Each module is 4 cm deep and 20 cm in diameter, with external alignment markings to allow centering of the phantom in the x, y, and z axes, and is used to measure different aspects of image quality.

Acute renal failure (ARF): Rapid loss of renal function caused by damage to the kidney, resulting in retention of waste products that are normally excreted by the kidney.

Adaptive array: Detector rows that have variable widths and sizes. Also called nonuniform or hybrid arrays.

Adrenal adenoma: Benign adrenal mass.

Advanced display functions: Display functions that include multiplanar reformation and three-dimensional reformation.

Afterglow: A brief, persistent flash of scintillation that must be taken into account and subtracted before image reconstruction.

Air embolism: Air that enters the bloodstream and can occur during an IV injection. Small quantities of air can be absorbed by the body; thus small air emboli may never be detected if patients are asymptomatic. However, large air emboli can cause seizures, permanent neurologic damage, or occasionally death. These large air emboli occur only as a result of human error.

Algorithm: A precise set of steps to be performed in a specific order to solve a problem. Algorithms are the basis for most computer programming.

Aliasing: Artifacts that result from insufficient projection data; cause fine stripes that appear to be radiating from a dense structure.

Analog-to-digital converter (ADC): Converts the analog signal to a digital format.

Anaphylactoid: Life-threatening reactions; symptoms include substantial respiratory distress, unresponsiveness, convulsions, clinically manifested arrhythmias, and cardiopulmonary arrest. These reactions require prompt recognition and treatment.

Anatomic landmark: Landmark, such as the xiphoid or the iliac crest, used as a reference point when planning the scout image.

Anatomic position: Characterized by an individual standing erect, with the palms of the hands facing forward. This position is used internationally and guarantees uniformity in descriptions of direction.

Angioplasty: Technique that is used to dilate an area of arterial blockage using a catheter with a small, inflatable, sausage-shaped balloon at its tip.

Anode: X-ray tube design includes a cathode, which emits electrons, and an anode, which collects electrons.

Anterior: Term used to describe movement forward (toward the face); also referred to as ventral.

Archiving: Saving studies on auxiliary devices for the purpose of future viewing.

Array processor: Now outdated, an array processor is a CPU design frequently used for CT image reconstruction. Also called a vector processor, this design was able to run mathematical operations on multiple data elements simultaneously. General increases in performance and processor design have made this design obsolete.

Arteriovenous iodine difference: Comparison of a Hounsfield unit (HU) measurement taken within the aorta to that of a measurement taken in the inferior vena cava. Used to assess the phase of tissue enhancement after the IV injection of contrast media.

Arteriovenous malformations: Composed of tangles of arteries and arterialized veins. In the brain there is tissue interposed between the vessels, but it is usually abnormal and often scarred from previous tiny hemorrhages; blood is shunted directly from the arterial system to the venous system. This shunting allows oxygenated blood to enter the veins. The flow is high and the pressure is elevated within the veins. The elevated pressure can cause the vessels to rupture, resulting in a hemorrhagic stroke.

Artifacts: Objects seen on the image but not present in the object scanned.

Atherosclerosis: The buildup of fat and cholesterol plaque.

Atrial fibrillation: A disorder of heart rate and rhythm in which the atria are stimulated to contract in a very rapid or disorganized manner rather than in an organized one.

Attenuation correction: Method for reducing artifacts in the PET image. In PET, loss of counts can occur because of anomalies in attenuation, scatter and random image noise, image artifacts, and image distortion. In a dedicated PET system, attenuation correction features are built into the process using a PET transmission scan. However, when PET/CT is used, data from the CT images can be used for attenuation correction of the PET emission data, eliminating the need for a separate, time-consuming transmission scan.

Attenuation profile: The system accounts for the attenuation properties of each ray sum and correlates it to the position of the ray.

Autochangers: Robotic storage systems that automatically load and unload optical discs. The devices are also called optical disc libraries, robotic drives, or optical jukeboxes.

Automated injection triggering: Injection methods that individualize the scan delay. Two methods exist–the injection of a test bolus and bolus triggering.

Automatic tube current modulation: An equipment option that will make changes in tube current (mA) based on the estimated attenuation of the patient at a specific location. The estimations are derived from scout views done in both the anteroposterior and lateral projections or from the previous slices. From these views, the mA will be programmed to vary by location along the length of the patient. The exact details of the option vary by manufacturer.

Axial scanning: Scan method in which the CT table moves to the desired location and remains stationary while the x-ray tube rotates within the gantry, collecting data; scans produced with the step-and-shoot method result in images that are perpendicular to the z axis (or tabletop) and parallel to every other slice, like slices of a sausage. Also called step-and-shoot scanning.

Back projection: Process of converting the data from the attenuation profile to a matrix.

Balloon angioplasty: Technique that is used to dilate an area of arterial blockage using a catheter with a small, inflatable, sausage-shaped balloon at its tip.

Bandwidth: Amount of data that can be transmitted between two points in the network in a set period of time.

Barium peritonitis: Barium leaking into the peritoneal cavity.

Basal ganglia: Part of the brain. The level of the basal ganglia contains territories supplied by the anterior (ACA), middle (MCA), and posterior cerebral arteries (PCA). Therefore, this is the level most frequently scanned for brain perfusion studies.

Beam attenuation: Phenomenon by which an x-ray beam passing through a structure is decreased in intensity or amount because of absorption and interaction with matter. The alteration in the beam varies with the density of the structure it passes through.

Beam pitch: Table movement per rotation divided by beam width.

Beam-hardening artifacts: Artifacts that result from lower-energy photons being preferentially absorbed, leaving higher-intensity photons to strike the detector array.

β–blockers: Pharmaceuticals used to reduce motion artifact on cardiac CTA images by temporarily lowering a patient's heart rate.

Biphasic injection: Injection technique in which two flow rates are used.

Bits: Binary digits.

Blood-brain barrier (BBB): A semipermeable structure that protects the brain from most substances in the blood, while still allowing essential metabolic function.

Blu-ray discs: Optical storage device; can be used for long-term data storage with a storage capacity of more than 500 gigabytes.

Bolus injection technique: A rapid injection of contrast material. A volume of contrast of 50 to 200 mL is injected at a rate between 1 and 6 mL/s. The contrast bolus can be delivered by hand (using syringes) or by a mechanical injection system.

Bolus phase: The initial phase that immediately follows an IV bolus injection. In the bolus phase of contrast enhancement, the arterial structures are filled with contrast medium and brightly displayed on the image. Contrast media has not yet filled the venous structures. Also called the arterial phase.

Bolus shaping: Manipulating the flow rate to change the characteristics of the time-density curves.

Bolus triggering: Method of individualizing the scan delay using the contrast bolus itself to initiate the scan. It uses a series of low-radiation scans to monitor the progress of the contrast bolus. Once an adequate level of enhancement is achieved, the table moves to the starting level and scanning begins.

Bow tie filters: Mechanical filter that removes soft, or low-energy, x-ray beams, minimizing patient exposure and providing a more uniform beam intensity.

Bytes: Unit of information storage composed of 8 bits of data.

Calcium score: The amount of calcification on cardiac CT.

Capture efficiency: Ability with which the detector obtains photons that have passed through the patient.

Cardiac gating: CT techniques that attempt to minimize cardiac motion in the study by selecting (or acquiring) images during cardiac segments with relatively low cardiac motion. ECG tracings are acquired with the scan acquisition.

Caudal: Term used to describe movement toward the feet; synonymous with inferior.

Centigray (cGy): A centigray (cGy) equals 1 rad. There are 100 rad in 1 gray (Gy).

Central processing unit (CPU): Component that interprets computer program instructions and sequences tasks. It contains the microprocessor, the control unit, and the primary memory.

Central venous access devices (CVAD): A venous catheter designed to deliver medications and fluids directly into the superior vena cava (SVC), inferior vena cava (IVC), or right atrium (RA).

Central volume principle: Principle that states cerebral blood volume can be calculated as the product of the total cerebral blood flow and the time needed for the cerebral blood passage: CBF = CBV/MTT.

Cerebrovascular accident: Term used to describe stroke; no longer favored because it implies a random, unpredictable, or uncertain nature to the condition.

Cerebrovascular reserve capacity (CVRC): Describes how far cerebral perfusion can increase from a baseline value after undergoing stimulation. It is essentially a "stress test" for the brain.

Stimulation is provided through the intravenous administration of a drug such as acetazolamide.

Chemotoxic reactions: Reactions that result from the physicochemical properties of the contrast media, the dose, and speed of injection. All hemodynamic (i.e., relating to blood circulation) disturbances and injuries to organs or vessels perfused by the contrast medium are included in this category. Contrast-induced nephropathy is an example of a chemotoxic reaction.

Clearance: The ability of the kidney to remove a substance from the blood.

Client-server network: Computers in this model are either classified as servers or clients. A server is a computer that facilitates communication between and delivers information to other computers. The server acts on requests from other networked computers (the clients), rather than from a person inputting directly into it.

Clinical information systems (CIS): Information systems that keep track of clinical data.

Clustered scans: The practice of grouping more than one scan in a single breath-hold.

Collimators: Mechanical hardware that resembles small shutters and adjusts the opening based on the operator's selection.

Compact discs (CD): Optical storage devices; can be used for long-term data storage. A CD has the storage capacity of 700 megabytes.

Compensating filters: Filters the x-ray beam to reduce the radiation dose to the patient; help to minimize image artifact and improve image quality.

Completed stroke: Preferred medical term used to describe an acute episode of interrupted blood flow to the brain that lasts longer than 24 hours. Also called an established stroke.

Computed tomography dose index (CTDI): Dose reported to the FDA; slices must be contiguous.

Computerized physician order-entry (CPOE): System that electronically transmits clinician orders to radiology and other departments.

Cone beam: The radiation emitted from the collimated x-ray source in multidetector row CT systems.

Cone-beam artifacts: Artifacts that relate to the cone-shaped beam required for MDCT helical scans. These artifacts are more pronounced for the outer detector rows. The larger the cone beam (i.e., more detector channels), the more pronounced the effect.

Contiguous: Method of acquiring slices in which one slice abuts the next.

Continuous acquisition scanning: Scanning method that includes a continually rotating x-ray tube, constant x-ray output, and uninterrupted table movement Also called helical, spiral, or volumetric scanning.

Contrast-detail curve: Result of measuring and charting the relationship between object size and visibility (contrast-detail response).

Contrast-detail response: The relationship between object size and visibility.

Contrast detectability: Ability of the system to differentiate between objects with similar densities. Also called low-contrast resolution.

Contrast media extravasation: The leakage of fluid from a vein into the surrounding tissue during IV contrast administration.

Contrast media-induced nephropathy (CIN): An acute impairment of renal function that follows the intravascular administration of contrast material, for which alternative causes have been excluded.

Contrast washout: An imaging characteristic regarding how quickly the iodinated contrast is washed out of the adrenal gland. It can be used to differentiate adenomas from metastases; relies on physiologic differences in perfusion.

Convolution: Process of applying a filter function to an attenuation profile.

Cooling systems: Cooling mechanisms included in the gantry, such as blowers, filters, or devices that perform oil-to-air heat exchange.

Core servers: Server computers that are integral to the functioning of the PACS.

Coronal plane: Body plane that divides the body into anterior and posterior sections.

Coronary artery bypass graft surgery (CABG): Commonly pronounced "cabbage," this surgical procedure is typically recommended when there is disease of the left main coronary artery or in three or more vessels, or if nonsurgical management has failed. Arteries or veins taken from elsewhere in the patient's body are grafted from the aorta to the coronary arteries to bypass atherosclerotic narrowings and improve the blood supply to the coronary circulation supplying the myocardium. The terms "single," "double," "triple," or "quadruple bypass" refer to the number of coronary arteries bypassed in the procedure.

Coronary artery disease (CAD): A condition that results when plaque builds up in the coronary arteries. A partial or total blockage results, and the heart muscle does not get an adequate blood supply. Also referred to as ischemic heart disease.

Coronary circulation: The movement of blood through the tissues of the heart. Blood is carried to the heart by the two coronary arteries and their branches. Cardiac veins remove deoxygenated blood and waste products.

Coronary stenting: Stents are made of self-expanding, stainless-steel mesh. They are mounted on a balloon catheter in a collapsed form. When the balloon is inflated, the stent expands and pushes against the inner wall of the coronary artery.

Corticomedullary phase: The phase of renal enhancement that follows the portal venous phase that typically occurs approximately 30 to 70 seconds after the IV administration of a bolus of contrast material.

Crosstalk: Image noise resulting from the scattering of x-ray photons by adjacent detectors.

CRT: Monitors used in radiology departments were all adaptations of the cathode-ray tube (CRT).

CT angiography: CT technique used to visualize the arterial and venous vessels throughout the body. Scans are performed in the helical mode with a high flow rate contrast injection.

CT arthrography (CTA): CT procedure in which a needle is introduced into a joint and contrast media is injected, outlining the joint capsule, ligaments, and articular surfaces.

CT brain perfusion: CT method that provides a qualitative and quantitative evaluation of cerebral perfusion. CT perfusion provides this information by calculating regional blood flow (rCBF), regional blood volume (rCBV), and mean transit time (MTT). Perfusion studies are obtained by monitoring the passage of iodinated contrast through the cerebral vasculature.

CT fluoroscopy (CTF): An add-on option for some scanners. Often used for CT-guided interventions. CTF allows for the near real-time capabilities of traditional fluoroscopy while maintaining the superior contrast resolution and 3D anatomic display of CT.

CT venography: Modification of CTA that is used for the depiction of venous anatomy. Scan parameters are quite similar to CTA, except images are acquired while contrast is in the venous enhancement phase.

CTDI phantoms: Phantoms used to measure the radiation dose delivered for various CT examinations. CTDI is an acronym for computed tomography dose index.

$CTDI_{100}$: Result when the CTDI is measured using a pencil ionization chamber. This 100-mm-long thin cylindrical device is long enough to span the width of 14 contiguous 7-mm CT slices. This provides a better estimate of MSAD for thin slices than that of the single-slice method.

$CTDI_{vol}$: The $CTDI_{vol}$ is a measure of exposure per slice and is independent of scan length. It is the preferred expression of radiation dose in CT dosimetry.

$CTDI_w$: The $CTDI_w$ adjusts for variation across the scan field of view by providing a weighted average of measurements at the center and the peripheral slice locations (i.e., the x and y dimensions of the slice).

Cupping artifacts: Artifact that results from beam hardening. It appears on the image as a vague area of increased density in a somewhat concentric shape around the periphery of an image, similar to the shape of a cup.

Data-acquisition system (DAS): Measures the number of photons that strikes the detector, converts the information to a digital signal, and sends the signal to the computer.

Delayed reactions: Reactions occurring between 1 hour and 1 week after contrast medium injection.

Detector: Element in a CT system that collects attenuation information. It measures the intensity of the transmitted x-ray radiation along a beam projected from the x-ray source to that particular detector element.

Detector aperture: Size of the detector opening.

Detector array: Entire collection of detectors included in a CT system; detector elements are situated in an arc or a ring.

Detector efficiency: Ability of the detector to capture transmitted photons and change them to electronic signals.

Detector pitch: Table movement per rotation time divided by the selected slice thickness of the detector.

Detector spacing: Measured from the middle of one detector to the middle of the neighboring detector; accounts for the spacing bar.

DICOM: Universally adopted standard for medical image interchange known as the Digital Imaging and Communication in Medicine.

Digital versatile discs (DVD): Optical storage devices; can be used for long-term data storage. A DVD has the storage capacity of up to 15.9 gigabytes.

Digital-to-analog converters (DAC): Changes the digital signal from the computer memory back to an analog format so that the image can be displayed on the monitor.

Direct axial plane: A direct plane is one that can be obtained by positioning the patient in a specific position. For the foot, the direct axial plane is defined as the plane parallel to the plantar surface of the foot.

Direct digital capture: Image acquisition from the CT scanner to the PACS in which CT data are transferred directly, which allows full spatial resolution and image manipulation capabilities (such as adjusting window width and level).

Discrete Fourier transform (DFT): A technique for expressing a waveform as a weighted sum of sines and cosines.

Display field of view (DFOV): The section of data selected for display on the image.

Display monitors: Output device that allows the information stored in computer memory to be displayed.

Display processor: CT component that assigns a group of Hounsfield units to each shade of gray.

Displayed contrast: The displayed contrast of an image is dependent on the window settings used for its display.

Distal: Term used in referring to extremities. Distal (away from) refers to movement toward the ends. The distal end of the forearm is the end to which the hand is attached.

Distance measurement: The system calculates the distance between two deposited points in either centimeters or millimeters.

Dorsal: Term used to describe movement toward the back surface of the body; also referred to as posterior.

Dose-length product (DLP): $DLP = CTDI_{vol} \times$ scan length. Although the DLP more closely reflects the radiation dose for a specific CT examination, its value is affected by variances in patient anatomy.

Double contrast technique: Injection technique used for arthrography in which both iodinated contrast and air are injected into the joint space.

Drip infusion: Technique used to administer contrast material in which an IV line is initiated and contrast medium is allowed to drip in during a period of several minutes.

Dual source: CT design that uses two sets of x-ray tubes and two corresponding detector arrays in a single CT gantry.

Dynamic range: Ratio of the maximum signal measured to the minimum signal the detectors can measure. The range of x-ray intensity values to which the scanner can accurately respond.

ECG-pulsed tube current modulation: Method developed to address concern about the radiation dose from retrospective ECG gating methods in CT. The tube current is automatically decreased during the systolic phase of the ECG tracing.

Edge gradient effect: Streak artifact or shading (both light and dark) arising from irregularly shaped objects that have a pronounced difference in density from surrounding structures.

Effective dose: A measurement, reported in Sv or rem, that attempts to account for the effects particular to the patient's tissue that has absorbed the radiation dose. It extrapolates the risk of partial body exposure to patients from data obtained from whole body doses to Japanese atomic bomb survivors. Although methods to calculate the effective dose have been established, they depend on the ability to estimate the dose to radiosensitive organs from the CT procedure. Also called effective dose equivalent.

Effective slice thickness: Thickness of the slice that is actually represented on the CT image, as opposed to the size selected by the collimator opening. In traditional axial scanning, selected slice thickness is equal to effective slice thickness. However, because of the interpolation process used in helical scanning, the effective slice thickness may be wider than the selected slice thickness. Also called the slice-sensitivity profile.

Electron beam imaging: Also referred to as EBCT or ultrafast CT. It differs from conventional CT in a number of ways. This system uses a large electron gun as its x-ray beam source. A massive anode target is placed in a semicircular ring around the patient. Neither the x-ray beam source nor the detectors move, and the scan can be acquired in a short time.

Electronic health record (EHR): Generic term for a digital patient record; in general usage, EHR and EMR are used synonymously.

Electronic medical record (EMR): Electronic health records (EHR) are often composed of electronic medical records (EMR) from a variety of sources, including radiology. However, in general usage, EHR and EMR are used synonymously.

Embolic stroke: Type of ischemic stroke resulting from a traveling particle that forms elsewhere and is too large to pass through small vessels and eventually lodges in a smaller artery.

Embolism: The formation, development, or existence of a clot within the vascular system that detaches from its original site.

Endoluminal imaging: A form of volume rendering designed to reveal the inside of the lumen of a structure. The technique is also called virtual endoscopy, virtual bronchoscopy, and virtual colonoscopy.

Enterprise-wide distribution: Distribution channels that encompass off-site outpatient clinics or allow on-call radiologists to review studies from home.

Equilibrium phase: The last phase of tissue enhancement after the IV injection of contrast media. It can begin as early as 2 minutes after the bolus phase or after a drip infusion. In this phase contrast media is largely emptied from the arteries, is greatly diluted in the veins, and has soaked the organ parenchyma. In this phase, intravascular structures and interstitial concentrations of contrast material equilibrate and decline at an equal rate. Also called the delayed phase.

Ethernet: Connections used to attach computers to the network, consisting of cables that are made up of twisted pairs of copper wire.

Excretory phase: The phase of renal enhancement that follows the nephrogram phase that typically occurs approximately 3 minutes after the IV administration of a bolus of contrast material and can last 15 minutes or longer.

Fan beam: The radiation emitted from the collimated x-ray source in single-detector row CT systems.

Fast Fourier transform (FFT): Discrete Fourier transform's inverse. FFTs are of great importance to a wide variety of applications, including acoustical and image analysis.

Fatty infiltration of the liver: The accumulation of fat in liver cells. It is also called steatosis. It is one of the most common liver abnormalities diagnosed by liver CT and can result from a variety of causes including alcoholism, obesity, diabetes, chemotherapy, corticosteroid therapy, hyperalimentation (i.e., total parental nutrition–intravenous feeding), and malnutrition.

Filter functions: Applied to the scan data before back projection occurs to minimize artifacts.

Fluorine-18 fluorodeoxyglucose: Radiotracer that has played a key role in advancing PET based on the fact that malignant tumors often favor the glycolytic pathway for metabolism.

Focal spot: Area of the anode where the electrons strike and the x-ray beam is produced.

Focused appendiceal CT: Protocol that limits the scan area to the lower abdomen and upper pelvis.

Fourier transform (FT): A method to study waves of many different sorts and also to solve several kinds of linear differential equations. Loosely speaking it separates a function into its frequency components.

Fourth-generation design: Scanner configuration that uses a detector array that is fixed in a 360° circle within the gantry. Sometimes referred to as rotate-only systems.

Frame grabbing: Analog method of image acquisition in which an image on the monitor is converted to a digital format, somewhat similar to a screen capture. Converting CT data in this way loses the original pixel's metrics.

Fully automated segmentation: The process of selectively removing or isolating information from the data set by a method that is fully automated by the software. Fully automatic segmentation methods are usually impractical because of image complexity and the variety of image types and clinical indications.

Gantry: Ring-shaped part of the CT scanner that houses many of the components necessary to produce and detect x-rays.

Gantry aperture: Opening in the gantry; range of aperture size is typically 70 to 90 cm.

Glabellomeatal line: Imaginary line used for positioning that connects the external acoustic meatus to the supraorbital margin. Also called the supraorbital meatal line.

Glomerular filtration rate (GFR): Describes the flow rate of filtered fluid through the kidney and is a measurement of kidney function.

Graves' disease: One of the main causes of hyperthyroidism.

Gray (Gy): SI unit of absorbed dose.

Gray scale: System that assigns a certain number of Hounsfield values to each shade of gray.

Half-life: Time it takes for half of the dose of a substance to be eliminated from the body.

Hand bolus: A rapid injection of contrast material delivered by hand, using syringes.

Hard disk: An essential component of all CT systems. It saves the thousands of bits of data acquired with each gantry rotation.

Hardware: Portions of the computer that can be physically touched.

Health Level Seven (HL7): An organization that works to develop universal standards for clinical and administrative data throughout the healthcare arena.

Heat capacity: Ability of the tube to withstand the heat.

Heat dissipation: Ability of the tube to rid itself of heat.

Helical interpolation artifacts: Result in subtle inaccuracies in CT numbers and can be easily misinterpreted as disease. These artifacts can best be avoided by using a low pitch whenever possible.

Helical interpolation methods: Complex statistical methods to, in effect, take the slant and blur out of the helical image and create images that closely resemble those acquired in a traditional axial mode.

Helical scanning: Scanning method that includes a continually rotating x-ray tube, constant x-ray output, and uninterrupted table movement Also called spiral, volumetric, or continuous acquisition scanning.

Hemangioma: Abnormal proliferation of blood vessels in the skin or internal organs.

Hemorrhagic stroke: Category of stroke caused by a tear in the artery's wall that produces bleeding in the brain.

Hepatic arterial phase: The first phase of enhancement typically occurring 15 to 25 seconds after the IV administration of a bolus of contrast material.

High attenuation: An x-ray beam is greatly impeded by an object; typically shown as light gray or white on an image.

High-contrast resolution: Ability of a system to resolve, as separate forms, small objects that are very close together. Also call spatial resolution or detail resolution.

High-frequency generator: Produces high voltage and transmits it to the x-ray tube.

High-osmolality contrast media (HOCM): Older iodinated agents, now less commonly used for intravascular injections. The osmolality of these agents ranges from approximately 1,300 to 2,140 mOsm/kg, or about 4 to 7 times that of human blood.

Histogram: A graphical display showing how frequently a range of CT numbers occur within an ROI.

Homeostasis: Literally translated as "standing or staying the same," in regards to the body, the minute-to-minute state of balance of water, electrolytes (such as sodium, potassium, chloride, and bicarbonate), and pH.

Hospital information systems (HIS): Information systems that focus on administrative issues, such as patient demographic data, financial data, and patient locations within the hospital.

Hounsfield units (HU): Measure of the beam attenuation capability of a specific structure. Also call pixel values, density numbers, or CT numbers.

HRCT: High-resolution CT of the chest is a technique used for the assessment of lung parenchyma in patients with diffuse lung disease such as fibrosis and emphysema.

Huber needle: A special noncoring hooked needle used to access an implantable port.

Hybrid arrays: Detector rows that have variable widths and sizes. Also called adaptive or nonuniform arrays.

Hydronephrosis: Obstruction resulting in dilatation, distention, and enlargement of the collection system in the kidney caused by ureteral stones.

Hyperosmolar: Having a greater number of particles in solution per unit of liquid, as compared with blood.

Hyperthyroidism: Condition in which thyroid hormone reaches a high level. In patients with a history of hyperthyroidism, iodinated contrast media can intensify thyroid toxicosis, and in rare cases it can precipitate a thyroid storm, which is a severe, life-threatening condition.

Hypertonic: Having a greater number of particles in solution per unit of liquid, as compared with blood.

Hypotensive stroke: Although rare, pressure that is too low can reduce oxygen supply to the brain enough to cause a stroke.

Idiosyncratic reactions: Unexplained reactions that are largely unpredictable, most often occurring within 1 hour of contrast medium administration, and are not related to the dose.

Image annotation: Information that appears on images. Can include facility name, patient name, identification number, date, slice number and thickness, pitch, table location, measurement scale, gray scale, and right and left indicators.

Image artifacts: Anything appearing on the image that is not present in the object scanned.

Image center: Specific area within the SFOV that will be displayed on the center of the image.

Image data: Once the computer has processed the raw data assigning one HU value to each pixel.

Image fidelity: Image accuracy.

Image magnification: When the displayed image is made larger. Uses only image data and does not improve resolution.

Image reconstruction: Use of raw data to create an image.

Image reformation: Image data are used to stacked cross-sectional slices and generate an image in a plane or orientation different from the prospective image. Also called image rendering.

Image rendering: Image data are used to stacked cross-sectional slices and generate an image in a plane or orientation different from the prospective image. Also called image reformation.

Imaging informatics: How information about medical images is exchanged within the radiology departments and throughout the medical enterprise.

Imaging planes: Imaginary planes that divide the body into sections.

Implantable ports: A single- or double-lumen reservoir attached to a catheter. The reservoir hub is implanted in the arm or chest subcutaneous tissue, and the catheter is tunneled to the accessed vein. No external device is visible. The outline of the device may be seen and felt as a small round elevation on the skin. Implanted ports are typically used for long-term intermittent access such as that required for chemotherapy.

Incidentalomas: Unsuspected adrenal masses that are found when CT studies are ordered as a result of unrelated symptoms.

Infarction: Areas of tissue death that occur because of a local lack of oxygen.

Inferior: Term used to describe movement toward the feet (down); synonymous with caudal.

Informatics: The collection, classification, storage, retrieval, and dissemination of recorded information.

Information technology (IT): The study, design, development, implementation, support, or management of computer-based information systems; particularly software applications and computer hardware.

In-plane resolution: Resolution in the xy direction.

Input device: Ancillary pieces of computer hardware designed to feed data into the computer. Examples include keyboard, mouse, touch-sensitive plasma screen, and CT detector mechanisms.

Interleukin 2: An immunotherapy used to treat some cancers.

Intermittent fluoroscopy: Method used to reduce the radiation dose during CT fluoroscopic procedures. Consists of alternately ceasing and beginning the radiation exposure rather than the continuous use of the fluoroscopic mode throughout the procedures.

International System of Units (SI): International System of Units (abbreviated SI from the French Le Système International d'Unités) is a system that is used internationally, both in everyday commerce and in science.

Intracellular lipid content: The amount of fat molecules a mass contains.

Intracranial hemorrhage (ICH): Bleeding in the brain caused by the rupture of a blood vessel.

Ionicity: Refers to whether the molecules in a contrast agent will separate into charged particles (i.e., ions) when dissolved in an aqueous solution. Ionic contrast agents are composed of molecules that will dissociate into ions when in solution. The molecules contained in nonionic contrast media do not dissociate.

Ischemic heart disease: A condition that results when plaque builds up in the coronary arteries. A partial or total blockage results, and the heart muscle does not get an adequate blood supply. Also referred to as coronary artery disease (CAD).

Ischemic stroke: Category of stroke caused by a blockage in an artery.

Isocenter: The absolute center of the gantry.

Isosmolar contrast media (IOCM): A contrast agent (Visipaque, GE Healthcare) with an osmolality equal to that of blood.

Isotonic: Having nearly the same number of particles in solution per unit of liquid as compared with blood.

Isotropic: Equal in all directions; a voxel that is cube-shaped.

Kidney stones: Gravel-like deposits that appear in the kidney. Also called renal calculi or renal stones.

Kilovolt-peak (kVp): Defines the quality (average energy) of the x-ray beam.

Kinetic energy: Energy of motion.

Laser light accuracy: Determination of the accuracy of the alignment of the laser light used for patient positioning.

LCD: Liquid crystal display technology used for monitors in radiology departments.

Limiting resolution: The spatial frequency possible on a given CT system at an MTF equal to 0.1.

Line pairs phantom: A phantom used to measure spatial resolution. This type of phantom is made of acrylic and has closely spaced metal strips imbedded in it.

Linear attenuation coefficient: Amount of the x-ray beam that is scattered or absorbed per unit thickness of the absorber; is represented by the Greek letter μ.

Linear interpolation: The simplest type of a mathematical method of estimating the value of an unknown function using the known value on either side of the function; frequently used in mathematics and science. Linear interpolation assumes that an unknown point falls along a straight line between two known points.

Linearity: The relationship between CT numbers and the linear attenuation values of the scanned object at a designated kVp value.

Local area network (LAN): Linked computers that are geographically close together.

Localizer scans: Digital image acquisitions that are created while the tube is stationary and the table moves through the scan field. Referred to by various names, depending on the manufacturer, such as scout, topogram, scanogram, and pilot.

Longitudinal plane: Body plane perpendicular to the floor.

Longitudinal resolution: Resolution in the z direction.

Lossless compression: Method of image compression in which the image that is then decompressed is an exact replica of the original.

Lossy compression: Method that introduces compression artifacts because not all data are restored; used to transmit images that do not need to be of diagnostic quality. This is sometimes referred to as "conversational" quality.

Low attenuation: An x-ray beam that is nearly unimpeded by an object; typically shown as dark gray or black on an image.

Low-contrast resolution: Ability of the system to differentiate between objects with similar densities. Also called contrast resolution or contrast detectability.

Low-osmolality contrast media (LOCM): Contrast agents introduced in the 1980s that contain much lower osmolality, from approximately 600 to 850 mOsm/kg, or roughly 2 to 3 times the osmolality of human blood.

Luminance: Brightness.

Magnetic tape: One of the oldest data storage options used to record computer data; consists of a long narrow strip of plastic with a magnetizable coating, most often packaged in cartridges and cassettes.

Manual MPR: This method requires that the operator input the criteria, such as the thickness of the MPR, the plane desired, and the number or incrementation of the resulting planar images.

Manual segmentation: The process of selectively removing or isolating information from the data set by the manual process in which the user identifies and selects data to be saved or removed.

Matrix: Grid formed from the rows and columns of pixels.

Maximum-intensity projection (MIP): 3D technique that selects voxels with the highest value to display.

Mechanical injection systems: Method of administering iodinated contrast media, intravascularly, using a mechanical injection system that controls the flow rate and volume. Also known as power injection.

Memory: Devices that store data. The three principal types of solid-state memory are read-only memory (ROM), random access memory (RAM), and write-once read-many times memory (WORM).

Metformin therapy: An oral medication given to non–insulin-dependent diabetics to lower blood sugar; also available in combination with other drugs.

Milliampere (mA): Measure of the tube current used in the production of x-ray energy. In conjunction with the scan time, it is the quantitative measure of the x-ray beam.

Milliampere-seconds (mAs): The product of milliampere setting and scan time.

Minimum-intensity projection (MinIP): 3D technique that selects voxels with the lowest value to display.

Modulation transfer function (MTF): Most commonly used method of describing spatial resolution ability. It is often used to graphically represent a system's capability of passing information to the observer.

Molecular imaging: Any methodology that investigates events at the molecular and cellular levels.

MTF graph: Charts that depict spatial frequency (object size) on the x axis and MTF along the y axis.

MTT: Mean transit time.

Multidetector row CT (MDCT): Scanner design in which there are many parallel rows of detectors. A single rotation can produce multiple slices.

Multiphasic injection: Injection technique in which two or more flow rates are used.

Multiplanar reformation (MPR): Two-dimensional reformation done to show anatomy in various planes.

Multiple image display: Function that allows more than one image to be displayed in a single frame.

Multiple scan average dose (MSAD): Total dose is the central slice radiation dose, plus the scatter overlap (or tails); dose calculated from multiple scans.

Near-line archiving: Storage systems in which data are readily, although not immediately, available. Examples include an optical jukebox or tape library.

Needle-holding devices: Devices that hold needles during a CT fluoroscopic procedure to avoid the hand of the clinician or assistant entering the CT beam.

Negative contrast agents: A contrast agent that is of a lower density than the surrounding structure, such as air or carbon dioxide.

Nephrogram phase: The phase of renal enhancement that follows the corticomedullary phase that typically occurs approximately 100 to 120 seconds after the IV administration of a bolus of contrast material.

Nephrolithiasis: Gravel-like deposits that may appear in any part of the urinary system, from the kidney to the bladder; used interchangeably with renal stones, renal calculi, kidney stones, and urolithiasis.

Nephropathy: Any condition or disease affecting the kidney; sometimes used synonymously with renal impairment.

Neutral contrast agents: Oral contrast agents that have an HU similar to that of water. Because they possess a lower density than the surrounding bowel, may also be referred to as a negative contrast agent.

Nonequilibrium phase: Follows the bolus phase; the contrast agent is still much brighter in the arteries than in the parenchyma of organs, but now the venous structures are also opacified. This phase begins approximately 1 minute after the start of the bolus injection and lasts only a short time. Also called the venous phase.

Non-tunneled catheters: Central catheters of a larger caliber than PICCs because they are designed to be inserted into a relatively large, more central vein such as the subclavian or jugular. Non-tunneled catheters usually have three ports, are open ended, and typically remain in place for a few days to 2 weeks.

Nonuniform arrays: Detector rows that have variable widths and sizes. Also called adaptive or hybrid arrays.

Nyquist sampling theorem: Because an object may not lie entirely within a pixel, the pixel dimension should be half the size of the object to increase the likelihood of that object being resolved.

Oblique planes: Body planes that are slanted and lie at an angle to one of the three standard planes.

Off-line archiving: Storage system in which data are kept in a less accessible location, requiring manual intervention to use.

180LI: A technique of interpolating helical scan data for SDCT systems using 180° linear interpolation.

Online archiving: Storage system using devices such as hard drives that are instantly accessible to the user.

Opacity value: Each voxel is assigned an opacity value based on its Hounsfield units. This opacity value determines the degree to which it will contribute, along with other voxels along the same line, to the final image.

Optical disc libraries: Robotic storage systems that automatically load and unload optical discs. The devices are also called optical jukeboxes, robotic drives, or autochangers.

Optical jukebox: Robotic storage system that automatically loads and unloads optical discs. The devices are also called optical disc libraries, robotic drives, or autochangers.

Organ dose: The estimated radiation dose to radiosensitive organs from CT procedures. These averages are used to calculate effective dose.

Osmolality: Property of intravascular contrast media that refers to the number of particles in solution per unit liquid as compared with blood.

Out-of-field artifacts: Inaccuracies in the image caused when parts of the patient are located outside the scan field of view. These artifacts occur because the anatomy outside the SFOV attenuates and hardens the x-ray beam, but is ignored in the image reconstruction process.

Output device: Ancillary pieces of computer hardware designed to accept processed data from the computer. Examples include monitor, laser camera, printer, and archiving equipment such as optical discs or magnetic tape.

Overbeaming: When x-ray penumbra falls outside the active detectors; this occurs when collimators are opened so that the same x-ray intensity reaches all of the detectors in an MDCT system.

Overlapping reconstruction: Incrementation is changed to produce overlapping images that are then used in multiplanar or 3D reformations.

Partial volume artifact: Artifact that can result when an object does not appear on all views. Inconsistencies between views cause shading artifacts on the image.

Partial volume effect: Process by which different tissue attenuation values are averaged to produce one less accurate pixel reading. Also referred to as volume averaging.

Peak aortic enhancement: The point after an IV injection when the contrast agent reaches the highest concentration in the aorta.

Peak organ enhancement: The point after an IV injection when the contrast agent reaches the highest concentration in a specified organ. The peak organ enhancement for organs such as the pancreas, bowel, and bladder occurs about 5 to 15 seconds after peak aortic enhancement.

Peer-to-peer (P2P) network: Networks in which each user has the same capabilities and any party can initiate communication. P2P networks exploit the diverse connectivity and the cumulative data capacity of network participants, rather than using a centralized resource.

Pencil ionization chamber: A special cylindrical dosimeter used in conjunction with a CTDI phantom to assess the radiation dose in CT.

Penumbra: In the context of stroke (rather than x-ray beam physics) penumbra is surviving tissue at the margin of infarcted tissue. Without successful intervention this tissue is destined for infarction, but is not yet irreversibly injured. It is the penumbra that may be salvageable with the administration of t-PA.

Percutaneous procedures: Interventional procedures in which access to inner organs or other tissue is done via needle puncture of the skin.

Peripherally inserted central catheters (PICC): A long catheter that is inserted through the large veins of the upper arm (i.e., cephalic and basilic veins) and advanced so that its tip is located in the lower third of the SVC.

PET transmission scan: The attenuation correction feature that is built into a dedicated PET system (i.e., one that does not include a CT component).

Pharmacokinetic factors: Pharmacokinetics includes the study of the mechanisms of absorption and distribution of an administered drug, the rate at which a drug action begins and the duration of the effect, the chemical changes of the substance in the body, and the effects and routes of excretion of the metabolites of the drug. In the context of iodinated contrast medium pharmacokinetic factors refer to contrast medium characteristics, including iodine concentration, osmolality, viscosity, volume, and flow rate.

Picture archive and communication system (PACS): One of two key elements that form the radiology department's information infrastructure. The term PACS encompasses a broad range of technologies necessary for the storage, retrieval, distribution, and display of images.

Pitch: Relation of table speed to slice thickness. It is most commonly defined as the travel distance of the CT scan table per 360° rotation of the x-ray tube, divided by the x-ray beam collimation width.

Pixel: Picture element. Two-dimensional square of data. When arranged in rows and columns, they make up the image matrix.

Polychromatic x-ray energy: An x-ray beam that is composed of photons with varying energies.

Portal venous phase: The phase of enhancement that follows the hepatic arterial phase, which typically begins at 60 to 70 seconds after the IV administration of a bolus of contrast material.

Positive contrast agents: Contrast agents that are of a higher density than the structure being imaged. Most contain barium or iodine.

Posterior: Term used to describe movement toward the back surface of the body; also referred to as dorsal.

Power capacity: Listed in kilowatts (kW). The power capacity of the generator determines the range of exposure techniques (i.e., kV and mA settings) available on a particular system.

Predetector collimators: Shape the beam and are located below the patient and above the detector array.

Premedication: Pretreatment, most often with steroids, to prevent reactions to contrast media.

Prepatient collimators: Limit the x-ray beam before it passes through the patient.

Progressive stroke: A time-limited event in which the neurologic deficits occur in a progressive pattern. Also referred to as a stroke in evolution.

Projection displays: 3D technique. Two common projection displays are the maximum-intensity projection (MIP) and the minimum-intensity projection (MinIP). The former selects voxels with the highest value to display; the latter selects voxels with the lowest value.

Prospective ECG gating: Method that uses a signal, usually derived from the R wave of the patient's ECG, to trigger image acquisition.

Prospective reconstruction: Image reconstruction that is automatically produced during scanning.

Protocol: Common set of rules and signals that computers on the network use to communicate.

Proximal: Term used in referring to extremities. Proximal (close to) may be defined as situated near the point of attachment. For example, the proximal end of the arm is the end at which it attaches to the shoulder.

Pulmonary circulation: The circulation pattern of blood flow that carries oxygen-depleted blood away from the heart to the lungs, and returns oxygenated blood back to the heart.

Quality factor (Q): A conversion factor that is applied to the absorbed dose that accounts for the different biologic effects produced from different types of ionizing radiation. The quality factor is 1 for the diagnostic x-rays that are used in CT. When the quality factor has been applied to the radiation absorbed dose, the new quantity is called the dose equivalent.

Quantum mottle: Occurs when there are an insufficient number of photons detected. It is inversely related to the number of photons used to form the image. Hence, as the number of x-ray photons used to create an image decreases, noise increases. Also referred to as quantum noise.

Quantum noise: Occurs when there are an insufficient number of photons detected. It is inversely related to the number of photons used to form the image. Hence, as the number of x-ray photons used to create an image decreases, noise increases. Also referred to as quantum mottle.

Radiation absorbed dose (rad): Unit of absorbed dose.

Radiation profile: Variations along the length, or z axis, of the patient; also referred to as the z-axis dose distribution.

Radiology information system (RIS): One of two key elements that form the radiology department's information infrastructure. The RIS is most often designed for scheduling patients, storing reports, patient tracking, protocoling examinations, and billing.

Radiopharmaceutical: Radioactive pharmaceuticals used in the field of nuclear medicine as tracers in the diagnosis and treatment of many diseases.

Random access memory (RAM): Type of computer memory that includes instructions that are frequently changed, such as the data used to reconstruct images. RAM is so named because all parts of it can be reached easily at random.

RAS coordinates: Directional coordinate system—an acronym for right-left, anterior-posterior, superior-inferior—used to determine image center.

Raw data: All measurements obtained from the detector array and sitting in the computer waiting to be made into an image. Also called scan data.

Ray: The path that the x-ray beam takes from the tube to the detector.

Ray sum: The detector senses each arriving ray and senses how much of the beam was attenuated.

RCBF: Regional cerebral blood flow.

RCBV: Regional cerebral blood volume.

Read-only memory (ROM): Type of computer memory that is imprinted at the factory and is used to store frequently used instructions such as those required for starting the system.

Real-time MPR: Refers to the feature that allows the operator to manually change (typically by moving a mouse) the image plane while the software continually updates the image. This feature permits the operator to use trial and error to obtain the ideal image plane. Also called interactive MPR.

Receiver operator characteristics: The subjectivity inherent in the method of evaluating contrast resolution that requires an observer to detect objects as distinct. Result can vary because different observers will often look at the same image and evaluate it differently.

Reconstruction algorithm: Determines how the data are filtered in the reconstruction process. The appropriate reconstruction algorithm selection depends on which parts of the data should be enhanced or suppressed to optimize the image for diagnosis.

Redundancy: Describes an arrangement in which two or more components perform the same task—if one element fails the duplication keeps the system functioning while the failed component is repaired. It can also refer to the duplication of data to provide an alternative in case of failure of one part of the process.

Redundant array of inexpensive disks (RAID): Storage solution that capitalizes on speed and reliability that divides, or replicates, data among multiple hard drives. These drives are designed to work together and appear to the computer as a single storage device.

Reference detectors: Included in the detector array and help to calibrate data and reduce artifacts.

Reference dose values: Values published by the ACR regarding the radiation dose that is acceptable for a variety of CT scans.

Reference image: Displays the slice lines in corresponding locations on the scout image.

Region of interest (ROI): An area on the image defined by the operator.

Region-of-interest editing: The process of selectively removing or isolating information from the data set. Also called segmentation.

Renal calculi: Gravel-like deposits that appear in the kidney. Also called renal stones or kidney stones.

Renal colic: Acute, usually severe pain that accompanies the passage of renal calculi from the kidney through the urinary tract.

Renal failure: The inability of the kidney to filter waste from the blood that can result in the accumulation of nitrogenous wastes (or azotemia).

Renal insufficiency: Renal function is abnormal but capable of sustaining essential bodily function.

Renal stones: Gravel-like deposits that appear in the kidney. Also called renal calculi or kidney stones.

Response time: Time required for the signal from the detector to return to zero after stimulation of the detector by x-ray radiation so that it is ready to detect another x-ray event.

Retrospective ECG gating: Method that acquires helical data throughout the cardiac cycle in which images are then reconstructed in specified portions of the cardiac cycle.

Retrospective reconstruction: Process of using the same raw data to later generate a new image.

Ring artifacts: Ring artifacts occur with third-generation scanners and appear on the image as a ring or concentric rings centered on the rotational axis. They are caused by imperfect detector elements—either faulty or simply out of calibration.

Robotic drives: Robotic storage systems that automatically load and unload optical discs. The devices are also called optical disc libraries, optical jukeboxes, or autochangers.

Roentgen (R): Unit of x-ray exposure in air.

Roentgen equivalents man (rem): When the quality factor has been applied to the radiation absorbed dose, the new quantity is called the dose equivalent. The unit for dose equivalent is the rem.

R-R interval: The distance between two R waves of a patient's ECG that represents one complete cardiac cycle.

Sagittal plane: Body plane that divides the body into left and right sections.

Sampling rate: Number of samples taken per second from the continuous signal emitted from the detector.

Sampling theorem: Theorem that states because an object may not lie entirely within a pixel, the pixel dimension should be half the size of the object to increase the likelihood of that object being resolved.

Scan data: All measurements obtained from the detector array and sitting in the computer waiting to be made into an image. Also called raw data.

Scan field of view (SFOV): The area, within the gantry, from which the raw data are acquired. Also called calibration field of view.

Scan parameters: Factors that can be controlled by the operator and affect the quality of the image produced. These factors include milliamperes, scan time, slice thickness, field of view, reconstruction algorithm, and kilovolt-peak. When using helical scan methods, the operator also has a choice of pitch.

Scan time: Time the x-ray beam is on for the collection of data for each slice. Most often it is the time required for the gantry to make a 360° rotation, although with overscanning and partial scanning options there may be some mild variation.

Scannable range: Degree to which a table can move horizontally. Determines the extent a patient can be scanned without repositioning.

Scanner-created MPR: Scanner protocols are programmed so that MPRs are automatically generated by the scanner software.

Segmentation errors: Errors in the reformatted image that are introduced when important vessels or other structures are inadvertently edited out of the data set.

Semiautomatic segmentation: Combines many of the benefits of manual and automatic segmentation techniques to selectively remove or isolate information from the data set.

Sequential CT: An imaging technique used for CT-guided interventions. The process requires a scan acquisition, needle placement, another scan acquisition, adjustment of the needle, another scan acquisition, and so forth until the needle is confirmed to be in the correct location.

Serial access memory (SAM): Type of computer memory that stores data that can only be accessed sequentially (like a cassette tape).

Serum creatinine (SeCr): Laboratory test that measures creatinine level in the blood; it is a fast and inexpensive way to assess renal function.

Shaded-surface display (SSD): 3D reformation method in which the voxels located on the edge of a structure are used to show the outline or outside shell of the structure; it includes only information from the surface of an object. It can be compared to taking a photograph of the surface of the structure. Also known as surface rendering (SR).

Sievert (Sv): Once the quality factor has been applied to the radiation absorbed dose the new quantity is called the dose equivalent. The SI equivalent unit is the sievert (Sv). There are 100 rem in 1 Sv.

Signal-to-noise ratio (SNR): The number of x-ray photons detected per pixel in CT.

Single-detector row CT (SDCT): Early systems, which contained only a single row of detectors in the z axis, obtained data for one slice with each rotation.

Slice misregistration: Occurs when a patient breathes differently with each data acquisition. This difference in breathing places the second group of scans in an incorrect anatomic position relative to the first set of slices. Valuable information may be missed because of this effect.

Slice-sensitivity profile (SSP): Thickness of the slice that is actually represented on the CT image, as opposed to the size selected by the collimator opening. In traditional axial scanning, selected slice thickness is equal to effective slice thickness. However, because of the interpolation process used in helical scanning, the effective slice thickness may be wider than the selected slice thickness. Also called the effective slice thickness.

Slice thickness: On a single-detector row system this is controlled by the width of the collimator opening. On a multidetector row system it is controlled by a combination of collimation and detector configuration.

Slice thickness accuracy: Determination of the accuracy of the slice thickness selected by the operator versus the width of the collimator opening.

Slice thickness blooming: When the slice thickness displayed on the image is wider than that selected by the operator.

Slip rings: Electromechanical devices that use a brushlike apparatus to provide continuous electrical power and electronic communication across a rotating surface, permitting the gantry frame to rotate continuously, eliminating the need to straighten twisted system cables.

Software: Instructions that tell the computer what to do and when to do it.

Spatial frequency: The number of line pairs visible per unit length.

Spatial resolution: Ability of a system to resolve, as separate forms, small objects that are very close together. Also call high-contrast resolution or detail resolution.

Spiral scanning: Scanning method that includes a continually rotating x-ray tube, constant x-ray output, and uninterrupted table movement. Also called helical, volumetric, or continuous acquisition scanning.

Split bolus: Contrast injection techniques in which the total contrast dose is split, often in half. The first dose is given, and a delay of about 2 minutes is observed. This allows time for structures that are slower to enhance to be opacified. The delay is followed by a second bolus containing the remainder of the contrast; scanning is initiated soon after the second injection is complete, using this second injection to more fully opacify the vessels.

Staging: The process of determining the extent and distribution of disease.

Stair-step artifacts: When smooth objects, such as the aorta, appear on the reformatted image to have edges that resemble a flight of stairs. They result when wide slices are used as source images.

Standard deviation: Indicates the amount of CT number variance within the ROI.

Standard precautions: Include the use of hand washing and appropriate protective equipment such as gloves, gowns, and masks whenever touching or exposure to patients' body fluids is anticipated. They are designed to reduce the risk of transmission of microorganisms from both recognized and unrecognized sources of infection in hospitals.

Standard uptake value: An index of glucose metabolism. The number represents the relative uptake of radionuclides in tissue.

Step-and-shoot scanning: Scan method in which the CT table moves to the desired location and remains stationary while the x-ray tube rotates within the gantry, collecting data; scans produced with the step-and-shoot method result in images that are perpendicular to the z axis (or tabletop) and parallel to every other slice, like slices of a sausage. Also called axial scanning.

Stroke in evolution: A time-limited event in which the neurologic deficits occur in a progressive pattern. Also referred to as a progressive stroke.

Subarachnoid hemorrhagic stroke: Stroke that occurs when there is bleeding into the subarachnoid spaces and the CSF spaces; usually caused by the rupture of an aneurysm.

Subject contrast: Relates to the inherent properties of the object scanned. For example, the lung is said to possess high subject contrast because it is primarily air-filled. The low attenuation lungs provide a background that makes nearly any other object discernible because of its dramatic difference in density.

Subjective side effects: Side effects experienced to some degree by most patients to whom contrast is administered. These often mild effects include the feeling of heat, nausea, and mild flushing.

Superior: Superior defines movement toward the head (up) and is used interchangeable with the term cranial or cephalic.

Supraorbital meatal line: Imaginary line used for positioning that connects the external acoustic meatus to the supraorbital margin. Also called the glabellomeatal line.

Surface rendering (SR): 3D reformation method in which the voxels located on the edge of a structure are used to show the outline or outside shell of the structure; it includes only information from the surface of an object. It can be compared to taking a photograph of the surface of the structure. Also known as shaded-surface display (SSD).

Systemic circulation: The circular pattern of blood flow from the left ventricle of the heart through the blood vessels to all parts of the body and back to the right atrium.

Table incrementation: Process of moving the table by a specified measure. Also referred to as feed, step, or index.

Table referencing: When the table position is manually set at zero by the technologist.

Tails: Areas of scatter radiation into the tissue of adjacent slices.

Temporal resolution: How rapidly data are acquired. It is controlled by gantry rotation speed, the number of detector channels in the system, and the speed with which the system can record changing signals.

Test bolus: Method of individualizing the scan delay that consists of administering 10 to 20 mL of contrast medium by IV bolus injection and performing several trial scans to determine the length of time from injection to peak contrast enhancement in a target region, such as the aorta.

Third-generation design: Scanner configuration that consists of a detector array and an x-ray tube that produces a fan-shaped beam that covers the entire field of view and a detector array. Sometimes referred to as rotate-rotate scanners.

Three-dimensional reformation: Reformation that seeks to represent the entire scan volume in a single image. Unlike 2D displays, 3D techniques manipulate or combine CT values to display an image; the original CT value information is not included.

360LI: A technique of interpolating helical scan data for SDCT systems using the 360° linear interpolation.

Threshold CT values: A predetermined CT value limit set by the operator in some types of 3D reformation techniques. The software will include or exclude the voxel depending on whether its CT number is above or below the threshold.

Thrombolytic therapy: The use of drugs to break up or dissolve blood clots.

Thrombosis: The formation, development, or existence of a clot within the vascular system.

Thrombotic stroke: Type of ischemic stroke caused from a blood clot or a fatty deposit within one of the brain's arteries.

Thyroid storm: A severe, life-threatening condition resulting when thyroid hormone reaches a dangerously high level, also known as thyroid toxicosis.

Thyroid toxicosis: A severe, life-threatening condition resulting when thyroid hormone reaches a dangerously high level, also known as a thyroid storm.

Time-density curves: Graphical representation that demonstrates the effect of varying contrast dose on aortic and hepatic contrast enhancement.

Tissue plasminogen activator (t-PA): A treatment for acute ischemic stroke. The treatment, known as tissue plasminogen activator (t-PA), was the first of its kind and revolutionized the way the medical community can respond to treating the 80% of stroke patients who experience ischemic strokes. To be effective t-PA must be administered within 3 hours of the first signs of stroke. This means that the stroke victim must be transported to the hospital, diagnosed, and administered the t-PA treatment before the 3-hour window has expired.

Topology: The geometric arrangement of a computer system. Common topologies include bus, star, ring, and tree.

Transient ischemic attack (TIA): Reversible episode of focal neurologic dysfunction that typically lasts anywhere from a few minutes to a few hours. Attacks are usually caused by tiny emboli that lodge in an artery and then quickly break up and dissolve, with no residual damage.

Transverse plane: Body plane horizontal to the floor.

Tube arcing: Undesired surge of electrical current (i.e., a short-circuit) within the x-ray tube. A common cause of equipment-induced artifact.

Tube current: Measured in thousandths of an ampere, or milliamperes, it controls the quantity of electrons propelled from cathode to anode.

Tunneled catheters: Central venous catheters that are inserted into the target vein (often the subclavian) by "tunneling" under the skin. This reduces the risk of infection because bacteria from the skin surface are not able to travel directly into the vein. Examples of tunneled catheters include Hickman, Broviac, and Groshong catheters.

Uncoupling effect: With digital technology, the image is not as directly linked to the dose, so even when an mA or kVp setting that is too high is used, a good image results. This effect can make it difficult to identify when a dose that is higher than necessary is used.

Undersampling: Insufficient projection data (for instance, when the helical pitch is greatly extended) that cause inaccuracies related to reproducing sharp edges and small objects and result in an artifact known as aliasing.

Uniform array: Detector rows that are parallel and of equal size.

Uniformity: The ability of the scanner to yield the same CT number regardless of the location of an ROI within a homogeneous object.

Uniphasic injection: Injection technique in which a single injection flow rate is used.

Ureterolithiasis: Gravel-like deposits that appear in the ureter.

Urolithiasis: Gravel-like deposits that may appear in any part of the urinary system, from the kidney to the bladder; used interchangeably with renal stones, renal calculi, nephrolithiasis, and kidney stones.

Valsalva maneuver: Technique that requires the patient to blow the cheeks out to distend the pyriform sinuses.

Ventral: Term used to describe movement forward (toward the face); also referred to as anterior.

Vermiform appendix: Small, tubelike structure projecting from the cecum; literally means wormlike.

View: A complete set of ray sums.

Virtual bronchoscopy: A form of volume rendering designed to reveal the inside of the airways. The technique is also called endoluminal imaging.

Virtual colonoscopy: A form of volume rendering designed to reveal the inside of the colon. The technique is also called endoluminal imaging.

Virtual endoscopy: A form of volume rendering designed to reveal the inside of the lumen of a structure. The technique is also called endoluminal imaging, virtual bronchoscopy (for airways), and virtual colonoscopy (for the colon).

Virtual private networks (VPN): Distribution channel used to make the Internet a safe medium for the secure transmission of clinical data. By definition, VPNs overlay another network to provide a particular functionality.

Viscosity: Physical property that may be described as the thickness or friction of the fluid as it flows. It is an important property that will influence the injectability of intravascular agents through small-bore needles and intravenous catheters.

Volume averaging: Process by which different tissue attenuation values are averaged to produce one less accurate pixel reading. Also referred to as partial volume effect.

Volume rendering (VR): A 3D imaging technique that creates a semitransparent representation of the imaged structure. An advantage of VR is that all voxels contribute to the image, allowing the image to display multiple tissues and show their relationship to one another.

Volumetric HRCT: Volumetric HRCT protocols use a helical mode to acquire images of the entire lung, rather than representative slices. Because these helical protocols cover the entire lung, they result in a more complete assessment of the lung.

Voxel: Volume element. Three-dimensional cube of data acquired in CT.

Wide area network (WAN): Computers that are farther apart and must be connected by telephone lines, cables, or radio waves.

Windmill artifacts: Appear only on MDCT helical systems and relate to the cone-shaped beam required. They appear as either streaks or as bright and dark shading near areas of large density differences (e.g., bone and muscle).

Window center: Mechanism that selects the center CT value of the window width. Also called window level.

Window level: Mechanism that selects the center CT value of the window width. Also called window center.

Window width: Mechanism that determines the quantity of Hounsfield units represented as shades of gray on a specific image.

Wired: Refers to networks that are linked by a physical connection.

Wireless: Refers to network that use radio waves to transmit data between computers.

Workstation-created MPR: MPR generated directly on the workstation. This allows radiologists the flexibility and interactivity to create images that are suited to the specific clinical situation.

Write-once read-many times memory (WORM): Type of computer memory in which data can be written to once, but read from many times.

Z axis: Plane that correlates to the slice thickness, or depth, of the CT slice.

Z-axis dose distribution: Variations along the length, or z axis, of the patient; also referred to as the radiation profile.

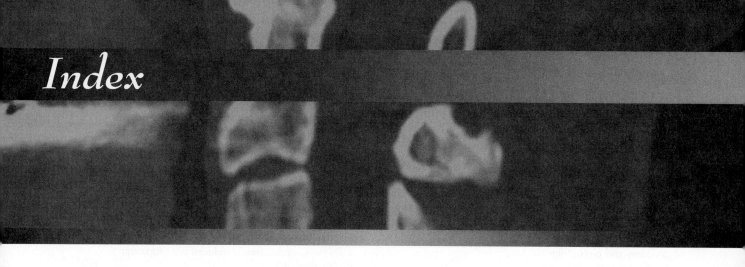

Index

Page numbers in *italics* denote figures; those followed by "t" denote tables.

A

Abdomen and pelvis imaging
  abdominopelvic anatomy, *214–219*
    female pelvis, *223*
    male pelvis, *220–222*
  acute appendicitis
    anatomy and function, 309–310, *309*
    clinical presentations, 311–312
    CT diagnostic protocols, 316t
    differential diagnosis, 312
    etiology and pathogenesis, 310–311
    imaging studies, 313–316
    incidence, 310
    laboratory tests, 312–313
    prognosis, 310
    signs, 312t
    symptoms, 311t
    ultrasonography *vs.* CT, 313t
  adrenal glands
    adrenal mass characterization, 306–308, *307*
    anatomy and physiology, 305–306, *305–306*
    disorders, 306
  general scanning method
    breath hold, 302
    contrast agent, oral, 300
    cross-sectional slices, 302
    display field of view (DFOV), 301–302
    intravenous contrast agents, 301
    low Hounsfield unit agents, 300
    patient positioning, 302
    routine scans, 302
    structures and abnormalities examination, 301t
    window setting, 301
  kidneys and ureters
    CT urography (CTU), 304–305
    renal mass evaluation, 304
  liver
    cavernous hemangioma, 302–303, *303*
    CT attenuation, 302
    fatty infiltration, 302, *303*
    hepatic arterial and portal venous phase, 303
    ROI measurement, 302, *303*
    tumors, 303–304
  pancreas, 304

  protocols
    abdomen pelvis aorta (post stent, nongated), 324–326
    adrenal mass (with delay), 331
    arterial venous liver, 326–327
    arterial venous pancreas, 327–328
    colonography, 330–331
    CT urogram, 333–334
    enterography, 329–330
    mesenteric, 328–329
    renal mass, 332
    renal stone, 332–333
    routine abdomen pelvis, 324
  urinary tract calculi
    causes, 317
    clinical presentation and differential diagnosis, 318–319
    diagnosis, 319–320
    epidemiology, 317
    stone types, 318t
    symptom, 318t
    terminology, 317
    urinary stones, 317–318
Acute appendicitis
  appendiceal CT protocols
    contrast-enhanced CT, 316
    CT diagnostic protocols, 316t
    focused technique, 315, *316*
    intravenous iodinated contrast agents, 315–316
    oral contrast material, 315
  appendicolith, *314*
  appendix
    air-filled appendix images, *315*
    anatomy and function, 309–310, *309*
    IV and oral contrast images, *315*
  clinical presentations, 311–312
  common CT findings, 313–314
  differential diagnosis, 312
  dilated nonopacified appendix, *314*
  etiology and pathogenesis, 310–311
  graded compression sonography, 313
  incidence, 310
  laboratory tests, 312–313
  prognosis, 310
  signs, 312t
  symptoms, 311t

Acute appendicitis (*Continued*)
  ultrasonography, 313
  ultrasonography *vs.* CT, 313t
Adaptive statistical iterative reconstruction, 27
Adrenal glands
  adrenal mass characterization, 308–309
    adenomas, 307
    adrenal incidentalomas, 306–307
    contrast medium washout, *307*, 308
    fine-needle aspiration (FNA) biopsy, 307
    intracellular lipid content, 307–308
  anatomy and physiology
    adrenal cortex, 306
    adrenal medulla, 306
    cross-sectional images, 305, *306*
    hormones, 305–306
    location, *305*
  disorders, 306

B

Beam attenuation, *5, 7*
  high attenuation, 5
  linear attenuation coefficient, 6, 6t
  low attenuation, 5
  negative contrast agent, 6
  positive contrast agent, 6

C

Cardiac CT
  cardiac anatomy
    cardiovascular system, 273–274
    cavities, 275, *276*
    endocardium, 275, *275*
    epicardium, 274–275, *275*
    location, *274*
    myocardium, *275*
    pericardium, 274, *275*
    valves and openings, 275, *276*
  cardiovascular disease (CVD), 273
  circulation, 276–277, *277–278*
  coronary angiography, 273
  coronary arteries branches, 277
  coronary artery disease (CAD), 273
  coronary artery grafts and stents
    angioplasty, 277–278
    atherosclerosis, 277
    coronary artery bypass graft (CABG) surgery, 277–278, *278*
    coronary stents, 278, *279–280*
    left internal mammary artery (LIMA) graft, 277, *279*
    right internal mammary artery (RIMA), 277
    saphenous veins, 277, *279*
    vessels choice, 277, *278*
  CT coronary calcium screening
    Agatston score, 286
    calcium volume score, 286
    calibration phantom, 286, *286*
    coronary artery calcification, 284, 286
    CT calcium scoring, 284, 286t
    limitation, 287
    MDCT, 286

technique
  β-blocker administration protocol, 281t
  breath-hold, 284, 285t
  challenges, 278–279
  contrast administration, 283–284, *284–285*
  ECG gating, 282–283, *282–283*
  pharmacologic heart rate control, 280–281
  pharmacologic vasodilatation, 281–282
  technical aspects, 285t
Chest, 204, *204–213*
Chronic sinusitis, 190
CIN (*see* Contrast media-induced nephropathy)
Collimators, 4
Compensating filters, 16
Contrast agents
  arteriovenous iodine difference (AVID), 148, *148*
  contrast arrival times, 150–151, 151t, *152*
  contrast medium
    characteristics, 155–156, 156t, *157*
    flow duration, 156
    flow rate, 158–159
    time-density curves, 157, *157–159*
    volume, 157–158, 158
  enhancement
    equipment factors, 160
    patient factors, 159–160, *160*
    pharmacokinetic factors, 155
  gastrointestinal tract (*see* Gastrointestinal contrast medium)
  intrathecal contrast administration, 139
  intravascular contrast agents (*see* Iodinated contrast agents)
  negative agent, 120
  phases
    bolus phase, 148, *148*
    equilibrium (or delayed) phase, 149, *149–150*
    nonequilibrium phase, 148, *149*
  positive agent, 120
Contrast media-induced nephropathy (CIN)
  clinical presentation, 133t
  dialysis and contrast media, 135
  incidence and risk factors, 133–134
  metformin therapy, 134
  prevention, 134
  renal anatomy and physiology, 129, 131
  renal function
    estimation, 131
    nephropathy, 132–133
    renal dysfunction, 132
    serum creatinine, GFR, 131–132, 132t
Cross-sectional images, 181–182
CT angiography (CTA)
  cervicocranial vascular evaluation, 242
  circle of Willis, 260–261
  pulmonary embolism, MDCT
    advantages, 271–272
    considerations, 272–273
    disadvantages, 272
  spine, 265–266
  vs. traditional angiography, 241–242
CT arthrography, 337
CT fluoroscopy (CTF), 345–346

CT urography (CTU), 304–305
CT venography (CTV), 242
  cranial venography, 261–262
  pulmonary embolism, 271
CT-guided biopsies
  complication, 346
  procedure, 346–347
  supplies, 346t
CT-guided fluid aspiration and abscess drainage, 346t, 347
CT/PET fusion imaging
  attenuation correction features, 356
  cancer location and metabolism, 348, *349*
  clinical procedures, 356
  coregistration, 355–356
  diagnostic accuracy, 355
  image aligning problem, 348
  structural information, 348
  technologist, 349
CTA (*see* CT angiography)
CTF (*see* CT fluoroscopy)
CTU (*see* CT urography)
CTV (*see* CT venography)

D
Data acquisition, *15*
  collimation
    predetector collimation, 16
    prepatient collimation, 16
  components, *15*
  cooling systems, 16
  detector electronics
    analog-to-digital converter (ADC), 20
    data-acquisition system (DAS), 20–21
    sampling rate, 21
  detectors, 17–18
  filtration
    bow tie filters, 16, *17*
    compensating filters, 16
  generators
    high-frequency generators, 15
    power capacity, 16
  helical scanning
    advantages, 50
    vs. axial scanning, 51–52
    detectors, 51
    dual-source CT, 56–57, *56*
    helical interpolation, 52
    pitch, 52–54
    raw data management, 51
    reconstructed slice thickness, 56
    scan coverage, 54–55, *54*
    scan speed, 50
    slice incrementation, 55, *55*
    slice thickness, 52, *52*
    slip rings, 50–51
    table movement and software, 51
    tube cooling, 51
    volumetric scanning, 50
    x-ray output, 51
  localizer scans
    anterior–posterior views, *41*
    cross-sectional images, 42
    digital images, 40
    display field of view (DFOV), 43, *43*, *44*
    image annotation, 42, *42*
    image localization, 40
    lateral views, *41*
    miscentered scans, 40
    tube positioning, 40, *41*
  patient table, 21
  scanner generation
    EBCT scanners design, 20, *20*
    electron beam imaging, 20
    fourth-generation design, 19, *20*
    ring artifacts, 19
    third-generation design, 19, *19*
  schematic of, *21*
  slip rings, 15
  step-and-shoot scanning
    advantages, 43–45
    applications, 50
    aspects, 43
    axial slices, 43, *45*
    disadvantages, 45
    multidetector row systems, 47–48, *47–49*, 50
    single-detector row systems, 45–46, *46*
    slice misregistration, 45, *45*
  x-ray source, 16
Data management
  hardcopy *vs.* electronic archiving, 94
  picture archive and communication system (PACS)
    data storage, 97–98
    electronic standards, 96
    image acquisition, 96–97
    image distribution, 98–99, 98t
    networking, 94–96, *95*
    workstation monitors, 97
Detectors
  absorption efficiency, 17
  afterglow, 17
  capture efficiency, 17
  characteristics of, 17, 18t
  detector array, 17–19, *18*
  dynamic range, 17
  efficiency, 17
  reference detectors, 17
  response time, 17
  solid-state crystal detector
    detector aperture, 18, *19*
    detector spacing, 18, *19*
  xenon gas detectors, 17–18, *18*
Display field of view (DFOV), 28–29, *29*
  abdomen and pelvis imaging, 301–302
  foot and ankle, 338
  knee, 337
  temporal bone, 194

F
Fluorine-18 fluorodeoxyglucose positron emission tomography
  (^{18}F FDG-PET) (*see* Positron emission tomography
  (PET))
Fourier transform, 23–24

G

Gantry, data acquisition (*see* Data acquisition)
Gastrointestinal contrast medium
   air or carbon dioxide, 138, *139*
   barium sulfate solutions, 136–138
   iodinated agents, 138
   water, 138

H

Hard disk, 24
Hounsfield units (HU), 6–7, *7*

I

ICH (*see* Intracranial hemorrhage)
Idiosyncratic reactions
   classifications, 126–127
   contrast media-induced nephropathy
      dialysis and contrast media, 135
      incidence and risk factors, 133–134
      metformin therapy, 134
      prevention, 134
      renal anatomy and physiology, 129, 131
      renal function, 131–133
   incidence and risk factors
      allergies, 127–128
      asthma, 127
      drugs, 128
      previous contrast medium reaction, 127
   prevention
      chemotoxic reactions, 129
      contrast reaction report form, *130*
      documentation, 129
      LOCM, 128
      premedication, 128, 128t
Image display
   cameras, 31–32
   display monitors, 31
   display options
      advance functions, 39
      distance measurements, 37–38
      histogram, 39
      Hounsfield measurement, 35–37
      image annotation, 38
      image magnification, 38–39
      multiple image display, 39
      reference image, 38
      region of interest (ROI), 35
      standard deviation, 37
   window settings, 35
      CT examination, 36t
      effect, image appearance, *32*
      gray scale, 32–33
      gray shade assignment, *34*
      liver display, *35*
      upper neck display, *36*
      window level, 33–34, *33–34*
      window widening, *34*
      window width, 33, *33*
Image pixel, 4–5
Image quality
   contrast resolution

mAs/dose, 68
   noise, 68
   patient size, 69
   reconstruction algorithm, 69
   scanner's low-contrast resolution, 68
   slice thickness, 69
   window setting effect, 69, *69*
   definition, 61–62
   evalution, criteria, 4
   scan geometry, 61
   scanning parameters
      field of view, 60–61
      kilovolt-peak (kVp) setting, 58
      milliampere setting, 58–59
      milliampere-second setting, 59–60
      pitch, 61
      reconstruction algorithms, 61
      slice thickness, 60
      tube voltage/kilovolt peak, 60
   spatial resolution
      DFOV selection, 64
      direct measurement, 62
      evaluation, modulation transfer function
         (MTF), 62–64
      focal spot size, 67
      in-plane *vs.* longitudinal resolution, 64
      matrix size, 64, *64*
      patient motion, 67
      pitch, 67
      pixel size, 64, *64*
      reconstruction algorithm, 66–67, *67*
      sampling theorem, 66, *66*
      slice thickness, 64–66
   temporal resolution, 69–70
Image reconstruction
   adaptive statistical iterative reconstruction, 27
   data types, 25
   display field of view (DFOV), 28–29, *29*
   equipment components
      computer components, 24–25
      hard disk, 24
      hardware and software, 24
   filter functions, 26–27
   image center, 30
   scan field of view (SFOV), 27–28, *28*
   temporal bone, 194
   terminology
      algorithm, 23
      Fourier transform, 23–24
      interpolation, 24
Imaging planes
   anatomic position, 9, *10*
   anterior, 9–10
   caudal, 9
   coronal plane, 10–11, *11*
   distal, 10
   dorsal, 9
   inferior, 9
   longitudinal plane, 10
   oblique plane, 10, *10*
   posterior, 9–10

proximal, 10
sagittal plane, 10
superior, 9
transverse plane, 10, 11
ventral, 9
Z axis, 4, *4*, 9
Imaging procedures and protocols
  abdomen and pelvis imaging (*see* Abdomen and pelvis imaging)
  examination protocols, 237–238
  musculoskeletal imaging (*see* Musculoskeletal imaging)
  neurologic imaging (*see* Neurologic imaging)
  routine scanning procedures, 238
  thoracic imaging (*see* Thoracic imaging)
Injection techniques
  American College of Radiology (ACR) recommendations, 142
  automated injection triggering
    bolus triggering, 162–163, 163, *163*
    test bolus, 160, *161–162*, 162, 162
  contrast enhancement
    contrast media volume, flow duration, flow rate, 156–159, *157–159*, 158–159
    contrast medium characteristics, 155–156, 156t, *157*
    equipment factors, 160
    patient factors, 159–160, *160*
    pharmacokinetic factors, 155
  contrast media delivery method
    drip infusion, 151
    hand bolus technique, 151–152
    mechanical injection system, 152–155, *153*, 154–155, 156t
  tissue enhancement phases
    arteriovenous iodine difference (AVID), 148, *148*
    bolus phase, 148, *148*
    contrast arrival times, 150–151, 151t, *152*
    contrast phase terms, 149, 150t
    equilibrium (or delayed) phase, 149, *149–150*
    nonequilibrium phase, 148, *149*
  vascular access
    aseptic technique, 143
    central venous access device (CVAD), 145
    indwelling catheter set, 143, *143*, 144–145
    non-tunneled and tunneled central venous catheters, 146–147, *147*
    peripherally inserted central catheters (PICC), 145–146, *147*
    placement, 144
    superficial veins, 143–144, *144*
    supplies, 143
    venipuncture technique, 143–144, 145
    venous access site, 143–144, *144*
Interventional CT
  CT-guided interventions
    CT fluoroscopy (CTF), 345–346
    sequential CT, 345
  CT-guided procedures
    CT-guided biopsies, 346–347
    CT-guided fluid aspiration and abscess drainage, 346t, 347
  high-density material image, 345

Intracranial hemorrhage (ICH), 240–241
Intravenous (IV) contrast enhancement
  brain, 183, *183–189*
  chest, 204, *204–213*
  neck, 198, *198–200*
  sinus, 190, *190–193*
  temporal bones
    axial plane, *196–197*
    coronal plane, 194, *194–195*
Iodinated contrast agents
  adverse effects
    central nervous system, 135–136
    contrast extravasation, 136
    mechanism, 125–126
    pheochromocytoma, 135
    pulmonary effects, 135
    thyroid function, 135
  delayed reaction, 136
  dose
    administeration practice, 124
    iodine concentration, 122–123
    overdosage affect, 123
    variation, 124, 124t
  idiosyncratic reactions (*see* Idiosyncratic reactions)
  lactation, 124, 125t
  pregnancy, 124, 125t
  properties
    clearance, 122
    ionicity, 122, 123t
    osmolality, 121–122
    viscosity, 122

K
Kidneys and ureters, 304–305
Knee CT, 337–338

L
Liver imaging
  cavernous hemangioma, 302–303
  CT attenuation, 302
  fatty infiltration, 302, *303*
  hepatic arterial and portal venous phase, 303
  ROI measurement, 302, *303*
  tumors, 303–304
Low-contrast resolution, 4

M
Matrix, 4
Mechanical injectors
  air embolism, 154–155
  contrast medium extravasation, 154, 154
  injection method, 155, 156t
  models, 153, *153*
  precautions, 155
  pressure limit, 153–154
  programmable, 153
  protocol, 155, 155
  saline test injection, 154
  visual indicators, 155
Molecular imaging method, 348 (*see also* Positron emission tomography (PET))

Multiplanar reformation (MPR)
  coronal plane, *85*
  CT attenuation, *84*
  curved reformations, *85*
  manual and real-time MPR, 84
  scanner-created MPR, 84–85
  workstation-created MPR, 85
Musculoskeletal imaging
  anatomy
    foot, *233–235*
    hip (left), *227–229*
    knee (left), *230–232*
    wrist (right), *224–226*
  CT scanning method
    advantages, 335
    IV contrast medium, 336
    multidetector row CT (MDCT), 335
    multiplanar reformations (MPR), 335
    patient positioning, 335–336
    reconstruction algorithm, 336
  foot and ankle, 338
  knee, 337–338
  protocols
    ankle/distal tibia, 344
    elbow, 341
    hip/proximal femur, 342
    knee/tibial plateau, 343
    shoulder/scapula, 339
    wrist, 340
  shoulder, 337
  wrist
    annotation system, 337
    fracture examination, 336
    patient positioning, 336, *337*
Myelography, 201

N
NCHCT (*see* Noncontrast helical CT)
Neuroanatomy
  brain, 183, *183–189*
  neck, 198, *198–200*
  sinus, 190, *190–193*
  spine, 201, *201–203*
  temporal bones
    axial plane, *196–197*
    coronal plane, 194, *194–195*
Neurologic imaging
  CT angiography (CTA)
    cervicocranial vascular evaluation, 242
    circle of Willis, 260–261
    spine, 265–266
    vs. traditional angiography, 241–242
  CT venography (CTV), 242
  head imaging method
    cross-sectional slices, window settings, 240
    CT *vs.* MRI, 241
    intracranial hemorrhage (ICH), 240–241, *241*
    motion-related artifacts, 240
    patient positioning, 239–240, *240*
    posterior fossa, 240
    thin slices, 240
    x-ray attenuation, 240, 240t

intradural and extradural abnormalities
    visualization, 242
  intrathecal contrast medium, 242
  neck protocols, 241
  protocols
    brain perfusion, 259
    CTV–cranial venography, 261–262
    head, 253
    neck (soft tissue), 262
    orbits, 257–258
    sella, 258–259
    sinus screen, 255–256
    skull base (posterior fossa), 253–254
    temporal bones, 254–255
    trauma facial bones, 256
  spine protocols, 242
    cervical spine, 263
    lumbar spine, 264–265
    thoracic spine, 264
  stroke
    CT brain perfusion scans, 248–251
    diagnosis and treatment, 247–248
    hemorrhagic stroke, 244–245
    hypotensive stroke, 245
    ischemic stroke, 243–244
    risk factors, 246–247
    symptoms, 245–246
  Valsalva maneuver, 241
Noncontrast helical CT (NCHCT), 319–320
Nonverbal communication
  objects, 106
  tactile, 105
  time and space, 105–106
  visual communication, 105
  vocal cues, 105

P
PACS (*see* Picture, archive, and communication system)
Pancreas, 304
Partial volume effect, 8
Patient communication
  barriers, 104–105
  benefits, 103, 104t
  nonverbal communication
    objects, 106
    tactile, 105
    time and space, 105–106
    visual communication, 105
    vocal cues, 105
  practical advice
    communication habits, 106–108
    listener's responsibilities, 106
    speaker's responsibilities, 106
Patient preparation
  assessment and monitoring vital signs
    blood pressure, 118–119
    body temperature, 117, 118t
    pulse, 117–118, *118*
    respirations, 118
  examination initiation, 110
  immobilization and restraint devices, 114, 117
  informed consent, 114, 115t–116t

medical history
    diagnostic information, 113
    laboratory values, 113, 114t
    patient safety, 111–113
    protocol selection, 113
  patient education, 113–114
  protocol selection, 110–111
  room preparation, 111
PET (*see* Positron emission tomography)
Picture, archive, and communication system (PACS), 238
  data storage, 97–98
  electronic standards, 96
  image acquisition, 96–97
  image distribution, 98–99, 98t
  networking, 94–96, *95*
  workstation monitors, 97
Polychromatic x-ray beams
  artifacts, 7
  beam-hardening artifacts, 7–8
  cupping artifacts, 8, *8*
Positron emission tomography (PET) (*see also* CT/PET fusion
    imaging)
  FDG uptake, imaging pitfalls
    benign pathologies, 354
    blood vessels, 354
    bone marrow, 354, *354*
    breast, 352
    diabetic patients, 350
    extravasation, 354, *355*
    gastrointestinal tract, 352–353, *353*
    head and neck, 351, *352*
    kidney and lower urinary tract, 353
    lung, 352
    meal timing, 350
    physical activity, 350
    reproductive system, 353
    skeletal muscles, 350–351
    thorax and myocardium, 351–352, *352*
    thymus, 352, *353*
  radiopharmaceutical
    fluorine-18 fluorodeoxyglucose (^{18}F-FDG) structure,
      349–350, *350*
    imaging method, 349–350
    photon annihilation, 349, *350*
  standard uptake value (SUV), 355
Post-processing techniques (*see also* Post-processing techniques)
  image reformation (*see also* Three-dimensional image
    reformation)
    artifacts, 91, *91*
    image noise, 91
    multiplanar reformation, 84–85
    reformatted images, 83–84, *83*
    segmentation errors, 90–91, *90*
    three-dimensional reformation, 86–89
  region-of-interest editing
    fully automated segmentation, 89
    manual segmentation, 89, *89*
    semiautomatic segmentations, 89–90
  retrospective reconstruction, 81–82
Pulmonary embolism
  D-dimer assays, 271
  deep vein thrombosis (DVT), 269

  embolus, 269
  MDCT, CTA
    advantages, 271–272
    considerations, 272–273, *273*
    CT venography (CTV), 271
    disadvantages, 272
  pulmonary angiography, 271
  pulmonary artery, 269–271, *270–271*
  systemic and pulmonary circulation, 269, *270*
  thrombosis, 269
  venous thromboembolism, 269
  ventilation-perfusion scanning (VQ scans), 271

Q
Quality assurance
  ACR CT accreditation phantom, 72, *72*
  basic rules, 71
  contrast resolution, 72
  image artifacts
    aliasing, 75–76
    beam hardening, 75, *75*
    edge gradient effect, 76, *76*
    helical and cone beam effect, 78–79
    metallic artifacts, 77, *77*
    motion, 76–77, *76*
    out-of-field artifacts, 77–78, *77*
    partial volume effect, 75, *76*
    ring artifacts, 78, *78*
    three-dimensional (3D) images, 80
    troubleshooting, 79t
    tube arcing, 78
  laser light accuracy, 72
  linearity, 73, *73*, 74
  noise, 72–73
  radiation dose, 73
  slice thickness accuracy, 72
  spatial resolution, 72
  uniformity, 73, *73*

R
Radiation dosimetry
  biologic effects of ionizing radiation (BEIR VII), 169
  CT *vs.* conventional radiography, 169, 169t
  dose geometry
    central scan dose, 167, *167*
    computed tomography dose index (CTDI), 168
    exit and entrance dose, 166, *166*
    multiple scan average dose (MSAD), 168
    rotational nature, 166, *166*
    z axis dose distribution, 167–168, *167–168*
  dose reducing strategies, 176t
    automatic tube current modulation, 176
    clinically indicated CT examination, 177
    CT examination customization, 177
    increased kVp avoidance, 176
    increased pitch, 176
    mAs adjustment, 176
    patient shielding, 177–178
    reconstruction method, 176
    repeat scans limitation, 176
    technical parameters, 177
    thin slices usage limitation, 176

Radiation dosimetry (*Continued*)
  factors affecting
    collimation, 171
    detector efficiency, 169
    filtration, 169
    localization scans, 171
    patient size and body part thickness, 171
    pitch, 170, 170t
    radiation beam geometry, 169
    radiographic technique, 171
    repeat scans, 171
    scan field diameter, 170–171
    slice width and spacing, 169–170
  measurement terminology
    absorbed dose unit, 165
    effective dose, 166
    equivalent dose (H), 166
    quality factor (Q), 166
    x-ray exposure unit, 165
  pediatric population
    dose reducing strategies, 176–177
    special consideration, 175
  radiation dose management and image quality
    extra images, 172–173
    health care education, 172
    high radiation dose, 171
    lack of awareness, 173–174
    low-dose radiation effects, 172
    scanning parameters, 172
  risk perception, 174
Raw data *vs.* image data, 9

S
Scan field of view (SFOV), 27–28, *28*
Scanner operation, 12
Scanner-created multiplanar reformation, 84–85
Scanning modes, 9
Scout image, 238, 242
Sequential CT, 345
SFOV (*see* Scan field of view)
Spatial resolution, 4
Split-bolus technique, 304
Stroke
  blood supply to brain, 243
  cerebrovascular accident (CVA), 243
  CT brain perfusion scans
    cerebrovascular reserve determination, 251
    contrast enhancement curves, 250, *250*
    CT angiography, 250
    hemodynamics measurement, 248
    image postprocessing, 249–250
    indications, 250–251
    quantitative data extraction, 250, *250*
    scanner, 248–249, *249*
    software, 248
    temporary balloon occlusion, 251
  diagnosis and treatment
    CT examination, 247–248
    tissue plasminogen activator (t-PA) therapy, 247, 248t
  hemorrhagic stroke
    arteriovenous malformation (AVM), 245

    intracerebral hemorrhage, 244–245
    occurrence, 244
    subarachnoid hemorrhage, 245
  hypotensive stroke, 245
  ischemic stroke
    definition, 243
    embolic stroke, 243–244
    lacunar stroke, 244
    thrombotic stroke, 243, *244*
  prevalence, 242
  risk factors
    alcohol and drug abuse, 247
    atrial fibrillation, 246
    cholesterol and other lipids, 246
    diabetes mellitus, 246
    heart disease, 246
    heredity, 246
    homocysteine and vitamin B deficiency, 246
    hypertension, 246
    migraine, 246
    obesity, 246–247
    smoking, 246
  symptoms
    hemorrhagic stroke, 246
    hypertensive stroke, 246
    major ischemic stroke, 245–246
    silent brain infarctions, 246
    transient ischemic attacks, 245
  thrombolytic therapy, 242–243

T
Temporal bones
  axial plane, *196–197*
  coronal plane, 194, *194–195*
Temporal resolution, 4
Thoracic imaging
  airways, 268
  cardiac CT
    cardiac anatomy, 273–278
    CT coronary calcium screening, 284–287
    technique, 278–284
  chest anatomy, 204, *204–213*
  clinical manifestation, 267
  CT bronchography, 268
  general scanning method
    intravenous (IV) contrast materials, 267–268
    patient positioning, 267
  high-resolution CT (HRCT), 268–269
  protocols
    cardiac calcium scoring (gated), 294
    chest abdomen, 292–293
    CTA–chest aorta (gated), 295
    CTA–chest for pulmonary embolism, 293–294
    CTA–coronary, 297–298
    CTA–heart general, 296–297
    CTA–pulmonary veins (gated), 298–299
    high-resolution chest CT, 290–291
    lung nodule, 289–290
    routine chest, 289
    tracheobronchial, 291–292

thoracic CTA, pulmonary embolism
    anatomy and terminology, 269–271
    diagnostic options, 271–273
    virtual bronchoscopy, 268
Three-dimensional image reformation
    endoluminal imaging, 88–89
    multiplanar reformation, 86
    projection displays, 86, *87*
    surface rendering (SR), 86
    volume rendering, 87–88, *88*
Tissue plasminogen activator (t-PA) treatment
    benefits, 247
    contraindications, 247, 248t

U
Urinary tract calculi
    calcium salt stones, 317
    causes, 317
    clinical presentation, 318–319
    cystine stone, 317
    diagnosis
        imaging modalities, 319t–320t
        noncontrast helical CT (NCHCT), 319–320
    differential diagnosis, 318–319
    epidemiology, 317
    noncontrast helical computed tomography (NCHCT), 317
    stone types, 318t
    struvite stones, 317
    symptom, 318t

terminology, 317
uric acid stones, 317

V
Vascular access
    aseptic technique, 143
    indwelling catheter set, 143, *143*
    patient management
        central venous access device (CVAD), 145
        indwelling venous catheter, 144–145
        non-tunneled central venous catheters (CVC), 146
        peripherally inserted central catheters (PICC), 145–146, *147*
        tunneled central venous catheters (CVC), 146–147, *147*
    placement, 144
    superficial veins, 143–144, *144*
    supplies, 143
    venipuncture technique, 143–144, 145
    venous access site, 143–144, *144*

W
Workstation-created multiplanar reformation, 85
Wrist imaging
    annotation system, 337
    fracture examination, 336
    patient positioning, 336, *337*

X
Xenon gas detectors, 17–18, *18*